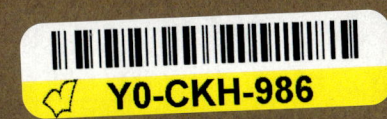

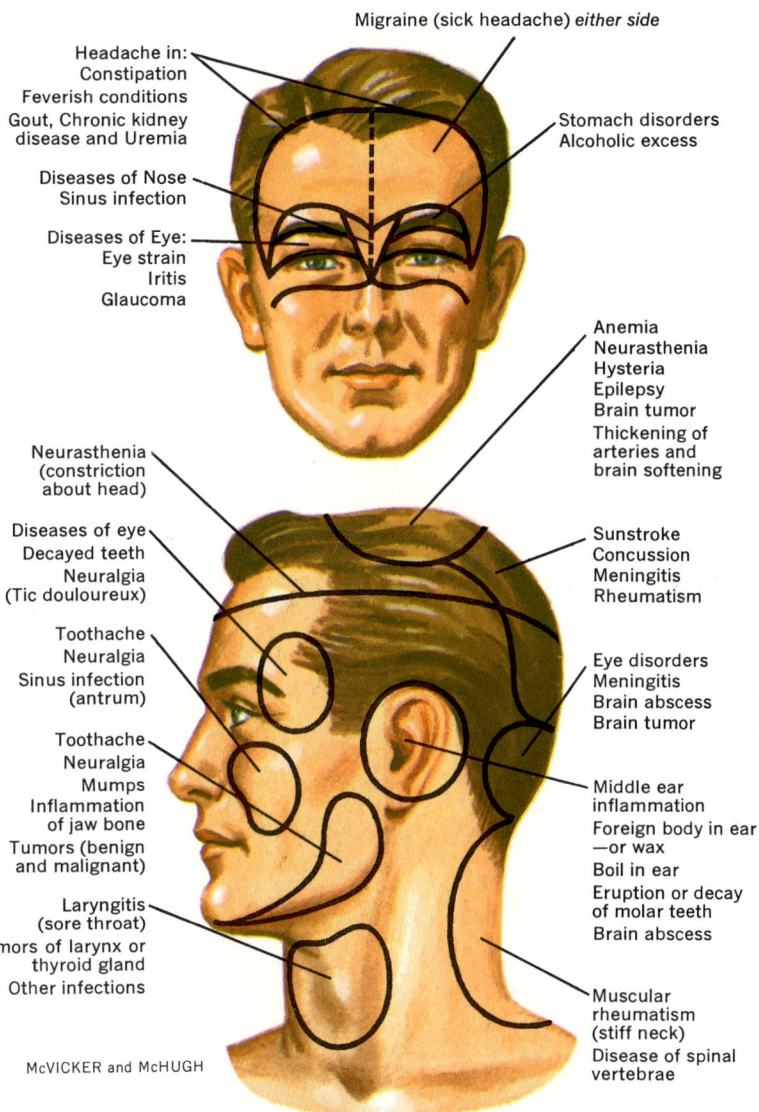

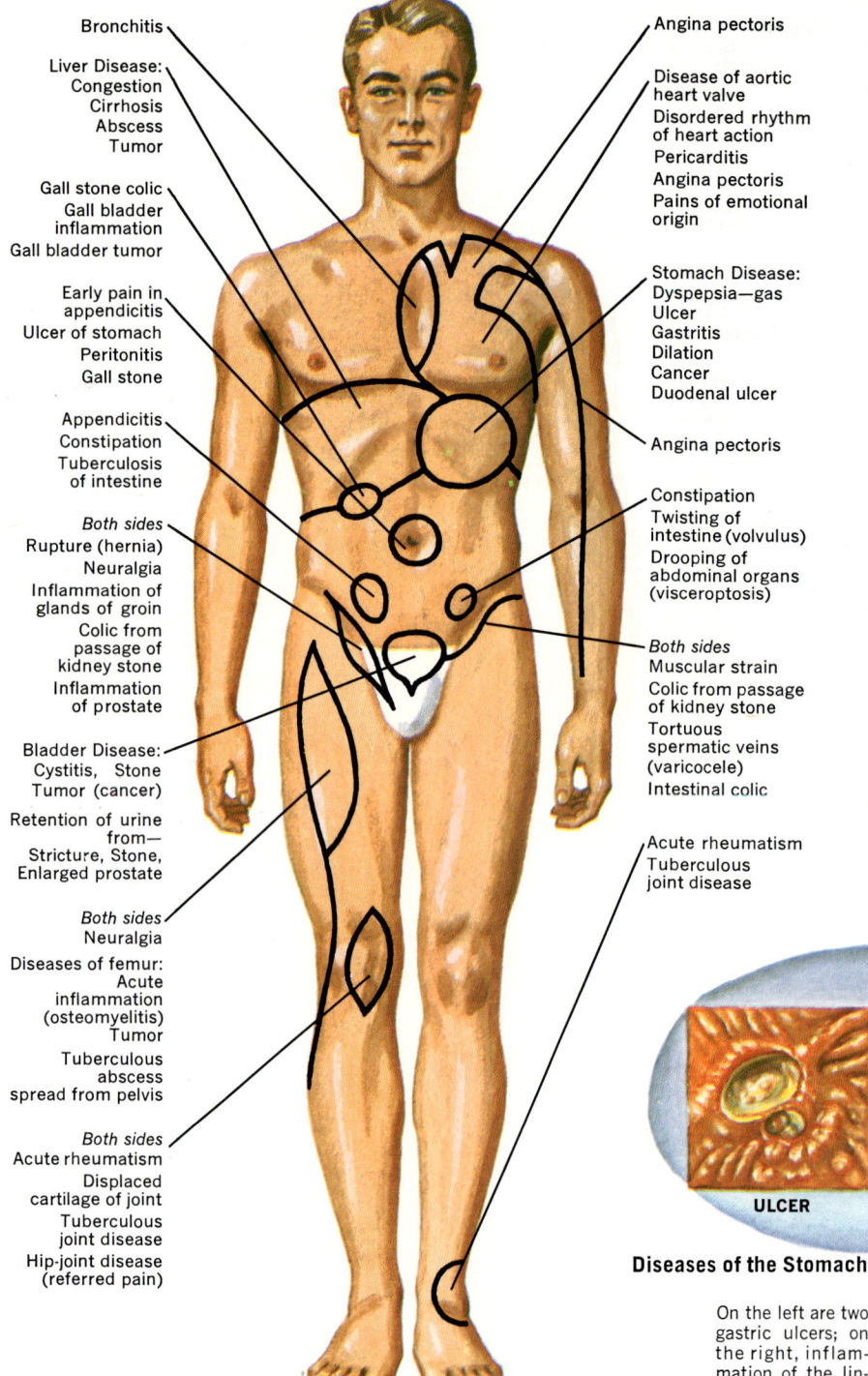

Diseases of the Stomach

On the left are two gastric ulcers; on the right, inflammation of the lining of the stomach

of Pain

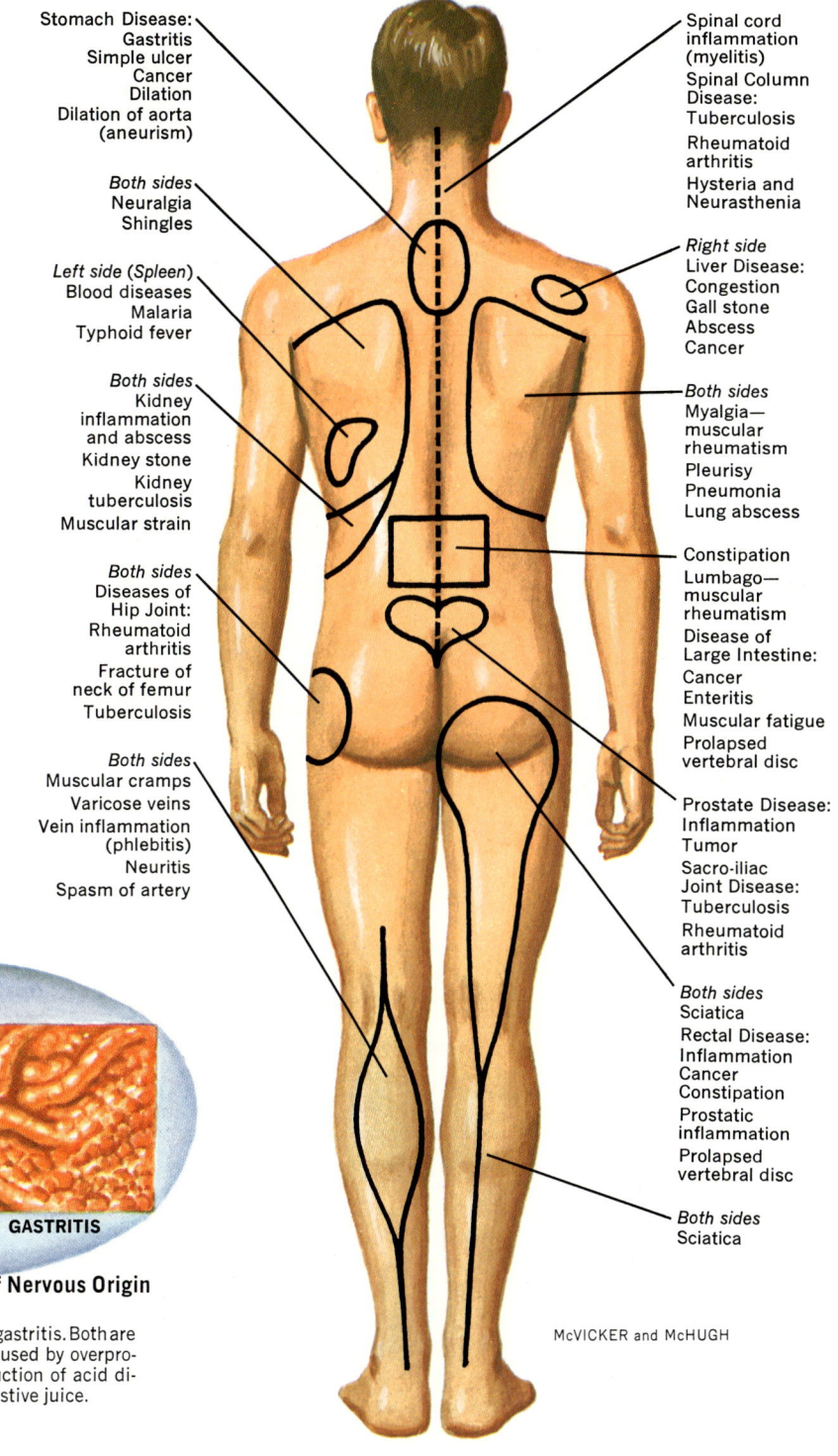

Stomach Disease:
Gastritis
Simple ulcer
Cancer
Dilation
Dilation of aorta
(aneurism)

Both sides
Neuralgia
Shingles

Left side (Spleen)
Blood diseases
Malaria
Typhoid fever

Both sides
Kidney
inflammation
and abscess
Kidney stone
Kidney
tuberculosis
Muscular strain

Both sides
Diseases of
Hip Joint:
Rheumatoid
arthritis
Fracture of
neck of femur
Tuberculosis

Both sides
Muscular cramps
Varicose veins
Vein inflammation
(phlebitis)
Neuritis
Spasm of artery

Spinal cord
inflammation
(myelitis)
Spinal Column
Disease:
Tuberculosis
Rheumatoid
arthritis
Hysteria and
Neurasthenia

Right side
Liver Disease:
Congestion
Gall stone
Abscess
Cancer

Both sides
Myalgia—
muscular
rheumatism
Pleurisy
Pneumonia
Lung abscess

Constipation
Lumbago—
muscular
rheumatism
Disease of
Large Intestine:
Cancer
Enteritis
Muscular fatigue
Prolapsed
vertebral disc

Prostate Disease:
Inflammation
Tumor
Sacro-iliac
Joint Disease:
Tuberculosis
Rheumatoid
arthritis

Both sides
Sciatica
Rectal Disease:
Inflammation
Cancer
Constipation
Prostatic
inflammation
Prolapsed
vertebral disc

Both sides
Sciatica

McVICKER and McHUGH

GASTRITIS

of Nervous Origin

—gastritis. Both are caused by overproduction of acid digestive juice.

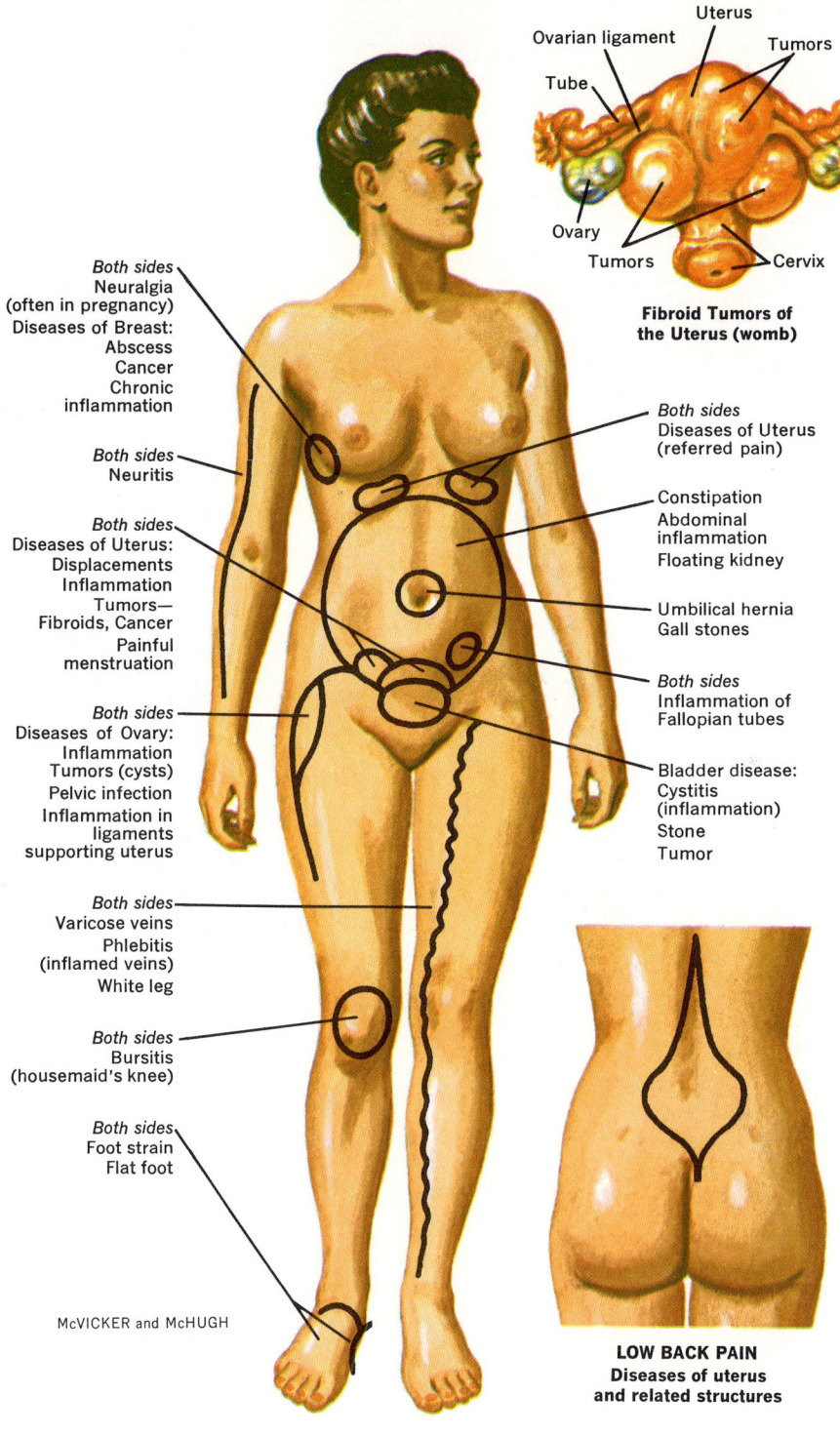

THE *N*EW ILLUSTRATED MEDICAL and HEALTH ENCYCLOPEDIA

Home Library Edition

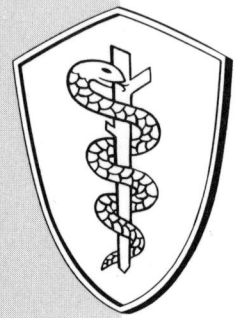

COMPLETE IN 4 VOLUMES

This 4 volume edition contains new entries, illustrations, anatomical charts and MEDIGRAPHS plus matter from THE MODERN FAMILY HEALTH GUIDE.

VOLUME 4

PNEUMONIA
••••••••••••
ZYME

INDEX

THE NEW ILLUSTRATED MEDICAL and HEALTH ENCYCLOPEDIA

EDITED BY

MORRIS FISHBEIN, M.D.

EDITOR, Medical Progress
EDITOR, Modern Home Medical Advisor
EDITOR, Excerpta Medica
CONTRIBUTING EDITOR, Postgraduate Medicine
MEDICAL EDITOR, Encyclopedia Book of the Year
FORMERLY EDITOR, Journal of the American Medical Association

With the Collaboration
of 27 Leading Specialists in
Medicine and Surgery

H. S. STUTTMAN CO., Inc. *Publishers*
New York, N.Y. 10016

HOME LIBRARY EDITION
THE NEW ILLUSTRATED MEDICAL AND HEALTH ENCYCLOPEDIA
Copyright © 1970 by H. S. STUTTMAN CO., INC.
Copyright © 1974 by H. S. STUTTMAN CO., INC.

All Rights Reserved

Matter from THE MODERN FAMILY HEALTH GUIDE
Copyright © 1959 by NELSON DOUBLEDAY, INC.

Anatomical Charts and MEDIGRAPHS
Copyright © 1970, 1964 by H. S. STUTTMAN CO., INC.

Library of Congress Catalog Card Number 70-78432

1974

PRINTED IN THE UNITED STATES OF AMERICA

24P-0674-35(515)

PNEUMONIA, an inflammation of one or both lungs. Many types of pneumonia have been distinguished, but usually when the word pneumonia is used without qualification, *lobar pneumonia,* in which one or more entire lobes are infected, is implied, and the causative organism is the *pneumococcus.* Other organisms may also produce pneumonia, such as the *streptococcus* and *staphylococcus,* which may cause *bronchopneumonia.*

The symptoms of a typical case of pneumonia may follow a slight cold or infectious disease or may appear suddenly without warning. A shaking chill may be followed by a sharp stabbing pain on the side of or in the chest, with coughing and expectoration of brown or bloody sputum. The pulse is rapid, the cheeks flushed, temperature rises sharply, and weakness and even prostration, headache, nausea, vomiting, and diarrhea sometimes ensue.

The person with pneumonia must be put to bed immediately, and carefully watched, since restlessness, sleeplessness, and even delirium may provoke the patient, despite his weakness, to try to get out of bed.

As the infection progresses, changes may take place in the lung itself. It may become filled with inflammatory material and solidify, causing shortness of breath and shallow noisy breathing. The blood cannot obtain sufficient oxygen and so the skin and mucous membranes may become bluish, a condition known as *cyanosis.* The patient must be placed in an oxygen tent to assist his breathing as well as correct the cyanosis.

During the acute stages of pneumonia, care must be taken to prevent complications, such as *heart failure, empyema, distention of the abdomen,* and *abscess.* The development of other diseases, including *pericarditis, endocarditis, meningitis,* and *arthritis,* must also be carefully prevented.

For a long time pneumonia was a dreaded disease with a high mortality

the disease and its causes Pneumonia is an acute infection of one or both lungs. At one time lobar pneumonia was the typical form seen. However, sulfa drugs and antibiotics have been so effective in dealing with it that this type is rarely seen today—although it still occurs. The exact diagnosis depends on the bacteria isolated, X ray evidence, and the visible symptoms.

The type of pneumonia most common now is virus, or atypical, pneumonia. Despite the name and the belief that a virus is involved, the precise cause is not known. It is this form of bronchopneumonia which is discussed here and described in the Medi-Graph.

symptoms The onset is usually slow. There are minor upper respiratory symptoms, low-grade temperature, chills and headache. Appetite is poor. The throat may be dry or scratchy. Pain beneath the breastbone is common along with a cough when the patient breathes deeply. After a few days the dry cough becomes looser, with thick sputum that may be streaked with blood. Temperature can rise as high as 104° in the first few days, but the fever generally drops back to normal about the 5th to 7th day.

Convalescence from pneumonia is slow and it may take weeks for a patient to lose his cough and his feeling of weakness. Very often patients have virus pneumonia in a form so mild they do not know they have it. There is no temperature, a mild cough, and some feeling of weakness. The presence of the disease is made known in such cases only when routine chest X rays are taken and the lung infection is revealed.

Virus pneumonia is not seen often in a severe form, but it can and does attack chronically ill, debilitated patients.

complications These are rare. Occasionally the membranes that surround the lungs fill with fluid. And infrequently, the brain and heart become involved.

prevention (or lessening of impact) Since the precise cause of this disease is unknown, there is no known method of preventing it. Cold shots and vaccines are available and are helpful to some, but they are not proven preventives. It can only be suggested that one should avoid exposure to infected individuals, follow a sensible diet, and get sufficient rest.

Pneumonia

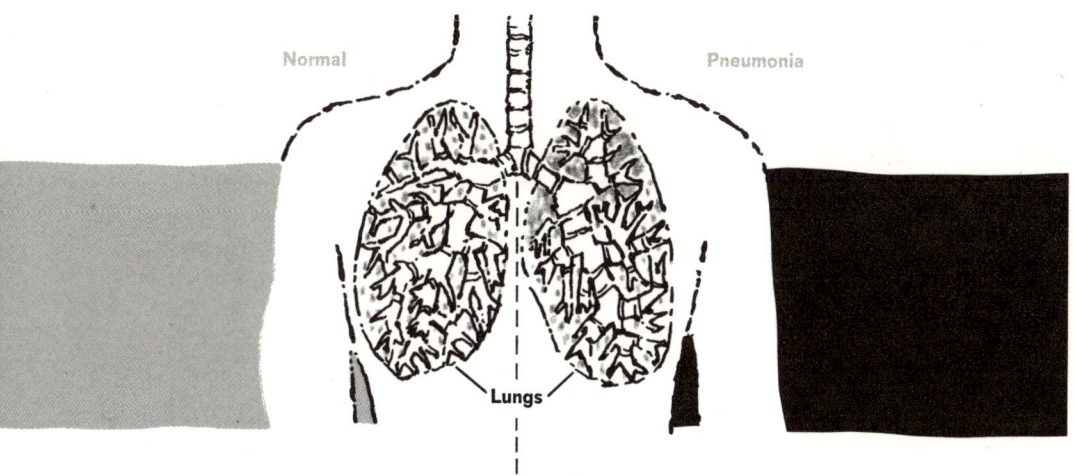

Lung is composed of millions of tiny little air cells surrounded by network of blood vessels. In normal breathing, lung flexibly contracts to force stale air out of cells, expands to bring in fresh air.

Lung is inflamed and congested by fluid or other material. This impairs ability of air cells to give off stale air, bring in fresh air.

Typical Symptoms of Virus Pneumonia

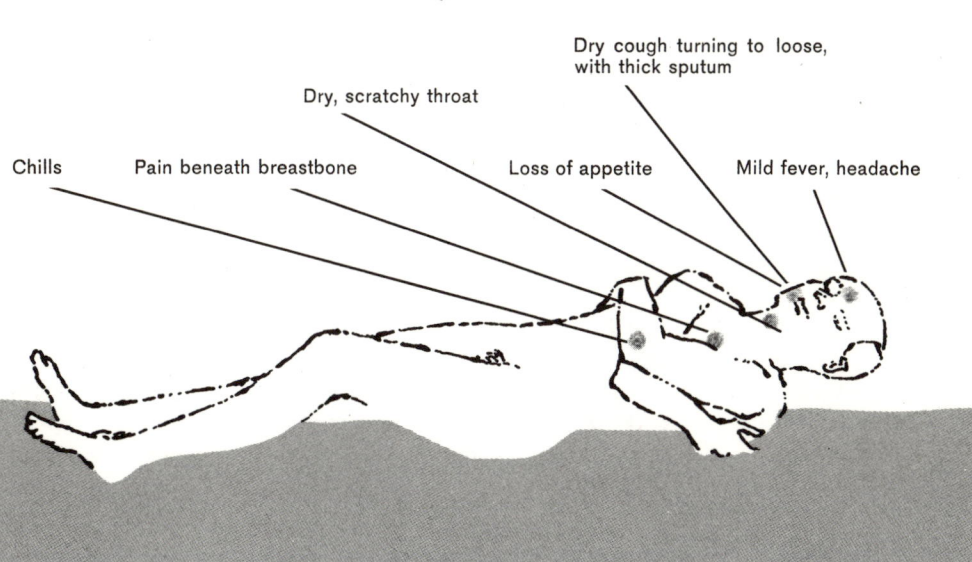

- Chills
- Pain beneath breastbone
- Dry, scratchy throat
- Loss of appetite
- Dry cough turning to loose, with thick sputum
- Mild fever, headache

1051

rate. Treatment depended on the use of serums, which were developed to combat specific infections, and the condition usually led to an acute stage with a definite "crisis," in which the patient appeared near collapse. After the crisis, a sharp drop in temperature followed and the patient fell into a deep sleep, with subsequent recovery in some cases.

Today the use of *sulfonamides* and *antibiotics,* such as *penicillin, terramycin, aureomycin, and streptomycin,* have decreased the development of lung abscess and empyema, and the death rate has fallen sharply. Good nursing care in pneumonia still continues to play a considerable part. The recovery period is especially significant. The patient should not get up from bed or engage in activity too early. A complete physical checkup, including a chest x-ray examination, is strongly advised following pneumonia.

The number of cases of *virus pneumonia* has sharply increased, at the same time that *bacterial pneumonia* has yielded to treatment with sulfa drugs and antibiotics. Although the nature of viruses is not completely understood, and few specific measures have been developed to combat them, it is known that virus pneumonia is produced by a number of specific types of virus. Virus pneumonia may vary from a mild or "walking" state to a serious condition requiring hospitalization. In a mild case the patient may not suspect that he has anything more severe than a slight cough and fever, which he may ascribe to a cold. In the more severe form, fever, sweating, malaise, headache, sore throat, weakness, and a dry hacking cough are involved.

Treatment of virus pneumonia includes bed rest, even in a mild case. Antibiotics are frequently effective in preventing complications. It is essential to treat the fever and cough; and in severe cases in which cyanosis is present, an oxygen tent may also be required. In general, virus pneumonia does not persist more than a few days to a week. However, convalescence, usually characterized by weakness, is often long and slow, and x-ray examination of the chest may reveal shadows for several weeks. *See* MEDIGRAPHS pages 863, 1051.

PNEUMONIC PLAGUE. *See* PLAGUE.

POISONING. Any substance which is capable of producing a harmful or deadly effect can be considered a poison. For most such substances there is both a safe dose and a poisonous dose, the severity of the effect depending on the amount taken and on the age and physical condition of the person involved.

Poisoning is an emergency situation; *the doctor should be called immediately,* and first aid given at once. Symptoms, although there may be no early ones, include nausea, vomiting, cramps, and stomach pains. If a *corrosive* poison has been taken, burns and stains may appear on and around the mouth and tongue. Headache remedies and sleep-producing drugs produce drowsiness, sleep, and sometimes unconsciousness.

In first-aid treatment for poisoning, two points are important. The first is that a poison diluted with a large amount of liquid is absorbed less quickly than in concentrate and vomiting can be induced more easily when the stomach is filled. Second, once the poison is removed from the body it can do no further harm and so in some types of poisoning it is imperative to induce vomiting repeatedly until the fluid ejected is as clear as when it was swallowed.

To dilute the poison and induce vomiting various liquids may be used: warm soapsuds, soda water made with common baking soda, or salt water. The liquid should preferably be lukewarm. It may be necessary to give six or seven or more glasses of liquid.

After the stomach is thoroughly cleaned out, an *antidote* may be given. A **universal antidote** which can be given for all cases of poisoning and which every household should keep on hand consists of the following: two parts powdered burnt toast, one part milk of magnesia, one part strong tea. The carbon in the toast absorbs poisons; the magnesium has a soothing effect on the mucous membranes of the stomach and a laxative action which also neutralizes acid poisons; and the tannic acid in the tea tends to neutralize caustic alkaline materials. A heaping tablespoon of Epsom salts also can be given.

Two important exceptions are alkali and acid poisoning. In these cases, vomiting *should not be induced,* to avoid danger of perforation. In first-aid treatment for *acid poisoning,* neutralize the poison with an alkali, such as baking soda, lime water, milk of magnesia, or chalk. Then give a demulcent, such as milk, olive oil, or egg white. The victim should be kept warm.

For *alkali poisoning,* neutralize the alkali with a weak acid such as dilute lemon juice or vinegar. Then give milk. The victim should be kept warm.

Shock is frequently present in all types of poisoning and must be controlled. The victim should be kept warm and if breathing stops, *artificial respiration* applied.

In poisoning from a sleep-producing drug, it is especially important that the stomach be washed out by whatever means possible, and a cup of strong coffee every half hour or so is also recommended. The danger that breathing may stop is particularly imminent and artificial respiration may be necessary.

There are a vast number of substances which when swallowed or inhaled can be poisonous, such as insecticides, polishes, sprays, cleaners. When poisoning is suspected, it is sometimes difficult to determine what the poisonous substance has been. If the victim is unable to give the information, perhaps an open bottle or his physical symptoms can help decide. In the case of some substance taken from a container, the container often but not always gives the remedy for poisoning. Some cities maintain special bureaus which give information about poisoning and its antidotes, including all the new products on the market which might conceivably be poisonous.

Following is a list of some of the more common causes of poisoning, with symptoms and treatment.

ACETANILID POISONING. *Acetanilid, phenacetin,* and *Pyramidon* are frequently constituents of headache remedies which, in sufficiently large doses, can cause death, especially in children. The person will have disturbed hearing or deafness, rapid breathing, blue lips and nails, nausea, vomiting, and sometimes convulsions, stupor, or coma. Vomiting should be induced unless the person is unconscious or has already vomited excessively. Then the universal antidote is given. Since respiratory failure is a dangerous possibility, artificial respiration may have to be given. When the doctor arrives, he may have the victim placed in an oxygen tent.

ARSENIC POISONING. *Arsenic* is present in many insecticides, rodent killers, paints, dyes, and cosmetics. Small doses of arsenic taken into the body over a long period produce irritation of nerve endings. The person who has swallowed an arsenic product will have burning pains in the throat and stomach, and the odor of garlic on his breath. Other symptoms may be vomiting and diarrhea and extreme thirst with a choking sensation. Vomiting should be induced, followed by an antidote of egg whites in water or milk, and the vomiting-antidote procedure repeated. Afterward strong coffee or tea is given, and then Epsom salts in water or castor oil.

BARBITURATE POISONING. The *barbiturates* include such well-known drugs as *Luminal, Seconal, phenobarbital, pentobarbital, Amytal, Dial, Ipral, neonal,* and *Evipal.* Either intentionally or unintentionally people sometimes take overdoses of "sleeping pills," which in many cases leads to death, and most states have laws governing purchase of these potentially harmful drugs. Symptoms of barbiturate poisoning include headache and confusion, bluish color of nails and lips, uneven breathing, drowsiness, stupor and coma. Vomiting should be induced. The chief problem is to maintain proper breathing and to control shock. Strong coffee or tea is given and artificial respiration if necessary. The doctor will make certain that the throat is free of mucus and that the victim is receiving enough air.

BENZENE POISONING. *Benzene,* a widely used solvent, is frequently a constituent of floor waxes, floor cleaners, varnish removers, and numerous other products. Benzene vapor is heavier than air, but when warmed it rises and spreads easily. A person who has inhaled benzene fumes will act, at first, as though intoxicated, appearing flushed, dazed, and staggering. He will become drowsy and gradually unconscious. He should immediately receive fresh air and be given artificial respiration if necessary. In case the benzene has been swallowed, the person will breathe with difficulty and have a slow pulse. Nausea and vomiting will probably occur and maybe convulsions. Vomiting is *not* to be induced, but strong coffee or tea given. The victim must receive fresh air and artificial respiration if necessary. The doctor will support the action of the heart with drugs. A victim of benzene poisoning must be particularly careful to receive adequate nutriments in order to build up the blood.

BORIC ACID POISONING. Infants have been seriously poisoned by mistakenly being given boric acid solutions instead of water, although boric acid in ordinary quantities is not a dangerous poison. Vomiting should be induced, coffee given as a stimulant, and large amounts of alkaline drinks to protect the kidneys.

COAL OIL OR KEROSENE POISONING. The first symptom of ingestion of kerosene is a burning sensation in the stomach, mouth, and throat, followed by nausea and vomiting with slow breathing and feeble pulse, and convulsions and coma. Strong coffee or tea should be given and artificial respiration if necessary. Vomiting should *not* be induced. If kerosene fumes have been inhaled, the person's face is flushed or his lips blue, and he has difficulty breathing. He should be removed from the area of the fumes into fresh air, and artificial respiration given if necessary. Persons who work in an atmosphere where they inhale great amounts of coal, oil, kerosene, or naphtha fumes develop symptoms of "naphtha jag," characterized by a sense of excitement and lack of self-control, followed by depression, headache, nausea, a roaring sound in the ears, irritation in the throat, and a trembling of the hands and arms. If sufficient fumes have been inhaled, shallow breathing, weak heart, convulsions, and death may ensue. The doctor may give antibiotics to prevent pneumonia, and blood transfusions may be required.

CYANIDE POISONING. *Cyanide,* used in the silver industry and in certain insecticides, is lethal in small quantities and acts with extreme rapidity. Hundreds of deaths occur each year from cyanide poisoning and in most cases it is difficult for the doctor to determine just how much cyanide has been taken. Treatment has been unsatisfactory because the poison is so rapidly fatal. *Antidotes* used are *methylene blue, glucose injections, amyl nitrate inhalation,* and *sodium thiosulphate* and *sodium nitrite injections.* Lavage with *potassium permanganate* is also part of current treatment.

The person who has swallowed cyanide has the odor of bitter almonds on his breath, is confused, and has a headache. Vomiting and diarrhea are present, followed by convulsions, unconsciousness, stoppage of breath. First-aid treatment includes inducement of vomiting and drinking large amounts of *hydrogen peroxide* in water.

LYE POISONING. *Lye* is a caustic alkali used as a cleansing agent in washing powder, drainpipe cleaner, and paint remover, and is a household menace, especially to children. The person who has swallowed lye has burns and stains on the mouth and a burning pain in the mouth, throat, and stomach. Vomiting occurs. Vomiting should *never* be induced. The alkali should be neutralized with a weak acid such as diluted vinegar or citrus fruit juice—as much as the person can drink. The doctor may reopen the throat passage so that the person can breath and swallow by using a rubber eyeless catheter which is gradually increased in size. Treatment to dilate the passage with this device may in some cases continue for as long as a year. The doctor may also give sedatives to relieve pain and treat the local burns.

MERCURY POISONING. *Bichloride of mercury* acts rapidly on the tissues of the body. In severe cases, the victim suffers pains in the abdomen, vomiting. Egg whites and milk help to inactivate the mercury. The doctor may give BAL for several days. It forms an easily excretable combination with the mercury.

NARCOTIC POISONING. The victim of narcotic poisoning is drowsy and may fall asleep, pass into a coma, and die. Vomiting should be induced and strong coffee given as a stimulant. It may even be imperative to move the person about forcibly to keep him awake and avoid respiratory failure. Artificial respiration may be required.

NICOTINE POISONING. *Nicotine* is a constituent of a group of insecticides. Ingestion of nicotine causes a hot burning sensation of the stomach; it is rapidly absorbed and may cause heart failure, convulsions, and respiratory failure. Initially the person is nervous and excited, then depressed. He may suffer vomiting and diarrhea, breathe deeply and rapidly, and have pale clammy skin. Vomiting should be induced, followed by hot tea and burnt toast, or the universal antidote. Artificial respiration may be necessary and the doctor may give oxygen inhalations.

STRYCHNINE POISONING. Some cathartics and tonics contain *strychnine*. Symptoms of strychnine poisoning are nervousness and excitement, stiff neck, and twitching muscles and convulsions. Vomiting should *not* be induced except immediately after the poison has been taken. Burnt toast is given and the victim kept in a quiet dark room. The doctor may control the convulsions with barbiturates and wash the stomach with *potassium permanganate solution* or *tannic acid*. Artificial respiration or oxygen may be necessary.

THALLIUM POISONING. *Thallium sulfate* is an ingredient of some depilatories. The symptoms are nausea, pain in the stomach, diarrhea, delirium, and convulsions. Vomiting should be induced and strong coffee or tea given.

TURPENTINE. Turpentine comes in straight form, and floor polishes may contain this potential poison. Symptoms are abdominal pain, nausea, vomiting, and diarrhea, and later excitement, stupor, and coma. Sometimes the urine contains whole blood. Treatment includes inducement of vomiting, followed by Epsom salts in water and large amounts of water to promote urination.

See also CARBON MONOXIDE; DEADLY NIGHTSHADE POISONING; FOOD POISONING; MUSHROOM POISONING; LEAD POISONING; METALLIC POISONS; INHALING OF DANGEROUS SUBSTANCES; OCCUPATIONAL HAZARDS IN INDUSTRY.

POLIOMYELITIS

POLIOMYELITIS, an inflammation of the anterior horn cells in the gray matter of the spinal cord. It is caused by a virus, the smallest living material. Viruses differ from bacteria mainly in that they cannot move by themselves and cannot live outside a living body. The virus of poliomyelitis is one of the smallest known. Man is affected almost exclusively although monkeys may be infected.

Poliomyelitis can exist in one of three forms. Many people have had poliomyelitis without realizing it, having contracted a mild case which rendered them immune to further attacks. Poliomyelitis may cause only a little diarrhea, stomach upset, cold, or muscle aches, which last for a few days. This is known as *abortive poliomyelitis*. If temporary paralysis of arms or legs occurs, the condition is known as *nonparalytic poliomyelitis*. The third type, *paralytic poliomyelitis*, may cause lasting damage or death if respiratory muscles are involved.

Epidemics of poliomyelitis usually occur during the warm months: July to October in the United States and the rest of the northern hemisphere, and February through April in Australia and other parts of the southern hemisphere. The virus is present in the nasopharynx and bowel movements and may be spread by sneezing, coughing, or by contamination of water or food with sewage. The poliomyelitis virus affects the cells of the spinal cord, brain, and other nervous tissue, leading to the familiar paralyses. Adults as well as children may be affected. Symptoms may be vague at first and include

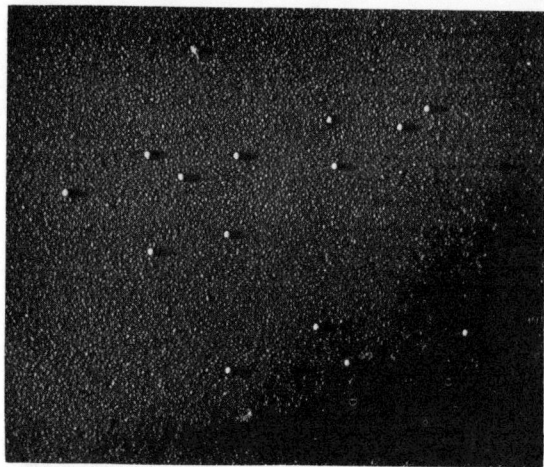

Poliomyelitis—The human polio virus magnified 100,000 times by the electron microscope. The viruses in this photograph were obtained from tissue cultures of monkey kidneys. The particles are about 28 millimicrons or one millionth of an inch in diameter.

fever, headache, spasms of the arms, neck, thighs, and weakness. Treatment, which is not yet wholly satisfactory, consists of exercising the affected muscle groups to prevent withering and shrinking from lack of use; employment of the iron lung to carry on respiration when the respiratory or breathing muscles are damaged, and other such supportive measures.

Many children have become permanent cripples as a result of polio, and many adults and children have died from it.

The development of the *Salk poliomyelitis vaccine* has been a particular blessing to all parents and children. The vaccine can produce immunity to the poliomyelitis virus, and this may last for many years. The vaccine is produced by growing virus on the tissue of the kidneys of monkeys. The virus is then denatured, or killed, making it safe for

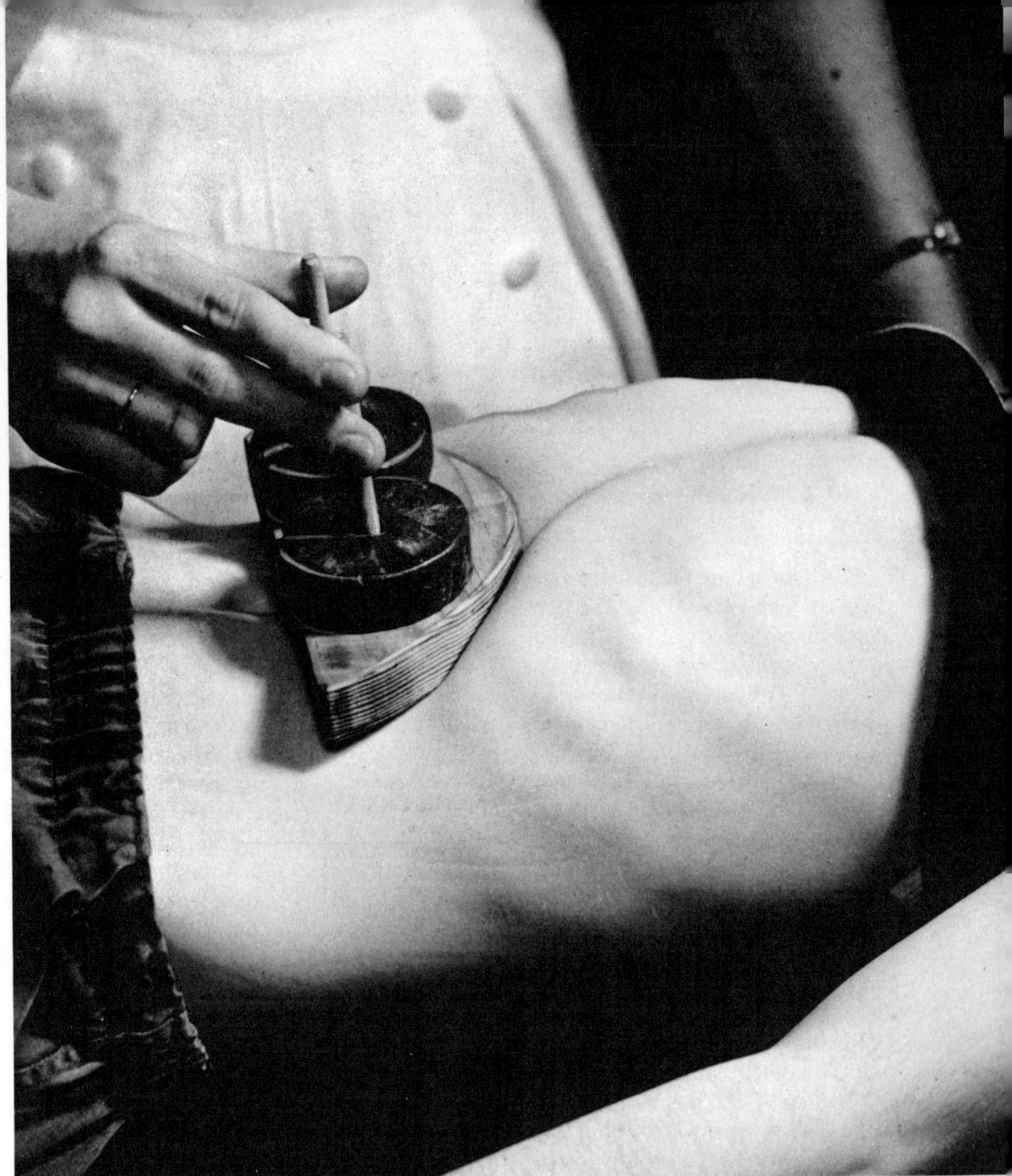

Poliomyelitis was for many years one of the most dreaded of all diseases, although in reality its incidence was comparatively infrequent. Its effects could include paralysis and permanent disability. While the Salk and Sabin vaccines are effective preventives, those disabled still require therapy. Exercising the muscles of the abdomen and diaphragm is an important part of the corrective treatment for those who have been crippled by poliomyelitis. The patient shown above and at right *(bottom)* is undergoing hydrotherapy, often useful in regaining muscular control. He is supported by floats at the head, hip, and right ankle. The victim swims, later walks again.

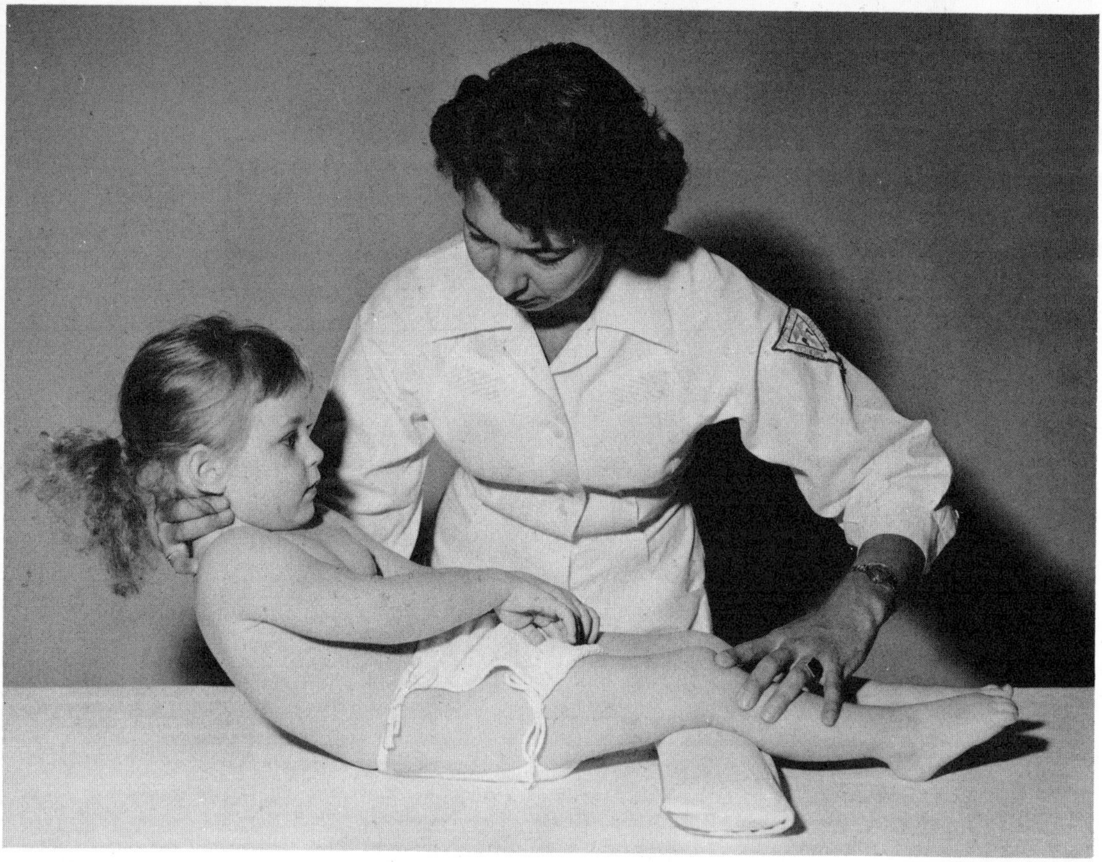

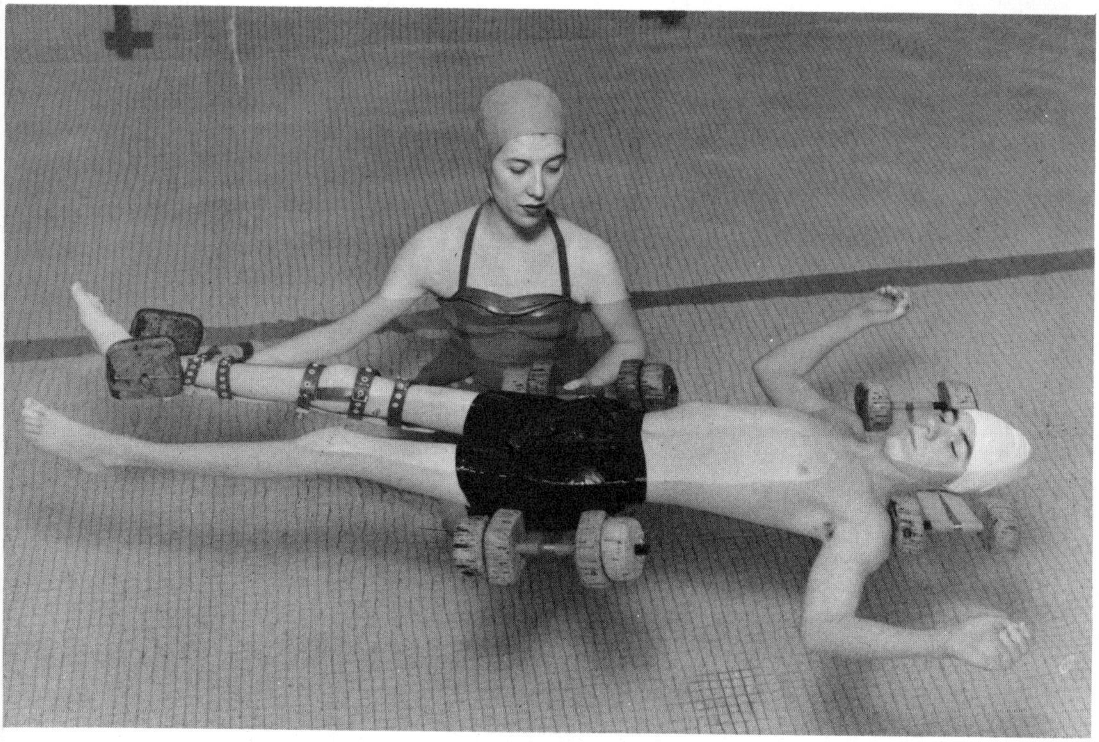

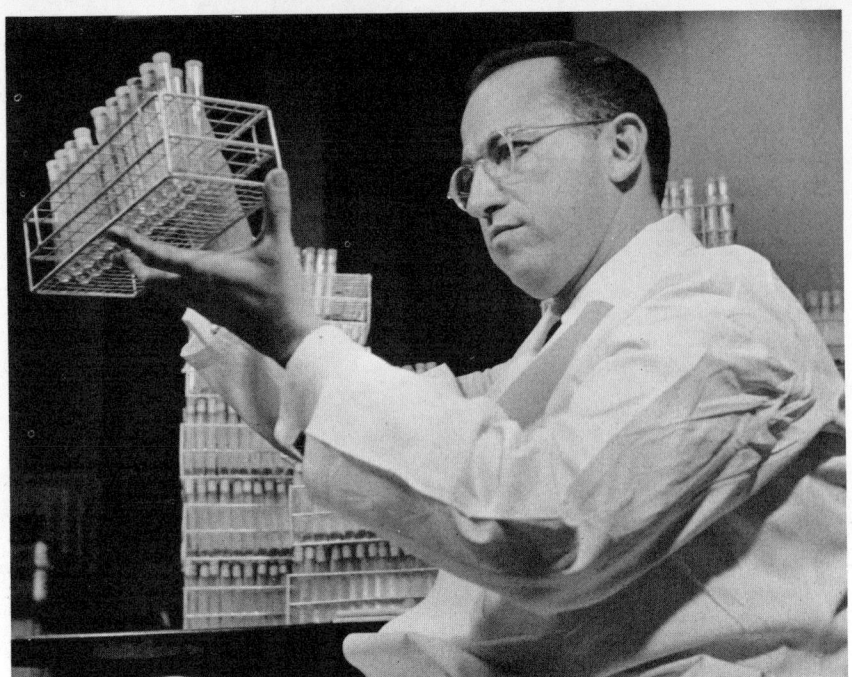

Dr. Jonas E. Salk developed the first effective vaccine against poliomyelitis. This vaccine (which is administered intravenously) together with the more recent oral vaccine developed by Dr. Albert B. Sabin has effectively eliminated the threat of this crippling disease. Dr. Salk is shown here at work in his laboratory and (opposite, bottom) administering the vaccine to an enthusiastic young man. Research toward discovering a cure for poliomyelitis began in earnest in the 1930's. It was necessary to isolate the virus responsible for the disease in order to develop a vaccine. Experimenters devised a method for growing the virus on the kidney tissue of monkeys. The virus was then killed by various methods, including the use of ultraviolet rays and formaldehyde. A vaccine was prepared from the killed virus.

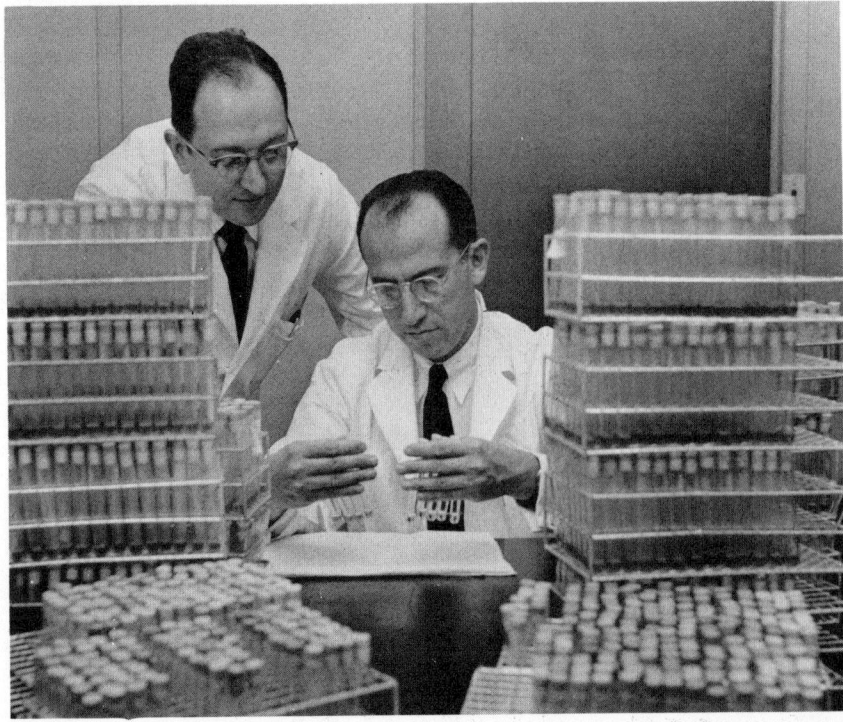

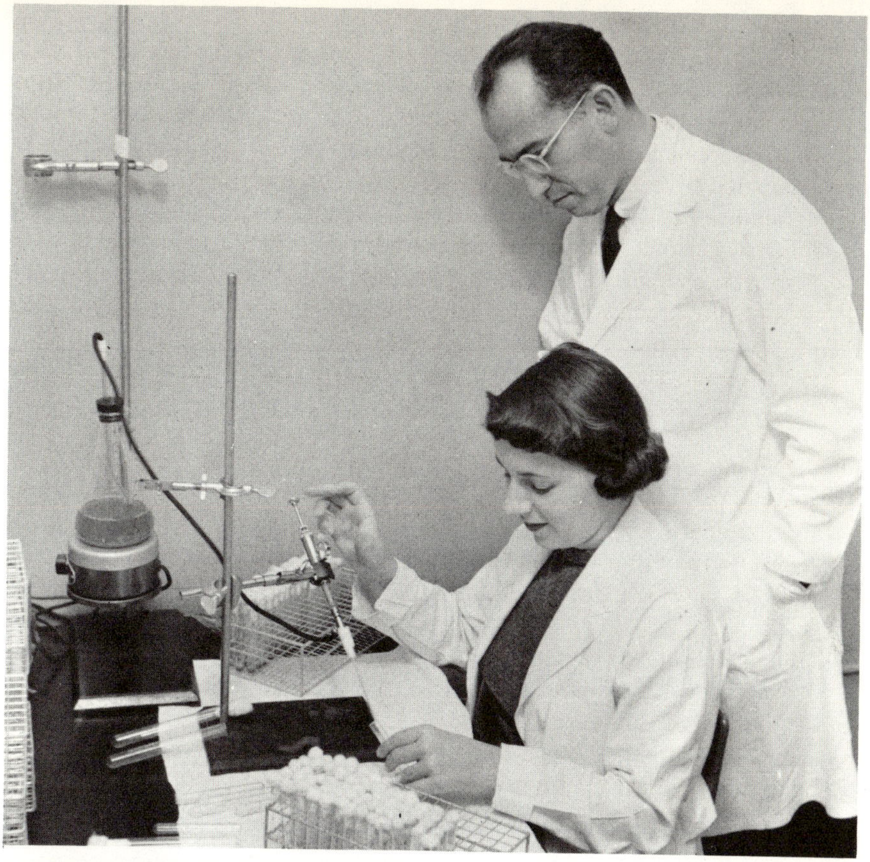

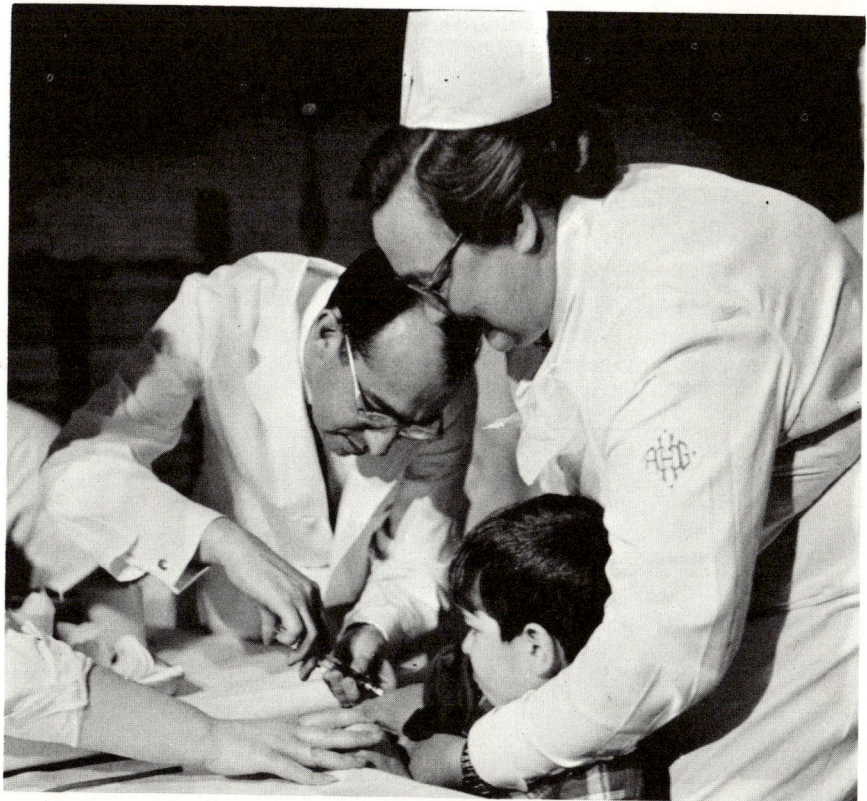

the disease and its causes Poliomyelitis, or infantile paralysis, is an acute virus infection of the central nervous system. It is spread in two ways: through the intestinal tract by means of food and water that have been contaminated by convalescent patients, healthy carriers, fleas, insects, pests, or animals; and through the secretions from the nose and throat of an infected person. The incubation period is 7 to 14 days, and the disease is usually over in 10 to 14 days. One attack gives lifelong immunity but only to the specific type of polio involved. Infants have a high degree of natural immunity. However, the disease hits hardest at young children. Youngsters with recent tonsillectomies seem to be particularly susceptible during epidemics.

symptoms The onset is usually sudden, with fever, headache, drowsiness, and irritability. The neck becomes stiff and the spine rigid. Muscles can be quite tender. By the third day the temperature may drop, only to rise again by the 5th day as muscle paralysis develops. While any group of muscles may be involved, usually it is those of the lower extremities or back.

Bulbar polio is a severe form in which the base of the brain is involved. In such a case, swallowing becomes difficult and speech and breathing are interfered with. It is often fatal.

A mild or "abortive" type of polio is also seen. All the early symptoms may be present, but no paralysis develops. Because the attack is so mild, diagnosis is difficult and often is never made.

complications There are secondary complications, particularly pneumonia and kidney infection. Other problems arise in relation to the areas involved and the degree of nerve damage, and these depend upon the severity of the illness.

prevention (or lessening of impact) Two effective vaccines are now available. One is the "killed" Salk vaccine which is given by injection. The other is the "live" Sabin vaccine taken by mouth. Anyone who starts on the Salk vaccine may continue with the Sabin provided each vaccine is taken exactly as recommended. In that way maximum protection is provided. Every infant should be routinely immunized. For that matter, unless otherwise advised by the physician, everyone should be protected by one or both of these vaccines.

Poliomyelitis (Infantile Paralysis)

After day or two of fever, headache and weakness, patient begins to develop such symptoms as:

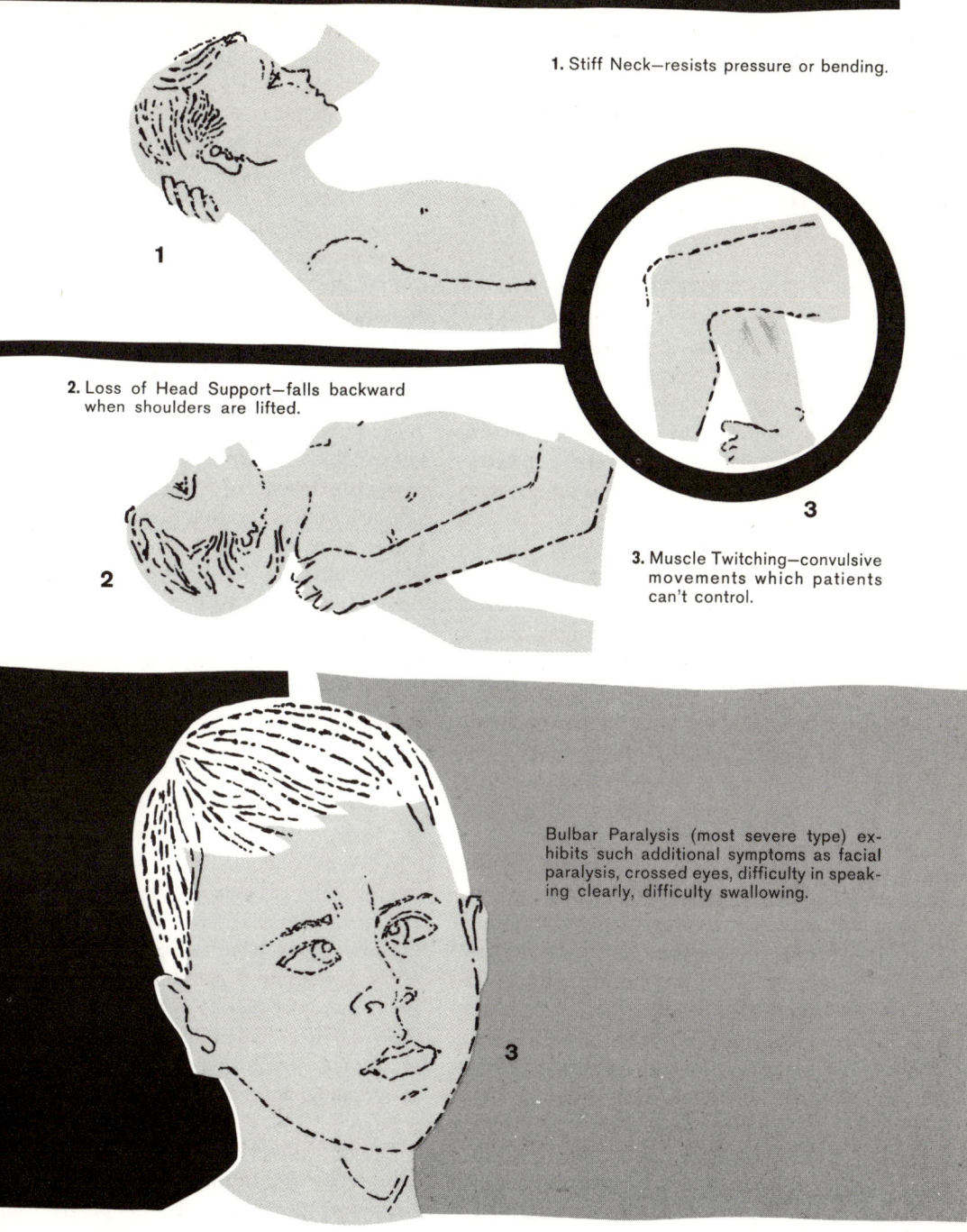

1. Stiff Neck—resists pressure or bending.

2. Loss of Head Support—falls backward when shoulders are lifted.

3. Muscle Twitching—convulsive movements which patients can't control.

Bulbar Paralysis (most severe type) exhibits such additional symptoms as facial paralysis, crossed eyes, difficulty in speaking clearly, difficulty swallowing.

1063

injection into human beings. Even though denatured, the vaccine can cause the human body to produce resistant substances, or *antibodies,* to poliomyelitis. All human beings should be vaccinated. See MEDIGRAPH page 1063.

POLYARTERITIS NODOSA. See COLLAGEN DISEASES.

POLYCYTHEMIA, a disease of unknown origin in which the production of red blood cells in the bone marrow is greatly increased. The average number of red blood cells is about five to six million per cubic millimeter of blood. In polycythemia, the number may reach as many as fifteen million red blood cells per cubic millimeter of blood. Usually white blood cells and platelets increase also, adding to the viscosity of the blood and affecting its flow to the brain and other parts of the body.

The symptoms in polycythemia may include dizziness, severe headache, and a feeling of fullness in the head. In some cases, fainting occurs and numbness and tingling in the hands and feet. The person may feel irritable and sluggish and have occasional spells of amnesia. Sometimes the vision is disturbed and there is a constant ringing in the ears. The spleen becomes greatly enlarged in order to act as a storage reservoir for the increased production of blood cells. The person's skin often has a bluish cast because of the prominence of small veins.

Treatment for overproduction of blood cells with the consequent enlarged spleen may be done by x-ray of the entire body. *Radioactive phosphorus* seems to be the most effective treatment, bringing relief for long periods.

When great overproduction of white blood cells and platelets also occurs, other drugs are effective. Blood-letting to relieve severe attacks of polycythemia is sometimes practiced, and has been found effective when *thromboembolism* is a complicating factor. In mild cases of polycythemia, *periodic blood-letting* may be the only treatment. However, there is danger of loss of iron and consequent anemia, in terms of hemoglobin content and oxygen-carrying capacity of the blood. Besides thromboembolism, hemorrhage and gout can also be complications of polycythemia. *See also* RED BLOOD CELLS, DISEASES OF.

POLYP, a nonmalignant tumor which hangs by a pedicle or stalk from the surface of a body cavity. Polyps vary widely in structure and nature, depending on their location. In the *ear,* a polyp consists of granular tissue caused by chronic irritation. A *nasal polyp* contains a soft overgrowth of mucous membrane and generally indicates disease of the underlying bone tissue. A *rectal polyp* is usually a glandular tumor. Polyps are frequently found inside the *sinuses* as inflammatory growth on mucous lining. A *gastric polyp* is a nonmalignant tumor in the stomach.

Surgery is generally employed to remove polyps. In the nose, the base must also be excised after the polyp

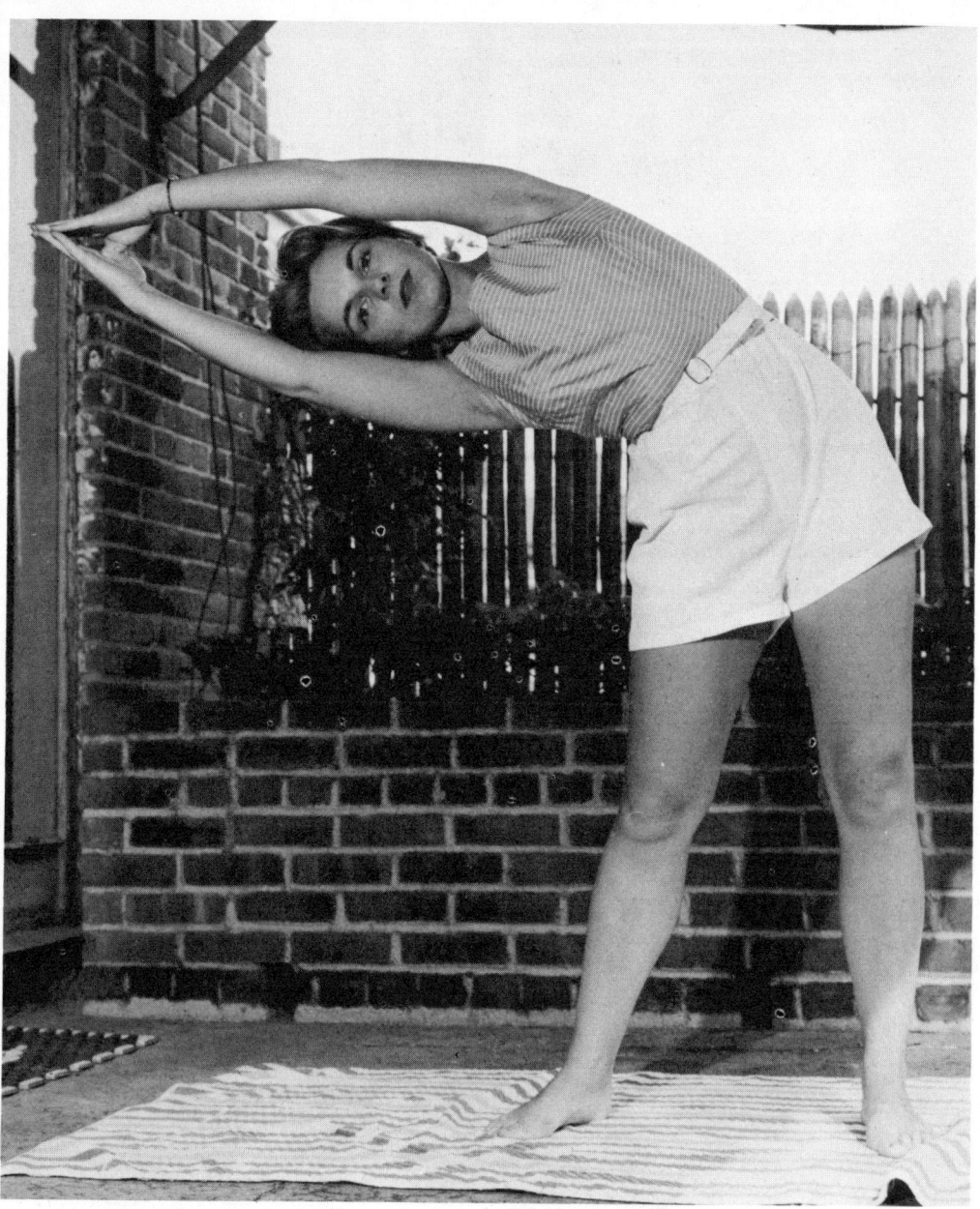

Physical exercises are very beneficial in maintaining a trim shape, firm tone and buoyant health. They are particularly advisable for the young mother during the months immediately following delivery. Some of the exercises appropriate to young mothers are shown on these pages. Above: a waist-slimming exercise. The woman stands erect, feet apart, arms overhead, palms together. She then bends as far as possible to one side, succeeded by a similar bend to the other side. This procedure is then repeated for ten times in both directions. After the body has become adjusted to this type of exercise, the number of repetitions can be increased to twenty or more in each direction. This exercise helps to reduce fat around the waist.

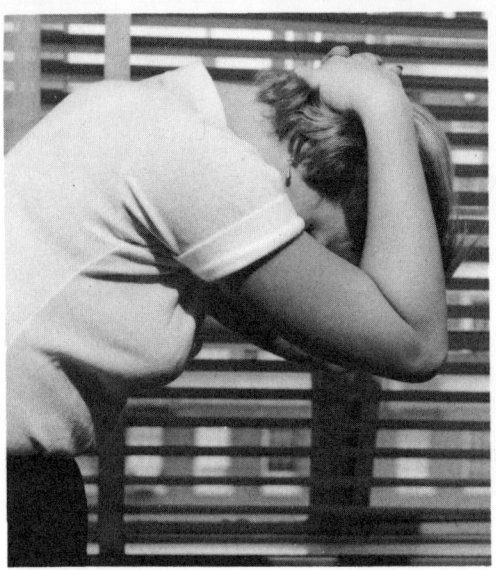
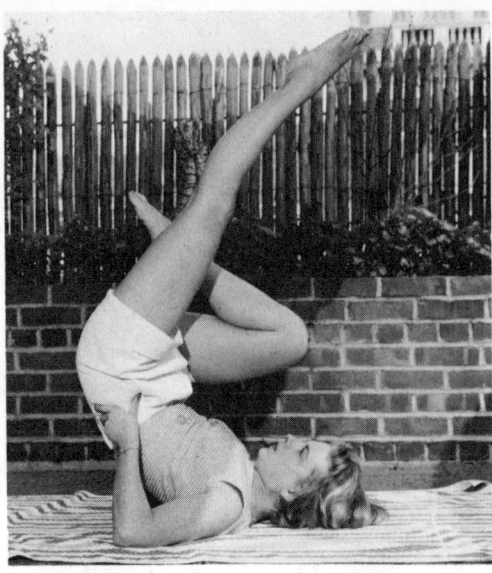

In the exercise shown above, left, the chin is first held high and the hands clasped behind the head. The head is then pulled down to the chest. This is repeated about fifteen times. This exercise strengthens arm and back muscles. Above, right, the woman lies on her back, arms at her sides, then bends her knees and draws them toward the chest until hips are off the floor and knees almost touch chin. This helps to slim the abdomen. A similar exercise below consists in raising the body from a supine to a sitting position and back for five or ten times. This also helps to slim abdomen.

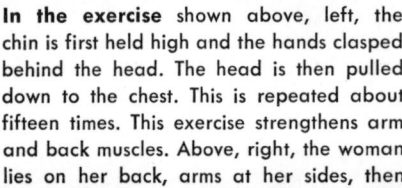

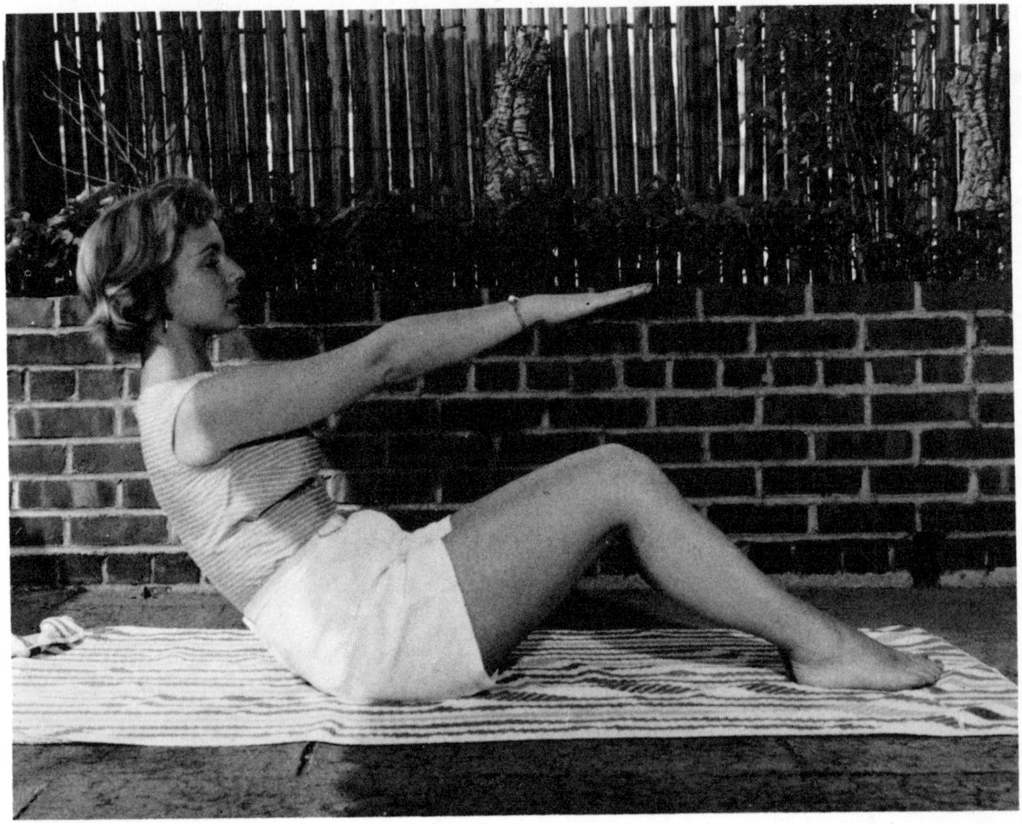

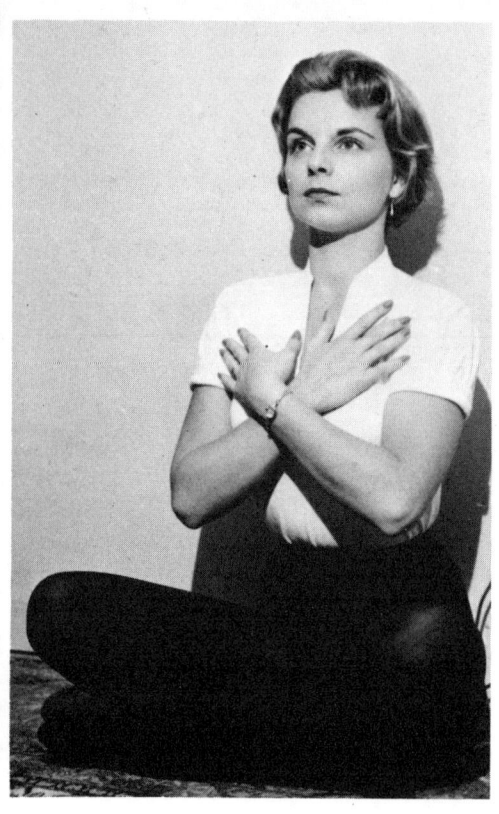

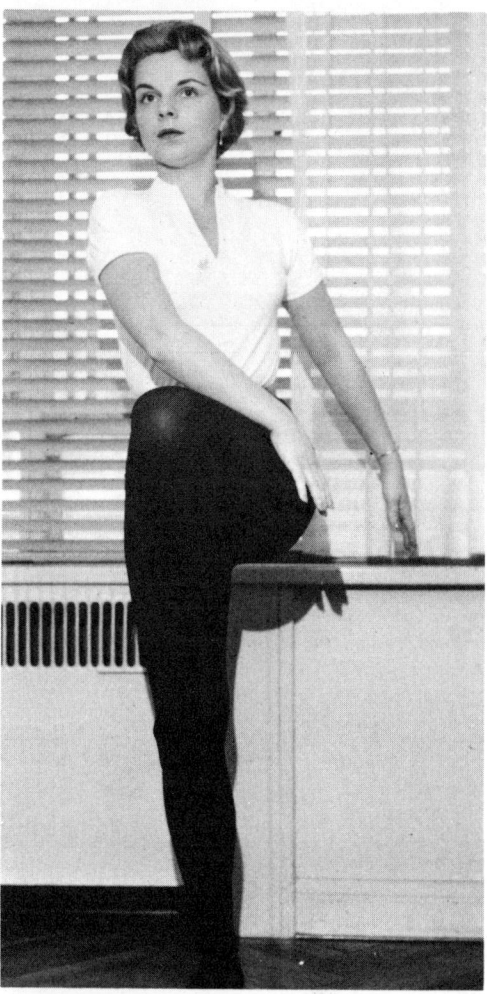

The exercises shown on this page are for the purpose of slimming the busts and thighs. Above, left, the woman sits crossed-legged on the floor, arms crossed and fingertips near shoulders. Stomach is pulled in and arms moved up and out *(below, right)*. Another bust-slimming exercise *(below, left)* consists simply in holding arms at shoulder length and clasping hands. The thigh-trimming exercise *(above, right)* involves standing erect, swinging arms to the left and bending knee toward the right shoulder.

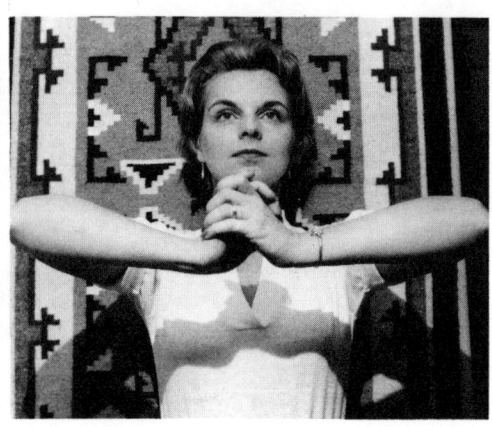

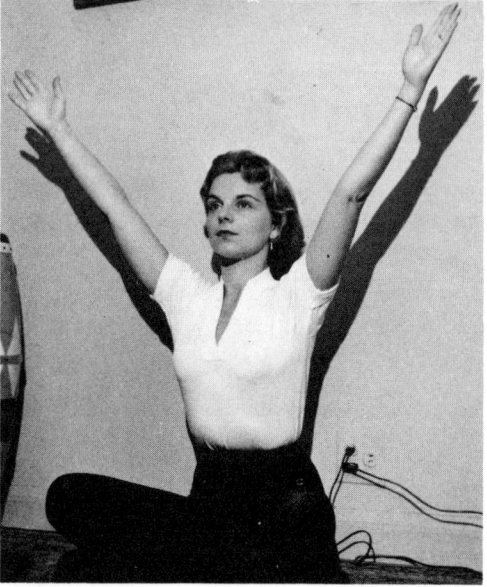

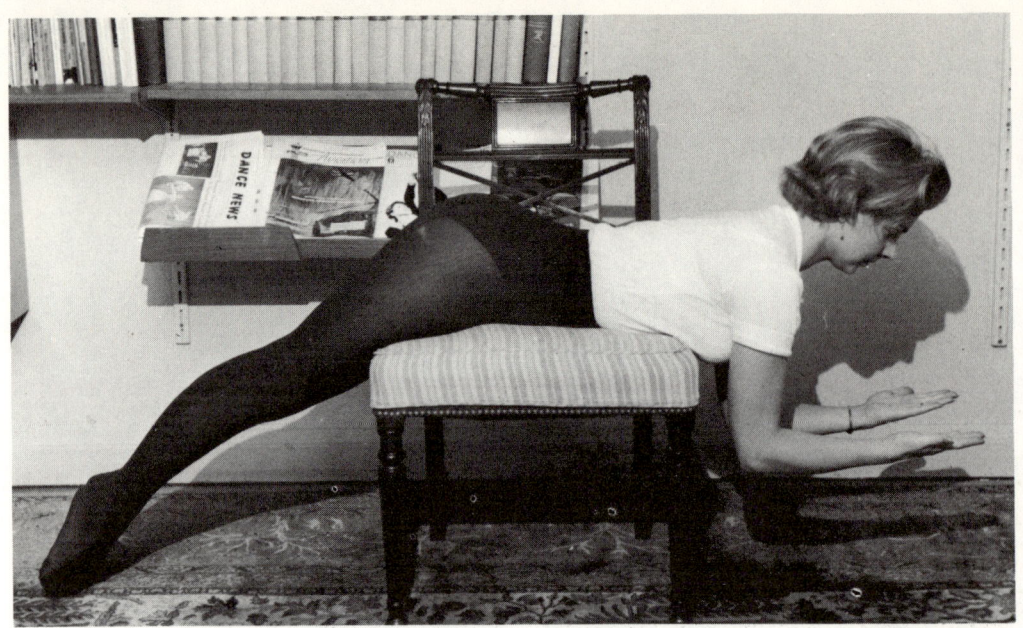

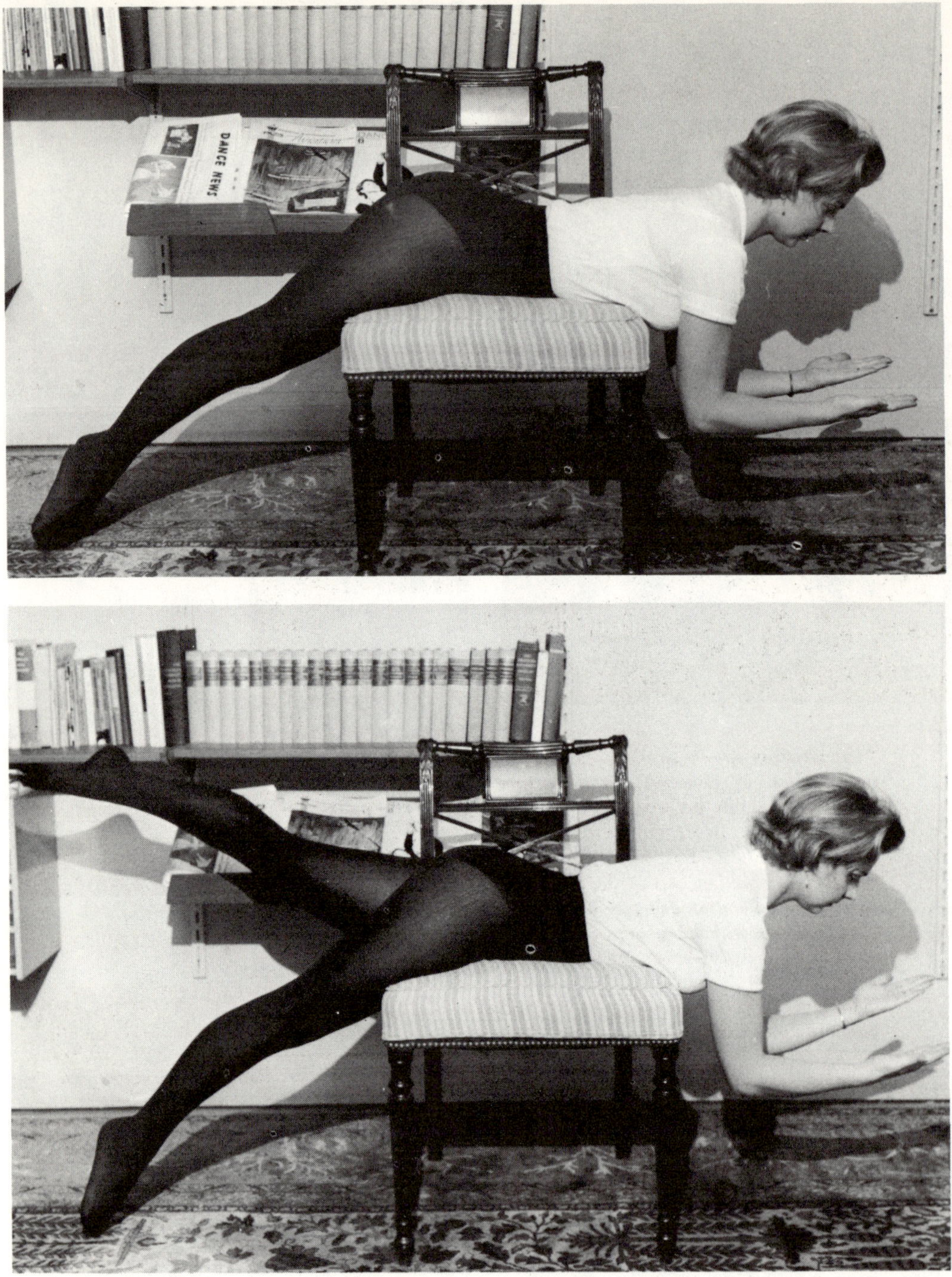

A good leg-slimming exercise is demonstrated here. First, the woman should lie prone, legs outstretched. Preferably, a chair of the sort depicted should be used. At the beginning of the exercise, the feet are touching the floor. The legs are then raised to a horizontal position. Each leg is then raised and lowered in succession.

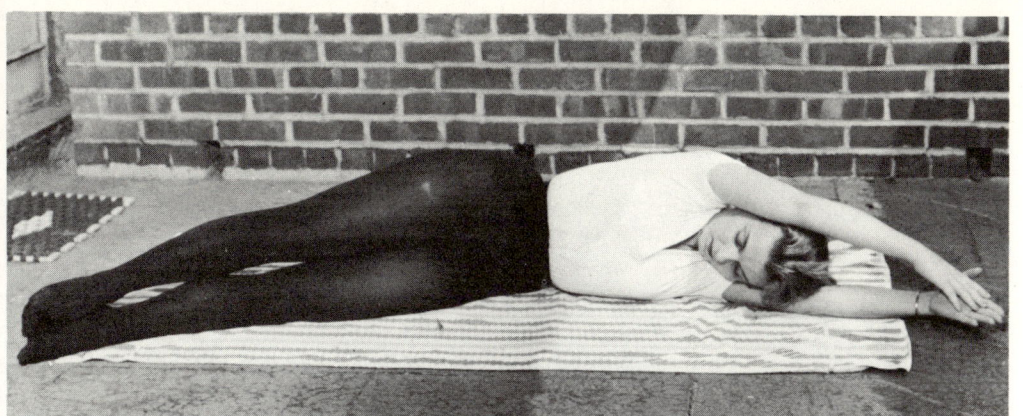

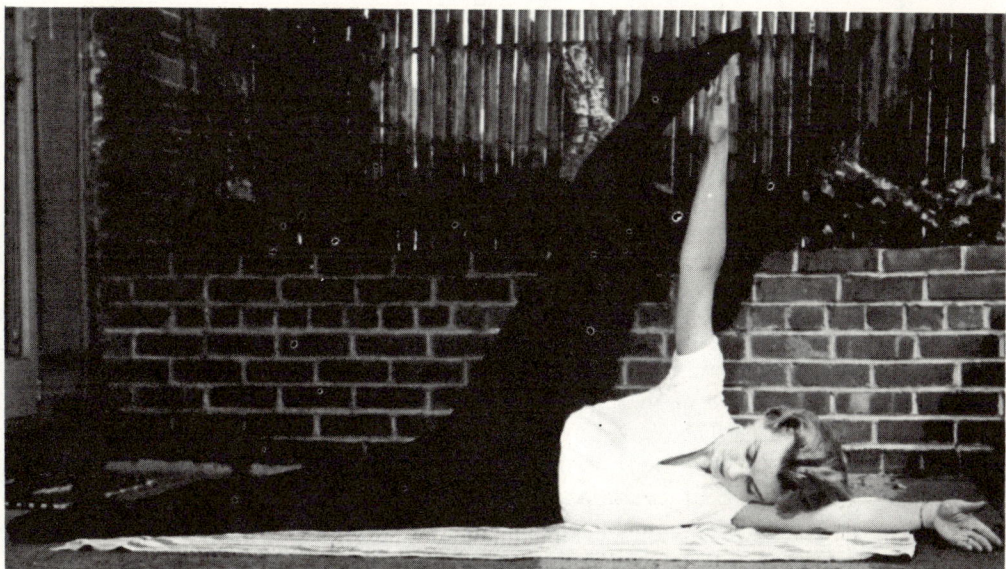

Another exercise for trimming the abdomen is shown here. The woman lies on her side, arms outstretched above the head, the body curved so that the toes can be seen. The arm and leg are then lifted until the fingers can touch the toes. This is repeated ten times, after which the woman changes to the other side and repeats the procedure with the other arm and leg. This exercise may be done outdoors, as shown here. Of course, one of the best exercises of all is playing with the baby!

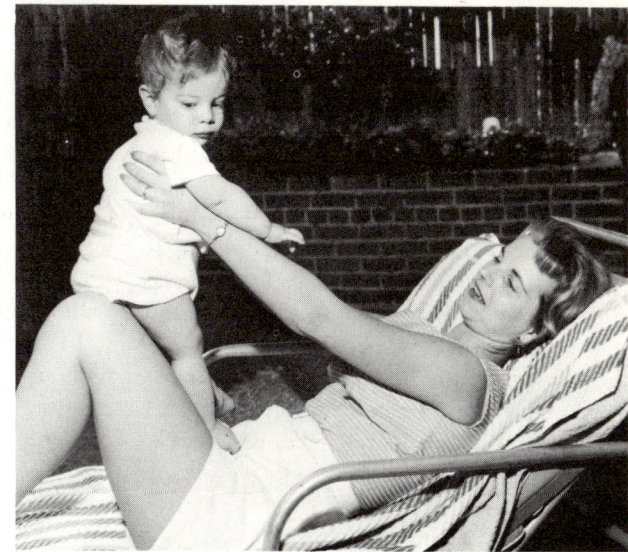

has been removed. Sometimes polyps occur in groups in the large intestine and must be removed and the entire area excised because of the danger that one may have become malignant. *Electric current* is often used to remove polyps in the *urethra*. Polyps on the walls of the uterus may not require treatment unless they endanger health. Rectal and gastric polyps also may become malignant and should therefore be removed.

PORES, DILATED. A dilated pore usually becomes filled with a plug of soggy material. If the material is squeezed out, the pore fills up again in about a month. Past treatment has usually included cauterization, freezing with carbon-dioxide snow, or surgical excision and closing. New research shows that a dilated pore results from growth of the lining of the hair follicle. The best way to eliminate the dilated pore permanently is by surgical excision and closing. Superficial measures attack only the surface of the dilated pore and will not eradicate it. *See also* ACNE; SKIN.

POST-NATAL CARE OF THE MOTHER. In the weeks following delivery, the mother should have an abundance of sleep and should be insulated from disturbing influences or situations. She should rest in a reclining position for definite periods of time in the morning and afternoon. While resting, it is advisable for her to lie on her abdomen for fifteen to twenty minutes at a time. During the first week, visitors and telephone conversations should be limited and those with colds or other infections excluded. If the mother herself has a cold, she should cover her mouth and nose with a handkerchief or mask when nursing or bathing the baby.

Systematic exercises should be initiated after delivery. During the first three or four days, these should be performed for only five minutes; the time allotted to them can gradually be extended.

For the woman with a lax abdominal wall, a supporting garment is most helpful. Showers or tub baths should be taken daily. In addition to the systematic exercises, walking is advisable. Strenuous physical activity, such as swimming, playing tennis or golf, and driving should be avoided for at least several weeks. Naturally, social functions should be kept to a minimum. *See also* CHILDBIRTH AND PRENATAL CARE; CHILD CARE.

POSTURE, position or bearing of the body. Good posture means that the body is held in the correct position when standing, sitting, lying down, or in motion.

In standing, the ideal posture is one in which the person stands tall and erect, the abdomen drawn in, the shoulders square and high, the chin straight back and held in, the weight properly distributed on the feet, and the curve of the back well within normal limitations.

In a correct sitting position, the body is erect and the head poised to bring the center of gravity in the line joining the bones of the hips.

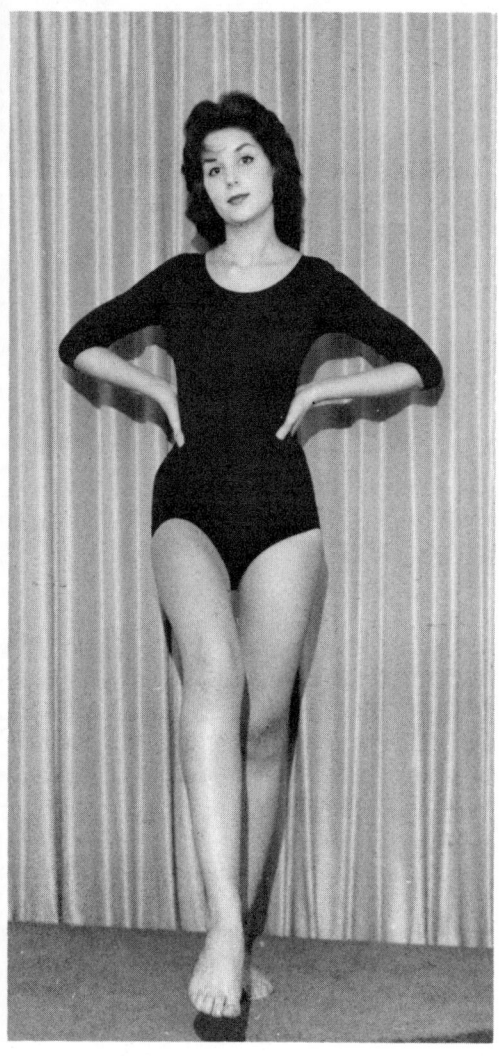 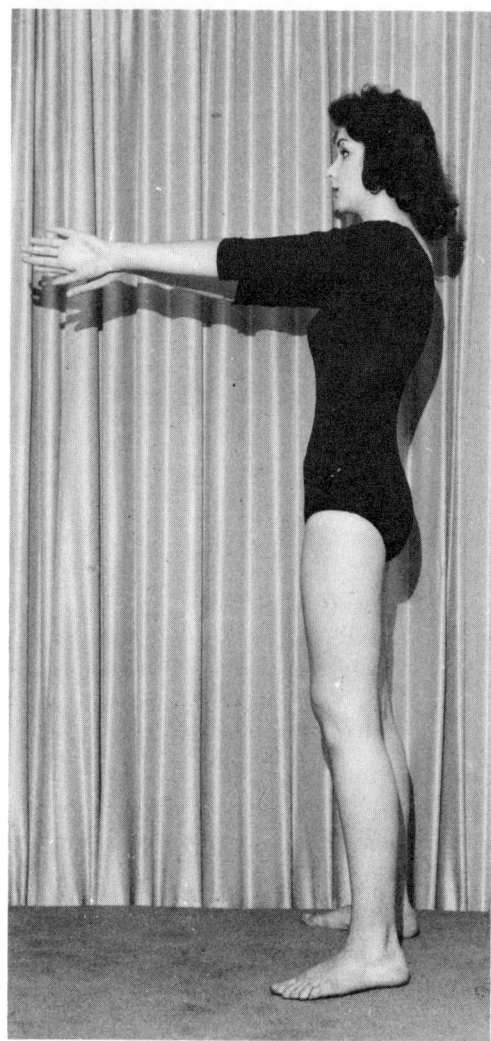

Good posture should be practiced at all times. It is easy to fall into poor posture habits, particularly as one grows older. A few simple posture exercises can help to correct these habits and ameliorate the crinks and pains in the back which often result from poor posture. While these exercises are especially useful for adults, it is advisable for parents and physical education instructors to teach them to children as well. If good posture habits are acquired early in life, the individual will be spared many back problems later on. A few simple figure exercises are all that is required to maintain good back tone and posture, provided these are observed daily. A five-minute workout is usually sufficient to accomplish this purpose. These exercises are beneficial not only for the back, but also for the chest, arms, and legs. Above, a chest exercise is demonstrated. The subject stands with feet apart, brings her arms together, the palms of the hands turned outward as shown, then swings the arms around in half circles. This is the most scientific chest exercise.

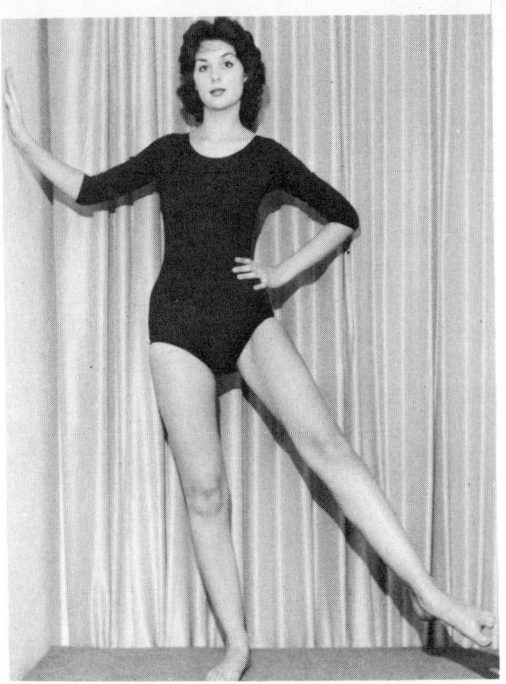
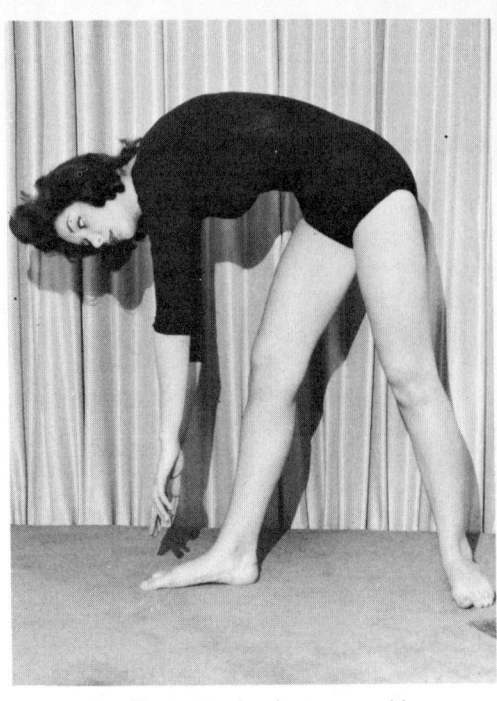

The exercise shown above at left is good for developing firm hips. The subject stands with one arm touching the wall and swings the opposite leg in a rhythmic pattern. Above, right, the well-known toe-touching exercise is effective in developing a stable back. Below, bending backwards is good for the circulation. The exercise at right involves a swinging action attained from bent knees and position shown on toes.

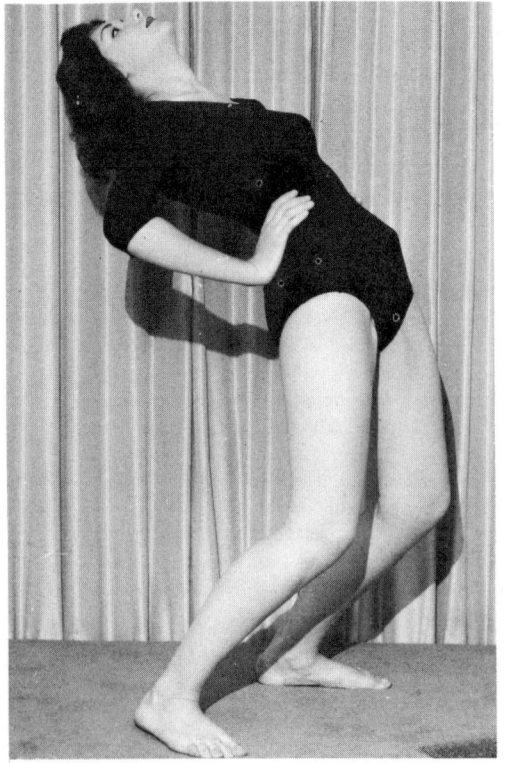
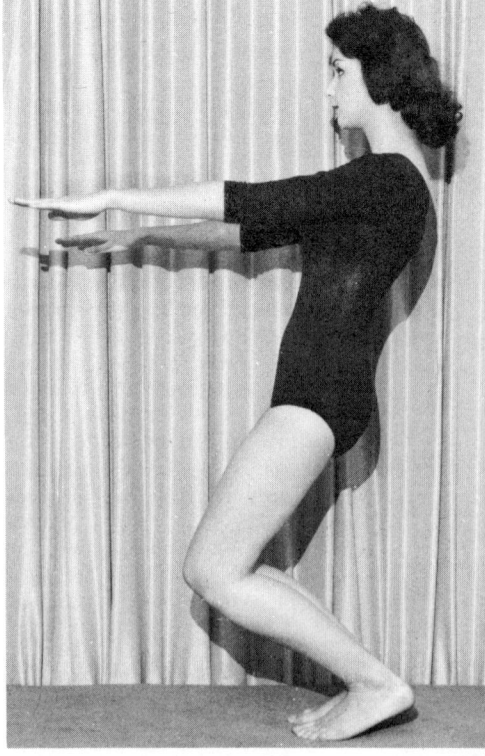

The exercise shown at the right is good for the thighs. While resting on the knees, the body is sprung up and down. The exercise depicted in the center photograph is beneficial to the abdominal muscles. Below, another abdominal exercise. The subject lies flat on the floor, then raises the trunk to a sitting position.

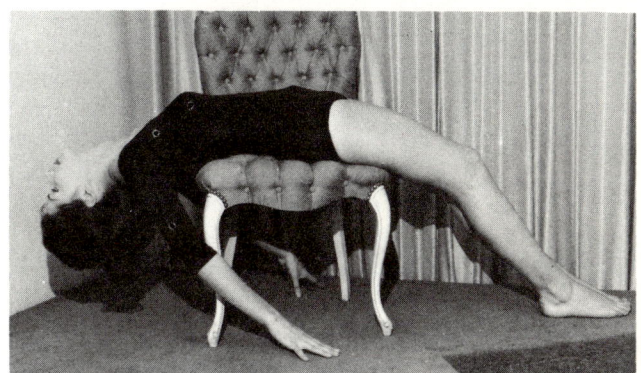

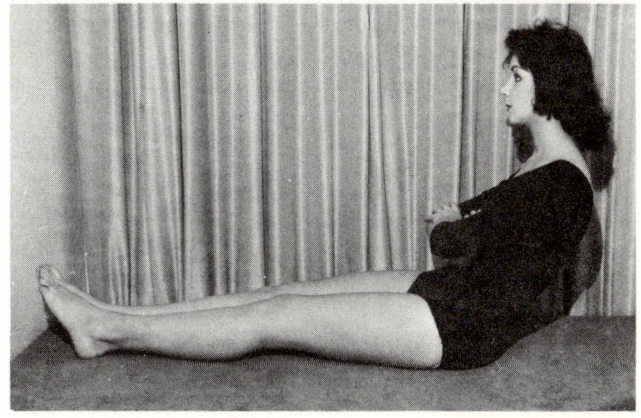

A constant bent posture or droopy position while at work or at rest results in stretching and relaxing of ligaments, with a tendency toward permanent sagging. As a result, the back becomes rounded and the chin pushed forward.

Good posture through life is desirable because it will prevent many disorders and help cure others. Both the home and school can cooperate effectively in training children to observe the rules of correct posture. Defects in posture can be corrected in preschool children if detected early enough. The teacher should always be alert to poor posture in pupils and take steps to single out cases for special attention. Physical exercise and posture training throughout school and college, and a program of physical exercise in adulthood are important to good health.

Faulty posture may be related to improper clothing and especially to the wrong kind of shoes. A definite relationship between flat feet, twisted spine, and other posture deformities and ill-fitting shoes has been established.

Exercises for Faulty Posture. The following exercises are recommended for correcting ordinary faulty posture:

1. The person with faulty posture should stand in front of a mirror. Another person should place his hand about one inch in front of the flat bone of the chest and push it forward to touch the hand, without swaying the body. He should try not to draw his shoulders back but keep them relaxed. Gradually the distance to which the chest is to be brought forward is increased by holding the hand farther away. Once the person is accustomed to the feeling of this exercise, he can do it without using a mirror. This posture should be repeated until it becomes easy and natural and can be maintained without strain or discomfort. The object is to achieve a proper relation between the thorax and the pelvis.

After this exercise has been repeated twenty times, the following exercises should be performed.

2. Raise arms forward, stretch them upward, rise on tiptoes, and inhale. Lower arms to the sides, slowly press the arms back, and exhale. This exercise, when done correctly, expands the chest, bringing in all the extensor muscles of the back and the levator muscles of the shoulders.

3. Stand with arms down and back, fingers interlocked, and palms out. Extend the neck, roll the shoulders back and turn the forearms so that the palms turn in, then down, and then out. Reverse to starting position and relax. This exercise is valuable for projecting the chest forward, stretching the shortened ligaments, and drawing in the abdomen. Care should be taken to have the chin back when the arms are brought down and turned out. When this exercise cannot be done with the fingers interlocked, a handkerchief tied in a loop may be substituted and held in the fingers.

4. Stand with the arms at the sides. Raise arms, stretch, inhale, bend forward, and rise. Lower arms, exhale. In this exercise the lungs are

filled when the chest is in the most favorable position for expansion. The breath is retained when the trunk is flexed, forcing the air into the cells of the lungs, under pressure. The bending and rising employs the extensor muscles of the neck and the retractor muscles of the shoulders.

5. Lie prone on a couch with the feet strapped, or on the floor with the feet caught on the edge of a bureau or other article of furniture. Clasp hands behind the head. Raise the head and extend the spine, pressing the elbows back. This exercise strengthens the back and shoulders. Follow with a deep breathing exercise.

6. Lie in the same position as in exercise 5, arms at the sides. Raise head, bring arms forward, and imitate the breast stroke.

In this exercise the spine is kept in static contraction, while the retractors of the shoulders are alternately contracted and relaxed.

Additional Exercises. Following are some simple exercises which help to strengthen the muscles of the back and abdomen and thus improve posture:

1. Lie on the back, hands back of the neck. Take a deep breath and raise chest high; keep chest up and exhale by pulling abdomen in.

2. In the same position, bend the knees and pull feet up. Pull abdomen in hard, and then relax.

3. Sit in a chair, trunk bending forward from the hips, keeping spine straight. This exercise may be done standing.

4. Stand with the heels four inches away from the wall but with the hips, shoulders, and head touching the wall; flatten the lower part of the back against the wall by pulling in the abdominal muscles. Holding this position, come away from the wall, with the weight well forward on the balls of the feet.

5. Stand with hands on hips, back flat, and chin in; raise one leg forward without bending the knee; lower it; repeat with other leg.

6. With head forward, clasp hands behind the head. Force the head back against their pressure, keeping chin in. This strengthens the muscles of the back of the neck.

7. Stand tall, holding the back straight. Rise on the toes, with arms extended forward and up, stretching the arms and the body.

PREFRONTAL LOBOTOMY. *See* PSYCHOSURGERY.

PREGNANCY AND PRENATAL CARE. *See* CHILDBIRTH AND PRENATAL CARE.

PREGNANCY, SIGNS OF. The signs of pregnancy are those changes which can be objectively observed by a woman, her doctor or both. Early in pregnancy these signs can be confused with other conditions but in the last half of pregnancy there can be little doubt about a woman's condition. Some of these signs do not occur in every pregnant woman. Others, however, always accompany pregnancy.

Changes in the skin. From the

beginning of pregnancy certain areas of the skin may become more heavily pigmented. At first the pigmentation is localized around the nipples and in a straight line down the middle of the abdomen. This is usually quite apparent about the end of the second month. Pigmentation in the form of blotches may appear on the face, hands, or other parts of the body. When they occur on the face they are sometimes termed the "mask of pregnancy." Wherever this pigmentation occurs, however, it is only temporary and disappears after childbirth.

In some pregnancies a skin condition known as *striae* is found. Pinkish lines are seen about the abdomen, breasts, and thighs, sometimes producing a sensation of itchiness and superficial tenderness. After childbirth the striae become white and almost unnoticeable.

Rarely, but in some pregnant women, fine hair appears on the surface of the body, particularly on the face. This almost invariably disappears soon after pregnancy.

Changes in the vagina and uterus. The lining of the vagina, which is a canal or tube leading from the uterus (womb) to the external orifice of the genital canal, and through which the child is born, becomes darkened early in pregnancy. The tip of the womb softens and the womb itself becomes softened and enlarged. A physician considering these changes along with symptoms reported by his patient sometimes can tell, with a fair degree of certainty, whether or not his patient is pregnant.

Changes in the breasts. Nature prepares the breasts of a pregnant woman for nursing her infant. Whether or not she chooses to breastfeed her baby is another matter. In any case, the supply of blood in the breasts increases and the blood vessels become apparent through the skin. Toward the end of the first month of pregnancy a pricking sensation and feeling of weight are experienced in the breasts. During the next few months, a secretion gradually forms which toward the last days of pregnancy becomes abundant and almost continuously discharges from the breasts. This is a whitish opaque substance called *colostrum*. The appearance of this substance is an indication that it is highly probable that the mother can successfully feed her baby.

A second breast change occurs about the eighth week of pregnancy and is a positive sign of conception. This is a new growth of tiny glands in the pigmented area around the nipples. These have the appearance of little protuberances and are known as *Montgomery's tubercles*.

Quickening. The baby is in fact a living creature from the instant of conception, but its movements are first sensed by its mother about the eighteenth week of pregnancy. This movement is called *quickening*—literally, coming to life.

Increase in size of abdomen. In a woman of average size, there is a slight bulge of the lower abdomen at about the third or fourth month of pregnancy. This alone, however, is not sure evidence of pregnancy because a tumor may cause a similar contour.

Fetal outline and movements. During the fifth month the baby's movement can usually be detected by the doctor, by touch or by direct vision. By exploring the abdomen by hand, he can outline the fetal parts. The outline and movements are positive signs of pregnancy.

Fetal heartbeat. When the fetus is four and a half months old, a doctor, listening through a stethoscope, can hear the baby's heartbeats. These are distinguishable from the mother's heartbeat because the fetal rate is very rapid—approximately 160 beats per minute early in pregnancy and a little slower later. This in itself is a positive sign of pregnancy. *See also* CHILDBIRTH AND PRENATAL CARE.

PREGNANCY, SYMPTOMS OF. Symptoms of pregnancy are those changes and sensations which become apparent to a prospective mother at the beginning of her pregnancy and during the weeks that follow.

Cessation of menstruation. Systemic disease or emotional disturbances may delay menstruation for five days or longer. When a woman has been fairly regular in her periods, however, a prolonged delay of ten or more days can be considered good evidence of pregnancy.

Frequency of urination. In the early stages of pregnancy, an increased frequency of urinations and a feeling of fullness of the bladder are usual. This is due to the pressure of the enlarging womb on the bladder and need not cause concern. This sensation disappears early in the pregnancy but returns during the last two months when the head of the baby is in the process of descending, preparatory to birth.

Nausea and vomiting. A large percentage of pregnant women experience neither of these symptoms: about one-third have nausea only, and one-third both nausea and vomiting. Some women experience these symptoms only in the morning, while others are troubled throughout the day. Nausea, when it does occur, usually starts about two weeks after conception but disappears in about four to six weeks. The intensity of this condition varies with different women. In some women it may persist for as long as three months but when recognized can be controlled by diet and medication recommended by the doctor.

Fatigue and constipation. During the early weeks of pregnancy an expectant mother sometimes complains of constipation and feels as if she were unable to get enough rest. Both these symptoms disappear, as a rule, in three to four weeks, in the absence of some complicating condition. *See also* CHILDBIRTH AND PRENATAL CARE.

PREMATURE BABIES. *See* BABIES, PREMATURE.

PRESBYOPIA, a form of *farsightedness* in which objects close to the eye may be seen only with difficulty. Farsightedness is a condition which normally develops with advancing years. First showing itself when the person is, perhaps, in his forties, presbyopia becomes progressively more acute until approximately the age of seventy-seven.

Among younger persons, the lens is elastic so that it can make itself quickly globular in order to see objects close at hand. With age, however, this elasticity lessens, the lens tends to remain increasingly flat, and the nearest point of clear vision becomes farther removed from the eye.

A person whose "point of convergence" is moving gradually farther from his eyes may boast of his ability to read auto licenses a block away but have to hold a book or newspaper at arm's length in order to read it.

In prescribing convex lenses for presbyopia, the oculist will take account of the patient's vocation. Thus, a linotypist should be able to see, with ease, at a distance of twelve or thirteen inches, whereas a pianist might require glasses which are not quite so strong.

The lenses, so prescribed, are not permanent and should be changed. The frequency of the changes can, in some instances, be limited, however, by the use of certain exercises suggested by the physician. *See also* EYE.

PRESCRIPTION, a written direction by which a remedy may be prepared and administered. Its four parts include: (1) the *superscription,* which consists merely of the letter R, with a line drawn across the second leg. This sign is an abbreviation for the Latin word *recipe,* meaning "take." (2) The *inscription,* which gives the ingredients to be used in preparing the remedy. (3) The *subscription,* which indicates how the remedy is to be compounded. (4) The *signature,* often preceded by the letter S, for the Latin *signa.* In this part the druggist is told what instructions to write on the outside of the container for the benefit of the patient.

Prescriptions at one time often contained a large number of ingredients, the doctor having prescribed something to cover all of the patient's symptoms. Today drugs are more powerful and more specific in their action and so the doctor usually limits the number and is likely to include only a few ingredients in a prescription. He is more concerned with controlling the source of the disease than with relieving all of the symptoms.

PRICKLY HEAT, medically called *miliaria,* an acute inflammatory skin rash, characterized by acute itching, which occurs when the skin fails to adapt itself to an increase in temperature and humidity. *Heat rash,* as it is also called, affects children more frequently than adults. Newcomers in a tropical locality will often cease to suffer from prickly heat as soon as their bodies have become adjusted to the new environment.

This rash consists of small elevations containing a watery fluid. They are found over pores and occur because the inflamed skin, usually pinkish, prevents the perspiration from emerging in the usual manner. Often these eruptions link with others to form stretches of unbroken rash.

Persons subjected to a hot and humid atmosphere often can avoid prickly heat by observing a few precautions. Heavy clothing should never be worn, especially by children. Frequent baths, followed by the use of a dusting powder, are desirable, and water or other liquids should be consumed in liberal quantities.

If an attack of prickly heat does occur, however, it will ordinarily yield to standard treatments such as the application of cool packs to the area. The skin should then be dusted with an antiseptic and nonirritating powder. Soap should be avoided since it is likely to irritate the rash. For cleansing purposes, a suitable oil is preferable, followed by the application of a soothing lotion.

If the rash persists, the person should consult a physician since the eruptions are a constant invitation to secondary infection.

PROLAPSE, the dropping of an internal body organ from its normal position, or the protrusion of the lining of a body cavity through a natural opening, or of an organ through a wound.

At childbirth, the stretching of the supportive tissues of the uterus may produce *prolapse of the uterus,* in which the womb falls from the normal position and the *cervix* is pushed far into the *vagina.* Severe prolapse can cause the womb to push the cervix through the vagina. This may provoke complications which require surgery. To correct prolapse by other than surgical means, various types of *pessaries* may be used, depending on the nature of the prolapse.

Prolapse through wounds occurs in the case of the bowels or the lung, when the abdominal or chest wall is penetrated. Another example of prolapse may be associated with a *perforated corneal ulcer,* where there is danger of *prolapse of the iris.*

PROSTATE, an organ in the human male located at the neck of the *urinary bladder,* surrounding the first part of the *urethra,* the passage through which *urine* is excreted and *semen* is ejaculated.

The prostate is partly glandular and partly muscular tissue. It produces a substance called *prostatic fluid* which is an important part of the semen, the substance that transports the male *sperm cells* into the female during sexual intercourse. Prostatic fluid is produced constantly and escapes through the urine. During sexual excitement, it increases in volume and is discharged into the urethra and thus into the semen at the time of ejaculation. The exact function of the prostatic fluid is not known, but it is believed to be related to the survival of the sperm in the female vagina.

The prostate is a gland with a minor function in reproduction and does not produce a hormone or other substance required in the body, nor does prostatic fluid enter the blood stream.

Inflammation or infection of the prostate is not uncommon and may be *chronic* or *acute.* Prostatic massage affords relief to men with chronic and subacute *prostatitis.* Acute

the disease and its causes PROSTATIC ENLARGEMENT The prostate is a gland located at the base of the bladder. This gland sometimes enlarges and continues to enlarge as a man gets older. The cause of this enlargement is not known; it affects about 30% of all men, married and single, by the time they reach 50 years of age; and there is no known relationship to other infections or to individual sex habits.
CANCER Cancer of the prostate accounts for 1 out of every 10 deaths from cancer in men. As with most malignant diseases, the cause is not known.

symptoms PROSTATIC ENLARGEMENT The symptoms of prostate enlargement are shown in the accompanying Medi-Graph. The patient urinates more frequently and feels the urge to urinate several times during the night. As the disease progresses and the prostate enlarges, the bladder becomes thin, weak, and less efficient. There is difficulty starting the stream of urine. Waste products are retained in the blood, leading to generalized weakness. In the final stage, the patient cannot pass urine at all.
CANCER Cancer of the prostate can be undetected until it has spread to involve other organ systems or bones, because very often there are no symptoms and no discomfort to the patient. Sometimes there may be mild discomfort on urination, or blood in the urine—as shown in the Medi-Graph. If there is pain, it is felt in the area just below the rectum. Sometimes the cancer is discovered when a prostate condition is treated surgically and routine biopsy reveals its presence. Bone pain in the lower back, or lung involvement which is discovered in a routine chest X ray, may be the first indication that the disease is already beyond control.

complications PROSTATIC ENLARGEMENT Complications in prostatic enlargement develop when obstruction, due to enlargement, prevents the free passage of urine and stagnant urine collects. There is back pressure and infection involving the ureter, urinary tract, and the kidneys. At a late stage of the illness, the patient may be in great pain because the bladder is so overstretched. Uremia may be an end result of this condition.
CANCER Complications in cancer of the prostate develop when the cancer is not diagnosed early and it spreads beyond the prostate, out of control.

prevention (or lessening of impact) PROSTATIC ENLARGEMENT Since there is no known method of preventing enlargement or cancer, men after 50 should have a physical check-up at regular six-month intervals, including a urine analysis and prostatic examination. Where enlargement is present, the doctor will advise treatment before urinary obstruction becomes a problem.
CANCER The prime hope in cancer of the prostate is early diagnosis.

Prostate Gland Enlargement

Cancer of the Prostate

Enlargement

1. Difficulty clearing bladder of urine
2. Swelling of Prostate Gland constricts urethral passage through it
3. Difficulty starting urination
4. Lessening of force and quantity of urine

Cancer

Symptoms similar to Prostate Gland Enlargement plus

A. Occasional drops of blood in urine

B. Pain in pelvis and thigh bones as cancer spreads

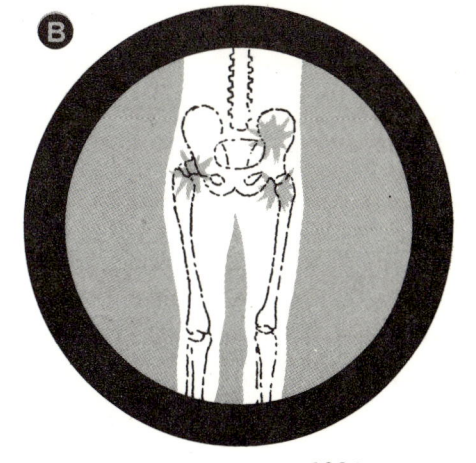

prostatitis can become extremely troublesome. The desire to urinate increases in frequency and urination is painful. An abscess may form in the gland and not only give great pain at the slightest motion but may break into the urethra or other nearby tissues and have to be treated surgically. *Antibiotics* and a *hot sitz bath* each evening are helpful in many cases of the various types of prostatitis.

The most frequent disorder of the prostate is its gradual *enlargement* in men over fifty. Sometimes this is first noticed in increasing difficulty of urination; in other cases the first sign may be desire, even during sleep, to urinate more often.

As the condition develops, a residue of voided urine tends to remain in the bladder. Eventually this will begin to decompose and irritate the whole bladder, leading to inflammation. One recourse now widely employed is the use of a *catheter* to assure complete evacuation; another is *surgical removal* of part or all of the prostate, and a third means is the use of *glandular substances* which restrain its overgrowth.

One of the most impressive recent advances in medicine has been the improved techniques for treating prostatic conditions. Surgery has advanced from a two-stage operation which had many fatalities to the use of a tube, passed into the prostatic area from outside the body, through which *electrical dissection* can remove enlarged tissue.

The prostate is especially subject to *cancer* and some authorities believe it the commonest cancer of men since it accounts for 10 per cent of the deaths from cancer. Cancer arises in the prostate frequently without any symptom or warning, but becomes evident in one of two principal ways. Difficulty in urination, much like that attending simple prostatic enlargement, may occur, and sometimes blood appears in the urine. Neither of these signs is conclusive proof of cancer, but since urinary irregularity may signal a highly dangerous and progressive condition prompt medical attention should always be given.

The other sign of prostatic cancer is pain in the bones of the pelvis and thigh. This is caused by the spread of the original cancer. Medical examination of the prostate gland, a simple procedure, and x-ray pictures of the bones will establish the diagnosis.

Today cancer of the prostate can be treated with great success if it is recognized while still localized—that is, before it has spread. A rather reliable means of insuring that if it does occur it can be recognized in time is regular prostatic examination by a doctor at six-month intervals for every man over fifty. The procedure is simple and quick and is a form of life insurance.

The only real cure of this condition is complete removal of the whole gland before cancer has spread to other areas. However, new methods developed in the past few years make it possible to prolong the lives of those in whom cancer has spread to the bones and to relieve their suffering. Removal of the testicles or administration of female sex hormones or both give many such patients twice the life expectancy they had before, as well as relief from acute suffering. *See also* REPRODUCTION SYSTEM. *See* MEDIGRAPHS pages 1081, 1311.

PROTEIN, one of a group of complex *nitrogenous substances* of high molecular weight which are found in various forms in animals and plants and are *characteristic of living matter.* In the chemical makeup of the body, proteins occupy a significant place, being essential in the maintenance of tissue and also a valuable source of energy. In the process of digestion, the complex proteins, which are largely *giant molecules,* split into simpler forms and finally into *amino acids.*

Amino acids contain *carbon, oxygen, hydrogen,* and *nitrogen* and some contain *sulphur.* Amino acids replace parts of body protein which are constantly being lost or destroyed through excretion. Some amino acids can be manufactured by the body from other substances but not in sufficient quantity to sustain life, so that the diet must contain essential amino acids if body growth and repair are to continue.

Proteins which furnish essential amino acids in large amounts are called *complete proteins.* Meat, largely composed of animal protein, contains the most nearly complete edible protein. Plant proteins are generally *incomplete,* and cannot supply the body with enough of certain essential amino acids. Eggs, fish, and milk are complete proteins.

Proteins have been classified into numerous groups, two of the significant ones being *albumins* and the *globulins.* Egg white is largely albumin, but also contains globulin. Blood plasma contains both. The ability of the blood to clot depends on *fibrinogen,* a globulin. Some of the *antibodies* which the blood develops to combat disease are also globulins.

Every diet should contain two or more portions of protein foods a day to prevent *amino acid deficiency.* A diet high in carbohydrates and low in protein fails to supply the body adequately with amino acids and *edema* can result. *See also* EDEMA; NUTRITION; VITAMINS; KWASHIORKOR.

PRURITIS. *See* ITCHING.

PSITTACOSIS, commonly called *parrot fever,* a disease not only of parrots, parakeets, lovebirds, canaries, pigeons, ducks, and other birds, but one also readily transmitted to human beings. Occasionally the infection is spread from one infected person to another.

The infection is caused by a virus which can be found in the nasal discharges and droppings of infected birds and which contaminate their feathers and cages. The virus enters the human body by inhalation. Psittacosis usually appears sporadically, but outbreaks have occurred among family groups, employees of pet shops, and laboratory workers.

In birds the liver and spleen are affected, but in men the lungs are usually involved. The disease is serious, especially in older persons.

Usually the disease begins seven to fifteen days after exposure to the infection with headache, sore throat, chills, fever, and backache followed by a dry cough. In severe cases the temperature may remain high for two or three weeks. The lungs are congested and sometimes a large amount of slightly blood-stained sputum may be expectorated. Convalescence begins with a drop in temperature and is generally lengthy in severe cases.

Psittacosis is one of the few virus diseases which yield to treatment with certain antibiotics. These also can prevent bacterial infections which often follow an attack. Expectorants and inhalants may be prescribed for dry coughs and sputum discharge. A person who has psittacosis is ordinarily isolated and anyone coming in contact with him is protected against discharges from cough or sputum. A wise precaution includes destroying the infected bird, and burning the cage and all materials that have been in contact with the bird.

PSORIASIS, a chronic inflammatory skin diease, and one of the ten most frequent skin ailments. It affects both men and women, and usually appears after the age of fifteen. It is non-infectious, but some families seem to have a tendency to it.

The cause of psoriasis is unknown. Numerous theories have been advanced, but as yet no cause has been definitely established. Some doctors believe it is of nervous origin, others think it may be related to difficulty in digesting fat, or to certain germs and viruses.

The first sign of psoriasis is generally an eruption of pinhead-size, bright red spots which group to form larger ones, finally becoming great patches of reddened skin. The healing begins from the center and leaves a red or reddish–brown stain. Also characteristic of psoriasis are thick, silver-white scales. When they are removed, small bleeding spots remain. There is seldom any itching nor is general health affected.

Eruption is usually on the elbows, knees, and backs of the arms and leg; occasionally the chest and abdomen are involved. Sometimes the lesions become infected and form pus. Fingernails and toenails and the palms of the hands and soles of the feet may be affected also.

Treatment requires patient careful management by the doctor and complete cooperation of the patient. Since the cause is unknown, treatment may be varied and tentative until the doctor arrives at the most effective method.

Psoriasis has been treated by diets, most of which seem to have been ineffective, with the possible exception of low-fat diets. *Tar bath treatments* have been helpful and many patients have improved with exposure to *sunlight* or *ultraviolet rays* following application of *special tar ointment.* Fowler's solution of arsenic, formerly used, has largely been replaced. Several special drugs have been developed for treatment of psoriasis. *Chrysarobin* is often effective when the palms of the hands and soles of the feet are involved.

Hormone injections have been tried; but unless peeling of the horny layer of the skin is excessive and widespread, there is not enough evidence of relation between glands and psoriasis to warrant the use of hormones.

Radiation therapy is often helpful in healing psoriasis, but cannot prevent its recurrence, and this treatment should only be used in special cases and with extreme care, since serious changes in the skin may occur.

Sedatives and *tranquilizing drugs* have been found effective, especially in those cases which seem connected with emotional stress.

The cytostatic drug *methotrexate* has given excellent results in many cases.

Psoriasis in children must be managed with special care, since there is danger of absorption of the tarry substances or other drugs, such as *ammoniated mercury* used in treating psoriasis of the scalp. For this type of psoriasis, shampooing with *salicylic acid,* ammoniated mercury, and other substances is sometimes effective. See MEDIGRAPH page 1087.

PSYCHIATRY, the branch of medicine dealing with the treatment of *mental and emotional disorders.* See PSYCHOSIS; NEUROSIS; MANIC-DEPRESSIVE PSYCHOSIS; PARANOIA; SCHIZOPHRENIA; MENTAL DEPRESSION; INVOLUTIONAL MELANCHOLIA; ELECTRIC SHOCK TREATMENT; PSYCHOANALYSIS; FEEBLE-MINDEDNESS; DELUSIONS; AMNESIA; APHASIA; HYPNOSIS; PSYCHOSOMATIC DISORDERS; BARBITURATES; PARESIS. See also PSYCHOLOGY.

PSYCHOANALYSIS, a method of psychotherapy originated by Sigmund Freud which attempts to determine the motivations of the personality in order to treat emotional disorders. Many psychiatrists, among them Jung and Adler, have worked in this field, modifying and changing the Freudian psychoanalytic method, so that many adaptations of psychoanalysis are now practiced. The technique is used in the study and treatment of a wide variety of emotional problems, particularly the *neuroses.*

Typically the patient in psychoanalysis meets with his analyst a minimum of two one-hour periods a week, and talks as freely and fully as possible about anything he chooses. In theory, the patient comes to realize more and more what in his past and present life is relevant and significant to his emotional problems. Gradually the psychoanalyst and patient come to recognize the roots and patterns of the patient's attitudes and actions. The goal is to create within the patient both an intellectual and emotional awareness of why he thinks and acts as he does. Often an *intellectual grasp* of the problems precedes an *emotional grasp*—i.e., he may *know* that he drinks to excess when he is worried, but still not have reached the point where this knowledge will *serve to help him.* Since neuroses have origins which reach far back into the patient's life, the patient often devotes a large part of his attention to early childhood and adolescence.

the disease and its causes This is a chronic, recurrent skin eruption which seems to run in families. The cause is unknown. Attacks are triggered by emotional stress or shock; children often develop it after a strep infection; sometimes it appears at the site of a skin injury. It is neither infectious nor contagious, and there is little or no itching. Both sexes, in all age groups, are subject to psoriasis—and it is more common in patients who drink a good deal of liquor.

symptoms The disease begins without any warning and with no generalized symptoms. Small, flat, red patches appear which may or may not show a tendency to peel. They spread by direct extension, and the surface shows thin, silvery white scales. All of the infected area is covered with these except for the narrow red rim. Itching, if present, is moderate. In 75% of the cases the scalp, knees, elbows, and back are involved, but it is not unusual to see psoriasis involving the nails. The disease may be limited to one or two patches or cover the entire body.

If the surface scales are removed, a raw, red surface is exposed, with minute bleeding points.

complications There are no serious complications. Secondary infection can follow severe nail involvement, in which case the nail itself may have to be removed.

prevention (or lessening of impact) There is no known method of avoiding this disease, and no known cure.

Good eating habits, the elimination of alcohol from the diet, vitamin therapy, and the maintenance of good health can help limit the severity of psoriasis flare-ups. Many medications to control the rash are available.

Psoriasis

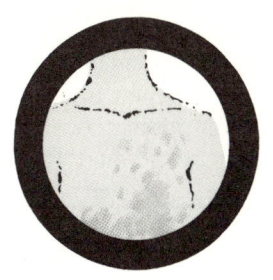

1. Starts as small red patches which enlarge and join together

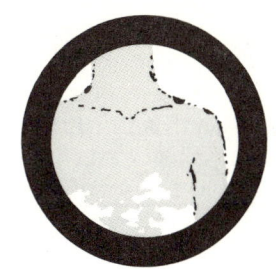

2. Patches usually become covered with silvery-white, scaly skin

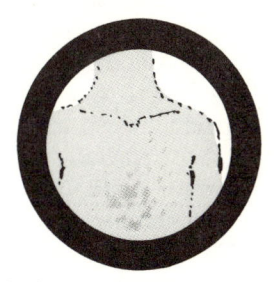

3. If scales fall off or are removed, red pinpoint area revealed underneath

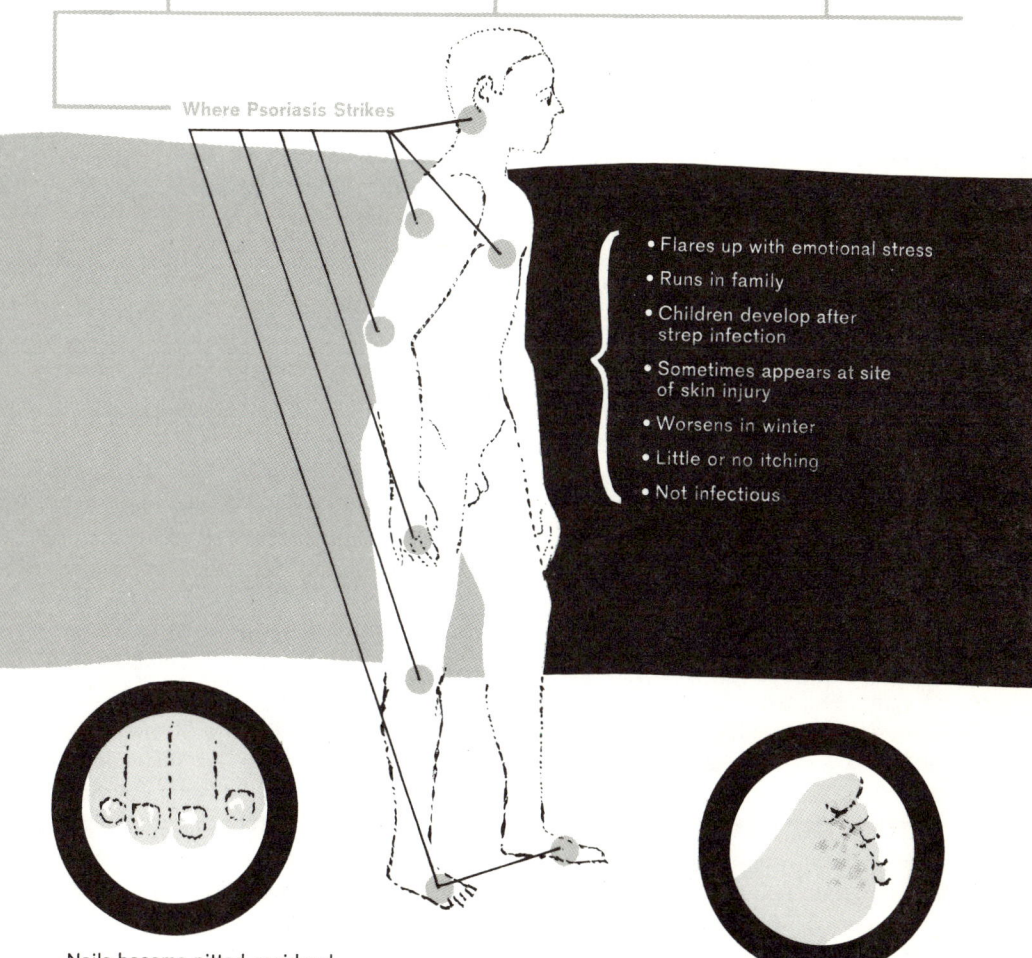

Where Psoriasis Strikes

- Flares up with emotional stress
- Runs in family
- Children develop after strep infection
- Sometimes appears at site of skin injury
- Worsens in winter
- Little or no itching
- Not infectious

Nails become pitted or ridged with yellow spots — Soles of feet (and sometimes palms) may develop infection

1087

Psychoanalysis can take from months to years, the patient deciding when he no longer needs the services of his psychoanalyst. Naturally, such extended treatment is exceedingly costly, and each patient must determine for himself whether the results obtained are worth the expense involved. Some psychiatrists reject the psychoanalytic method, preferring more effective methods such as chemotherapy or hypnosis.

PSYCHOLOGY, the systematic study of *behavior,* particularly the study of human behavior with reference to the *cultural environment*; the investigation of *individual responses* to *given stimuli.* It is to be distinguished from *psychiatry,* which is the medical treatment of mental and emotional disorders.

PSYCHOSIS, a severe mental disorder which manifests itself in abnormal behavior, reactions, and ideas. The victim is no longer able to cope with his environment.

A *psychotic* differs from a *neurotic* in that the latter has succeeded in making some adjustment to his environment—the inadequate nature of the adjustment being itself the neurosis. *See also* MANIC-DEPRESSIVE PSYCHOSIS; NEUROSIS; PARANOIA; SCHIZOPHRENIA.

PSYCHOSOMATIC DISORDERS, illnesses which result from the interaction of mental and physical processes, rather than from any specific organic factors. The emotional element in sickness has been recognized since ancient times. However, the role of emotional factors and their connection with diseases has been established as an accepted area of medical study only in this century.

Psychosomatic disorders may result from multiple causes where the *emotional stimulus* is combined with other factors, such as a *physical predisposition.* In ailments like *asthma* or *colitis,* for example, the site of the difficulty may be physically predisposed, while the *catalyst* is emotional in nature.

Psychosomatic disturbances may take place in any of the involuntary organs of the body, including the digestive tract, the respiratory region, the heart and circulatory systems, the genitourinary system, the endocrine glands, and the skin.

Certain forms of allergy are also greatly influenced by emotional factors. In some instances chronic cases of asthma have been helped by psychotherapy. *See also* NEUROSIS; PEPTIC ULCER.

PSYCHOSURGERY, an operation recommended only in cases of otherwise incurable *psychosis,* in which the nerve fibers leading to the frontal lobes of the brain are severed—also known as *prefrontal lobotomy* or *leukotomy.* Violent or intractable patients can sometimes be rendered docile and harmless by this operation. However, every other method of therapy should be exhausted without success before resorting to such a radical procedure. *See also* ELECTRIC SHOCK TREATMENT; HYPNOSIS.

PSYCHOTHERAPY. *See* PSYCHIATRY; PSYCHOANALYSIS.

PTOMAINE POISONING. See FOOD POISONING.

PUBERTY, the period in which the physical form of the child is gradually transformed into that of the young adult. These changes are far-reaching. Physical growth is usually rapid and the transition from child to tall gangling youth sometimes seems to occur almost overnight. Girls are a bit more precocious than boys in this change. The physical changes of adolescence frequently begin about the age of eleven (sometimes earlier) with girls but are likely to begin at thirteen with boys. Girls maintain this relatively advanced position in relation to boys during most of the high school years, but by the time college years are reached the difference is no longer apparent. Girls tend to prefer association with boys a bit older than themselves and this tendency is likely to persist into adulthood. Eventually they are likely to marry men a bit older than themselves.

Growth in height is the most obvious of the far-reaching physical changes of the youth during adolescence. Full height may be achieved as early as the fourteenth year, yet some young people continue to grow taller into the early twenties. This depends, among other considerations, on the timing and rate of development of the *endocrine glands,* which include the *ovaries* and *testes* (the *gonads*). The hormones secreted by these glands bring about many of the maturational changes of puberty and at the same time inhibit growth in height. If puberty is rapid and the physical changes completed early, growth stops early. If there is a lag in the maturing of the gonads, growth in height may be prolonged.

Girls at puberty begin to develop the contours of young womanhood. The breasts develop, the hips broaden, and they lose the earlier likeness to the more boyish figure of childhood. The internal organs essential to a womanly life—the uterus especially—develop and the first *menstruation* is the definite signal of approaching maturity. This sometimes occurs as early as age ten but may not occur until thirteen of even fourteen years of age. Girls should be prepared for this event. This preparation can best come from the mother, who should inform her daughter in direct terms about body structure and function. Otherwise, incorrect and distorted information may be received from other girls or may be fantasied.

The approach of adolescence is heralded by the development of the *secondary sexual characteristics.* The development of axillary and pubic hair are obvious examples. With boys, the beginning development of the beard calls for an initial effort at shaving; soon heavier growth of the facial hair calls for regular grooming. The genitals of the boy approach adult size and *emissions* indicate the development of the testes and achievement of fertility. The deepening of the voice, most noticeably in boys, is another obvious secondary characteristic.

The skin of the adolescent undergoes characteristic changes. Sweat glands of more mature form develop; the skin becomes more oily. Often *acne* appears, especially in fair-skinned individuals, and when severe causes the adolescent much distress. The adolescent is most sensitive to anything that can be interpreted as a defect or blemish. Under some circumstances, adolescent acne may cause intense emotional suffering. While the condition is only temporary, psychiatric advice and aid may be needed if careful cleansing of the skin alone does not keep it under control.

The development of sexual fertility and the concomitant sexual urges in the adolescent boy lead almost inevitably to the practice of *masturbation*. The adolescent's first sexual experience is usually masturbatory. Adolescents are unlikely to require explanations or interference from adults concerning masturbation, and parents should never attempt to alarm them with unfounded tales of injurious consequences (which in fact are nonexistent) or with feelings of guilt or remorse. The adolescent boy is highly potent sexually and biologically quite capable of fatherhood, but emotionally is still very ill-prepared to assume such a role, even if society were to sanction it, which it seldom is willing to do before the boy is at least 18 years old. Masturbation is thus the only sexual outlet at the boy's disposal in which he can indulge without the involvement or distress of others.

The girl's reaction to the bodily changes that occur and to menstruation normally is one of satisfaction and pride. She begins to feel that—like the older girls she admires and (if she has a good relationship with her mother) like her mother—she is approaching the dignity of young womanhood. This pride in self can only occur, however, if by example and by proper teaching in her own home she is able to anticipate that her approaching womanliness brings healthy promise for the future. Many adolescent girls are anxious and confused by the changes of adolescence. A girl may childishly attempt to deny or hide her physical development if she has not been helped to understand and accept her approach to adult femininity. Sometimes masturbation becomes a practice. Disturbed attitudes of women toward the role of wife and mother are not infrequently reflected in the uncertainties of their daughters during adolescence about these roles. The healthy mother brings to her daughter her own assurance that the sexual, family, and social role of wife and mother are sources of profound gratification.

Boys gain much satisfaction and pride from becoming large and strong, capable of physical performances that they admire in others and for themselves. The boy who early develops the physique of the football player is likely to have an easier time, in certain respects, than the boy whose physical development is minimal. If he actually remains below average in size and strength, he is likely to suffer. Most boys sharply compare themselves with others, are most sensitive to anything that might indicate they are less capable than their friends, particularly in sports. Boys are sensitive about breadth of chest expansion, strength of arms, and may be concerned about general appearances. Some of them go to extremes to overcome what they consider physical defects. Whether hips are too broad, legs too skinny or too fat, breasts too flat or too rounded are matters of undue concern for many uncertain adolescents.

At times, boys and girls must be dealt with directly about their competitive feelings as reflected in apprehension about their own powers or appearance. The adolescent, when given proper opportunity, will ask questions about bodily changes; he will reveal his uncertainty and anxiety about his ability to measure up to others of his age. Since most adolescent anxieties center about the problem of his capacity to meet the demands of adult life, an approach to the seemingly simple matter of how he feels about his own body and appearance will frequently lead to a frank facing of deeper-lying concerns about his sexual impulses, his social and vocational uncertainties. *See also* ADOLESCENCE.

PUBLIC HEALTH. Most countries today maintain government agencies concerned with the regulation and conservation of public health. In the United States, the FOOD AND DRUG ADMINISTRATION is charged with this responsibility. The FDA establishes standards which must be met by all food, drug, and cosmetic manufacturers, and periodically inspects their facilities and analyses their products. The agency also specifies the amount and nature of additives that may be used in foods, and regulates the manufacture of agricultural pesticides. The Food and Drug Administration is now part of the Department of Health, Education and Welfare.

PULMONIC STENOSIS, SURGERY IN. Pulmonic stenosis is an obstruction in the valve between the heart and the artery which carries blood into the lungs. Formerly the only treatment attempted was the construction of an artificial bypass to detour the blood around the obstruction. This operation was of limited value, adding a man-made malformation to the already imperfect heart. While this operation was done entirely outside the heart, the new technique involves corrective surgery within the heart itself. The surgeon inserts a miniature knife through a tiny slit in the heart wall, and working by touch, eliminates the obstruction in or near the valve. *See also* HEART SURGERY, ARTIFICIAL.

PULSE, the intermittent change in the shape of an *artery* due to an increase in the tension of its walls following the *contraction of the heart.* The impulses which the beating of the heart sends through the arteries can be felt at various places on the surface of the body. The artery usually selected for examination of the pulse is the *radial artery* lying over the *radius bone* at the *wrist.* A finger is placed on this artery and the number of beats per minute re-

1091

PUNCTURE WOUND

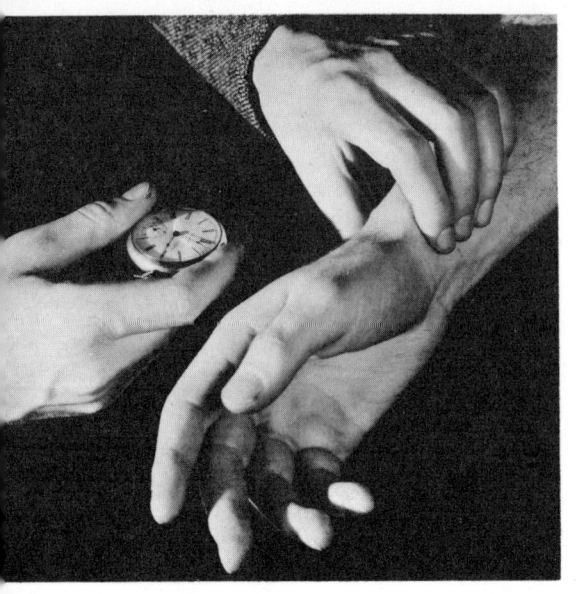

Pulse—Proper technique for taking the pulse. With the index finger, not the thumb, the pulse beat is found on the thumb side of the wrist and the beats are counted for a full minute.

corded. A machine which measures pulse rate has also been developed.

In adults, the number of pulsations per minute varies from 67 to 72. In infants, the rate is 120 to 140 in the first few weeks of life, slowing gradually to 100 to 120.

Excessive rapidity of pulse rate is called *tachycardia,* and excessive slowness is called *brachycardia.* In fever, the pulse rate increases from 8 to 10 beats per minute for each degree of temperature rise above normal. After exertion the rate increases but usually returns to normal within a few minutes. Many long-distance runners have pulse rates as low as 40 to 65.

Normal pulse is regular, the beats occurring in the same intervals. In *auricular fibrillation,* the pulse is ex-

PURPURA HEMORRHAGICA

tremely irregular. The force of the pulse may also vary in disorders associated with a depressed physical state and with certain ailments of the blood vessels. *See also* ARTERIOSCLEROSIS; BLOOD PRESSURE; HEART.

PUNCTURE WOUND. *See* WOUNDS.

PURGATIVE. *See* CATHARTICS.

PURPURA HEMORRHAGICA, a condition caused by a decrease to below normal in the number of *blood platelets,* which are factors in *coagulation.* When a shortage of blood platelets occurs, *bleeding* will begin almost spontaneously, particularly from the mucous membranes in the nose and mouth. Bleeding underneath the skin is frequent, giving the appearance of bruises.

The number of platelets may be lessened as a result of some action on the *bone marrow,* in which the cells that form the platelets are manufactured. Fewer platelets may result from a decrease of the cells or from a toxic action that destroys these blood cells more rapidly than they are formed. Sometimes it is associated with *sensitivity to drugs,* such as the sulfonamides, quinine, barbiturates, or with the *toxicity* that results from the action of *certain types of disease,* such as measles, tuberculosis, and infectious mononucleosis. In many women, a lessening of the platelets occurs at *menstruation.*

Purpura hemorrhagica is seen most frequently in persons between the ages of twelve and twenty-five,

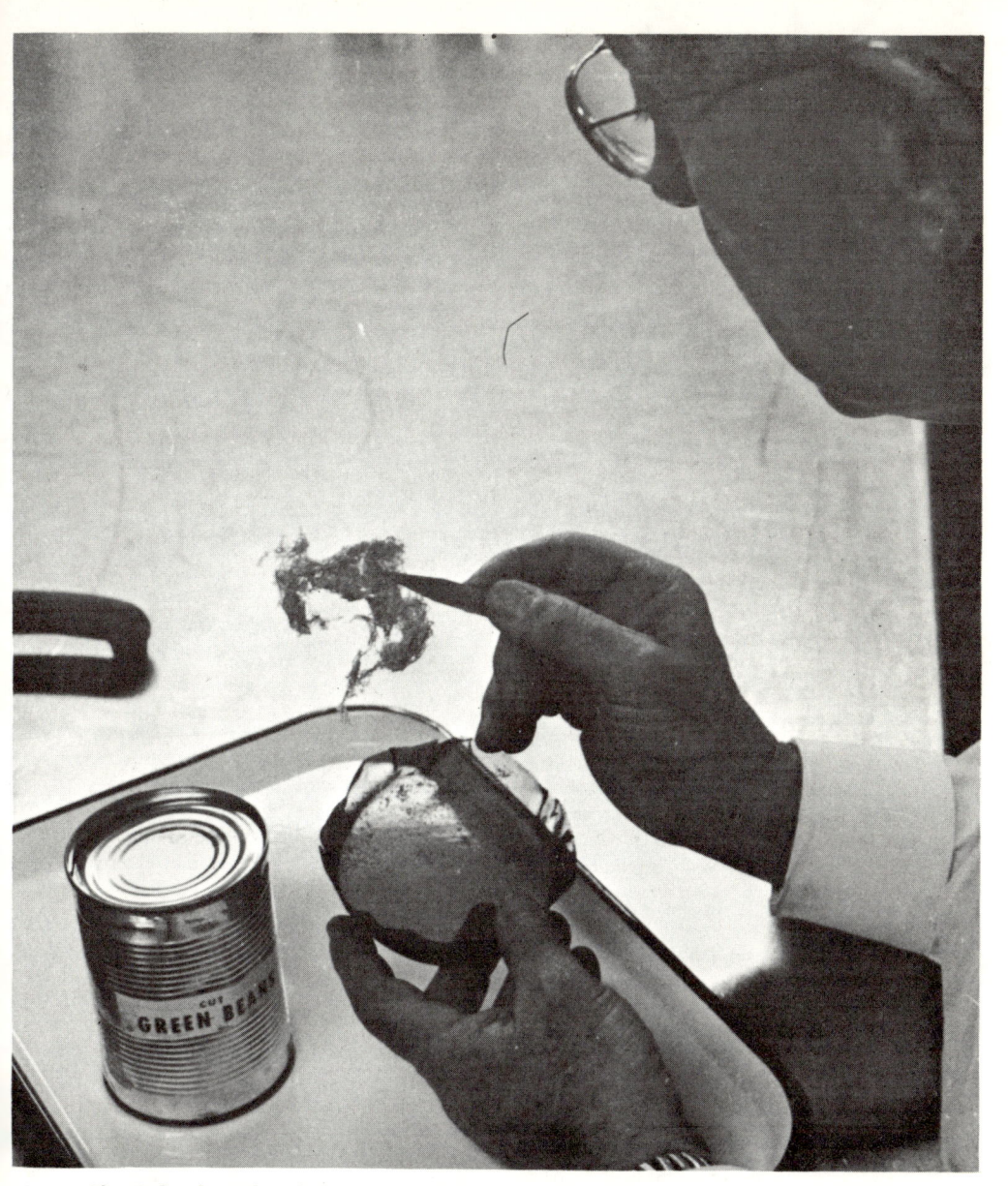

The Federal Food and Drug Administration is concerned with the protection of the consumer. A scientific and law enforcement agency of the government, it is responsible for the laws passed by Congress pertaining to the purity, safety, effectiveness, and labeling of foods, drugs, cosmetics, and chemicals. FDA inspectors and scientists in eighteen districts are constantly at work assembling data and evidence for the purpose of enforcing the Food, Drug, and Cosmetic Act, the Hazardous Substances Labeling Act, and other Federal laws pertinent to these and related fields. The data and evidence are evaluated by headquarters personnel in Washington, D.C. Whenever products in interstate commerce are found to be adulterated or misbranded, the agency takes remedial or punitive action through the Federal Courts. Such action is designed to protect the public health. Above, a can of beans is inspected.

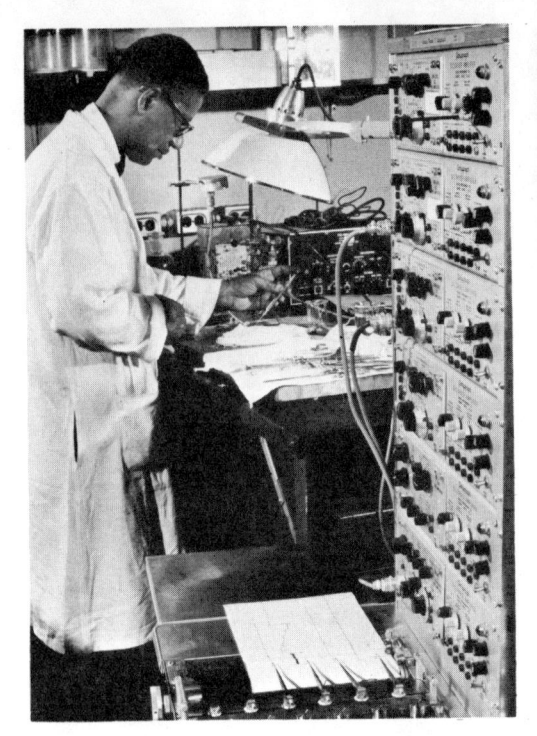

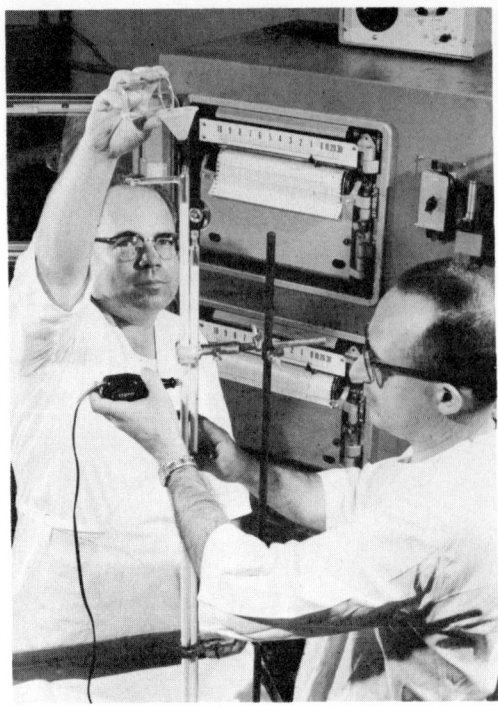

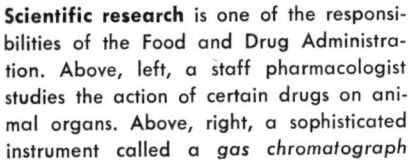

Scientific research is one of the responsibilities of the Food and Drug Administration. Above, left, a staff pharmacologist studies the action of certain drugs on animal organs. Above, right, a sophisticated instrument called a *gas chromatograph* measures minute amounts of food additives and other chemicals. Below, Federal inspectors are shown at work in a food-processing plant. All such facilities are subject to periodic inspection by government officials. In this way, the public is assured protection.

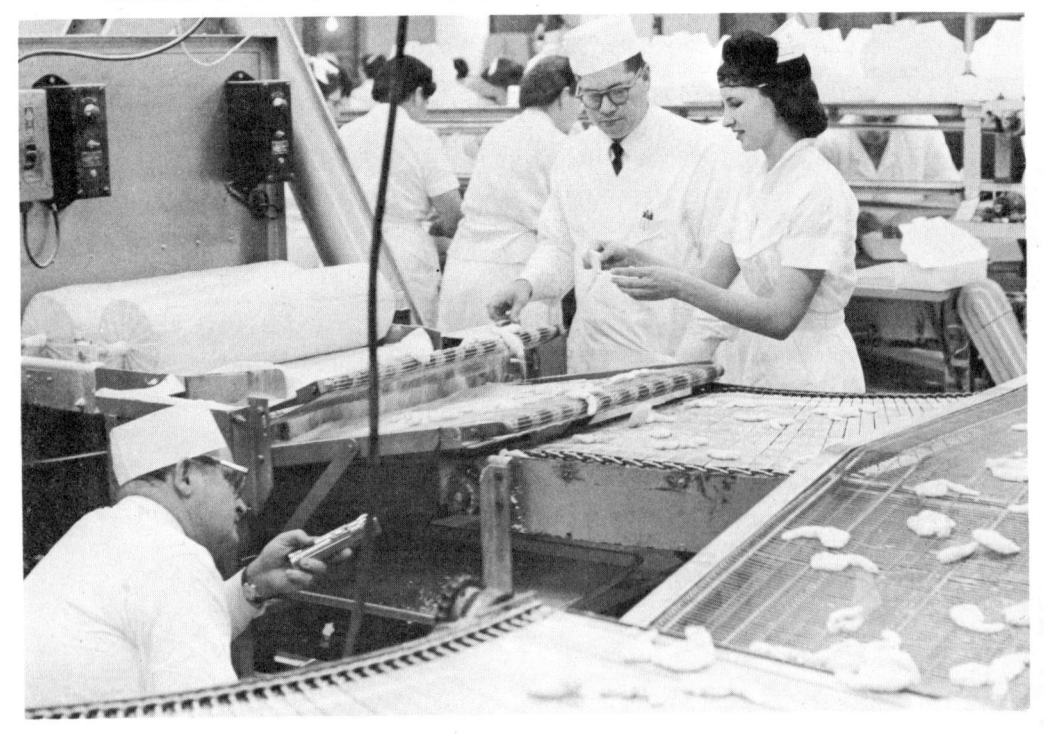

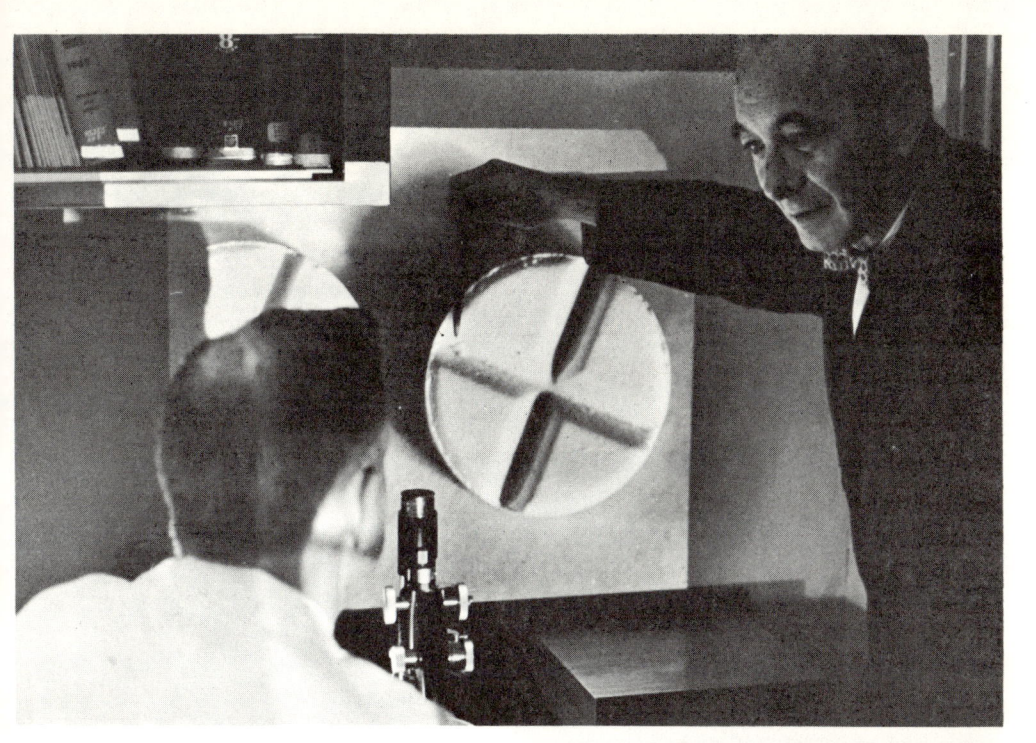

Above, government inspectors examine a shipment of drugs with sophisticated machinery. Drugs are characteristically marked by the machines that make them. Scientists have devised methods to identify drugs found in illegal channels. Colors used in foods, drugs, and cosmetics must be safe to be lawful. At right, a scientist separates the components of a color in a tube. Each component is then identified to determine if it meets Federal certification requirements. Below, an inspector checks a pill-coating machine.

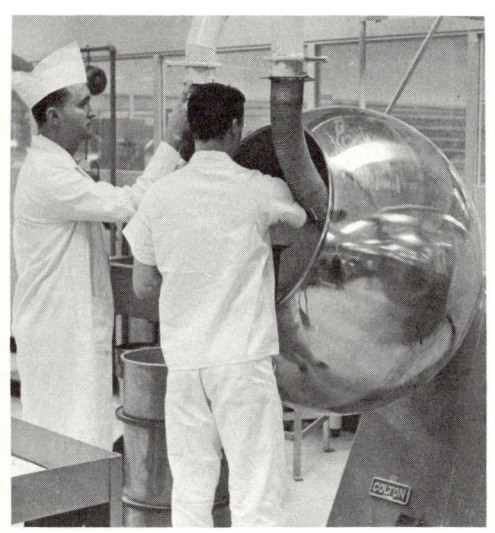

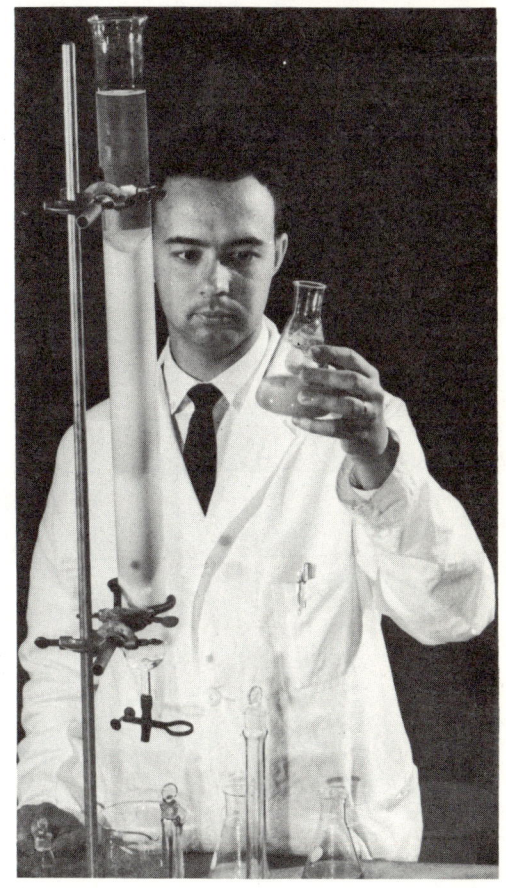

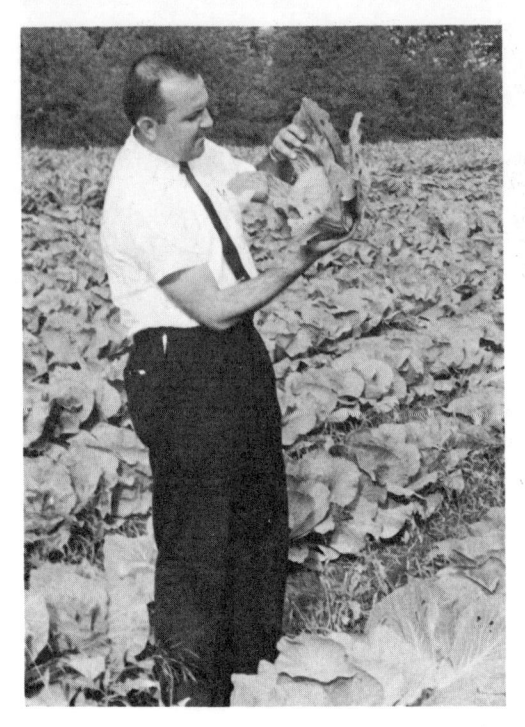

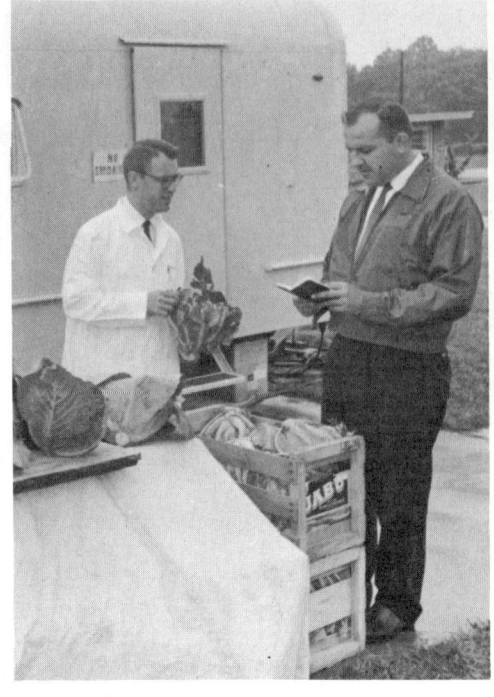

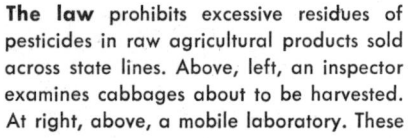

The law prohibits excessive residues of pesticides in raw agricultural products sold across state lines. Above, left, an inspector examines cabbages about to be harvested. At right, above, a mobile laboratory. These are sometimes moved into harvest areas so that samples of raw agricultural products can be quickly analyzed. Below, a railroad car of wheat is inspected for any possibility of chemical contamination.

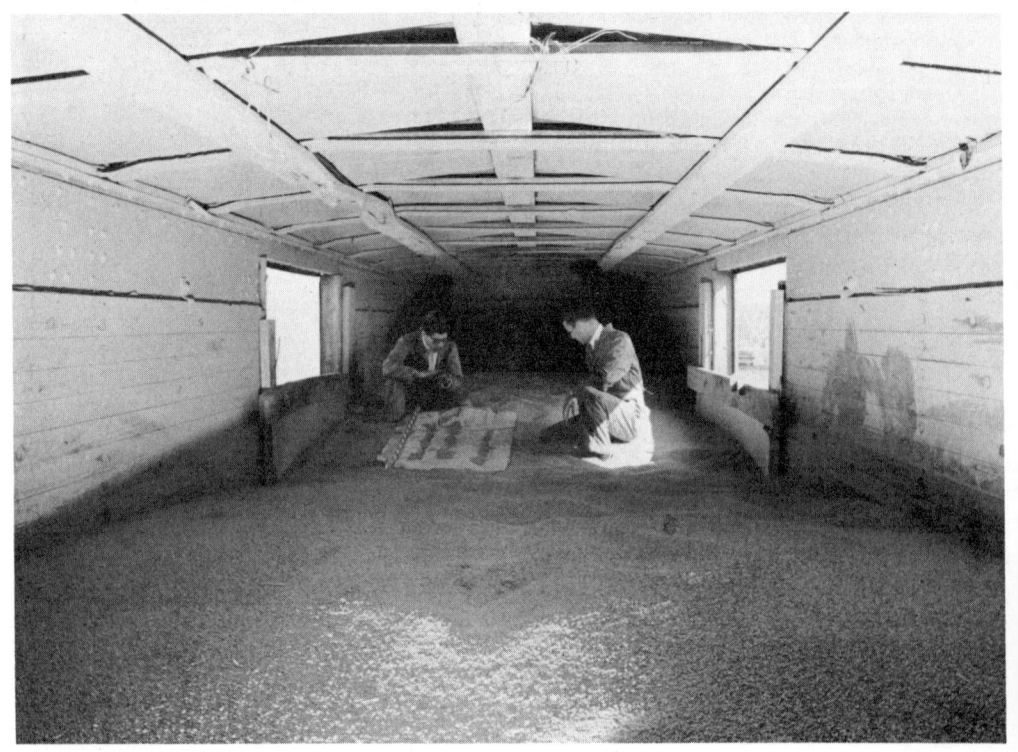

although it may occur at any age. The condition may develop gradually so that the onset cannot be determined accurately. Some acute cases are so severe that there is danger of bleeding to death within a few days or weeks. In others, the condition may be chronic, varying in severity throughout the person's life.

Many different procedures have been used to treat patients suffering from purpura, often with the hope of at least improving the condition, since a cure is not always possible. One of the simplest and most direct methods is injection of blood into the body, either intravenously, into the muscles, or under the skin. *Transfusion of whole blood* is one of the most helpful treatments. The use of *ACTH, cortisone,* or *hydrocortisone,* in connection with transfusions or alone, has been found to modify rapidly the bleeding tendency in many cases. Sometimes *removal of the spleen* by surgical operation has been helpful and is now an accepted technique of treatment. *Injection of hormones* in connection with the operation depends on the individual case. In many instances, a new chemical, *vitamin K_1,* supplements other supportive measures, such as *replenishment of iron.*

Most of the management of treatment of purpura hemorrhagica is considered experimental for the individual case, and for each patient a study should be made to determine the presence of an *allergy to a protein,* and whether or not the disturbance in platelet production is related to such sensitivity. The *removal of allergens* and *use of antihistamines* and other supportive measures has generally been helpful in the treatment of disorders caused by allergies.

PUS, the thick, creamy, yellowish product of inflammation, found in abscesses. It consists chiefly of serum and white blood cells. The color varies with the causative microorganism. A discharge containing or forming pus is called *purulent.*

PYELITIS, an inflammation of the *pelvis* or lower part of the kidney. In pregnancy, chills, fever, and pain between the hips and ribs may be indicative of pyelitis. See also KIDNEYS; NEPHRITIS. See MEDIGRAPH page 1311.

PYELONEPHRITIS, the most common type of kidney infection, involving both the pelvis of the kidney and the kidney itself. See also KIDNEYS; NEPHRITIS.

PYEMIA, an infection due to the presence of pus-producing germs in the blood stream and the formation of abscesses where these organisms lodge. See also BACTEREMIA.

PYLORUS, the valve which releases food from the *stomach* into the *duodenum.* Ulcers may form in the pylorus with subsequent scarring and constriction. Babies are sometimes born with an enlargement of the muscles which form the pyloric valve. This causes obstruction of the passage of food and spasms which result in vomiting. The child will lose weight rapidly since he cannot retain food. The usual treatment for a congenital malformed pyloric valve is a surgical division of the muscle.

PYORRHEA, usually refers to an inflammation of the *gums* and outer covering of the roots of the teeth when it reaches the purulent stage. It is easier to prevent than cure and rarely occurs when good general care is taken of the teeth and gums. Beginning with tender bleeding gums the inflammation advances until the teeth become loosened from the supporting gum. The dentist follows a regular course of treatment. If started early enough, treatment is effective, but when there is extensive bone loss and shifting of teeth in their sockets little can be done, and removal of the teeth affected is advised in order to save the rest. *See also* GINGIVITIS; TEETH.

Q

Q FEVER, often called *nine-mile fever,* an infection which resembles *influenza* or *virus pneumonia.* It is caused by a *rickettsial organism,* a microorganism smaller than bacteria but larger than a filterable virus, and is transmitted to man by *ticks* that live on infected animals. Q fever was first recognized in Australia, where it occurred among workers in packing houses and dairies and among foresters. Almost at the same time, a group of laboratory workers in Montana contracted it. The outbreaks were apparently due to inhalation of dust contaminated with rickettsiae or by dried feces of infected ticks.

Q fever begins with *fever, headache, chills, malaise,* and *weakness.* Mild cases last a few days, but more severe attacks may persist for two to three weeks; the condition usually ends in complete recovery. Treatment ordinarily consists of *good nursing care* and *use of appropriate drugs* early in the course of the illness.

Q fever can also be acquired by contact with infected milk or dairy products, and proper pasteurization of milk is a significant factor in preventing the spread of Q fever.

QUACKS, individuals who falsely claim to possess medical knowledge which enables them to cure or treat disease. Fortunately today legislation has been passed which limits their activity, whereas formerly they had complete freedom to advertise through newspapers and radio, and to prepare and sell medicines.

The quacks are marked by certain definite characteristics. They claim knowledge that they do not possess. They put after their names long appendages of degrees, most of which were never conferred on them by any university. They make exaggerated claims as to their ability to cure disease. They do not even hesitate to guarantee a cure if that seems necessary to secure a patient. They are likely to charge far more than the traffic will bear or else to build up a tremendous group of followers by charging just a trifle to thousands of people. Finally, they always claim to be able to perform functions in the field of healing which are far beyond the ability claimed by others.

The public can tell a good doctor by the fact that he is just the opposite of the list of attributes that has just been mentioned. A good doctor will have graduated from a good medical school, he will have had an internship in an approved hospital, he will be a member of leading medical organizations, and he will be a member of the staff of a reputable hospital. If he is a specialist, he will have the certificate of one of the certifying boards in the various specialties. He will not be an advertiser. He will not pass out handbills. He will not have a big electric sign in front of his office. He will never guarantee a cure or promise to cure a serious disease in one or two treatments. He will be a reputable citizen of his community.

QUARANTINE, the limitation of freedom of movement of persons or animals who have been exposed to a communicable disease, for a period of time usually equal to the longest incubation period of the disease to which they have been exposed. The word *quarantine* comes from the Italian word for *forty*. During the Middle Ages, ships were detained for forty days before entering port in an attempt to avoid spread of the *plague*.

Today most countries are constantly on the alert to guard against disease-bearing persons or animals entering the country. For example, in Great Britain a dog cannot be brought into the country until after a quarantine period to assure that the dog does not have *rabies*.

Persons *actually sick* are *isolated*, not *quarantined*. Every infectious disease has a particular period of quarantine and of isolation. For example, a child with scarlet fever is isolated, and members of the family are quarantined.

QUICKENING, the first feeling of fetal movements by a pregnant woman. These first noticeable movements of the unborn child usually appear during the sixteenth to eighteenth week of pregnancy.

QUININE, an alkaloid obtained from the bark of the *cinchona* plant, is a drug used specifically in the treatment of *malaria*. In solution quinine may be taken orally, in another form it may be injected but usually it is taken as a salt, *quinine sulphate,* in the form of capsules, pills, or tablets. It is also used as a tonic and as bitters, and has been helpful in cases of *neuralgia* and certain forms of muscle weakness.

Quinine should be taken only under a doctor's supervision, as overuse may have a toxic effect. *Atabrine,* a substitute, is also prescribed as a specific against malaria.

Another derivative of the bark of cinchona is *quinidine,* a drug that is valuable in treating heart ailments in which rapid or irregular beating of the heart is a symptom. It slows down heart action and lengthens the time of conduction of the heartbeat. It has been found particularly beneficial in treating fibrillation of the heart muscle.

QUINSY, a sore throat caused by an abscess in the tissues around the tonsils. Pain is generally localized on one side. The person has great difficulty in swallowing and talking, the breath becomes unpleasant, the tongue thickly coated, and the sense of taste and smell may be affected and almost lost.

Rest in bed is imperative and the physician will prescribe antibiotic drugs at once to relieve pain and control infection. Sometimes he will incise the abscess to release the accumulation of pus. *See also* TONSILS. *See* MEDIGRAPH page 1269.

R

RABBIT FEVER. *See* TULAREMIA.

RABIES, or *hydrophobia,* a virulent infectious disease of animals, caused by a *filterable virus,* and transmitted to other animals and human beings by the bite of an infected animal. It occurs in dogs, cattle, horses, wolves, cats, bats, and other animals. The *dog* is most frequently attacked by rabies, as well as being the most common transmitter to human beings of the disease.

The first signs of rabies in a dog are irritability and restlessness, followed by difficulty in swallowing and paralysis, which makes the mouth hang open and causes drooling of saliva. In the final stages of rabies, an infected dog will howl, snap, run about, and bite. Eventually it becomes paralyzed, has convulsions, and dies. The disease rarely reaches the last stages, since the animal is usually spotted beforehand and killed.

Rabies is caused by a virus which occurs in the saliva of an animal several days before serious symptoms become evident. When this virus enters the body of a human being, either from the bite of an animal or in another way, the virus affects the nervous system and eventually reaches the central nervous system, including the spinal cord and brain. Bites on the face, lips, and hands are of particularly urgent gravity because the point of inoculation of the virus is nearer the brain.

Epidemics of rabies have appeared in the United States from time to time. Reports of cases of rabies resulting from the bite of bats led to the discovery that many of the millions of bats inhabiting the Carlsbad Caverns of New Mexico either are or have been infected with rabies.

Because of the grave possibility of rabies, a definite course should be followed after any dog bite. The animal should be kept confined for at least ten days and watched for signs of rabies.

As a first-aid measure, a wound incurred from a dog bite should be washed immediately with a strong warm soap solution. Punctures and lacerations should be washed to the depth of the wound, using a blunt-tipped syringe. If a person is bitten on the face or hands, the doctor will begin to give *antirabies vaccine* at once, since the rabies virus reaches the brain and nervous system so rapidly. The vaccine most commonly available is the *Semple vaccine*. Sensitivity reactions to serum must be guarded against, however, and a valuable adjunct to vaccine treatment is *antirabies serum,* especially for bites about the head, or severe wounds of the hand. Vaccine is also given when visible wounds are known or suspected of having been made by the teeth of the animal, when preexistent cuts and sores may have been contaminated by fresh saliva, and when small children who have had contact with the animal are too young to give reliable testimony.

The doctor will usually discontinue treatment if the biting animal is alive and well after seven days of observation. Without treatment, the onset of rabies usually follows the bite of an infected animal in from twenty to ninety days, and during this period the symptoms may include restlessness, apprehension, and irritation and tingling at the site of the bite. When the disease begins, a slight huskiness of the voice is followed by a sense of choking, since the muscles of swallowing and breathing go into spasms. The infected person may refuse to drink water, because of the pain that accompanies swallowing. Once the disease has developed, it is fatal in from two to ten days, the average being three days.

The best general measure to prevent rabies is to have all puppies receive *rabies inoculation* as soon as possible. Most cities and communities have strict regulations regarding this, as well as a rule requiring that all dogs outside their home be on a leash. It is best to avoid strange dogs. Antirabies vaccine is essential in cases of bite by such animals, especially if they escape and cannot be observed. Unfortunately, the injections, given in the abdomen, are extremely painful. Temporary pain is, of course, preferable to fatal convulsions. Both can be obviated by avoidance of unknown animals.

RADIATION, the therapeutic use of *roentgen rays* or *radium*. The term is also used to denote divergence from a common center of *sensations* and *stimuli*.

Radiography describes the use of *x-ray* as well as *roentgenography,* which derives its name from Wilhelm Roentgen, the inventor of the x-ray.

Radiation treatment is widely used in medicine and includes the exposure of part or all of the body to x-rays, or specific spots to radium and newer *radioactive isotopes*.

The advent of atomic energy and use of radioactive materials in industry and medicine has posed many new problems because of the possi-

1103

ble disastrous effect of radiation on living tissue. The United Nations Scientific Committee on the Effects of Atomic Radiation has been established to study this problem. *See also* X-RAYS; RADIOACTIVITY.

RADIATION SICKNESS, a condition caused by overexposure to radiation, as in *radiotherapy* or the explosion of an *atomic bomb*. The symptoms of radiation sickness are mild to severe nausea, fatigue, diarrhea, internal bleeding, and gradual loss of white blood corpuscles.

Everyone is constantly exposed to minute amounts of radioactive materials that occur naturally in the environment. However, this radiation is so small in amount that it does not have any significant effect on the body. Also, a certain amount of radiation may come from x-ray tubes or from the taking of various radioactive isotopes. For that reason various means have been developed for determining the presence of radiation in the atmosphere. These include the exposure of photographic film and devices like the *Geiger counter*.

It is now known that there is much less residual radiation from an atomic blast than was at first believed. But a ground or water burst leaves a great amount of radioactivity behind in the spray or dirt that spreads contamination as it falls to earth. However, even if absorbed in considerable amount, radiation is not always fatal.

There is no immediate way of determining whether one has been exposed to radiation. Signs of radiation sickness appear later; how much later depends upon the amount absorbed. If the absorption is great, symptoms may appear within a few hours. The initial signs are nausea and shock. In the first day or two, the shock may be followed by vomiting, diarrhea, and fever. There will be no pain, but the patient suffers from discomfort, depression and fatigue. This is often followed by a period of relative well-being and then by severe illness and death.

Excessive radiation exposure damages the body's blood-forming organs and causes a reduction in the number of blood cells. Subsequent internal hemorrhage is due to the *destruction of the thrombocytes,* a blood platelet, and *increased permeability of the blood capillaries.* As a result, all bleeding, even from small cuts, is difficult to stop. *Loss of appetite* and *falling hair* are also frequent symptoms of radiation sickness.

In moderate cases of radiation sickness symptoms appear only after several days—in some cases two or three weeks. During this time the mouth and gums bleed and there is also internal bleeding. Temporary sterility often results, but permanent sterility is not common because the dosage necessary to sterilize the male sex gland is close to what would constitute a fatal dosage. In women, also, radiation may produce transient sterility; permanent sterility is rare. The effects of radiation on the *sex chromosomes* and hence on *future generations* remains in the field of speculation, but much evidence has been accumulated to

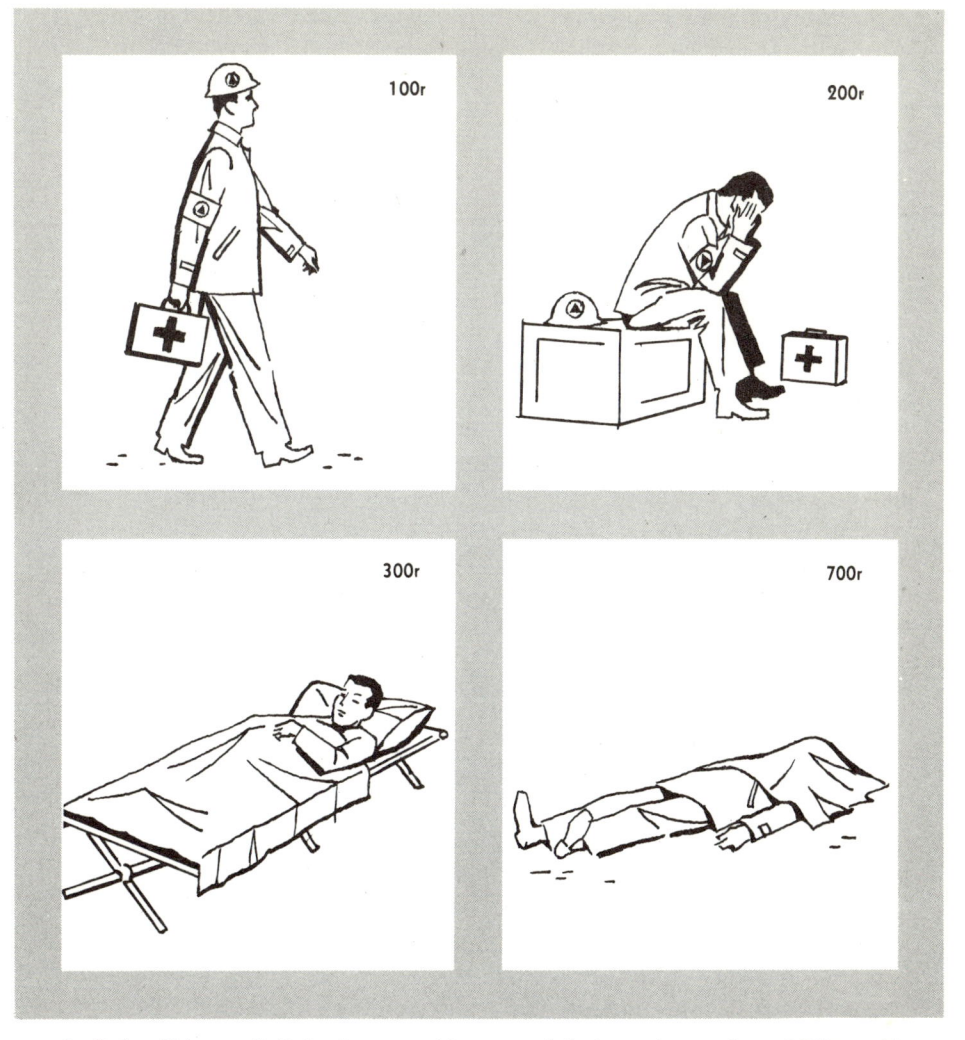

Radiation Sickness—Radiation is measured in *roentgens*. The damage that radiation can inflict upon the human body depends upon the radiation intensity, the length of exposure to it, and the age and health of the exposed person. Over a period of two days, a dose of 200r would make some people sick, but cause no deaths; a dose of 300r would make most people sick, and cause some to die. A dose of 700r in the same period would normally cause death.

demonstrate that these effects are often profound and highly deleterious. Radiation poisoning on a widespread scale, such as would occur in a thermonuclear war, would seriously threaten the continued propagation of the human race for many centuries, and might well be dangerously inimical to the very existence of the species for more than a few generations. These grave hazards render it imperative that thermonuclear war be avoided at all costs, even quite apart from consideration of the many millions who would be killed outright in such a conflict.

Exposure to radiation is best treated by the *transfusion of whole blood,* the *use of antibiotic drugs* to control infection, and *forced nutrition,* especially with foods rich in sugar and protein. See also ATOMIC ENERGY AND MEDICINE; FALLOUT PROTECTION; ATOMIC BOMB.

RADIOACTIVE GOLD. Radium emanation from seeds of radium encased in glass tubes and implanted in tumors has been used to treat the growths. Now *radioactive gold* is being used in a similar way. Patients have been treated by implantation in a tumor of a thread of radioactive gold sealed in a thin, inactive tube. Most of the patients for whom this was done were reported to have benefited from the treatment. See also RADIATION; RADIOACTIVE IODINE; RADIOACTIVITY; CANCER, TREATMENT OF.

RADIOACTIVE IODINE. Physicians have given radioactive iodine for periods of six months to four years to patients with advanced stages of heart disease. These people had *angina pectoris* or *congestive heart failure* and some of them a combination of the two conditions which were painful and which made it difficult for the heart to maintain the circulation. The effect of the radioactive iodine was to reduce the output of the hormone from the *thyroid gland.* As a result, the heart beat more slowly and its work was lessened. Fifty-three per cent of 231 patients in one example were classed as having made excellent progress and an additional 33 per cent made good progress. Only 14 per cent were found not to have improved. See also RADIATION; RADIOACTIVE GOLD; RADIOACTIVITY. See MEDIGRAPH page 1265.

RADIOACTIVE ISOTOPES. See RADIOACTIVITY.

RADIOACTIVITY. Medicine long ago began to study the potentialities of radioactive substances for research and in the treatment of disease. According to an educational bulletin of a leading life insurance company, the x-ray apparatus is one of the first standard implements of medicine to undergo change in keeping with radiological advances. A portable x-ray unit has been developed which employs *radioactive thulium,* a rare earth metal, as its source of radiation. A small amount of this substance encased in lead, which affords full protection to personnel, produces *radiographs* without the use of electricity, water, or darkroom facilities. The unit, which weighs only 40 pounds, is simple to operate and produces a finished radiograph ready for inspection in five to ten minutes.

The *radioisotopes,* at least 150 of which are now in use, are perhaps the most notable by-products of the current atomic energy program. One isotope, *artificially radioactivated iodine,* has provided a most sensitive indicator of thyroid gland activity. The activity has heretofore been largely determined by the *basal metabolic test.* A much more accurate determination of thyroid activity can now be achieved by measuring the gland's uptake of radioactive iodine.

Many isotopes have been used to apply radiation for treatment both externally and internally. A notable example is *cobalt-60* for deep therapy of cancer. The great energy of the radiations emitted by this substance is evidenced by the fact that their penetration of body tissues is approximately the same as that of the radiation from a 2-million-volt x-ray machine. It has been estimated that $47 million worth of radium would be required to do the work of a large cobalt-60 source.

The first "cobalt bomb" was manufactured in the Chalk River Plant of the Canadian Atomic Commission. This agency also supplied hospitals in the United States and Europe with "cobalt bombs."

A unique beam has been developed which provides energy capable of obliterating completely the pituitary gland of rats. Thus, it may someday be possible to perform "surgery" by radiation.

Valuable as the isotopes are in retarding the growth of some forms of cancer and arresting a few diseases, they are still basically investigative tools rather than therapeutic agents.

The isotopes, which carry their radioactivity wherever they go in the body, are revealing new facts about vital processes. *Iron* can be "tagged" and its integral part in the production of red blood cells elucidated by following the activated mineral. The average length of life of a red corpuscle has been established by labeling the iron in the cell's *hemoglobin*.

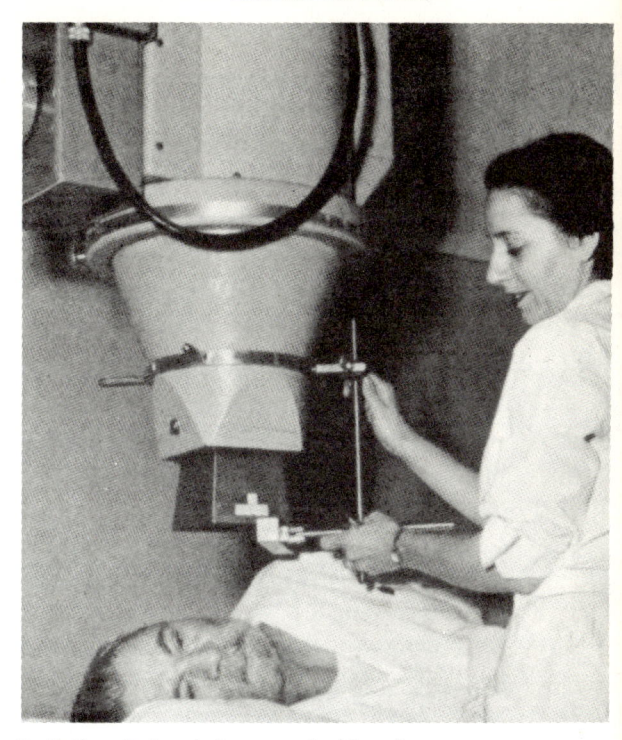

Radiation—Patient being treated with radiocobalt for cancer of the tonsil. The machine is adjusted so the rays will strike the diseased area. Proper doses of radiocobalt will interfere with the growth of cancerous tissue but will not affect healthy tissue.

An average lifetime of about 44 days was found.

Studies with isotopes are being conducted on what happens to the chemical elements in food when they are transformed into tissue or energy —the process called *metabolism*. The role of *cholesterol*, the fatty molecule believed to be partly responsible for arteriosclerosis, is likewise becoming better understood with the aid of isotopes. More is being learned about how the body uses sugar. When sugar is not metabolized properly, *diabetes* usually results. The course of sugar through the body is followed by incorporating *radioactive carbon* into the sugar molecule.

In drug therapy, the isotopes have been put to many uses. Knowledge of how medicinal substances act in the body has been fragmentary and inexact. How does the body use a drug? Where does it accumulate? What "breakdown" or end products does it liberate? How long does a drug remain active?

These questions could not be answered precisely before the advent of the isotopes because biological and chemical methods available were not sufficiently sensitive. With the isotopes, the course of a drug can be followed through all the body's organs and tissues, and through the urine and feces. The sensitivity of this new technique is revealed by experiments in which 1 milligram of *digitalis* was traced, over a period of 35 days in a human subject to whom this "heart drug" was administered. This delicate method will provide new facts about the way drugs behave in the body.

Mosquitoes, including those types that transmit *malaria* and *yellow fever,* can now be tagged with isotopes. *Radiostrontium,* for instance, when put into water in which larvae of the malaria-transmitting mosquito are developing, is taken up by a peculiar gland, analogous to the kidney of a mammal. The radioactive substance concentrates in this gland and remains there permanently throughout the life cycle of the insect. The behavior and growth of the mosquito, incidentally, are not in the least affected by the slight amount of radioactivity which the insect harbors in its body.

The migratory habits of the mosquitoes can be determined—and this is a prime factor in the spread of any contagion transmitted by insects. Then, too, it is possible to learn from the "tagged" mosquitoes more about their span of life, the places where they prefer to breed, how far they may fly, or whether they are carried by natural forces, such as winds, from one locality to another. Data thus obtained can be used in planning more effective programs for controlling diseases borne by insects, especially in those regions of the world that are still ravaged by the winged vectors of infection. *See also* RADIATION; CANCER, TREATMENT OF.

RADIUM, a highly radioactive element found in *pitchblende* and other mineral deposits. It was identified in 1898 by Pierre and Marie Curie, French scientists. The rays which radium gives off have an effect on the growth of human tissue, and radium has been effectively used in treatment of skin diseases of various types, including cancer, tumors, growths on the skin, and in hemorrhage and infections.

Radium is generally employed in the form of one of its salts, since they are more stable than the element itself. Various types of tubes are required for the insertion of radium into body cavities and tumorous tissue. *Platinum* or *gold needles* may be used, or tiny *glass tubes* called *seeds,* which are filled with *radon,* a gaseous emanation of radium, and inserted into tumors, in some cases permanently.

RÂLE, a French word meaning *rattle* and referring to the various sounds that are heard in the lungs when the doctor examines them with a *stethoscope*. Many adjectives have been employed by doctors to describe these sounds, such as coarse, medium, fine, moist, and dry.

RAT-BITE FEVER, an infection, characterized by *fever, nervous symptoms, malaise,* and *serious disability,* which is contracted from the bite of a diseased rat, or, less commonly, a cat, dog, weasel, squirrel, or pig, which injects a *spiral bacillus* into the body of the person bitten. The bacteria live in the noses and throats of rats without disturbing them, but cause a variety of febrile diseases when injected into human beings.

Another condition like rat-bite fever is *Haverhill fever,* so named because the first epidemic which was studied occurred in Haverhill, Massachusetts. Since that time, other cases have been reported in different parts of the United States. It is also caused by the bite of a rat or sometimes, by food contaminated with an organism similar to that transmitted through the bite.

Rat-bite fever has been found in practically every part of the world, and occurs most often in infants and children. Not every rat carries the infection. In the United States the large and vicious *Norway* or *sewer rats* are the most frequent carriers.

The incubation period of rat-bite fever ranges from one to four weeks. When the disease begins, fever comes and goes, fluctuating from time to time, and occasionally a skin rash appears. Haverhill fever has a much shorter incubation period and the fever does not increase and recede. The joints are involved, but if any skin rash is present, it is minor.

Rat-bite fever is treated with *penicillin, streptomycin,* or the *tetracyclines*. Other drugs are given to relieve headache and malaise. Most patients recover, particularly if the condition is diagnosed early and the treatment is prompt. Anyone bitten by a rat should immediately have the wound treated by a physician, who will cauterize the wound and treat it with a strong antiseptic. In case of abscess, he will incise and drain the wound; and if the puncture is deep, he may take prophylactic measures against *tetanus*. He will check to determine that *rabies* or *plague* are not present. See also RABIES; PLAGUE; TETANUS.

RAT CONTROL. Rats cause tremendous property loss each year, as well as being carriers of diseases, such as *rat-bite fever, bubonic plague* (through the rat flea), *Weil's disease* or *hemorrhagic jaundice, tapeworm, ringworm, food-poisoning* (through bacteria) and a form of *typhus*. The elimination of rats is therefore an essential part of any public health program and of concern to the private home owner or building proprietor. The best means of preventing rats is to make a building rat-proof by plugging openings, clearing away debris, and other measures. Once rats

RAYNAUD'S DISEASE

are established, they may be hunted or trapped, but use of poison is usually the most practical means of getting rid of them.

The ideal poison is one that will kill rats but which is harmless to animals and man. Many poisons have been tried, with varying degrees of success. A compound known as *ANTU* is effective. It affects dogs, cats, and other pets only mildly; a single dose will kill a half-pound rat quickly, but have little effect on a dog weighing ten pounds. One pound of ANTU is sufficient to kill 200,000 rats. Finely ground corn or wheat is mixed with ANTU and sprayed or dusted on cut-up vegetables, tomatoes or potatoes, as bait. After the rat has taken a small quantity of the poison, its lungs fill up with body fluid and it dies by suffocation.

Other poisons, of varying toxicity, are also employed, such as *zinc phosphate* and *thallium sulphate*. However, rats quickly learn to be wary of food containing these poisons.

Two newer poisons have been developed, *warfarin* and a related compound, *toumarin*. They are also mixed with edible bait and when ingested by rats the poisons attack the blood and act as *anticoagulants*. The rats bleed to death internally in from five to six days. *See also* RAT-BITE FEVER; PLAGUE; JAUNDICE; TYPHUS FEVER.

RAYNAUD'S DISEASE, a disease of the arteries in the extremities, characterized by periodic numbness and loss of blood in the hands and feet. *See* MEDIGRAPH page 1113.

RED BLOOD CELLS, DISEASES OF

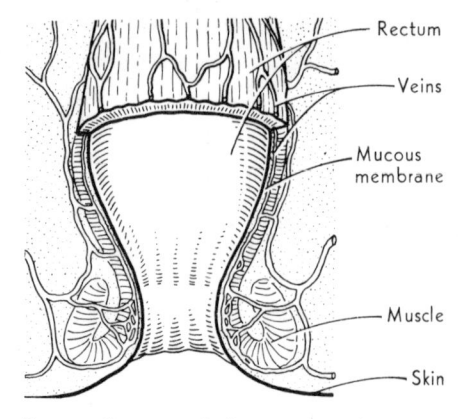

Rectum—Structure of the rectum and anus. The anus is the external opening at the end of the rectum. Strong ring-like muscles surround the anal opening and are able to close it. The rectum is a common site for cancer. Cancer of the rectum may develop in either sex, but the incidence is greater in men.

RECTUM, the lowest segment of the digestive tract, about six to eight inches long, terminating in the *anus* or lower opening through which solid waste matter is evacuated from the body. The large intestine, immediately above the rectum, first acts on the indigestible residue which remains when food has been digested and then passes it on into the rectum. When this occurs, the body, by a specific mechanism, indicates to the brain that expulsion of the waste through the anus is necessary. This is the urge for movement of the bowels. *See also* DIGESTIVE SYSTEM; INTESTINES; HEMORRHOIDS. *See* MEDIGRAPHS pages 301, 743.

RED BLOOD CELLS. *See* BLOOD.

RED BLOOD CELLS, DISEASES OF. The red cell of the human being is a disc measuring about three ten-thousandths of an inch in diameter. Normally there are approximately 5 million per cubic millimeter of blood. These cells are produced in the bone marrow of the body. The rate or type of production of red cells may be examined by removing a small amount of marrow. This is easily accomplished by inserting a needle into an accessible bone such as the breastbone or hip and drawing out the marrow with a syringe. Slides are then prepared and examined under a microscope. A red cell has a normal life span of 120 days. A lengthening of this life span is unknown. There are many diseases in which the life span of the cells is shortened, however, and these are known as *hemolytic anemias*.

The red color of the cell is due to a substance known as *hemoglobin*. Hemoglobin is an iron-containing pigment which has the vital job of transporting oxygen from the lungs to the tissues and removing the waste gas, carbon dioxide, from the tissues to be excreted via the lungs.

When a red cell dies, hemoglobin is broken down into its component parts. The iron is utilized again for red cell production. A portion of the hemglobin is converted to *bilirubin*, a yellow pigment. If there is a rapid breakdown of red cells, the bilirubin may pile up in the blood stream and the patient becomes yellow or jaundiced.

Symptoms of *anemia* generally are the same, independent of the type of anemia, but vary according to the severity of the disorder. Weariness, weakness, dizziness, ringing of the ears, spots before the eyes, pallor, and headaches are the most prevalent symptoms. If the anemia is severe, shortness of breath, rapid pulse, fainting, and even coma may ensue.

Probably one of the most common types of anemia is that due to a lack of iron. Iron is not excreted from the body. An iron deficiency in adults occurs for only two reasons: loss by bleeding and improper diet. In women, *iron deficiency anemia* is not uncommon. Loss of iron during menstrual bleeding, pregnancy, and breast feeding an infant may be quite severe. If a pregnant woman does not have sufficient iron stores, she will not be able to provide her child with iron. As a result, the infant may develop severe anemia at about the fourth to sixth month of life. The treatment is generally simple, consisting of supplying additional iron in pills or a liquid preparation. Iron may produce mild intestinal disturbances in some patients; this can usually be avoided, however, by giving the medication during meals. For men, an iron deficiency anemia indicates bleeding from a source such as the intestinal tract. The cause of bleeding must be determined because treatment of the anemia may only mask a primary disease.

Megaloblastic anemia encompasses a variety of anemic disorders due to a deficiency of either *folic acid* or *vitamin B_{12}*. When vitamin B_{12} or folic acid are not available to the marrow, production of red cells is deficient and abnormal. Red cells are larger than normal but the

1111

the disease and its causes This is a disease of the arteries of the hands and feet in which the fingers or toes become bloodless and white under certain conditions. Emotional upsets can bring about an attack. Cold weather, and even putting the hands in cold water, can also produce the change in color that is characteristic of Raynaud's disease. It occurs much more often in women than men, usually in the age group 20 to 40.

Occasionally Raynaud's disease occurs in association with other organic arterial diseases or with scleroderma (in which thickened, hard, rigid patches of skin develop), or cervical ribs (extra ribs in the neck which interfere with circulation), or with acute neck injuries.

symptoms When a patient with Raynaud's disease is exposed to cold, the fingers or toes may become bloodless and white. There is usually not much pain, but numbness is common. When warm again, the affected parts lose their white color and change from blue to red before turning normal. Between attacks, the fingers and toes appear normal. But when attacks are continuous or prolonged, small areas of gangrene can develop.

complications The only serious complication is gangrene, which is rare and most unusual. When it occurs, amputation may be necessary.

prevention (or lessening of impact) The patient with Raynaud's disease must take steps to prevent the development of gangrene and do what can be done to prevent attacks. She should keep her body and limbs warm. Any infection or associated illness should be treated. Emotional problems, which are thought to trigger attacks, should be handled professionally.

With proper care, Raynaud's disease rarely presents any serious problems.

Raynaud's Disease

Attacks precipitated by cold (low temperature)...

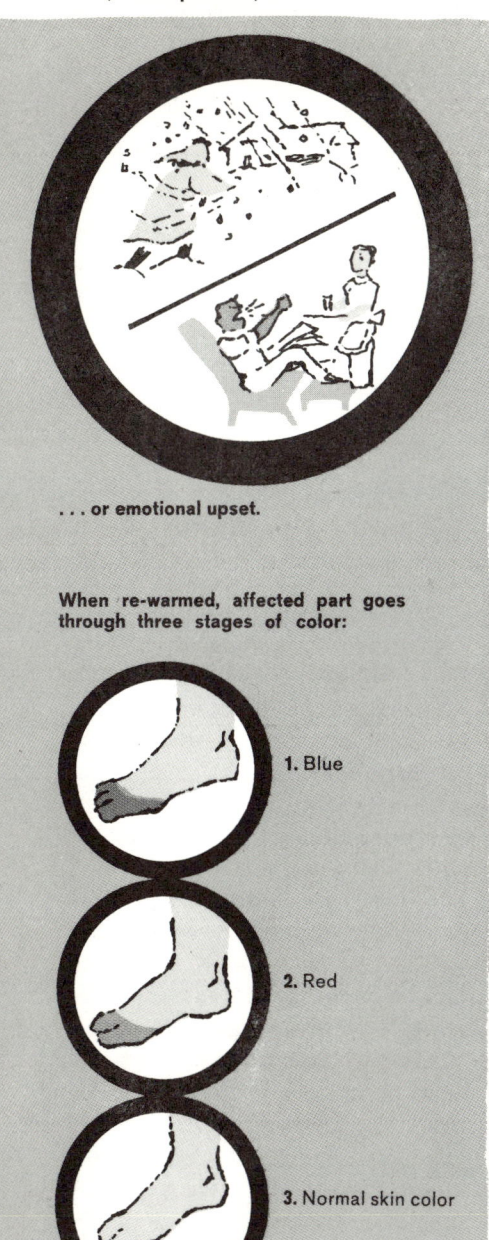

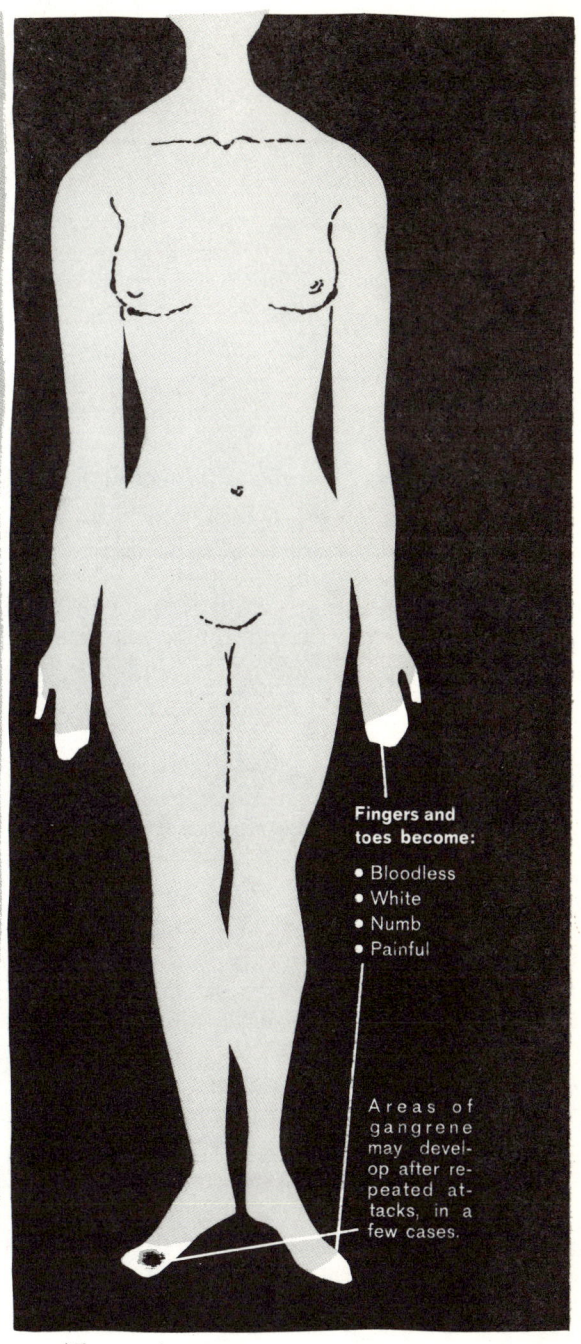

...or emotional upset.

When re-warmed, affected part goes through three stages of color:

1. Blue
2. Red
3. Normal skin color

Fingers and toes become:
- Bloodless
- White
- Numb
- Painful

Areas of gangrene may develop after repeated attacks, in a few cases.

RED BLOOD CELLS, DISEASES OF

rate of production is definitely slower so that anemia occurs. *Pernicious anemia* is the most common affliction in this group of disorders. In this disease, a substance called *intrinsic factor,* which is produced in the stomach, is absent and consequently the vitamin B_{12} is not absorbed. *Pernicious anemia* is accompanied by severe nervous system changes and if the disease is not diagnosed and treated early these changes may become permanent. Other megaloblastic anemias may occur during infancy, pregnancy, and in severe prolonged intestinal diseases such as *sprue.*

The *anemia of chronic infection* is similar to that caused by deficiencies. In chronic infections such as *tuberculosis,* the anemia does not respond to iron therapy. Toxic substances released by the infection inhibit the incorporation of iron into the red cells and also release of red cells from the marrow. The only remedy is treatment of the infection. A similar type of anemia accompanies chronic *kidney disease* and *cancer.*

Hereditary spherocytosis or *familial hemolytic jaundice,* is an inherited abnormality of the red cell in which there is a defect in the ability of the red cell to utilize sugar. The red cells take on a spherical shape and have a definitely shortened life span. The disease may be cured by removing the spleen. The spleen traps these abnormally shaped red cells and there they are rapidly destroyed. After *splenectomy,* a defect in utilizing sugar can still be observed but its survival is normal.

Mediterranean anemia, thalassemia, or *Cooley's anemia,* is another inherited disease of the red cells. It is primarily due to an inability to produce hemoglobin and the red cells become abnormally thin. Its mild form may closely resemble an iron deficiency anemia. In its severe form, the person is jaundiced, has an enlarged liver and spleen and severe anemia. *Transfusion* is the only treatment known to be effective.

Sickle cell anemia is an inherited genetic abnormality of the red cell in which its hemoglobin is faultily constituted. The red cell may take on the shape of a *sickle* or a *quarter moon.* The cells have a short survival time and consequently an affected person is anemic. The disease is also characterized by acute pain in the extremities.

A symptomless form of the disturbance exists in which the tendency to form sickled cells is present but not enough of the abnormal *sickle cell hemoglobin* is present in the red cell to produce symptoms. Persons with this condition are said to have *sickle cell traits* and to be *sickle cell carriers.* If a man and woman with sickle cell traits marry, their children possibly may develop a sudden and severe form of sickle cell anemia.

Hemoglobin consists of 574 separate amino acids. Experiments at the National Institutes of Health and other laboratories have shown that the peculiar shape of the red blood cells in sickle cell anemia is caused by an abnormal looping bond between two amino acids which in turn causes the hemoglobin to form in slender strands. Many such abnormal strands of hemoglobin strung together are responsible for the elongation of the red blood cell.

The abnormal bonds form when the oxygen level of the blood stream falls, and the elongated (sickle-shaped) red blood cells that result accumulate in the smaller capillaries, particularly those of the arms and legs.

It has been found that by placing the victim in a sealed chamber and raising the atmospheric pressure, the abnormal bonds can be broken—at least temporarily—and relief from pain obtained. A permanent cure for the disease, however, will evidently depend on further advances in the science of genetics.

Acquired hemolytic anemia is a form of rapid destruction of red cells within the body. It is not inherited and may be secondary to another disease. In this disturbance, a substance is produced which attacks and destroys red cells. Frequently a reason cannot be found for production of this destructive substance. Occasionally a tumor which produces the substance may be found. Acquired hemolytic anemia is not uncommon in malignant diseases such as *leukemia* and *lymphoma*. Hormones such as *ACTH* and *cortisone* or *splenectomy* may be beneficial.

Aplastic anemia is a disorder in which red cells are not produced. It is usually found after overdosage of *radiation* and exposure to certain toxic substances such as *arsenic* and *benzene*. The number of white cells and platelets also may be decreased.

Polycythemia is a condition in which there is an overabundance of red cells. In one form, known as *polycythemia vera,* there is usually an increase of all cellular elements of the blood. The red cell count is between 7 and 10 million per cubic millimeter. The blood volume may be increased from a normal of 5 quarts to as much as 10 quarts. A person with polycythemia usually has a reddish glow to his skin. The spleen frequently is enlarged and high blood pressure may be noted. The symptoms are due to the large amount of blood which is thicker than normal and therefore cannot move through the blood vessels with normal speed. The most common complication is *spontaneous clotting of the blood* within the blood vessels. Proper treatment can be accomplished by frequent examination and blood letting. Many pints of blood may have to be withdrawn to bring the total blood volume to a normal level. The use of radioactive substances has become important in treating this disease. Such agents as *radioactive phosphorus* will inhibit the marrow production of cells and thereby tend to maintain a normal red cell level. The choice of treatment depends on the individual case. The most important factor is patient-doctor cooperation with frequent visits to the doctor so that the blood volume may be stabilized at a normal level. The cause of this disorder is not yet known.

Secondary polycythemia is usually not as severe as *polycythemia vera*. It affects persons living at high altitudes and those with severe

RED BLOOD CELLS, DISEASES OF

pulmonary or cardiac disease. Polycythemia in these cases is a result of *oxygen deficiency*.

Certain aspects of the red blood cell are divided into many systems of so-called *blood groups*. The most important system is known as the *ABO system*. Another system which has received much study recently is the *Rh system*. Blood groups are *antigenic;* that is, if blood is injected into a person who has blood of a different group from that of his donor, a substance will be produced which will attack and destroy cells containing the donor's specific blood group. For example, a person having blood type A has an antibody to blood type B. In the ABO system, antibodies occur naturally; that is, persons with blood type A have anti-B; blood type B has anti-A; and type O has anti-A and anti-B. The *Rh system* divides blood into two groups, *positive* and *negative*. About 85 per cent of the population is Rh positive and 15 per cent Rh negative. Antibodies due to differences in Rh factor are not *naturally* present. Injection of blood containing an Rh factor into the system of a person who has no Rh factor (Rh negative) will *stimulate* the body to production of an anti-Rh antibody. A first injection of Rh positive red cells will sensitize a person but produce no harmful effects; a second injection of cells will be destroyed by the Rh antibody.

In *hemolytic disease of the newborn (erythroblastosis fetalis)* the mother is Rh negative and the father is Rh positive. The child will be Rh positive in this type of mating. Should some of the red cells of the child get into the mother's circulation, the mother will become sensitized to Rh positive blood. During a second pregnancy, the already sensitized mother may again receive Rh positive cells and the antibody then will be produced in sufficient quantity to get back into the child's circulation and damage the infant's red cells. These damaged red cells have a short life span and as they are rapidly destroyed the amount of *bilirubin* produced from the released *hemoglobin* begins to pile up. The child becomes *jaundiced* and *anemic*. The bilirubin in a newborn can pass into the spinal fluid and become deposited in the brain and may produce serious and irreversible brain damage. As only 15 per cent of the population is Rh negative, not every pregnant Rh negative woman will have a child with hemolytic disease of the newborn. The husband may be Rh negative also, in which case the child would not have the Rh positive blood group. The child's cells must get into the mother's circulation and this does not always occur. The doctor will check the blood types of both parents and if the proper conditions for the disease exist, he will check the level of any anti-Rh antibody which may develop in the mother throughout the course of the pregnancy. Should the child have *erythroblastosis fetalis*, it may have to undergo an exchange transfusion which removes the bilirubin and the dangerous antibody. Not every child will need this form of treatment since the severity of the disease varies from case to case. Cases of hemolytic disease of the newborn due to the ABO blood groups have been reported; however, they are usually very mild and require no treatment. *See also* BLOOD; BLOOD TYPES; LEUKEMIA; ANEMIA; ANEMIA, PERNICIOUS; RADIATION SICKNESS; POLYCYTHEMIA.

REDUCING DIET. *See* DIET, REDUCING; OBESITY.

REFLEX, an involuntary movement or *reaction* to a *stimulus,* removed from the point of action. Many reflex actions take place in the body as part of its ordinary functioning or in connection with disease. The *knee jerk,* an example of a reflex action, is absent in many diseases of the brain and spinal cord. The *oculocardiac reflex* is a slowing of the heartbeat that follows compression of the eyeball. A slowing of five to thirteen beats per minute is the normal decrease. When a substance is put on the back of the tongue, the *swallowing reflex* takes place. *Laughter* is a reflex to *tickling,* and when a person starts on hearing a loud noise, a *startle reflex* is provoked.

REGRESSION. The progress of *regression* in older people, sometimes referred to as *second childhood,* can be reversed in many instances, according to leading authorities. Many of these symptoms of *senility* result from a state of panic in the aged person when he feels that he has been rejected by society. Whether or not the feeling of neglect and isolation is real or imagined, the person reacts by building up tighter psychological defenses against his environment, or by losing all of his usual defenses. In either case, regression takes place.

The amount of regression varies, and in some cases is extreme. The stage of past psychological development to which the senile person regresses provides a clue to neurotic disturbances which may have lain dormant throughout his life. Treatment must be designed to deal with specifically diagnosed psychiatric conditions. *See also* SENILITY; SENESCENCE.

REHABILITATION. Until recently a disabled person was allowed to remain in a bed or a chair with little or no effort made to restore him to useful function. Those whose condition was considered hopeless were tragically ignored. A person with paralysis or loss of speech from a stroke or disabled because of a fractured hip was allowed to die without much effort to bring about his recovery. Often attempts were not made to give him mental comfort and encouragement. This situation has changed. Although many conditions are still recognized from which recovery is unlikely, much improvement and peace of mind can be obtained for patients suffering from these disorders.

One important way to stimulate recovery is to prevent long bed rest. Patients are urged to get out of bed soon after an operation, sometimes even on the day of surgery. In heart conditions or strokes, however, bed rest for longer periods of time may be essential. As soon as signs indicate that activity of a disease has ceased, the ailing person is required to get out of bed. Any complications are avoided and recovery is stimulated. After getting up, he must be encouraged to take part in as much directed activity as possible within the limits of his strength.

An ill person must be encouraged to feel that he will recover. If the invalid feels that recovery is imminent, he will respond accordingly and results are more apt to be satisfactory. Pleasant surroundings, ample air, and a view of the outside all provide contact with the world. A varied diet, consisting of well-prepared foods served, invitingly, is most necessary.

In the event of paralysis or loss of use of an arm or leg from a fracture, active steps must immediately be taken to restore function of affected parts. A physical therapist should promptly start such corrective treatment. Heat by *diathermy,* either from direct application or produced mechanically, often is necessary and motion of the affected part must be continued. Massage, continued movement by a therapist or by the patient himself, and electrical stimulation of the affected part all are helpful. Casts should be removed as soon as possible and physical therapy should be commenced. When needed, assistance and aids for walking are provided. If speech is impaired, a speech therapist may often work wonders. *See also* OCCUPATIONAL THERAPY.

RELAPSING FEVER, one of a group of specific infectious diseases caused by *spirochetes;* it is characterized by recurring attacks of high fever. The disease is transmitted by the bite of *ticks, lice,* and sometimes *bedbugs.*

Usually relapsing fever begins with sudden chills followed by a fever which may go as high as 105°F and remain at a high level for several days, and headache and weakness may occur. At the crisis there is often danger of collapse. After a few days the patient suddenly appears to recover, but in a week or so becomes ill again.

To treat relapsing fever, bed rest is essential, particularly during the period of high fever. Sponge baths and the use of *salicylic acid* and *sedatives* help make the patient more comfortable. Antibiotics, such as *aureomycin, terramycin,* and *chloromycetin* have been found the most effective drugs in controlling this disease.

REPRODUCTION SYSTEM. The human sexual reproduction system, which consists of the generative apparatus, is discussed here with reference to its anatomy and to conception.

Male sexual anatomy. The male sexual apparatus consists of the *penis, scrotum, testicles,* and several internal glands such as the *prostate.*

The *testicles*—the male *gonads*—are the most crucial component of the male sexual system. These extraordinary glands determine and govern the *maleness* of the individual: the secondary sexual character-

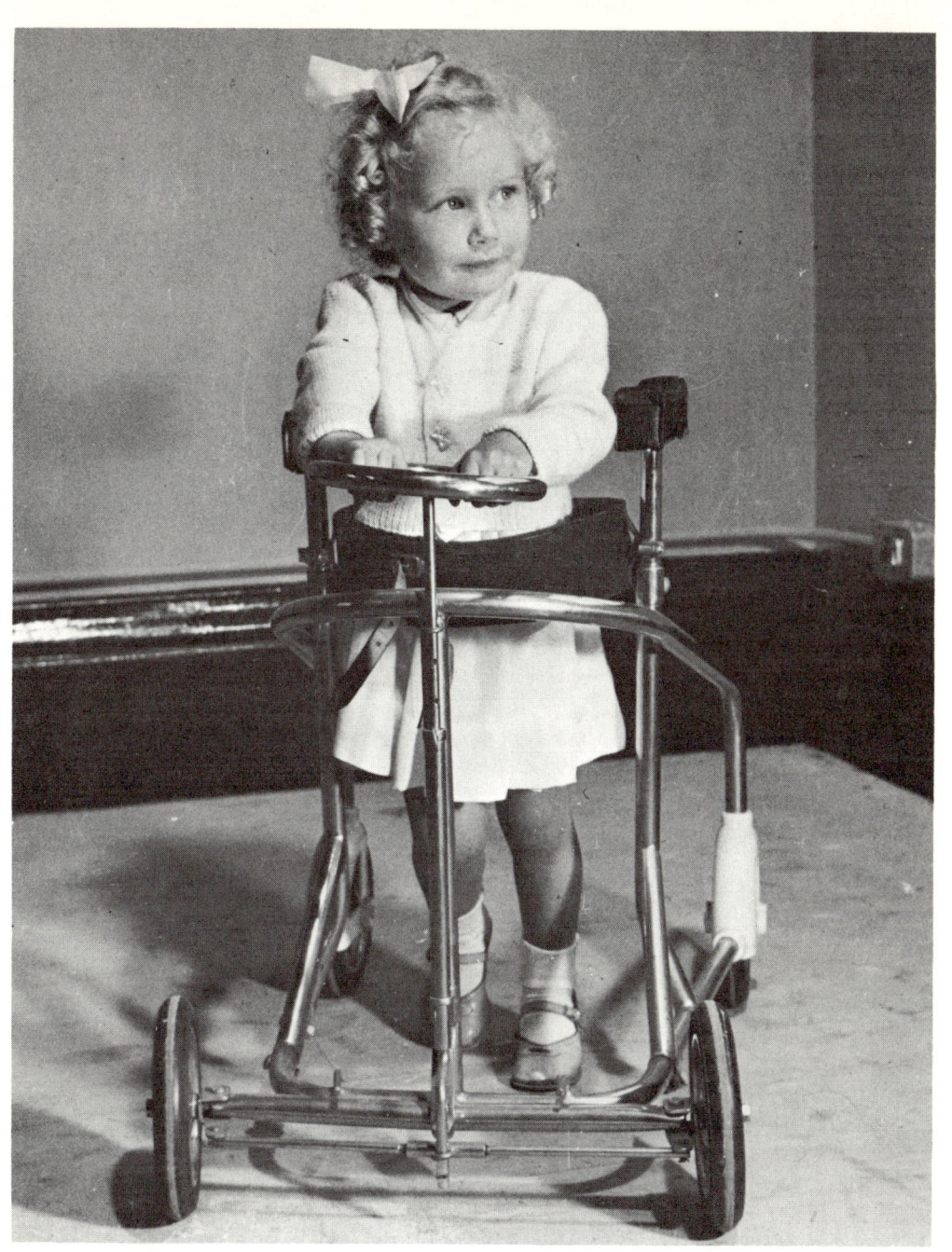

The former practice of confining those having been ill or subject to various infirmities to long periods of immobility has been largely discarded in favor of the encouragement of as much ambulation and physical activity as feasible. Those afflicted with paralytic diseases, like the young lady above, are provided with supports, braces, and similar accoutrements to facilitate mobility. It is now known that activity is conducive to recovery and well-being, and certainly to the patient's satisfaction.

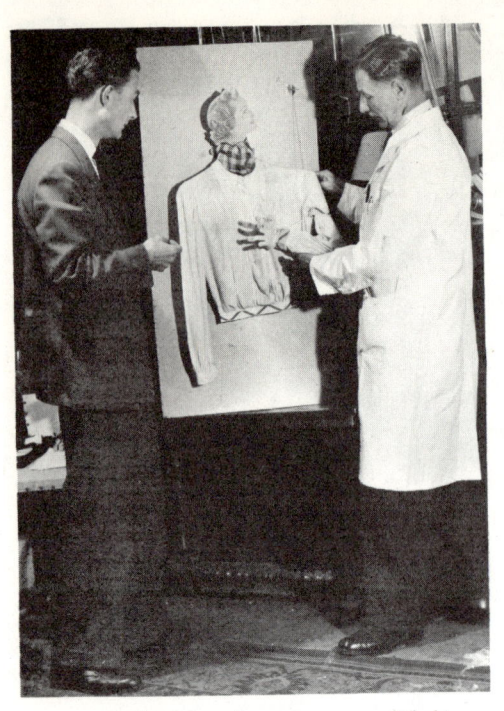

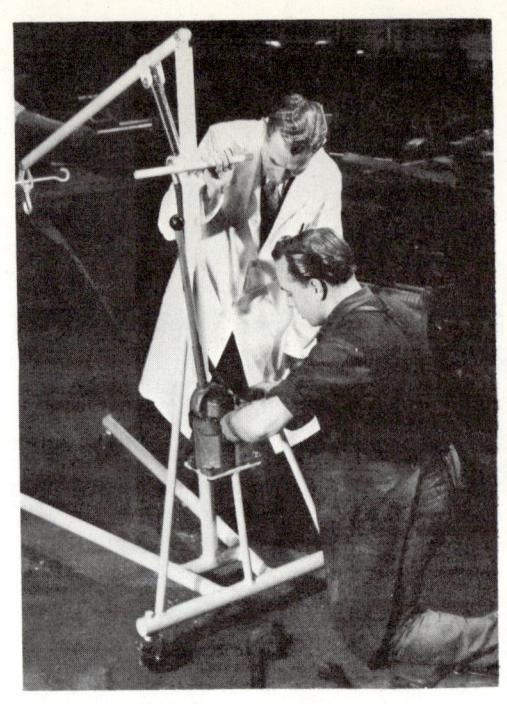

A physician discusses a case with his patient with the aid of a dummy model *(above, left)*. A final check is given to a hydraulically operated mobile patient hoist *(above, right)*, a device which enables a nurse to lift even the heaviest patients. Below is shown a scale model of a unit designed to enable paralyzed patients to lift themselves into or out of bed. These and similar devices can accelerate recovery.

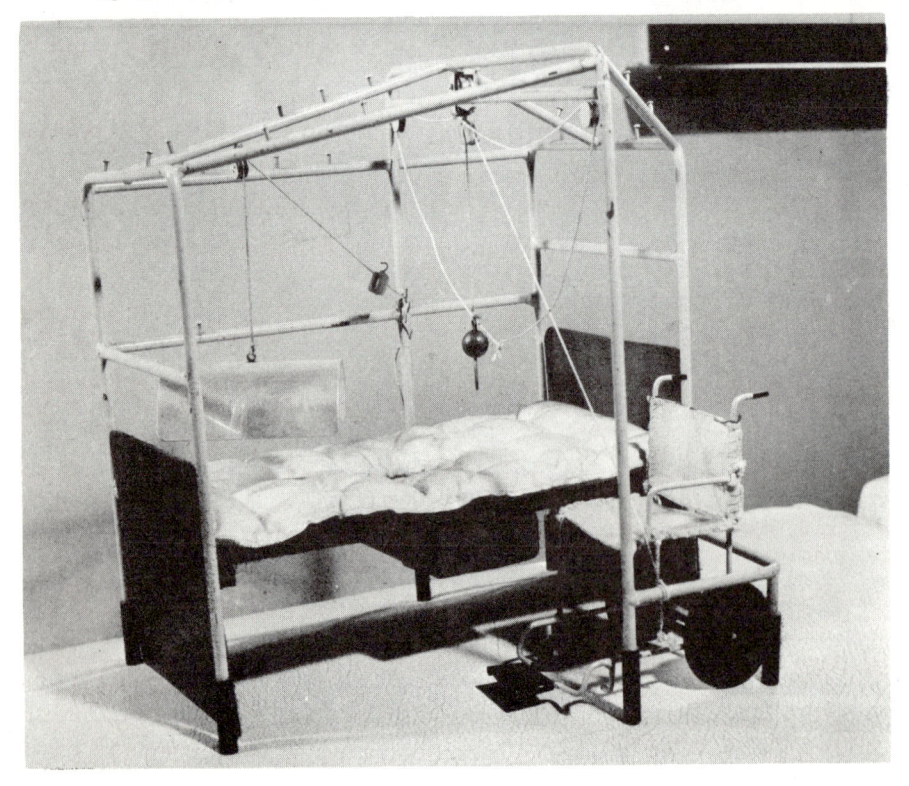

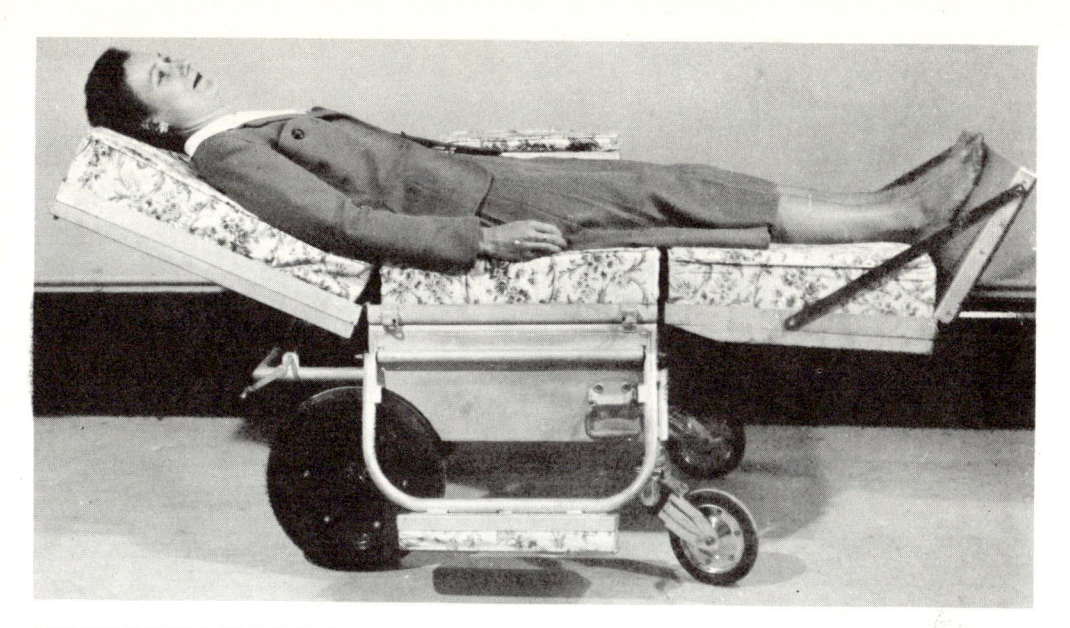

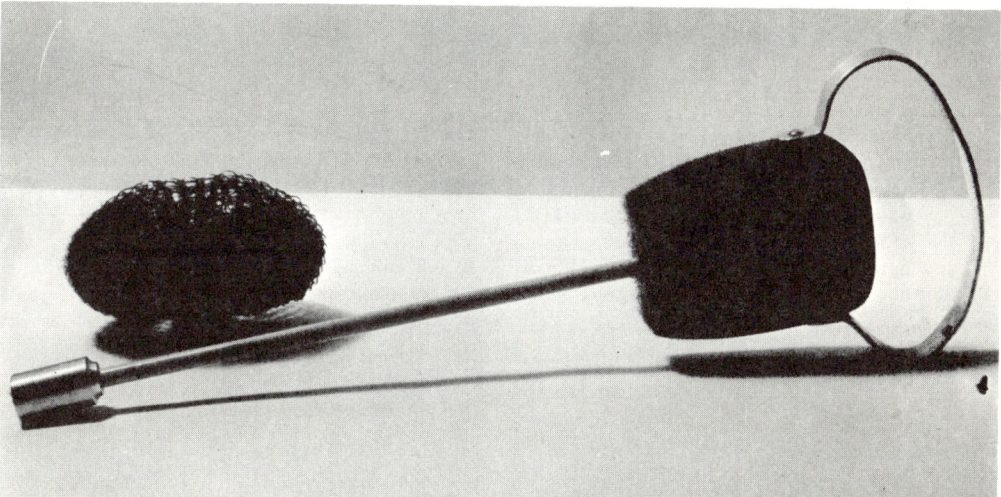

At top is shown a special threefold unit designed for the use of the immobilized patient. It serves as a wheelchair, armchair, and bed. Center: individuals disabled by arthritis or other crippling diseases can cope with dishwashing and scouring by means of this device, which can hold interchangeable parts. Bottom: this device can be held by a crippled hand to anchor meat, fish, or vegetables while the sound hand cuts and trims.

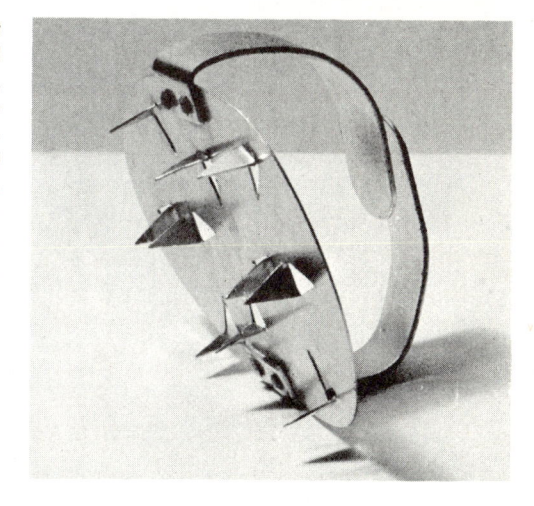

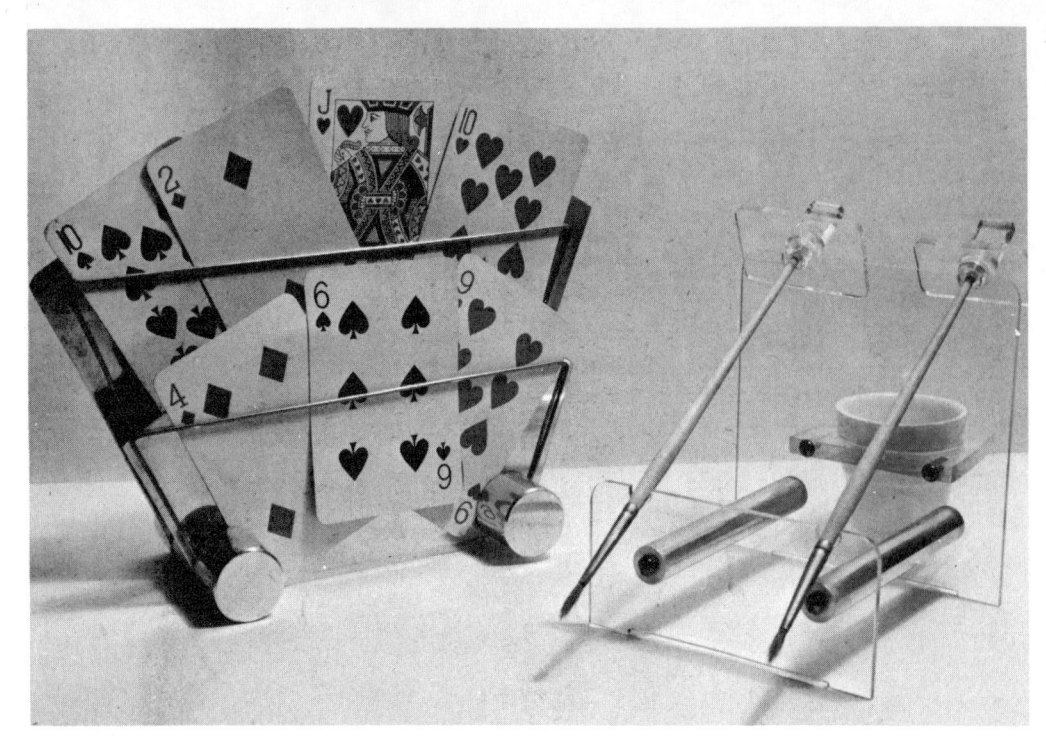

Many devices have been invented to assist the handicapped. Above, a special cardholder *(left)* and a mouth painting set which enables those who have lost the use of their arms to paint. Below, left, specially designed eating utensils; right, a special long-handled comb. Opposite page: a support for the glass enables a handicapped girl to drink unassisted *(top, left)*. A walking aid *(top, right)* helps those suffering from paralysis of the legs to move about. Bottom: A little girl too weak to stand by herself can still play while supported by this ingenious device.

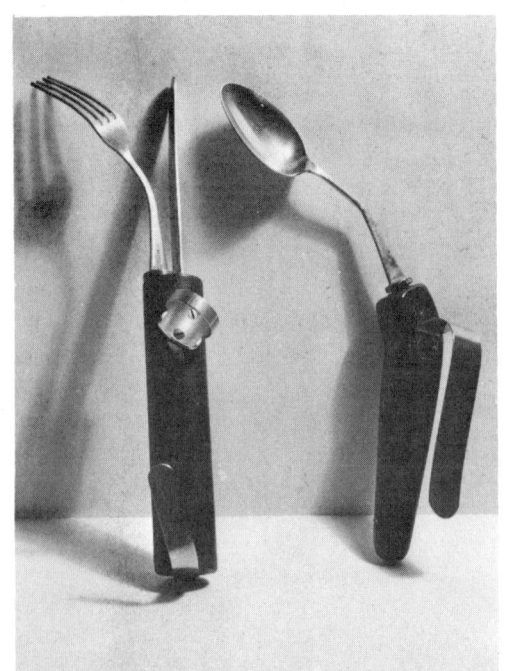

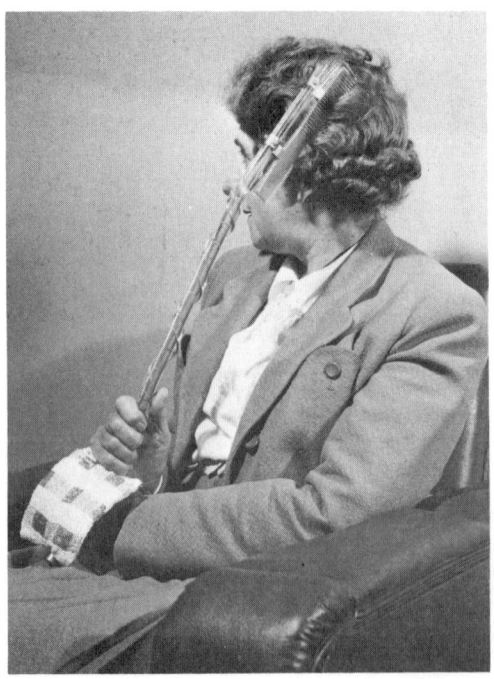

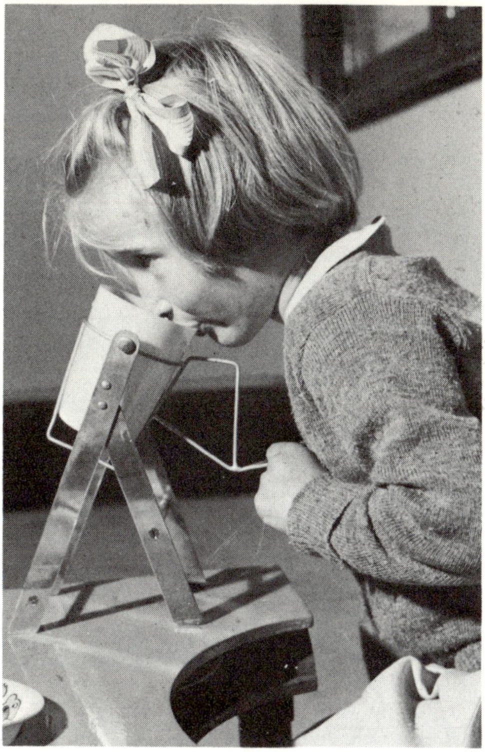

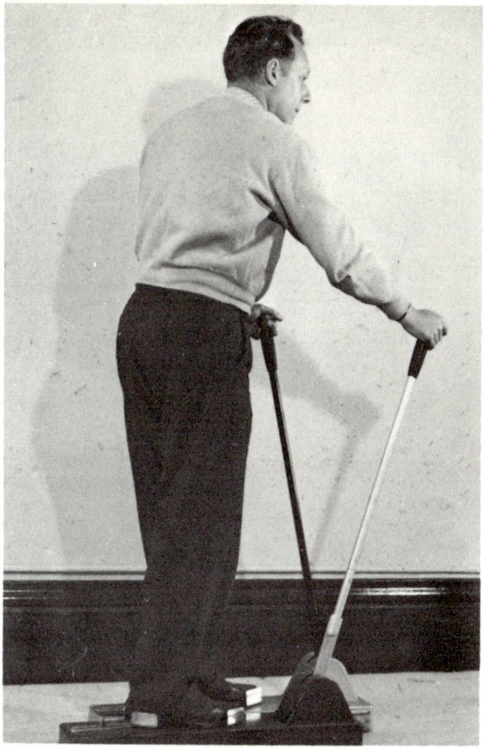

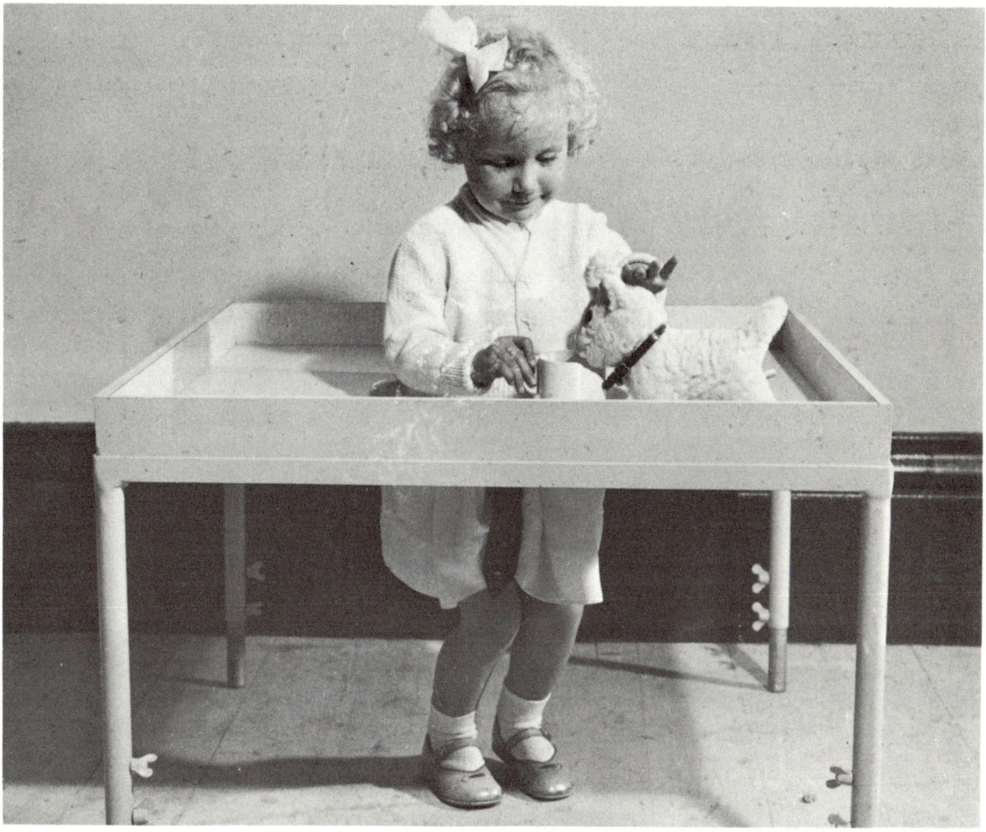

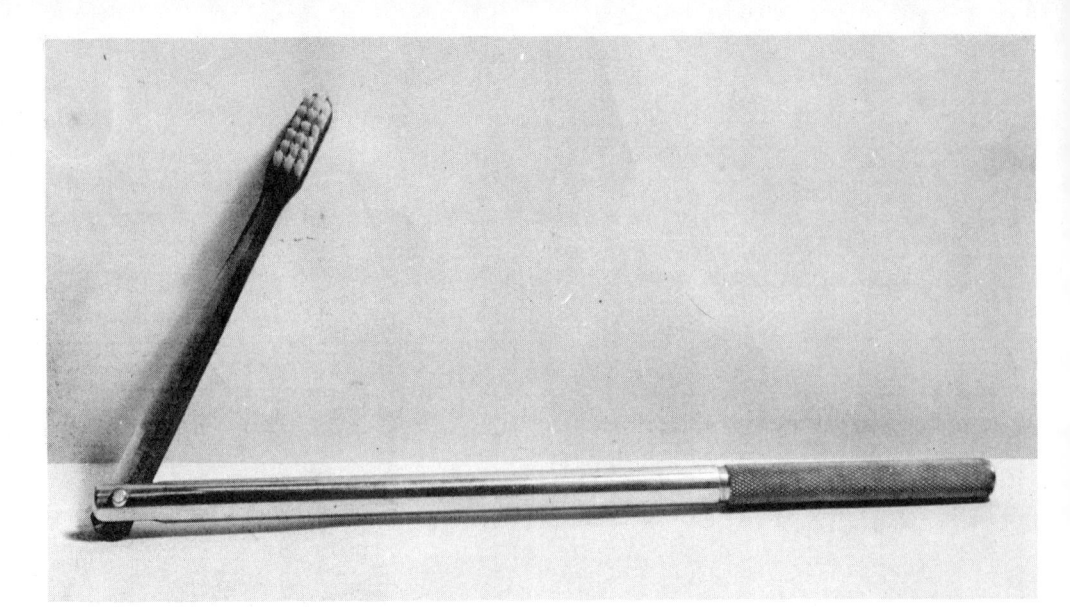

Above: a swivel toothbrush for those with stiff wrists. Below, a victim of paralysis feeds herself with the aid of special arm-supporting devices. Mr. Emil A. Andrae, inventor of all the devices shown on these pages, is at left. Opposite page: A severely disabled patient is lowered into a special tank for exercise. The pulley system can be handled by a single nurse. The nurse massages the weakened muscles of the patient in the tank, which is large enough to allow free body movement.

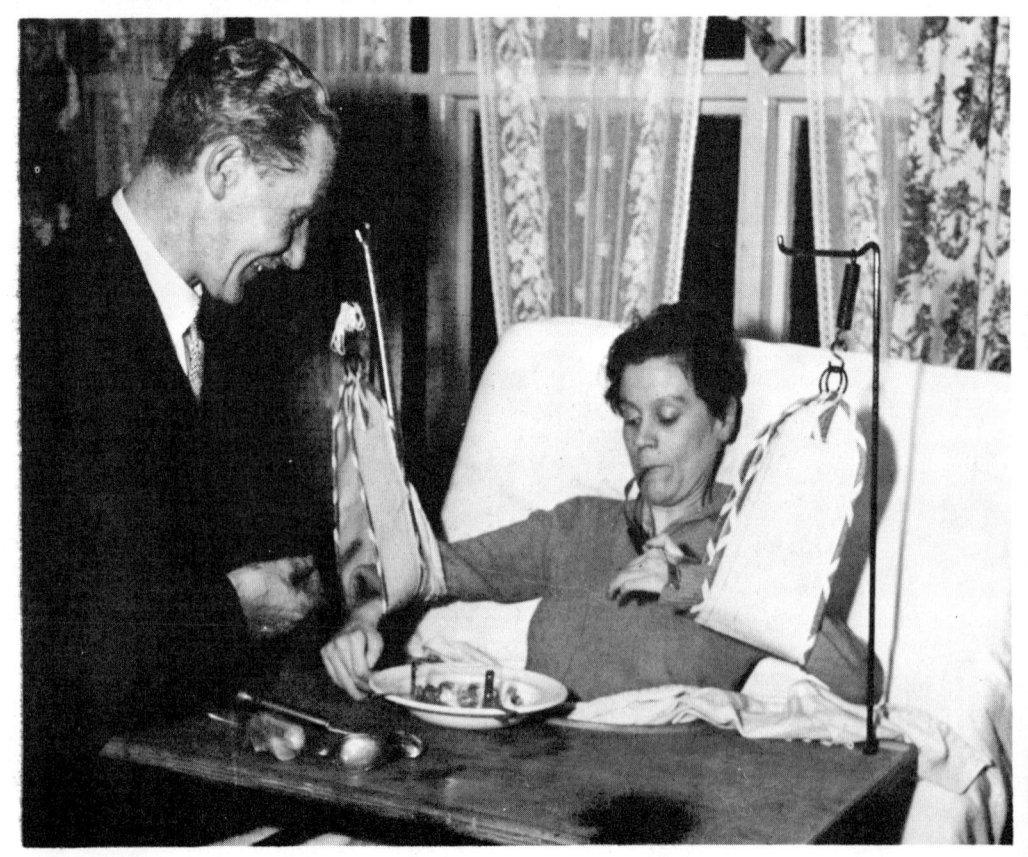

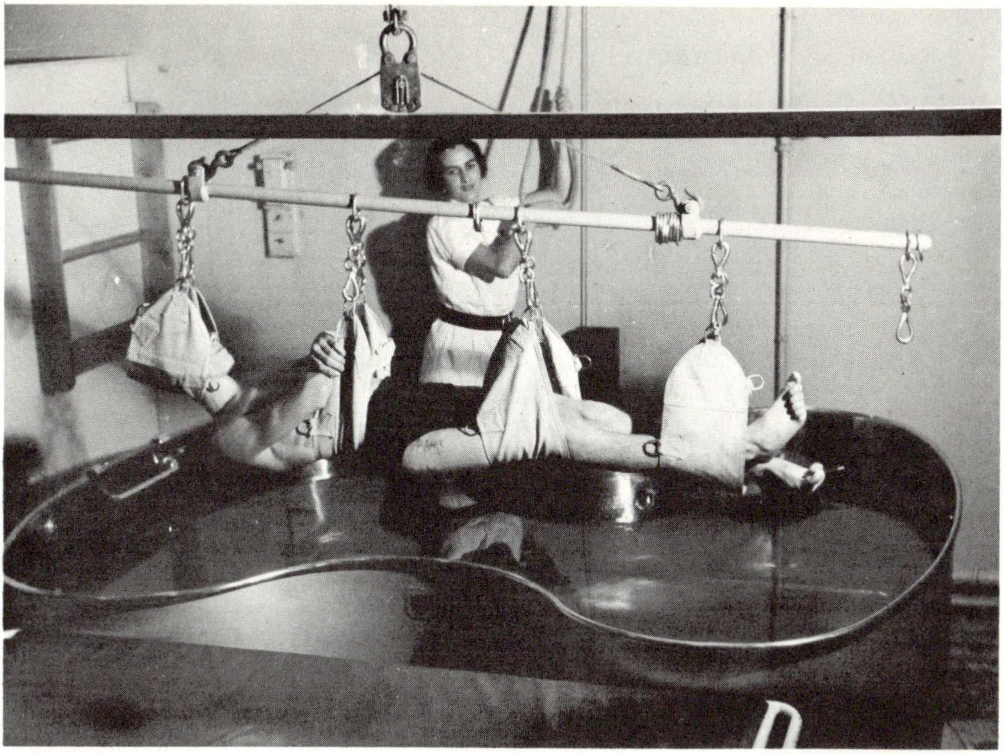

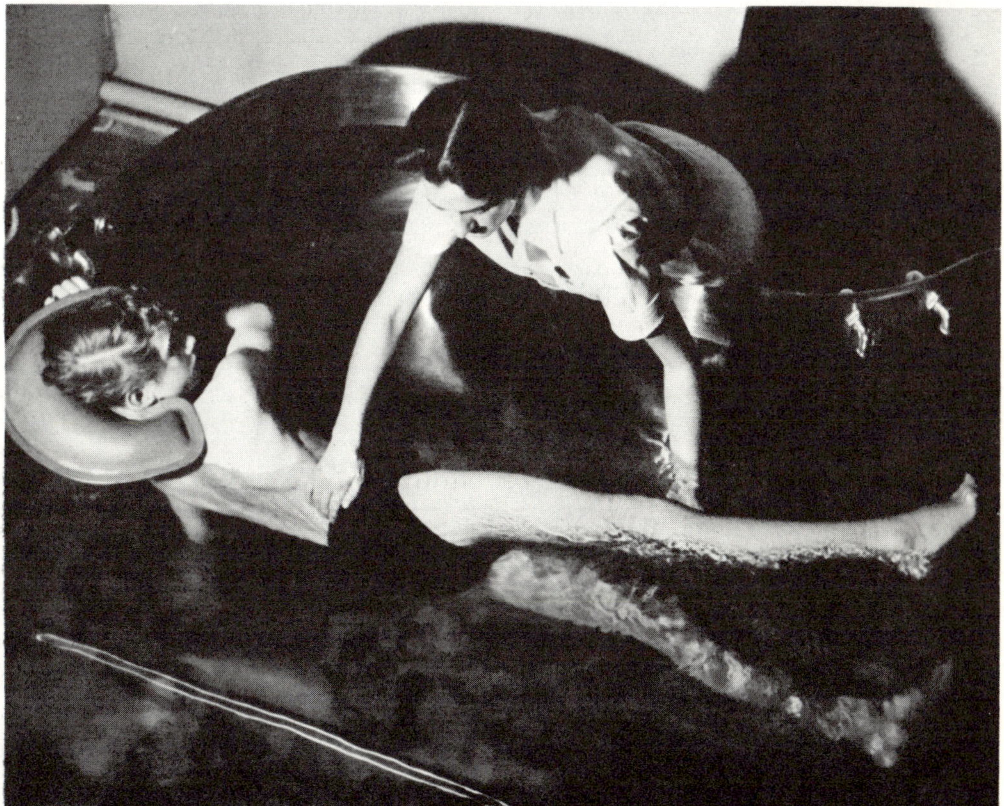

istics such as the beard, deep voice, heavy bones and narrow pelvis, and control his ability to procreate. Deprived of the testicles, as in *castration,* the individual cannot procreate, and may lose some of the secondary characteristics—or fail to develop these characteristics at all if the castration occurs before puberty.

The testicles, which lie outside the body proper in a thin-skinned sac called the *scrotum,* consist of a large number of tubular structures called *seminiferous tubules,* and of cells between the tubules called *interstitial cells.* The seminiferous tubules, from puberty to senility, are constantly producing *sperm cells (spermatozoa),* the male reproductive cells. Production of these sperm cells is the primary purpose of the testicles, and their conveyance to the female reproductive tract is the primary purpose of the whole male sexual system.

The *interstitial cells* produce the male hormone *testosterone* (and possibly other male hormones) which enter the blood stream and determine the male secondary sex characteristics. The *seminiferous tubules* all empty into the *epididymis,* a coiled tube partly covering the testicle which serves as a temporary storage area for the new sperm. The epididymis in turn empties into a long narrow duct called the *vas deferens* or *seminal duct,* through which the sperm cells pass to a larger storage area called the *seminal vesicle.* The seminal vesicles, in addition to serving as a storage place for sperm, also secrete a sticky viscous substance which aids in the preservation of the sperm and facilitates its further transport along the remainder of the seminal duct.

The seminal duct finally empties into the *urethra,* a channel which normally serves to convey urine from the bladder to the outside (hence the whole system is also called the *genito-urinary tract*). At this point, the urethra is surrounded by the *prostate* gland, which secretes another sticky white substance into the seminal fluid containing the sperm. This further facilitates the transport and preservation of the sperm. This final combined fluid is called *semen.*

The urethra passes into the erectile organ called the *penis.* Two small glands called *Cowper's glands* or the *bulbo-urethral* glands occur in this area. When sexual activity takes place, these small glands secrete an alkaline fluid which neutralizes any traces of urine which might still remain in the urethra. The acid urine would otherwise be highly injurious to the sperm cells. During sexual activity, special muscles close off the urethra from the bladder, making it impossible for any fresh urine to enter the urethra while sexual activity lasts.

The *penis,* through which the urethra travels, serves as the organ of intromission into the female *vagina* for depositing the semen in the female reproductive tract. Under the impetus of sexual desire or excitement, the highly flexible tissues of the penis become engorged with blood, and the normally flaccid organ assumes a rigid, greatly enlarged position called an *erection.* The state of erection permits the penis to be

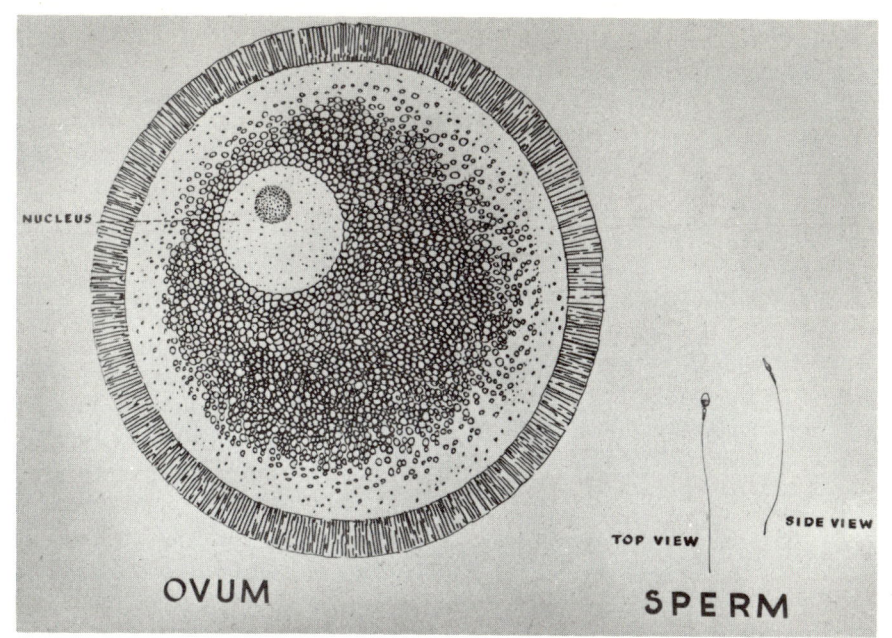

REPRODUCTION SYSTEM

OVUM

NUCLEUS

SPERM

TOP VIEW SIDE VIEW

Reproduction System—The sex cells. The *ovum* (egg) is much larger than the *sperm*. The inherited characteristics of the individual are carried in the head of the sperm and nucleus of the ovum. One sperm will attach itself to the egg wall; it loses its tail and its head penetrates into the interior of the egg. When the head fuses with the nucleus of the egg, fertilization occurs and the first cell of a new individual is formed. Early stages of development. We begin to grow into a new human being as soon as the egg is fertilized. Development takes place by repeated cell divisions into two cells, four cells, eight cells, until a stage is reached that resembles a mulberry; this is the *morula* stage. A hollow ball of cells results a few divisions later, known as the *blastula*. One side of this begins to push in like denting the side of a tennis ball, and eventually the whole mass begins to elongate, with the dent growing into a hollow tube which later forms the digestive tract.

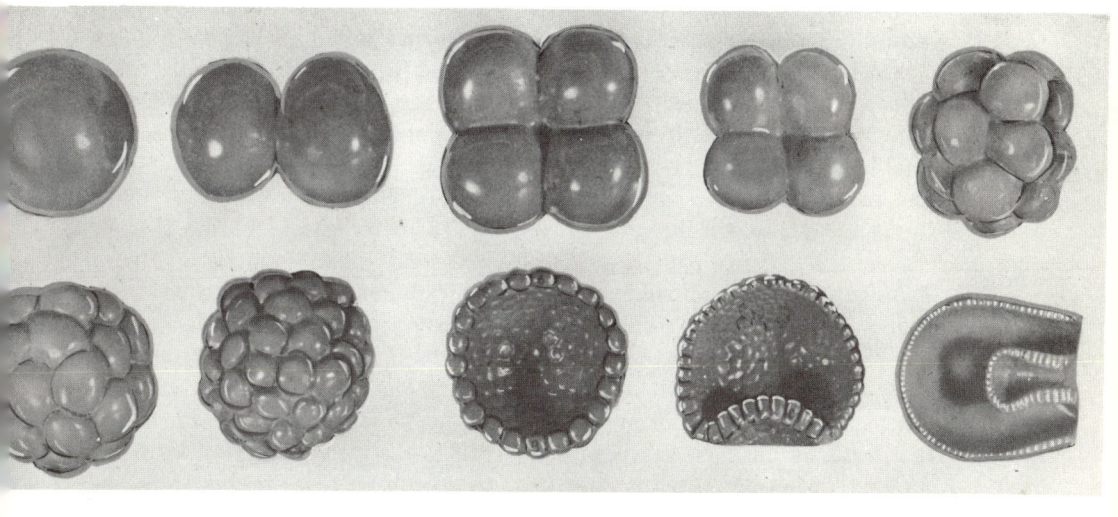

1127

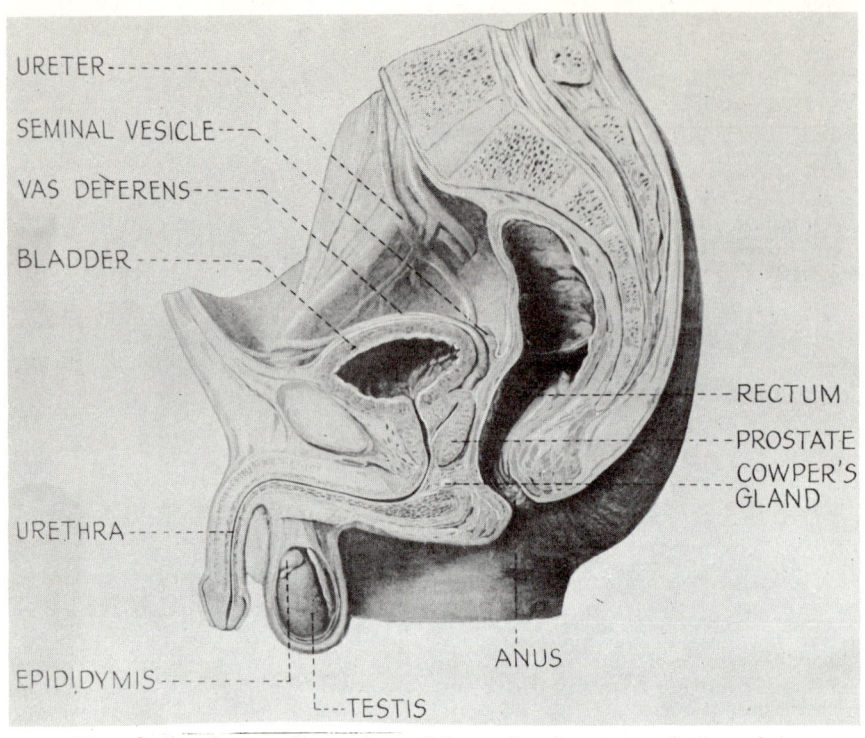

Reproduction System—The anatomy of the genito-urinary system in the male.

inserted deeply into the vagina. The friction of the vaginal tissues against the penis—normally highly pleasurable to both partners—causes muscular spasms to occur in the penis and along the seminal tract, finally resulting in the *ejaculation* of the semen into the vagina, an event known as *orgasm* in which the pleasurable sensations are greatest. Following orgasm, the blood drains from the penis and it resumes its flaccid state. Every ejaculation contains several hundred million sperm cells; only one of these can fertilize the female egg cell, resulting in a new human being; the others die after a few days. Fertilization does not occur at all if no egg is present in the female tract.

Female sexual anatomy. The female sexual apparatus consists of the *ovaries, uterus, oviducts, vagina,* and several small associated organs. The *ovaries*—the female *gonads*—perform functions analogous to those of the testicles in the male: they germinate the female reproductive cells, and govern the female secondary sex characteristics such as the high-pitched voice, absence of a beard, development of the breasts, and wide pelvis.

The female reproductive cells, called *eggs* or *ova* (singular *ovum*) develop in the interior of the ovaries within fluid-filled sacs called *follicles*. As an ovum matures, it attaches itself to the wall of the follicle. When the ovum becomes fully mature, the

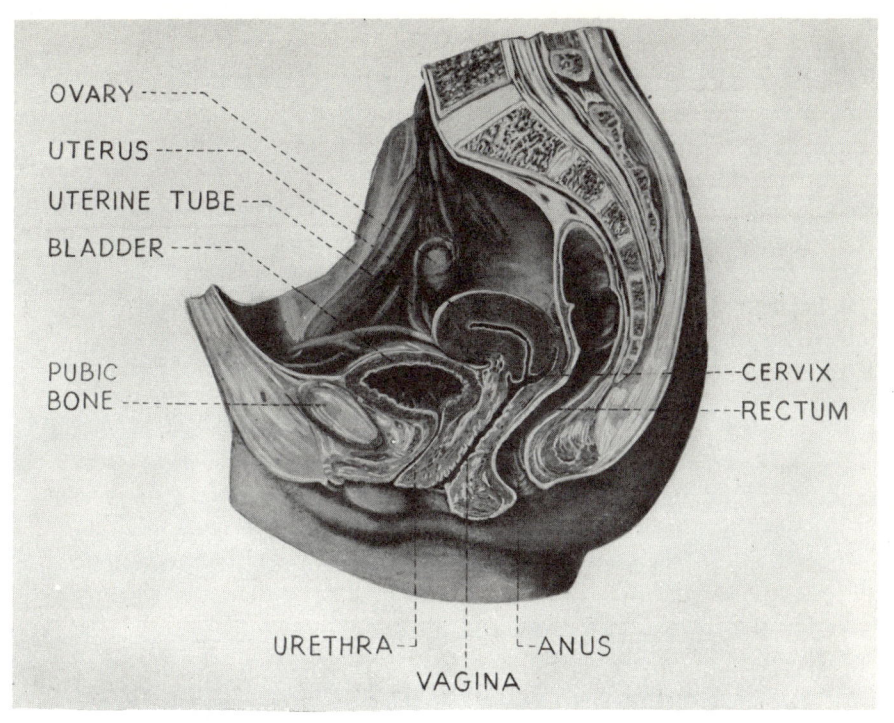

Reproduction System—The anatomy of the genito-urinary system in the female.

wall of the follicle bursts and the ovum escapes with the liberated *follicular fluid*—a process called *ovulation*. It then passes into the *oviduct* where it may be fertilized by a male *spermatozoon* if sexual intercourse has taken place.

The ovaries produce the female hormones or *estrogens*. These include *estradiol,* which specifically determines the female secondary sex characteristics, and *progesterone,* which brings about physiological changes in the uterus to prepare it for the reception and nurture of a fertilized egg cell—viz., a new human being. Progesterone is secreted into the uterus for about a week each month following the release of the ovum or ova.

As in the male, the production of reproduction cells and the secretion of sex hormones begins at puberty—usually about the age of eleven or twelve in the female. However, in the woman the sex glands cease these functions considerably earlier than in the male, usually between the ages of forty-five and fifty. This phenomenon is known as the *menopause.*

The *uterus* or *womb,* an organ capable of tremendous expansion, is where the fertilized egg develops into an embryo, a fetus, and finally a fully developed infant ready for birth. The *vagina* is the channel leading from the uterus to the outside of the body. It serves a twofold function: first, to admit the male penis into the female body so that semen may be deposited in the female reproductive tract, and—if conditions are propitious—an egg be fertilized; second, to serve as a channel for the birth of the developed infant, allowing it to emerge from the uterus into the outside world. Several small glands lubricate the vagina during sexual intercourse, facilitating the intromission of the penis and the passage of the semen. During intercourse, sensations of sexual pleasure occur in the vagina analagous to those the male experiences in the penis.

The entrance to the vagina resembles a small pair of vertical lips and is called the *labia minora*. Outside this is a larger pair of lips called the *labia majora* which encloses not only the entrance to the vagina but also the mouth of the urethra—through which urine is expelled—and, in front of that, the *clitoris*. The clitoris is a small fleshy projection which, in sexual excitement, may become erect, like a tiny penis. These external female sex organs are known as the *vulva*.

In young virgins, the opening of the vagina is covered by a thin membrane called the *hymen*. This disappears soon after intercourse is undertaken, and not infrequently even before.

Conception. Conception of a human being is an intricate event. In intercourse, the sperm cells are deposited near the mouth of the womb. These sperm cells may travel further, enter an oviduct, where one of them may meet with and fertilize one of the female egg cells. At once, by process of self-division, the fertilized egg cell—called a *zygote* (in reality a new living individual)—will begin to grow, feeding mainly on the food which it finds within itself.

Leaving the oviduct, this fertilized egg cell fastens itself to the inner wall of the womb. Soon, between the wall and the cell, the *placenta* develops. This is the channel of communication between mother and child, but the blood of the two never intermingles. Each, in the placenta, will have its own separate blood vessels. Other materials, however, such as fluids and gases, are passed from mother to child through the walls of these blood vessels, a process known as *osmosis,* which permits the mother to supply the child with such essentials as food, water, and oxygen. The child may also use this channel to rid itself of waste.

The placenta, together with membranes developed during pregnancy, is eliminated after the birth of the child, in the "afterbirth."

Genetics. The new human being exists as soon as the sperm cell has fertilized the egg cell, at which time the sex is determined.

All females are composed of cells each of which contains *46 chromosomes*—the infinitesimal protoplasmic bodies which govern the chemical (genetic) make-up of the individual, and determine such factors as the color of the hair, eyes and skin, the features of the face, the intelligence, etc. *Two* of these chromosomes govern the *sex* of the female and are labeled for convenience as *X chromosomes.*

The cells of males normally also

contain *46 chromosomes, two* of which are specifically *sex* chromosomes. One of these—as in the female—is an *X chromosome,* but the other exhibits a distinct genetic composition and is labeled a *Y chromosome.*

Thus, females are said to possess an *XX* genetic make-up (because they have *two* X sex chromosomes in each of their cells), and males are said to possess an *XY* genetic make-up (because each of their cells contains *one* X sex chromosome and *one* Y sex chromosome).

However, the *reproductive* cells —the *ova* and the *spermatozoa*— contain only *one* sex chromosome each, sharply differentiating them from all other cells in the body. In the female—since *all* of her sex chromosomes are X chromosomes —the one sex chromosome in any given reproductive cell (ovum) will *necessarily* be an X chromosome. In the male, any given reproductive cell (*spermatozoon*) may on the other hand contain *either* an X chromosome or a Y chromosome. (The spermatozoa are produced by division of other, nonspecialized cells in the walls of the seminiferous tubules. Any *one* spermatozoon may thus be formed with *either* an X or a Y chromosome obtained probably by sheer chance from its parent cell, which contained *both* an X and a Y chromosome.)

If the ovum—carrying (necessarily) an X chromosome—should happen to be fertilized by a spermatozoon *also* carrying an X chromosome, the resultant individual will inherit only X chromosomes from both parents and will thus be an *XX* individual, or *female.* If, on the other hand, the ovum should happen to be fertilized by a spermatozoon carrying a Y chromosome, the resultant individual will inherit an X chromosome from the mother but a Y chromosome from the father, and will thus be an *XY* individual, or *male.* As can readily be seen, it is the genetic make-up of the *father's fertilizing spermatozoon* which determines the sex of the offspring.

Equally obviously, there is no conceivable way to predict in advance what the sex of a child will be, and no way whatever in which the sex could be pre-controlled. There is simply no possible way of determining or ordaining which *one* of the *several hundred million* spermatozoa in an ejaculation will fertilize the ovum (even assuming there *is* an ovum conveniently available for fertilization!). Even if we could miraculously pick out one of these sperm cells from the many millions of other sperm cells around it, declare that this one would be the cell to fertilize the ovum, and then somehow see to it that it did *in fact* fertilize the conveniently available ovum, it would still be exceedingly difficult to ascertain with certainty whether this one given sperm cell were carrying an X or a Y chromosome. As it is, there is no conceivable way of performing any of these miracles. For better or worse, sex determination must remain in the field of chance.

It has recently been discovered that certain males—notably some of those prone to antisocial or criminal activity—possess an *extra* Y chromosome in their cells. Viz., they are *XYY* instead of normal *XY* males. Certainly, not all criminals are thus genetically abnormal; nor are all XYY males necessarily doomed to a life of crime. But it has been estimated that one in 300 men may possess this genetic abnormality, caused by the inexplicable presence of *two* Y chromosomes in the father's fertilizing spermatozoon. Several studies among prison inmates in the United States and Great Britain revealed an incidence of as high as 4 per cent of this genetic aberration. In addition to aggressive and violent tendencies, the XYY men tended to be tall, to have acne, and to be of low intelligence.

It has also been determined that certain women have an analogous genetic abnormality in which their cells contain *three* X chromosomes instead of the usual two—in other words, they are XXX females. Sometimes, the possession of three X *sex* chromosomes in women is associated with another abnormal phenomenon known as *mosaicism,* in which the total number of *all* chromosomes in the cells—normally 46 in each cell—varies markedly in different cells. Thus, while all human beings normally have 46 chromosomes in each and every individual cell of his or her body (of which two are sex chromosomes), the victims of mosaicism may have as few as 45 chromosomes in some cells, or as many as 48 chromosomes in other cells. The extent of mosaicism in the general population has not been determined, but it has been noted that there is a high incidence of mosaicism among *schizophrenics.* The exact relationship between schizophrenia and mosaicism remains to be determined.

These discoveries open up a whole new area of study in the fields of genetics, psychiatry and criminology. *See also* CERVIX; CONTRACEPTION; ECTOPIC PREGNANCY; FALLOPIAN TUBES; HETEROSEXUALITY; HOMOSEXUALITY; HORMONES; IMPOTENCE; MASTURBATION; MENSTRUATION; MENOPAUSE; ORGASM; OVARIES; PENIS; CHILDBIRTH AND PRENATAL CARE; PUBERTY; RHYTHM METHOD; SENESCENCE; SEXUAL INTERCOURSE; STERILITY; TESTICLES; URETHRA; UTERUS; VAGINA; VULVA. *See* MEDIGRAPHS pages 995, 1081.

RESERPINE, a new alkaloid drug which has proved useful against high blood pressure and in relieving the symptoms of acute mental disorders. The substance is derived from *rauwolfia serpentina,* a root from which extracts have been used in India for many centuries for a variety of medical purposes. Reserpine is a specific substance isolated from the root and believed to be the active principle to which the therapeutic effects are due. In India rauwolfia is a widely used sedative and has been employed against *snakebite* and other conditions for many centuries. *See also* BARBITURATES.

RESPIRATORY DISEASES, those disorders which affect the act of breathing with the lungs or the apparatus, the organs, tissues, and membranes, involved. The respira-

RESUSCITATION

tory system in the human being is chiefly composed of two lungs and the air passages which lead to them. See also COMMON COLD; LUNGS; PNEUMONIA; TUBERCULOSIS. See MEDIGRAPHS pages 273, 275, 279, 703, 863, 1047, 1051.

RESUSCITATION, the prevention of asphyxial death by *artificial respiration.* Unconsciousness is always an emergency situation. It can occur from inhalation of carbon monoxide, drowning, poisoning, electric shock, and other causes. Although various devices for artificial respiration are effective, manual artificial respiration is usually the most readily available, and unconsciousness requires immediate first-aid treatment.

The average person breathes from sixteen to twenty times a minute. However, most authorities believe that in artificial respiration a greater number of movements are necessary, since the patient will take in less than the normal amount of air in each breath. Some recommend that the rate be between twenty-four and forty movements per minute.

Until recently the most commonly practiced method of resuscitation was the *Schaefer technique,* named for the British physiologist who devised it. Another method, the *Holger method,* was then adopted by the American Red Cross, the American Medical Association, and other agencies. This procedure has now been augmented by mouth-to-mouth resuscitation.

The Holger method. The unconscious person is placed face down, with the hands on top of each other, the forehead resting on the hands with the face turned slightly to one side, and the elbows extended outward. The operator kneels on one or both knees in front of the head of the victim. He places his hands under

Resuscitation—The arm lift-back pressure method of manual artificial respiration (after Holger Nielsen). A, placing hands for arm lift. B, arm lift, the operator rocking backward. C, placing hands for back pressure. D, back pressure, the operator rocking forward.

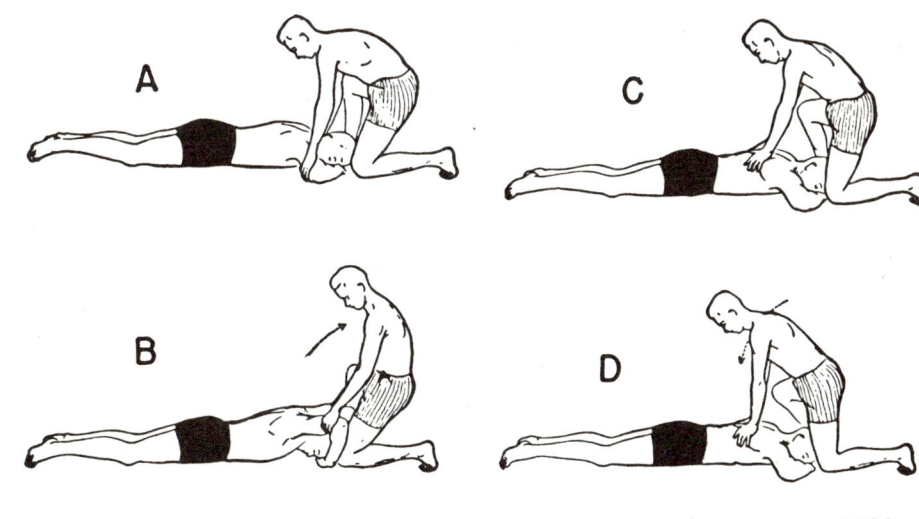

1133

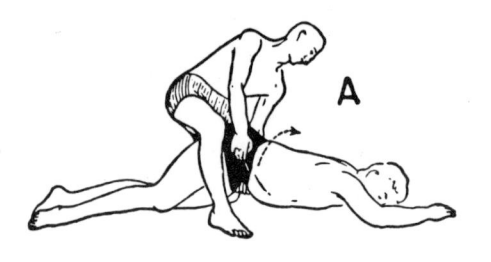

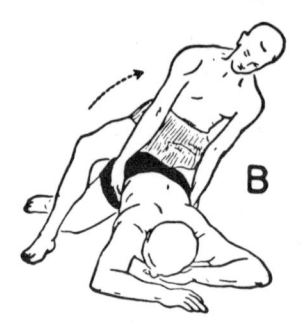

Resuscitation—The hip roll-back pressure method of manual artificial respiration. The operator, kneeling astride the subject, uses the knee on which he is kneeling as a fulcrum on which to roll the victim. A, side view of hip roll. B, front view of hip roll.

the victim's arms, above the elbow, and rocks backward drawing the arms upward and toward himself. The arms are elevated until firm resistance is met, then replaced on the floor. The operator then moves his hands to the back, just below the shoulder blades, and rocks forward, exerting pressure on the back. The operator's arms are kept straight during both the lift and the pressure phases, and the complete cycle is repeated about ten to twelve times a minute.

Hip lift. The unconscious person is placed in a prone position. The operator kneels on one knee near the victim's hip, straddles the victim, and places the other foot near the opposite hip. He places his hands under the hips, and raises the pelvis vertically upward four to six inches. The hips are then replaced on the ground and the cycle is repeated.

Resuscitation—The hip lift-back pressure method of manual artificial respiration. This method combines alternate lifting of hips with pressure on mid-back below shoulder blades. A, placing hands for hip lift. B, hip lift. C, placing hands for back pressure. D, back pressure.

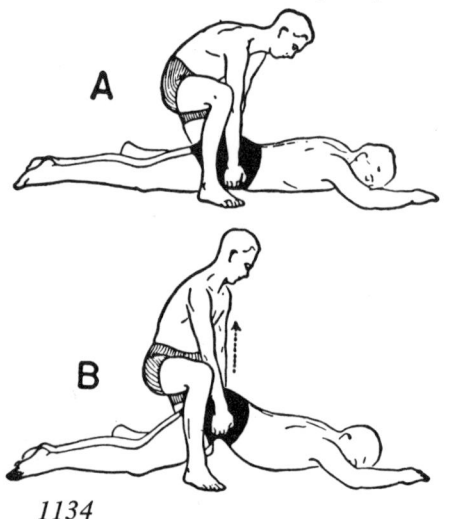

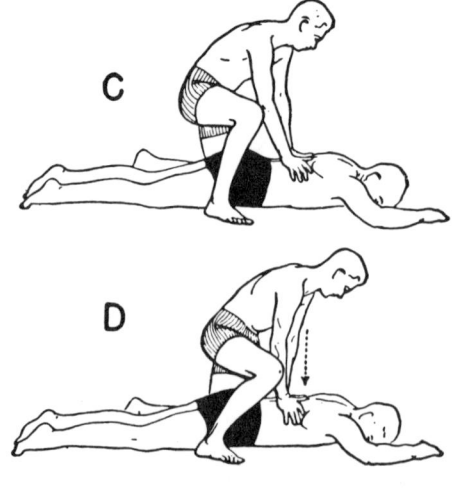

1134

RESUSCITATION

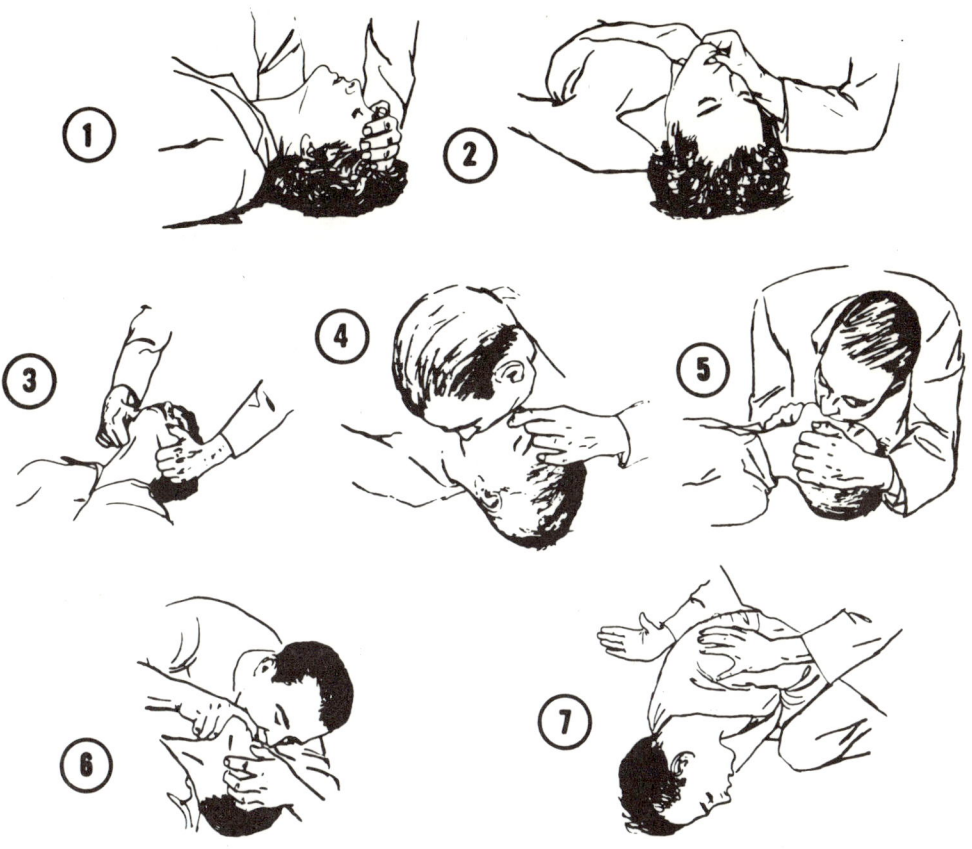

Resuscitation—The mouth-to-mouth method of artificial respiration. After removing foreign matter, if any, from mouth, tilt subjects head back so chin points upward (1). Thrust jaw into jutting-out position to clear base of tongue from throat (2, 3). Place wide-open mouth tightly over victim's mouth, pinching victim's nostrils shut (4); victim's nostrils may also be closed by operator's cheek (5). Mouth-to-nose method may be used by closing victim's mouth and breathing into victim's nose (6) instead of into mouth. If after first blowing efforts there is no air exchange, and recheck of head and jaw position does not induce breathing, victim should be turned quickly on side and given sharp blows between shoulder blades to dislodge foreign matter (7). Victim's mouth should then be rechecked for obstructions. For an adult, the rate should be 12 breaths, vigorously administered, a minute.

The hip lift is performed twelve times per minute. Lifting the hips produces active inspiration, as a result of several mechanisms: (1) When the hips are elevated, the abdominal contents sag downward toward the floor and result in an intra-abdominal negativity that tends to draw the diaphragm downward. (2) Because of the ligamentous attachments between the viscera and diaphragm, the downward movement of the abdominal organs is followed by a similar action of the diaphragm. (3) Elevating the hips hyperextends the spine and increases the intercostal spaces of the lower ribs.

RESUSCITATION

Hip lift-back pressure. The hip lift-back pressure method combines alternate lifting of the hips, as described, with pressure on the midback just below the shoulder blades, with the fingers spread and the thumbs about an inch from the spine. As the operator lifts the hips he rocks backward, and as he exerts back pressure he rocks forward. In each phase he keeps his arms straight, so that the work of lifting and pressing is distributed over the shoulders and back, rather than being imposed primarily on the arms.

Hip roll-back pressure. This is a modification of the hip lift-back pressure method in which a roll is substituted for the lift in order to increase the ease of performance. The operator kneels astride the prone subject as described for the hip lift method. Instead of lifting both hips, he uses the knee on which he is kneeling as a fulcrum on which to roll the victim. The operator keeps his arms straight, and rolls himself in the same direction in which he rolls the victim. Great care must be exercised to insure that the victim is rolled up onto the operator's knee or thigh, so that both hips are raised from the ground.

Mouth-to-mouth method. The Red Cross has revived an ancient method of artificial resuscitation as the best way of reviving infants and children whose breathing has stopped. This method is known as *mouth-to-mouth resuscitation,* and replaces the back pressure-arm lift method.

Following are steps in the mouth-to-mouth technique:

Resuscitation—Mouth-to-mouth method of artificial respiration for infants and small children. After the child's mouth and air passages are cleared of foreign matter, the child should be placed on his back and the lower jaw lifted from beneath and behind into jutting-out position (1). Then place your mouth over both the child's mouth and nose, breathing into them at the rate of about 20 breaths per minute (2). If the child's air passages remain blocked, he should be held up a moment by the ankles (3) or bent over one arm (4) and given a few sharp pats between shoulder blades to dislodge any obstructions.

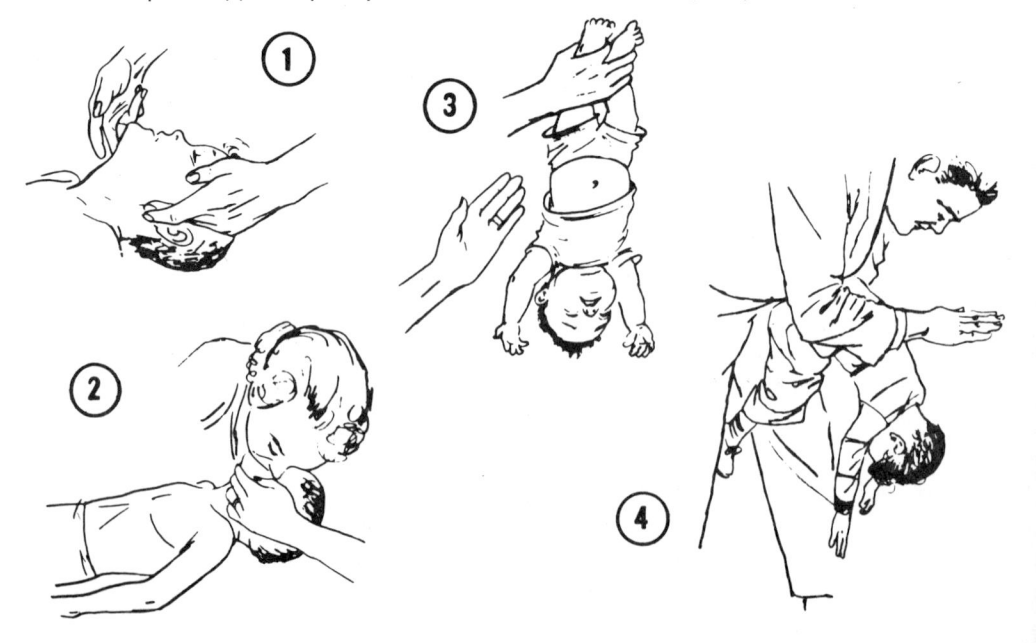

1. Clear the mouth of foreign matter with the middle finger of one hand, and with the same finger hold the tongue forward.

2. Place the child in a face-down, head-down position, and pat him firmly on the back with the free hand. This should help dislodge any foreign object in the air passages.

3. Place the child on his back and use the middle fingers of both hands to lift the lower jaw from beneath and behind so that it "juts out."

4. Hold the jaw in this position, using one hand only.

5. Place your mouth over the child's mouth and nose, making a relatively leakproof seal, and breathe into the child with a smooth steady action until you observe the chest rise. As you start this action, move the free hand to the child's abdomen, between the navel and the ribs, and apply continuous moderate pressure to prevent the stomach from becoming filled with air.

6. When the lungs have been inflated, remove your lips from the child's mouth and nose and allow the lungs to empty. Repeat this cycle, keeping one hand beneath the jaw and the other hand pressing on the stomach at all times. Continue at a rate of about twenty cycles a minute. If at any time resistance to breathing into the child is felt and the chest does not rise, repeat second step, then quickly resume mouth-to-mouth breathing. See also FIRST AID.

RETINA, the light-receptive layer of the eye and terminal expansion of the optic nerve. Vision is accomplished by the passing of light rays through the eye to the retina, the nervous tissue at the back of the eye.

A serious disorder is *detachment of the retina,* a condition in which small areas of the retina separate from the underlying coats usually as the result of injury, infection, or tumor and, sometimes, as a result of a disease, such as *tuberculosis.* An operative procedure has been developed in retinal detachment.

Inflammation of the retina is called *retinitis,* which may be due to infection, hemorrhage, or other types of injury. Sometimes it is associated with inflammation of the kidneys or hardening of the blood vessels.

Retinoblastoma is a malignant tumor of the retina, occurring in infancy or early childhood. In some instances tumor of the retina is present at birth. This disorder rarely occurs in persons more than ten years old. See also EYE.

RETROLENTAL FIBROPLASIA. Investigations of *retrolental fibroplasia*—scarring behind the lens of the eye, which causes blindness to develop in premature babies after birth—indicate that concentration of oxygen available to the tissues may be a causal factor. Doctors are now cautioned against giving too much oxygen to prematurely born babies in view of the danger of the development of an oxygen deficiency when the infant is returned to normal concentration. For this reason special attention is being given to the amount of oxygen available in different forms of modern incubator. In experiments with the offspring of

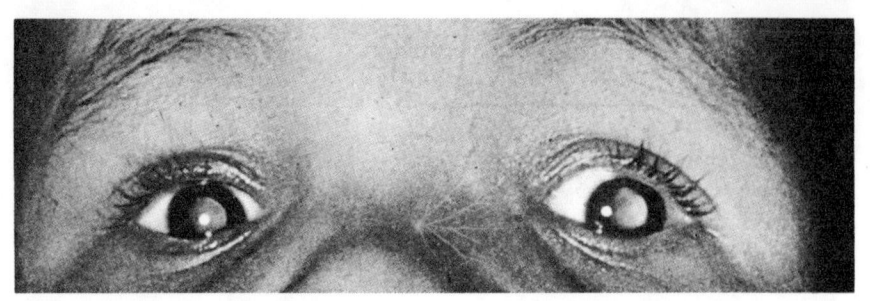

Retrolental Fibroplasia—A disease of premature infants which causes blindness is called *retrolental fibroplasia*. The disease is fully developed in this 2-year-old child. Note the white membranes in the pupils of the eyes. Retrolental fibroplasia appears most prevalently in premature infants of low birth weight. The eyes appear normal and do not differ from the eyes of other premature infants who do not develop the disease. But at one month to six weeks of age the blood vessels in the eyes enlarge and the first stage in the development of retrolental fibroplasia begins. The cause of retrolental fibroplasia is believed to be the injudicious use of oxygen during the early weeks of postnatal life.

mice previously subjected to an oxygen deficiency, one group of investigators produced changes in eye tissues similar to those that occur in retrolental fibroplasia.

RHEUMATIC FEVER, a *febrile disease* characterized by *painful migratory arthritis* and a *predilection to heart damage* leading to *chronic valvular disease*. It most frequently attacks young people between the ages of six and nineteen and, although no longer the leading cause of death in this age group, is among the foremost health problems. In at least one-fifth of all cases of rheumatic fever, the most serious associated condition is the attack on the heart. Rheumatic fever usually appears following infections of the nose and throat, but it may also be associated with *ear infection, scarlet fever, St. Vitus' dance* and other similar ailments related to *streptococcal infection*.

Great progress has been made in understanding and controlling rheumatic fever with the advance in control of infection and the near-conquest of streptococcal disease. However, the exact cause has not yet been determined nor the primary problem of prevention solved.

When rheumatic fever involves the heart, inflammatory changes occur in the muscles which affect the strength of the heart and cause it to dilate, and thus the heart does not function properly. Often rheumatic fever develops insidiously. The so-called *rheumatic lesions* may affect the joints, producing symptoms similar to "growing pains," and sometimes severe pain related to infection of the lymph gland is present. Mild fleeting pain may be felt in the tendons or muscles and pain in the heels is not infrequent. Twitching and mental hallucinations such as accompany St. Vitus' dance are sometimes symptoms.

More than half of the patients with rheumatic fever have had *tonsillitis* or sore throat from one to four weeks before the rheumatic symptoms appear. These symptoms may appear gradually or suddenly, and are usually associated with overexertion or chilling. The temperature rises to 102°F to 104°F, the pulse becomes rapid, there is profuse sweating, pain in the joints, and prostration. Joints most subject to stress and strain are affected first and pain seldom begins in all the joints at once. Sometimes the joints swell with fluid.

Pain and the other symptoms can usually be controlled by a doctor. The detection of the first signs of the heart disease associated with rheumatic fever is somewhat more difficult. When patients come under hospital care early, *electrocardiograph tests* will show at once transient abnormalities in the heart. The obvious signs of heart damage, such as irregularity, rapidity, pain, changes in size, and accumulations of fluid in the heart sac, appear later and are easily detected by the doctor. When the heart enlarges and its action is impaired, the sounds of the heart change and the pulse generally reflects the condition of the heart. Also typical of rheumatic condition are nodes which appear under the skin and an outbreak of rash.

The valves of the heart may be affected. Small nodules form on the valves and interfere with normal function. The nodules eventually disappear, leaving scars and causing the valve to develop unusually large numbers of blood vessels. If attacks of rheumatic fever recur, the patient may develop *hardening* of one of the valves. The blood is also affected. The white cells increase with the infection and the sedimentation rate of the red blood cells mounts, receding as the patient improves. Sometimes infection of the kidneys and the intestinal tract or severe pain similar to that of an attack of appendicitis accompany rheumatic fever.

At a point in an attack of rheumatic fever, the activity lessens and the infection becomes relatively inactive. When the condition becomes stabilized, the doctor usually reexamines the blood and heart and retests the white blood cell count and the rate of sedimentation of the red blood cells. Electrocardiograph tests are given and the vital capacity of the patient checked to determine the condition of his lungs. The doctor decides whether or not the patient can undertake mild activity. If the pulse rate continues high, even when the patient is asleep, or if the pulse does not return to its normal rate promptly following slight activity, it is too soon for the patient to resume activity. These tests also indicate the likelihood of partial or complete recovery.

The child with rheumatic heart disease or with any congenital ailment is especially susceptible to secondary infection, and continued treatment with antibiotics is essential. Persons with rheumatic fever are treated during the active stage of the disease by a variety of procedures. While these procedures are palliative, few are absolutely specific against rheumatic fever. *Sulfa drugs, penicillin, ACTH,* and *hydrocortisone* have all been used, but it has not been proved that any of these have conquered rheumatic fever.

the disease and its causes Rheumatic fever is a generalized infection caused by a bacterium or group of bacteria of the streptococcus family. It affects many different organ systems, including the central nervous system, the lungs, peritoneum, joints, and heart. The most likely point for the bacteria to enter the body is the throat, frequently the tonsils. The indication is that it is a sensitivity reaction in the patient which, under certain conditions, is responsible for the illness.

The disease occurs most often in young adolescents, equally divided between the sexes, and may involve several members of the family. It may also involve several families at a given time. Even epidemics have been reported. Crowded or unsanitary conditions seem to favor its occurrence.

symptoms There is usually a sore throat for a week or two before the onset of such symptoms as sudden fever of 101° to 104°, accompanied by profuse sweats and pain in the joints. This pain usually involves the large joints, traveling from one to another. The joint becomes painful, red, hot, and swollen. As one improves and returns to normal, without damage, another becomes involved. There may be prolonged, unexplained fever without any other symptoms. Early in the illness there may be frequent unaccounted-for nosebleeds. St. Vitus' Dance frequently heralds the onset of rheumatic fever. In 1 out of 10 cases there is a rash on the arms, over the back, chest, abdomen, or armpits.

complications Patients can recover completely from rheumatic fever. However, many suffer lifelong heart damage. Periodic flare-ups of this infection can increase the severity of the heart disease. Complications depend on the extent of damage. In very severe cases the damage can be overwhelming and the patient dies of heart failure. Rheumatic heart disease is discussed more fully under that heading.

prevention (or lessening of impact) There is no effective preventive for rheumatic fever. One should avoid contact, if possible, with people ill with a streptococcus infection. At the sign of a sore throat proper drug care should be taken, particularly where there is a history of rheumatic fever. Early recognition and prompt treatment can cut down complications.

In the convalescent period, patients with heart involvement must take extra care and resume activities at a slow pace dictated by the family doctor. Since rheumatic fever frequently recurs, it is important to check with the doctor at regular intervals, and particularly during periods of other infections, or preceding elective surgery or extensive dental work.

Rheumatic Fever

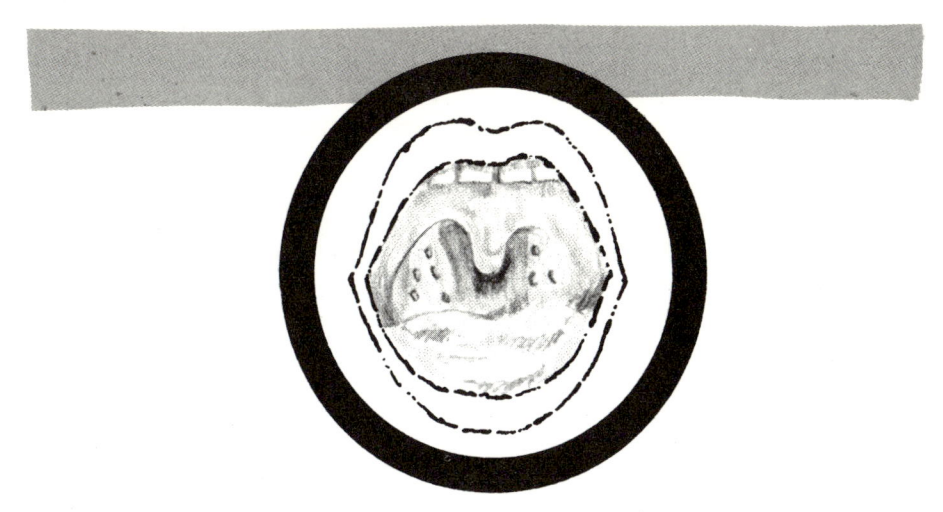

Usually preceded by tonsillitis or sore throat.

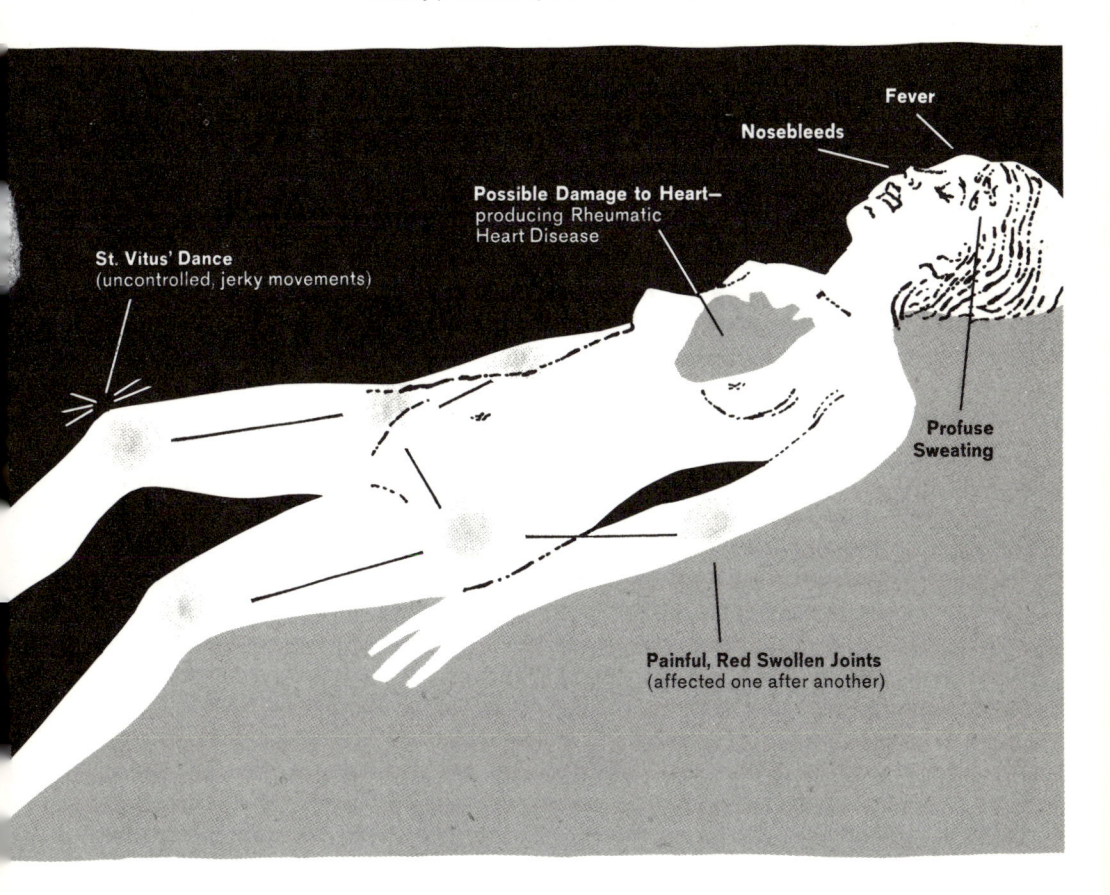

Fever

Nosebleeds

Possible Damage to Heart—producing Rheumatic Heart Disease

St. Vitus' Dance (uncontrolled, jerky movements)

Profuse Sweating

Painful, Red Swollen Joints (affected one after another)

the disease and its causes Some two-thirds of the known cases of rheumatic heart disease have a history of rheumatic fever, and it is generally accepted that acute rheumatic fever invariably involves the heart. In the course of such an attack the heart valves (most often the mitral and aortic) become scarred, usually quite rigid and contracted, and sometimes calcified. The accompanying Medi-Graph illustrates how the valves are affected.

In rheumatic heart disease the entire heart is involved—the pericardium, the myocardium, and the endocardium. There are often irregular heart rhythms which patients describe as a jumping sensation in the chest, or a sensation of having the heart skip a beat. Most so-called palpitations are of no consequence, but when they occur in an organically damaged heart, the doctor will want to study them carefully.

symptoms Symptoms depend upon several factors, including the presence of active rheumatic infection and associated heart failure. After the first attack of rheumatic fever there may be no symptoms for years. An adult may learn he has a heart murmur in a routine physical examination years after he has recovered uneventfully from a rheumatic fever siege. If the patient has had only minor heart valve damage he will probably have been living a normal, functioning life without signs of discomfort or disability.

The diagnosis is made by examination, electrocardiographic studies, and heart X rays.

complications It is the complications which are usually the clue to the presence of rheumatic heart disease. A serious one is the recurrence of rheumatic fever infection and further involvement of the heart and heart valves. Recurrence increases the destructive changes in the valve previously involved and puts additional strain on an already weakened heart muscle.

Despite the availability of antibiotic drugs, a not infrequent and serious complication is bacterial endocarditis—an infection of the lining membrane of the heart. Congestive heart failure and pericarditis, discussed elsewhere in this book, are other serious complications.

Emboli or blood clots discharged from the heart to distant parts of the body can often cause a condition that resembles stroke, if the brain is involved, or cause certain gangrenous changes when the lower extremities are involved.

prevention (or lessening of impact) As described in the section on rheumatic fever, it is important for a patient who has had this disease to take special care of himself. If the heart is not involved after rheumatic fever, a patient can in time do just about what he pleases. But appropriate antibiotics should be taken, as prescribed, when he undergoes minor surgical procedures or has dental extractions. If rheumatic heart disease symptoms develop, the doctor will decide upon a suitable program of activity.

Rheumatic Heart Disease

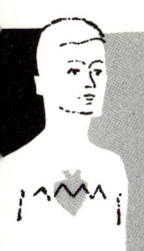

Most rheumatic heart disease develops between ages of 5-20

Rheumatic fever predisposes toward development of rheumatic heart disease — but many cases develop without history of rheumatic fever

Palpitations or jumping sensation in chest are sometimes sign of rheumatic heart disease

Normal Heart Action

1. Blood from body comes to heart through veins

2. Right heart pumps blood to lungs to get rid of carbon dioxide

3. Blood returns to heart after picking up oxygen supply in lungs

4. Freshened blood pumped out to body through Great Artery (aorta)

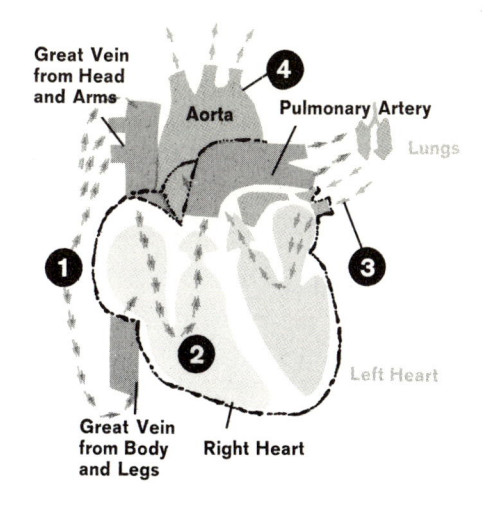

Mitral Valve Affected

1. Scar tissue from Rheumatic Fever obstructs mitral valve or prevents it from closing properly

2. Blood backs up putting increased pressure on left auricle

3. Pressure feeds back through pulmonary veins and arteries to right ventricle. It may eventually become enlarged and fail

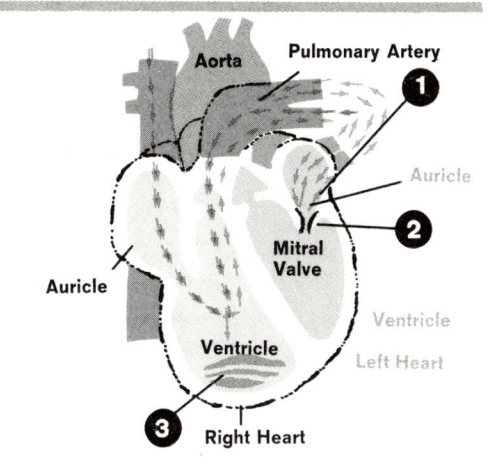

Aortic Valve Affected

1. Scar tissue from Rheumatic Fever obstructs aortic valve or prevents it from closing properly

2. Instead of pumping through aorta to rest of body, blood backs up, putting increased strain on left ventricle

3. Left ventricle may eventually become enlarged and fail

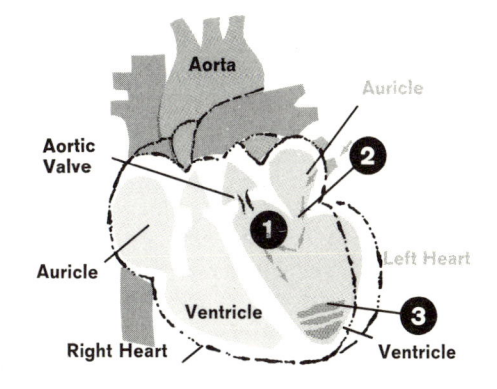

1143

Drugs of the *salicylate group* are especially useful in controlling such symptoms as fever, pain, and swelling in the joints. However, although these drugs do relieve the painful symptoms, they do not cure the disease itself. ACTH and *cortisone* have been lifesaving in controlling inflammation.

When the heart is especially involved, extra care must be taken to avoid every possible strain. *Continuous bed rest,* for weeks or even months, for the duration of the active stage is absolutely imperative. It is the one treatment of which doctors are certain.

Gradual resumption of physical activity must be carefully controlled. For example, the person is allowed to sit in a chair half an hour twice a day for one week; the next week, fifteen minutes more a day, if there have been no untoward symptoms; and, at the end of two weeks, perhaps he may be permitted to go to the bathroom by himself. Then moderate exercise may be allowed for fifteen minutes a day for two or three weeks; and perhaps, after five or six months, normal activity can be resumed, if the person's condition permits.

Unfortunately rheumatic fever has a tendency to recur after it has apparently gone. The doctor must determine, after the active stage has passed, whether or not the heart has been permanently damaged, and the person must continue to be reexamined at regular intervals to make certain that new activity has not begun and that he is in good health. For example, every sore throat should be treated immediately with antibiotics and sulfonamides.

Since complete bed rest, preferably outdoors in an open pavilion or on a protected porch, is so vital, children with rheumatic fever are best cared for in special sanatoriums where they may remain as long as necessary under the best possible conditions of ventilation, rest, sunshine, and nutrition.

If the person with rheumatic fever is anemic, special diets may be given which are high in protein, minerals, and vitamins. Infected tonsils and adenoids should be removed during the quiet periods of the rheumatic fever. All such operations are implemented with sulfa drugs or penicillin or other drugs to prevent secondary streptococcus infection.

The vast majority of children with rheumatic heart disease can and should attend regular schools and engage in a normally active life. In many large cities special schools are maintained for children with handicaps of the heart. In one report on the care of rheumatic fever, the following recommendations for treatment of children with inactive cases of rheumatic fever were made:

1. Take measures to improve the general health and resistance of the child.

2. Observe the patient regularly for signs of recurrence and for alterations in cardiac status.

3. Encourage physical activity to the limit of the child's capacity. Only a small percentage of children at adolescence are found to have sufficient permanent disease to preclude normal activity.

4. Provide vocational guidance and occupational training for the relatively small group who cannot engage in normal physical activity.

5. Discourage parents and teachers from making a chronic invalid of the child. Educational authorities should learn that the vast majority who attend regular school when the disease is inactive can and should engage in normal school ilfe.

6. Minimize exposure to upper respiratory infections, if possible, by improving living conditions—for example, by avoiding overcrowding in the home, particularly in bedrooms —and by controlling the spread of infection through school and family contacts. *See also* HEART. *See* MEDIGRAPHS pages 717, 1031, 1141, 1143.

RHEUMATISM, an overall term used to indicate diseases of muscle, tendon, joint, bone, or nerve resulting in discomfort and disability. More than 7,500,000 people in the United States are affected by it, which makes it the most widespread chronic disease and several times more frequent than tuberculosis, diabetes, or cancer. Of those affected, 400,000 are completely helpless; 800,000, despite treatment, are partly crippled; and the rest have chronic pain and discomfort. Rheumatism has been called one of the principal health problems in the United States.

The most common form of rheumatism is *rheumatoid arthritis*. Other forms are *degenerative joint disease, spondylitis, bursitis, fibrositis, myositis, neuritis, lumbago, sciatica,* and *gout*. These are all primarily afflictions that affect persons after the age of forty. *Rheumatic fever,* which often involves the heart, is essentially a disease of childhood, attacking children between the ages of five and fifteen. *See also* names of specific diseases mentioned above. *See* MEDIGRAPHS pages 135, 285, 947, 989, 1031, 1143.

RH FACTOR. *See* BLOOD TYPES.

RHINITIS, any inflammation of the nasal mucous membrane. One of the chief forms is the *common cold*. Rhinitis is largely the result of infection, but may be due to sensitivity to various substances. *See also* COMMON COLD; HAY FEVER; OZENA.

RHINOPHYMA, a form of acne, involving the blood vessels and sebaceous glands in the nose, which results in swelling and formation of great nodules. Rhinophyma is a disfiguring condition, sometimes called *toper's nose* or *whiskey nose*. Little can be done to alleviate it, except by plastic surgery.

RHINOPLASTY, a plastic operation on the nose.

RHUBARB, an herb which contains certain substances which act as a purgative. It was once widely used medically as a laxative in certain forms of constipation involving the intestines. As a purgative it is still popular because of its action of first cleansing the bowels and then checking any tendency to diarrhea. The mixture of rhubarb and soda is a rather widely known home remedy.

RHYTHM METHOD, a term used to indicate a method of birth control which avoids the use of artificial contraceptives and relies instead on abstention from sexual intercourse during the period of the woman's ovulation. Since pregnancy can only occur during the period of ovulation, it can be prevented by abstention on the days when ovulation occurs. This is ordinarily between 12 and 16 days after the onset of the previous menstruation. Because the cycle of ovulation may vary, it is necessary to keep exact records of menstruation and body temperature in order for the rhythm method to be successful. Body temperature rises slightly during ovulation.

The unfertilized ovum survives for only about twenty-four hours following ovulation. Therefore, if the parties abstain from relations during this period, pregnancy can be avoided. The difficulty is determining exactly when ovulation occurs. In order to do this, it is essential for the woman to keep an exact record of the onset of menstruation for a period of six to twelve months, and a record of the basal body temperature for the same period.

The basal body temperature curve is obtained by taking the temperature *immediately* upon awakening each day. Although a thermal shift occurs with ovulation, it does not actually pinpoint the moment of ovulation. But careful attention to the temperature curve can give a good general idea as to when ovulation has occurred. The curve is low in the first half of the ovulatory cycle and higher in the last half. The temperature remains high until the day before or the day of the onset of menstruation, when a sharp drop normally occurs. When the temperature has been high for several days, it can be assumed that ovulation has occurred. *See also* BIRTH CONTROL.

RIBOFLAVIN, the scientific term for the vitamin commonly called *vitamin B_2*. A deficiency of riboflavin may produce general body weakness and various skin disorders. The tip and margin of the tongue become sore and inflamed, painful cracks and fissures occur at the corners of the lips, and the face becomes greasy and scaly. The eyes are particularly sensitive to riboflavin deficiency and the cornea becomes cloudy and ulcerated, the mucous membranes inflamed, and the vision may be permanently impaired.

Management of riboflavin deficiency demands that the patient be given preparations containing large amounts of all major vitamins since a diet deficient in riboflavin is almost always deficient in other vitamins. The diet should then be permanently modified to contain adequate amounts of high riboflavin foods, such as liver, yeast, milk, eggs, whole-grain cereals, and greens. *See also* NUTRITION; VITAMINS.

RIBS, the curved, elongated bones which extend from the backbone around to the front of the chest. There are twenty-four ribs, twelve on each side of the rib cage. The upper seven are directly attached to the breastbone and are known as the *true ribs*. Of the remaining five, or *false ribs,* each of the upper three is attached to the rib above. The last two, called *floating ribs,* are not attached to other ribs.

The ribs act as a protective case for the organs in the chest. They may be injured by direct violence, such as blows, but are often fractured by the chest, under compression, as when a vehicle runs over the body. Frequently a fractured rib heals, simply by being properly strapped in place. An x-ray should be taken in every case where there is even a suspicion of a broken rib. Acute pain, increased by breathing, is usually a sign of a broken rib.

In some cases an extra rib, found high up on the chest, may cause pain because of pressure on the tissues. This is known as a *cervical rib*.

RICKETS, a deficiency disease that affects infants and children and is characterized by a failure of *calcium salts* to be deposited in sufficient quantity in growing cartilage and newly formed bone in the body. Deformities and other symptoms result from the failure of the bones to develop properly; they include growth of nodules on the ribs, development of potbelly, and bending bones. The child with rickets often sits with his thighs slightly spread apart, with one leg crossed over the other. The hands are placed on the floor or on the thighs, to assist the backbone in holding the body erect. The pull on the tissues by the muscles and the ligaments plus the softness of the bones cause bending, so that bowlegs and knock-knees are characteristic. Rickets also leads to delayed eruption of temporary teeth, and to deformities of the unerupted permanent teeth.

Since rickets is caused by insufficient amounts of *Vitamin D, calcium,* and *phosphorus* during the age when growth is rapid, and since the failure to receive sufficient amounts of one vitamin is likely to be associated with the failure to receive sufficient amounts of other vitamins and minerals, treatment involves a proper diet which includes them.

Parents should make certain that children, even in the nursing period, receive sufficient amounts of vitamins A, C, and D. They should also receive adequate amounts of calcium in the diet, best taken as milk, to insure proper and healthy growth. Cod liver oil, cod liver oil substitutes, vitamin D milk, and other dietary supplements are successful methods of preventing development of rickets in children and infants.

In severe cases of active rickets, large doses of vitamin D are administered, and in cases that do not yield rapidly, massive doses are given. The extent of rickets can be diagnosed, and the progress of treatment checked by x-ray. The diet must also contain sufficient amounts of calcium and phosphorus, which are necessary for the body to properly use vitamin D. *See also* NUTRITION; VITAMINS. *See* MEDIGRAPH page 1149.

the disease and its causes Rickets is a disease which results from a deficiency of vitamin D in the diet of infants (usually under the age of two). The only natural sources of this vitamin—which controls the deposition of calcium in the bones—are sunlight and certain foods such as eggs, sardines, tuna, herring, and salmon. Breast-fed infants get a fair amount of vitamin D from their mother's milk, but it needs to be supplemented with commercial preparations such as cod liver oil, or with milk to which vitamin D is added.

At present, in this country, the disease most often affects children who live under slum conditions where they are exposed to little sunlight.

symptoms The onset of rickets is very slow, and very often the symptoms are so slight that the disease is overlooked. The infant is restless and seems to be uncomfortable without cause. There may be thickening over the ankle and wrist joints, painful areas on the body, sweating, low-grade fever, weakness, and poor growth. Pressure on the skull deforms it easily because it remains soft. Softening of the bones also causes deformities of the legs (bow legs) and pelvic and chest deformities. Fractures (broken bones) are common. The child is also more susceptible to respiratory infections, such as colds, grippe, pneumonia, etc.

Adults with so-called chicken and funnel breasts probably had rickets in infancy.

complications The disease is rarely fatal in itself, but secondary infections are frequent and can result in death. Spasms of the larynx occur occasionally as well as convulsions. Tetany (a disease brought on by the influence of calcium in the blood) with convulsive spasms of the hands and feet, can be another complication.

In general, serious complications of rickets affect later life. A woman with a deformed pelvis can be severely handicapped during pregnancy. A patient with poor chest expansion due to rickets can be handicapped when he has a respiratory illness.

prevention (or lessening of impact) The simplest way to prevent rickets is to take supplementary doses of a commercial product high in vitamin D. Fortified vitamin D milk should be used when there is a need. Exposure to sunlight can be of some help. A pregnant mother should make certain to include adequate amounts of calcium and vitamin D in her diet.

When the diagnosis is established and corrective measures are indicated, care must be taken to prevent deformity of the bones involved. A deformity which has already developed may have to be corrected orthopedically.

Rickets

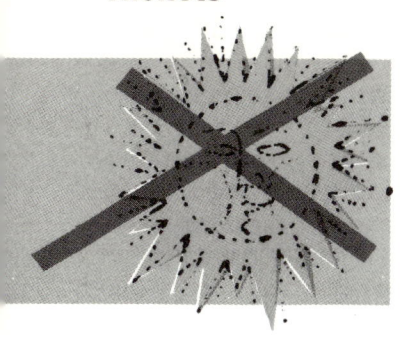

Develops in infants due to lack of Vitamin D

Sunlight prime source of Vitamin D, Mother's milk, egg yolk and cod liver oil can also supply infant's needs

Develops in Infants Between 3rd-18th Months

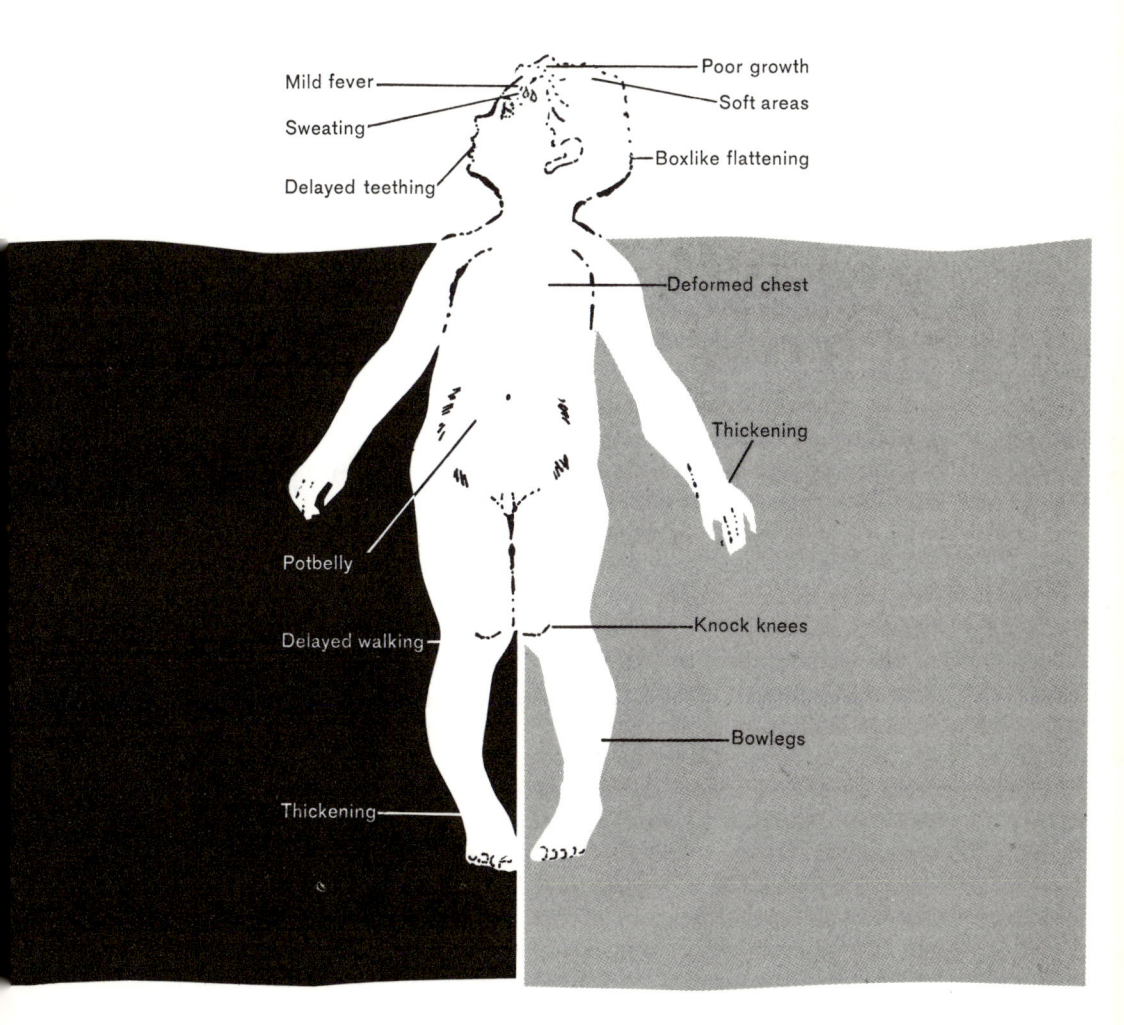

- Mild fever
- Sweating
- Delayed teething
- Poor growth
- Soft areas
- Boxlike flattening
- Deformed chest
- Thickening
- Potbelly
- Delayed walking
- Knock knees
- Bowlegs
- Thickening

RICKETTSIAL DISEASES, illnesses caused by one of the *Rickettsial organisms.* Rickettsiae are a family of microorganisms which have characteristics in common with both the *filterable viruses* and *true bacteria.* Under the microscope they have many shapes, but most of them resemble tiny rods. They were named after Dr. H. T. Ricketts of Chicago, who first isolated such an organism while he was studying *Rocky Mountain spotted fever* and *epidemic typhus fever.* In the course of these experiments Dr. Ricketts contracted typhus and died.

The rickettsiae are transmitted from man to man by an intermediate host, usually blood-sucking ticks, lice, or fleas. They generally pass into the blood stream of man through the bite of the insect, but infection may also be caused by excrement of the insect deposited on the skin.

The organism is responsible for at least four groups of diseases in human beings: *typhus fever, the Rocky Mountain spotted fever group, scrub typhus,* and *Q fever.* A person who has had a disease in a particular rickettsial disease group will have complete immunity to other diseases of the same group but will not be immune to those of the other groups.

Treatment, prevention, and control of the rickettsial diseases have made great strides with the development of large-scale *antirickettsial vaccines,* improved methods for mass delousing with DDT and other new insecticides, and with some of the newer antibiotics. *See also* names of specific diseases.

RICKETTSIALPOX, a disease caused by *Rickettsia acari,* a mild infection first identified in New York City in 1946.

The infection is transmitted by a small colorless *mite* which infests *house mice* and *small rodents.* About a week or two after the bite of an infected mite, a firm reddish blister appears at the site of the bite. It dries, forms a small black ulcer, and in two or three weeks the scab drops off, leaving a small scar. It is not painful. Rickettsialpox is characterized by fever, chills, sweats, headache, muscle pains, and loss of appetite, which last about a week. The eyes are sensitive and light hurts them. A rash appears on the body, sometimes involving the mucosa of the mouth, which also disappears in about a week.

Rickettsialpox is sometimes confused with *chickenpox.* However, it is not a childhood disease, and may occur in all age groups. Eradication of house mice and consequently the carrier mites helps to control the disease. *See also* RICKETTSIAL DISEASES.

RINGWORM, a ring-shaped infection, the most common of the superficial *fungus diseases,* once believed to have been caused by a worm, and hence formerly called *tinea,* the Latin word for worm. The infection is also found in dogs, cats, and other domestic animals, and is spread by contact with infected sources.

Normally the skin carries several species of fungi which remain inactive until they are aroused by conditions favorable for their growth, such as lowered resistance, excessive perspiration, heat, moisture, or friction. The fungi then attack the hair follicles of the scalp or beard, the nails, and certain nonhairy skin surfaces. The infection results in unsightly troublesome sores which stubbornly resist treatment.

Ringworm usually starts with small, red, slightly raised, round or oval sores which gradually enlarge and become redder. Blisters often follow, with some itching and burning. They generally start healing in the center, while the infection spreads outward in circular fashion.

Many ringworm infections, especially those found in children, are highly contagious. Public schools and children's hospitals take the utmost precautions to prevent the spread of the infection when a case is reported.

Ringworm of the scalp, or *tinea capitis,* is a common highly contagious infection, found most frequently in children. The hair loses its luster, becomes brittle and breaks off easily. The scalp becomes covered with grayish scaly patches and short stumps of diseased hair. The more severe forms consist of boggy inflamed sores which contain pus. Temporary baldness in stubborn cases may become permanent.

Treatment is directed primarily toward preventing the spread of the infection. The involved areas must be kept clean and dry and protected from any friction. The scalp should be shampooed daily with *tincture of green soap* and a good *fungicide.* The hair should be clipped short and the cuttings burned. In resistant cases the hair and its roots are removed by a physician. Combs, brushes and caps used during this period should be sterilized or destroyed and the fingers and nails of infected persons kept clean to avoid a secondary infection and to prevent spreading the ringworm by scratching.

The sooner a ringworm infection is recognized and proper treatment begun, the more rapidly will the spread of the infection be halted and the disease eradicated.

Ringworm of the groin, or *tinea cruris,* an eruption which generally affects the skin of the inner thighs or under the arms, may be found in both sexes, though more commonly in males. The eruption varies from light brown scales in mild cases to bright red patches in the active stages, with well-defined raised borders. There is intense itching, which is worse at night, and the condition is aggravated by obesity, excessive sweating, and lack of cleanliness.

Ringworm of the groin is one of the most common fungus diseases in the tropics where it was sometimes incorrectly called *dhobie itch.* It has also been known as *gym itch* and *jockey itch.* The disease is sometimes contracted around swimming pools and bath houses from infected clothing and towels. The eruption often subsides during cold weather, the infected skin becoming dry, flaky, and stained. Usually, however, it recurs with warm weather.

As in all cases of ringworm, the utmost precaution should be taken to prevent the spread of the infection. Frequent bathing, following by liberal use of dusting powder, and daily change of underclothing are essential. The infected person should sleep alone, and bed linens and personal laundry should be sterilized.

Treatment depends on the acuteness of the condition. For chronic cases the specialist often prescribes ointments containing *bismuth* or *salicylic acid*. The infected area must be kept clean and dry at all times, and reinfection by scratching or wearing contaminated clothing must be avoided.

Ringworm of the body, or *tinea circinata,* is another form of the infection, found in the nonhairy skin. This eruption begins as a small red sore and enlarges outward. The dry type tends to become scaly and the moist type forms little blisters or pus sacs. It usually begins on the exposed parts of the face and neck and later spreads to the trunk, forearms and legs. It is generally acquired from household pets.

This type of ringworm yields readily to treatment. The infected area is scrubbed with *tincture of green soap* to remove the crusted debris, and mild ointments of *salicylic acid* and *sulphur* are sufficient to control the condition.

Favus (tinea favosa). Although favus, another type of ringworm generally attacks the scalp, and is often limited to that region, it is caused by a different fungus than the one responsible for *tinea capitis*. Favus is caused by a vegetable parasite known as *Trichophyton schoenleini,* named for the German physician who first discovered it, Johann Lukas Schönlein. Climatic and social conditions may be factors in the transmission of this disease. It is relatively rare in the United States, but occurs more commonly in China, Central Asia, the Balkans, and Germany. Children are much more susceptible to the infection than adults.

Favus begins as a small, scaly, inflamed sore which is soon covered with a sulphur-yellow, cup-shaped adherent crust, or *scutulum,* through which sparse short hairs project. The hairs are brittle, dull, and lusterless, and break off easily. A "mousy" odor is usually present.

If the condition is treated early, little permanent baldness or scarring results. Cases of long duration may occasionally show large patches of slightly reddened and scaly areas of baldness.

Treatment is similar to that for *tinea capitis*. The hair is closely clipped, the crusts removed, and the scalp thoroughly shampooed. Antiparasitic ointments and lotions are applied, and the infected hairs are pulled out. The hair should be kept short and local treatments continued for at least a month after the scalp seems to be cured.

Ringworm of the nails, *tinea unguim,* or *onychomycosis,* may be associated with infection of the hair, as in *favus,* or it may appear independently. It is not uncommon among nurses, who acquire the infection by contact. The condition begins on the undersurface of the nail, which becomes dull and ridged, and is raised off its bed by a cloudy grayish patch extending toward the nail root.

Treatment consists of removing the infected nail and applying antiparasitic medication during the entire period of growth of the new nail. Recurrences are common, especially among those whose work necessitates wetting the hands often, for example, washers, soda dispensers, fur skinners, canners, and housewives.

For *ringworm of the beard,* see BARBER'S ITCH. See also ATHLETE'S FOOT. See MEDIGRAPH page 665.

RIO GRANDE FEVER. See UNDULANT FEVER.

ROCKY MOUNTAIN SPOTTED FEVER, an infectious condition caused by a rickettsial organism similar to the one that causes *typhus,* and transmitted to man by the bite of the *wood tick* or the *dog tick.* Spotted fever was known to the Indians of Montana and Idaho long before Caucasian settlers came. It has appeared in recent years in most parts of the country. Similar tick-borne diseases are the *boutonneuse fever* of the Mediterranean, *South African tickbite fever,* and other varieties found in Brazil, Colombia, Mexico, and Canada.

Three species of man-biting tick carry spotted fever in this country: the *common wood tick* of the northwestern states, the *dog tick* in the East, and the *Lone Star tick* of Texas. The ticks, which attach themselves to animals in wooded areas, pick up the rickettsiae and remain infected for life. The eggs and newly hatched ticks also carry the parasite and pass it on from generation to generation. Human beings are infected by the tick bite or from a skin wound contaminated by crushed ticks or tick feces. People have been known to be infected by crushing ticks with their fingers while removing them from dogs. In the West, where the wood tick is the carrier, more men have contracted the fever than women. In the East, where the infection is transmitted by the dog tick, women and children are more often affected.

About two days to two weeks after a person has been infected, the symptoms appear. A few days of malaise, chilly sensations, and loss of appetite are followed by headache, chills, severe pains in the back and muscles and the large joints. The face is flushed, the eyes are sensitive to light, a dry cough often develops, and the temperature may rise to 105°F and in severe cases even higher. On the third day a rash develops. Occasionally it is preceded by a mottled appearance of the face, neck, and upper chest, almost like that in measles. The rash spreads to the wrists, ankles, and back; then to the forehead, arms, and legs; and finally to the chest and abdomen. The rash begins to fade as the fever drops. Restlessness and insomnia often develop. The disease tends to be milder in children than in adults. One attack of spotted fever generally gives immunity for a long period. Second attacks may occasionally occur after a lapse of eight years or longer.

Early diagnosis and treatment with *antibiotics* can reduce the fever in a few days and prevent or minimize

ROCKY MOUNTAIN SPOTTED FEVER

the more severe disturbances which follow the fever.

The most effective protection for persons exposed to spotted fever is *vaccination,* preferably in the spring, before the ticks become numerous. A series of three injections establishes immunity for about a year, but must be repeated annually. People in tick-infested areas should wear one-piece outer clothing and high boots. The entire body should be inspected daily for ticks, especially about the hairline of the neck and the pubic hairs. The tick is slow to attach itself, and starts feeding only some time after it has become attached. Children should be examined twice daily, since in their play they may become especially exposed. Ticks should be removed with great care, to avoid crushing them and thus contaminating the spot to which they have become attached. The site of attachment should be disinfected with soap and

Rocky Mountain Spotted Fever—Rocky Mountain spotted fever is transmitted through the wood tick. The female tick transfers the organisms to the offspring through her eggs. The nymph feeds on the blood of rodents, and the adult tick infects dogs and man. Care should be taken to protect pets from wood ticks.

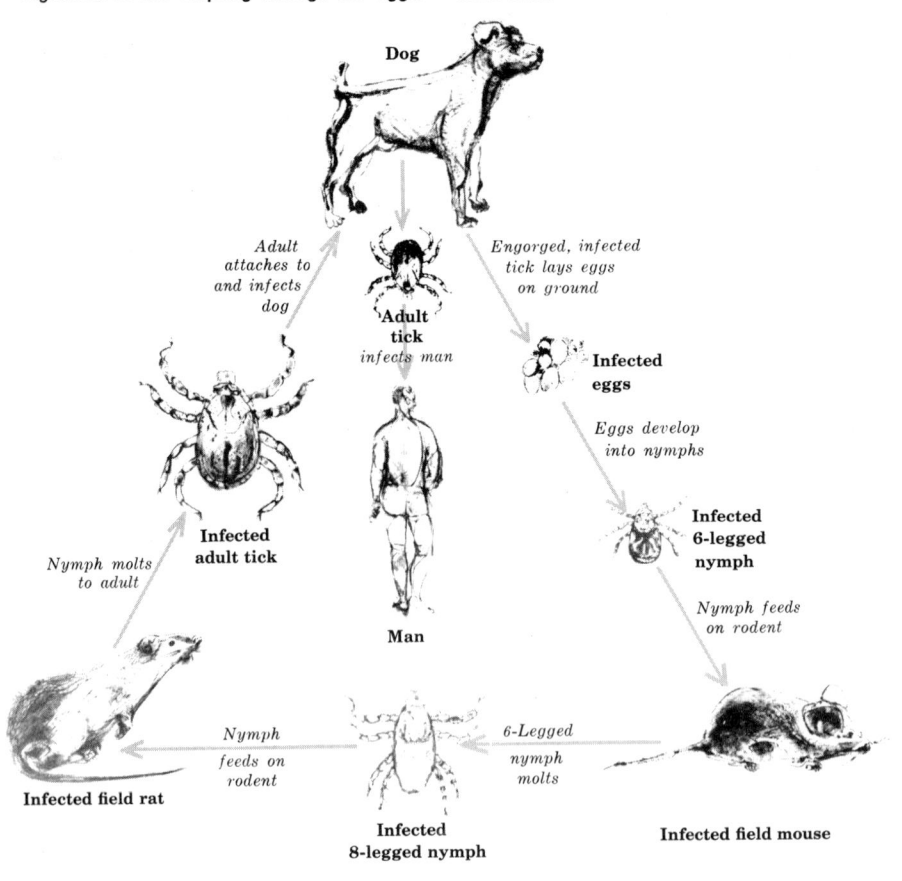

water, and the wound swabbed with a toothpick dipped in crude phenol or the most potent household antiseptic available. A dab of *ether, chloroform*, or *acetone* will usually cause the tick to drop off. If not, *forceps* or *tweezers* should be used gently, with care taken not to leave the mouth of the tick embedded in the skin. Ticks should never be removed with the bare fingers. Dust sprays containing an insecticide may be used to remove ticks from livestock and dogs, but should not be applied to cats, which lick their fur and may be poisoned. *DDT* and *chlordane*, applied directly to the ground and to low vegetation, are both effective in controlling wooded areas infested by ticks.

ROUNDWORM. *See* WORMS.

RUBELLA, another name for *German measles*. *See* GERMAN MEASLES.

RUBEOLA, another term for *measles*. *See* MEASLES.

RUPTURE. *See* HERNIA.

S

SACROILIAC, the joint at the base of the spine, between the *sacrum* and the *ilium*.

SACRUM, a triangular-shaped bone formed by the five *sacral vertebrae* fused together at the lower end of the spine. Inflammation of the joint between the sacrum at the back and the pelvis at the front produces pain which is sometimes mistaken for *sciatica*. *See also* SPINE.

SADISM, a sexual perversion in which the individual obtains pleasure from inflicting pain on others. The term is derived from the Marquis de Sade, a Frenchman who lived about 1800 and wrote several books about sexual cruelty. *See also* MASOCHISM.

ST. VITUS' DANCE. *See* CHOREA.

SALIVA, the opalescent, tasteless, weak alkaline fluid secreted chiefly by the salivary glands which open in the mouth under the jaw in front of the ear and under the tongue. The lining of the mouth also secretes saliva.

Saliva contains an enzyme which acts in the digestion of starch to change it into sugar. It serves also to moisten and soften food in the chewing process, and to keep the lining of the mouth moist. *See also* XEROSTOMA.

SALK VACCINE. *See* POLIOMYELITIS.

SALPINGITIS, inflammation of the uterine or Fallopian tubes, due to infection. *See also* FALLOPIAN TUBES.

SALT, chemically a substance resulting from the combination of an acid and a base. In nontechnical usage, however, it usually refers to the white powdery condiment *sodium chloride,* commonly used to season foods.

1156

The average person consumes about half an ounce of salt daily. This is usually adequate; but in extreme heat, when perspiration is heavy, more than the usual amount of salt is lost by the body and a deficiency can result, characterized by weakness, cramplike pains, and nausea. The increase in salt consumption necessary to relieve the deficiency is small—one extra pinch of salt is usually enough.

About three ounces of salt are present in the body of an adult person at any one time. The body's use of salt and its elimination are believed to be regulated by the *cortex* of the *adrenal glands,* the small bodies which secrete *cortisone.*

The human body uses salt to supply the *chlorine* required to synthesize *hydrochloric acid,* a significant digestive substance secreted by the stomach. *Pepsin* performs its digestive function only in the presence of hydrochloric acid.

The amount of salt in the diet may be related to various conditions which affect the kidneys and blood pressure, and low-salt and salt-free diets are prescribed in such cases. A reduction in salt, perhaps the usual half ounce decreased to a tenth of an ounce, may be desirable in *dropsy* or *edema,* in which fluid accumulates in the tissue.

Sodium chloride has various medical functions. Salt is injected when fluid which has been lost from the body by bleeding must be replaced. A strong salt solution is a good *emetic* and a weak solution is a mild *gargle.*

SANDFLY FEVER, an infectious viral disease, resembling *dengue fever* in many of its symptoms. It is of short duration and occurs most frequently in the Mediterranean area It is caused by the bite of the sandfly, *Phlebotomus paptasii.* The condition is also known as *pappataci fever, three-day fever,* and *phlebotomus fever.* See also DENGUE.

SAN JOAQUIN FEVER. *See* COCCIDIOIDOMYCOSIS.

SARCOMA, malignant tumor, most frequently involving nonepithelial tissue, which includes fibrous and connective tissue, cartilage and bone. Cancer in the skin, arising from the layers below the epidermis, occurs only in children. Sarcoma of the nerve cells is known as *fibroneurosarcoma.* It is also found in lymphoid and fatty tissue. Sarcoma may be detected and diagnosed by microscopic examination of a piece of the tumor, a procedure called a *biopsy.* See also CANCER.

SATYRIASIS, a morbid condition in the male analagous to *nymphomania* in the female, in which the individual is afflicted with insatiable sexual urges. It is usually attributable primarily to psychological disturbances. Such persons can be dangerous if not given proper psychiatric treatment. *See also* NYMPHOMANIA.

SCABIES, popularly known as the *itch* or *seven-year itch* follows invasion of the skin by the microscopic *itch mite,* which is no more than a fiftieth of an inch long, and whose name is *Acarus scabiei.*

The mites live on the surface, but the eggs of the female are laid under the skin. The female mites burrow under the skin and may remain for a long time, traveling along a tunnel of some length and laying eggs in the burrow. The young develop within a few days, then come to the surface where they repeat the cycle.

Several areas of the body seem to be favored by the mites. Most often they burrow on the inside of the fingers, near the webs. Other locations are the insides of the toes, the ankles and knee joints, the front of the armpit, the breasts of girls and women, and the outer sex organs of boys and men. The face never seems to be attacked.

The body becomes sensitized to the insects and intense itching results. Numerous blisters may form, and scratching may result in infection.

To rid the body of the itch mites, the most effective treatment includes bathing in hot water every day, followed by the use of *sulphur ointment.* For patients sensitive to sulphur, ointments containing other drugs, including *benzene hexachloride* which is less irritating than sulphur, may be prescribed.

Underclothing and bedding must be changed daily until all danger of further hatching of the eggs is removed. Extreme care must be taken that the infested person not infect other persons with whom he comes in contact. *See* MEDIGRAPH page 851.

SCARLET FEVER, an acute infectious disease characterized by a scarlet skin eruption. It occurs most frequently in fall or winter, and in children between the ages of five and twelve. Children less than one year old seldom contract it, probably because they have received antisubstances in their blood from the mother which afford protection.

The period of incubation is approximately three days following contact with an infected person. The symptoms are a painful sore throat, chill, nausea, and vomiting. The pulse rate increases, the temperature may rise as high as 104°F, and the child may suffer a severe headache.

The rash first appears in pinpoint spots of bright red, usually on the chest and neck, and then gradually over the rest of the body. Although this rash attacks the body more often than the face, the face often shows red spots, if only because of the high fever. Although the rash may continue only two or three days, it will take a week or more before the skin regains its normal color. Ten days to two weeks after the onset of scarlet fever, peeling of the skin begins. Large pieces of skin may come away from the feet and hands or drop off in scales, and other parts of the body can be affected, such as the teeth, fingernails, and sometimes the hair. The tongue develops a pitted scarlet appearance which gives it the name *strawberry tongue.*

Although scarlet fever often proves to be a relatively mild infection, it may have serious complications. The kidneys are frequently involved, or the ears, glands, and joints, so that this disease can do serious damage.

Scarlet fever is occasionally contracted by drinking milk or by contact with wastage thrown off from an infected person. The peeled skin is harmless, unless it happens to carry secretions from the nose or throat of the patient.

Many persons may have had the disease in a mild form at an earlier time, when it was erroneously diagnosed or ignored, and thereby gained immunity. This may help to explain why scarlet fever appears to be only mildly contagious. One attack of the illness seems to assure almost certain immunity.

Scientific understanding of scarlet fever has advanced greatly in recent years, and both diagnosis and treatment have improved. The *streptococcus* is the cause of the disease, and wherever the germ grows, poison or toxin is produced. If this poison is injected into the skin of someone who has never had scarlet fever, a severe reaction will be noted. In those persons who have had the disease and are immune, there will be no reaction.

When a small amount of this poison is rendered harmless and is injected into a person who has never been infected, he will then be able to resist the disease. However, this preventive toxoid is administered only to a person who has been exposed, or who works in the vicinity of people with scarlet fever, or during epidemics. The most effective technique to prevent spread of scarlet fever is to avoid contact with infected persons, particularly when discharge from the nose, throat, or ears is active.

As long as the fever persists, a mild diet is recommended. Once the fever has subsided, however, soft foods are usually given until the peeling period begins, when milk and fresh vegetables are added as well as food rich in vitamins, minerals, and protein.

Treatment demands that as little effort as possible be placed on the kidneys and heart, since they are already receiving from the toxin itself an attack almost greater than they can endure. Ordinarily the patient is required to remain in bed at least three weeks and must be protected from chill and cold. Sponge baths of tepid water may be given. A mild gargle may relieve sore throat, and one of the newer antibiotics will be even more effective. The person who cares for the patient should preferably be someone who has already had the disease, since he is directly exposed to germs. Reactions of the heart and kidneys and ears must be carefully watched. Occasionally when the ear is infected the ear drum is punctured so that the pus can be drained before the internal ear is involved.

Since the advent of *sulfa drugs* and *penicillin,* serious complications from scarlet fever have become rare. The drugs are also highly effective against the germ itself so that scarlet fever is no longer such a serious threat. *See* MEDIGRAPHS pages 1143, 1161.

the disease and its causes Scarlet fever is a contagious disease caused by certain types of streptococcus bacteria. It is spread in many ways—by direct contact with infected patients, by healthy carriers, by contaminated food or milk, or by contaminated objects. The incubation period is 2 to 5 days. The disease occurs most often during the colder seasons and begins in the throat. Young children are affected most, but infants under a year are generally immune.

symptoms Scarlet fever develops rapidly, with a sore throat, temperature as high as 104°, and swollen neck glands. The back of the throat becomes covered with red spots, and the patient develops a pitted "strawberry" tongue which is really the minute swellings of the tongue glands. From 12 to 36 hours after the onset of scarlet fever, a red rash which is described as "blushing goose flesh" develops. Pressure of a finger on the skin leaves an easily visible white mark. When the rash fades about a week later, it is followed by a flaking of the skin on many parts of the body. Sometimes the teeth, fingernails, and hair are affected.

Attacks of scarlet fever may be very mild, presenting a slight quick rash and resembling simple tonsillitis; or they may be severe, with high fever, vomiting, and delirium. In severe cases there may even be bursting of small blood vessels under the skin. One attack of scarlet fever seems to assure almost certain immunity to future attacks.

complications The more serious complications affect the kidneys and the heart. Nephritis, which is a kidney ailment, may appear about the third week of the illness. One indication of nephritis is the patient's urine, which turns a reddish color.

The heart changes are related to and resemble rheumatic fever. Sometimes severe arthritis is seen with scarlet fever. Ear infections are common, as well as swollen glands with occasional abcess formations.

prevention (or lessening of impact) The severity and complications of scarlet fever can be reduced greatly by prompt and adequate treatment with penicillin. This drug is also used effectively in preventive care. A scarlet fever antitoxin is available, but often it is not recommended because so many people react severely to it. Many people are immune simply because they had the disease in a mild form at an earlier period and it was not recognized for what it was. The Dick test, which checks whether or not a person has immunity to scarlet fever, is often given by the doctor to those who may be exposed to the disease.

Scarlet Fever (Scarlatina)

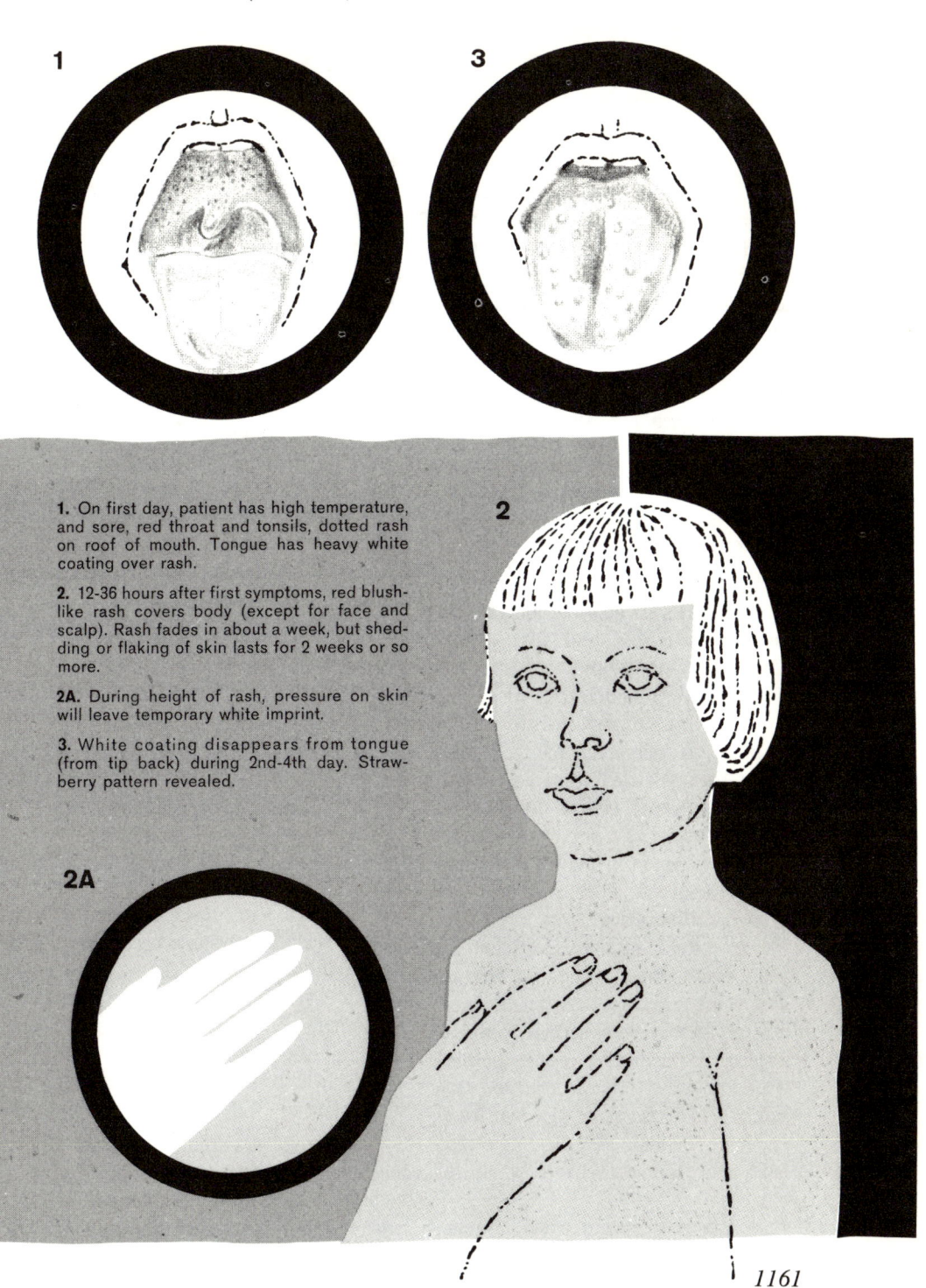

1. On first day, patient has high temperature, and sore, red throat and tonsils, dotted rash on roof of mouth. Tongue has heavy white coating over rash.

2. 12-36 hours after first symptoms, red blush-like rash covers body (except for face and scalp). Rash fades in about a week, but shedding or flaking of skin lasts for 2 weeks or so more.

2A. During height of rash, pressure on skin will leave temporary white imprint.

3. White coating disappears from tongue (from tip back) during 2nd-4th day. Strawberry pattern revealed.

1161

SCHISTOSOMIASIS. See BILHARZIASIS.

SCHIZOPHRENIA, a severe mental disorder, a major *psychosis,* which involves a loss of contact with reality and a temporary or permanent disorganization or disintegration of personality. *Schizo* means *splitting, phrenia* means *mind,* and so the term *schizophrenia* refers to a *splitting away of the mind from reality.* Schizophrenia is the most common form of mental illness and one-fourth of all hospitalized mental patients fall into this category.

The schizophrenic person rejects the outside world and turns to his own self-created world. His actions are made in accordance with this imagined world and so are difficult to interpret. His speech may be garbled and unintelligible and his actions completely inappropriate to his external situation, since they are motivated by his fantasy world and his inability to perceive reality in the normal way.

Schizophrenia is not one disease but rather a set of complex symptoms which encompass many forms of mental disorder. The causes are extremely difficult to treat. Factors which would appear pertinent in some cases do not apply to others. The schizophrenic is a person who has apparently been unable to find a way of adjusting to some painful situation and so has rejected the outside world in favor of his own inner version. Organic factors are also believed to be related to schizophrenia.

In the past few decades, understanding and treatment of schizophrenia has greatly improved and the rate of partial or complete recovery is higher. Expert psychiatric care is essential, preferably as soon as possible. *See also* MANIC-DEPRESSIVE PSYCHOSIS; PARANOIA; PSYCHOSIS; NEUROSIS; PSYCHIATRY; REPRODUCTION SYSTEM, *Genetics.*

SCIATICA. See SCIATIC NERVE; SCIATIC NEURITIS.

SCIATIC NERVE, the large long nerve which supplies the muscles of the thigh, leg, and foot and the skin of the leg. It runs the entire length of the leg with many branches and subdivisions. The nerve can be irritated or compressed at any point. *See also* SCIATIC NEURITIS.

SCIATIC NEURITIS, also frequently called *sciatica,* inflammation of the sciatic nerve, the longest nerve in the body, which passes from the lower part of the spinal column downward to the leg along the rear of the thigh. The term *sciatica* is often applied to cover a variety of ailments having no involvement with the sciatic nerve. True sciatica is *sciatic neuritis,* and pain is felt in the thigh and other areas associated with the sciatic nerve. Sciatic pain accompanies numerous conditions, and may be due to a number of factors which adversely affect the sciatic nerve.

The part of the spinal cord where the nerve originates may be disturbed, for example, by a slipped or ruptured disc, or by an inflammation in the vertebral bones. An abnormal condition in a nearby blood vessel may cause it to press on the nerve. Acute and prolonged constipation is sometimes responsible because the accumulation in the bowel exerts pressure on the nerve or because the body absorbs unexcreted toxic substances to which the nerve reacts. External conditions or occurrences may precipitate a sciatic disturbance, such as a bad fall or severe contortion of the body, or prolonged exposure to cold and dampness.

Because of the number of possible causes and the numerous possible ramifications which sciatic neuritis may have, it is, like headache and backache, an apparently simple discomfort which masks a potentially complicated situation. Diagnosis of the specific cause of a particular case of sciatic neuritis demands the attention of a skilled physician. The pain is only a symptom and the source of it must be determined before proper treatment can begin. The physician will first ascertain whether the pain involved is due to a sciatic condition or some other cause. He will check the sacroiliac joint, the spine for curvature, the back for bones out of position, the legs for muscle spasms or disordered muscles and tissue.

Treatment may begin with simple measures to relieve the immediate discomfort: bed rest, placing the body in the position with the least possible strain on affected parts, or use of heat to reduce pain. The doctor will examine the patient's diet and his daily activities, making sure that the diet is nutritionally adequate and that the patient's job, exercise, and general environment do not aggravate his condition. He may, for example, recommend that a patient who works in a cold damp

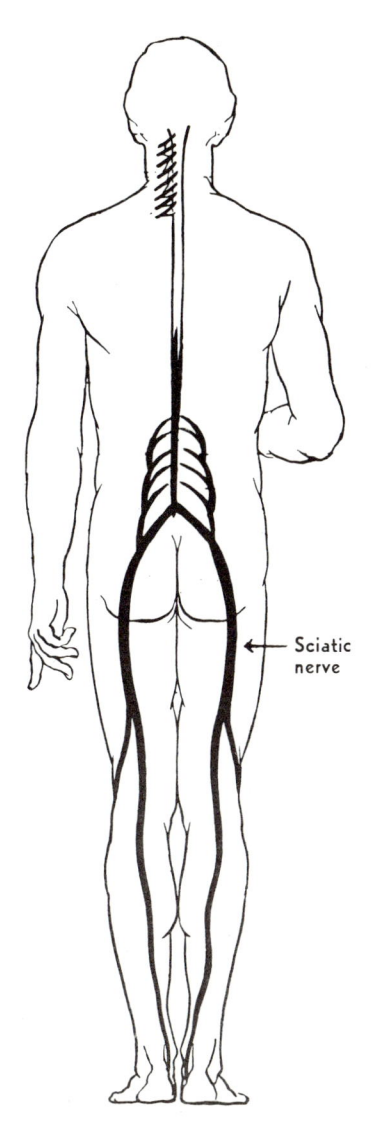

Sciatic Nerve—Diagram shows the sciatic nerve passing out of the spinal column, down the back of the thighs and onward to the leg. The sciatic nerve is the longest nerve of the body. Pains from inflammation of this nerve are usually felt in the back of the thigh.

place change his job. Injection of one of a variety of medicinal substances into the sciatic nerve or the surrounding areas is sometimes advisable and may bring good but not permanent results. Other measures are available for specialized treatment. *See also* SLIPPED DISC. *See* MEDIGRAPH page 947.

SCLERODERMA, a disease in which all the layers of the skin become hard and rigid. A grave affliction, *scleroderma* attacks women more often than men, usually between the ages of twenty and forty. Localized scleroderma often appears and disappears spontaneously in children.

Before the disease becomes apparent, the victim may for some time have complained about alterations in the circulation of his blood. Soon the hands and feet take on a bluish tinge, which changes later to white or yellow. At the same time the tissue itself becomes increasingly hard and rigid. Eventually both arms and legs—and even the entire body—may become hard as stone.

Almost nothing is known about the cause of scleroderma. Obviously, gross damage is done to the tissues, as well as to the superficial blood vessels, but the nature of the toxin is unknown. Some authorities have suggested that the cause may be traced to glandular changes and others believe that the nervous system causes the condition.

Treatment has included use of the *electric needle,* use of *ointments* and *massage,* and a *change of climate.* Modern drugs have been tried, such as *sodium paba, cortisone,* and *ACTH.* Little success has been recorded, however, either in the control or the cure of this serious and strange disease. *See also* COLLAGEN DISEASES. *See* MEDIGRAPH page 1113.

SCLEROSIS, a hardening of part of the body due to overgrowth of fibrous tissue. The term is applied particularly to *hardening of the nervous tissue* from atrophy or degeneration of the nerve elements, and to *thickening of the arteries* caused by growth of fibrous tissue and deposits of fatty substances and calcium salts. *See also* ARTERIOSCLEROSIS.

SCOLIOSIS. *See* SPINAL CURVATURE.

SCROTUM, the exterior pouch underneath the *penis* containing the *testicles.* It consists of translucent elastic skin, and of muscle fibers and membranes covering the testicles, *epididymides* and *spermatic cords* (the muscular cords surrounding the efferent seminal ducts).

The temperature of the scrotum is lower than that of the internal body, permitting the testicular production of sperm cells, a function impossible at the higher temperatures inside the body. The testicles normally descend into the scrotum shortly after birth. Under warm conditions, the skin of the scrotum loosens, drawing the testicles *away from* the heat of the body; conversely, under cold conditions, the scrotum tightens, drawing the testicles *toward* the body's

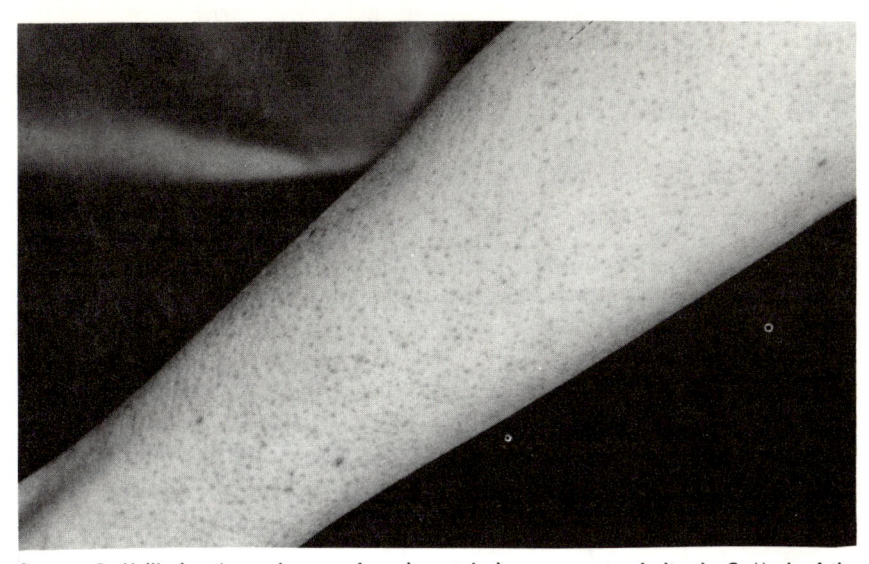

Scurvy—Perifollicular hemorrhages of early scurvy. Scurvy results from a deficiency of vitamin C. Fresh cabbage and citrus fruits contain large amounts of vitamin C. Much of the vitamin C content in foods is destroyed when the foods are cooked or exposed to the air.

warmth. *See also* TESTICLES; UNDESCENDED TESTES; PENIS; REPRODUCTION SYSTEM; SPERMATIC CORDS.

SCRUB TYPHUS, the common name in America for a rickettsial infection known also as *tsutsugamushi, Japanese river fever,* and *mite typhus.* It is widespread in Asia and southwestern Pacific areas, and is carried to man by *field mice* infected by *mites* or *chiggers.*

Scrub typhus was a serious problem for military medicine during World War II, when thousands of cases broke out among troops stationed in the Pacific region.

The illness follows the course of the rickettsial infections, with headache, fever, chill, and insomnia. A characteristic symptom is the small ulcer, or *eschar,* which develops where the mite is attached to the skin. About the fifth day a red rash appears on the trunk. The ulcer and rash are generally absent in Asiatic peoples. Temperature drops by the end of the second week, and is followed by slow convalescence. One attack will give immunity for many years.

Appropriate antibiotics produce an immediate drop in temperature, and general improvement ordinarily occurs in twelve hours. Vaccines have not yet been developed to prevent the disease. Mite repellents such as *phthalates,* or *benzyl benzoate,* smeared by hand on clothes and exposed skin surfaces, are effective. These drugs should not be used on or around sensitive skin areas such as the eyes or the perineum. *See also* RICKETTSIAL DISEASES.

SCURVY, a serious nutritional disorder caused by a lack of vitamin C. It is characterized by extreme

the disease and its causes Scurvy is a dietary deficiency disease which results from a lack of vitamin C. It is becoming rare, particularly in adults, because a person must go without this vitamin for several months to develop the disease. However, it is not uncommon in infants who are fed a diet without enough citrus fruit or tomato juice.

Vitamin C is found in high amounts in orange and lemon juice, fresh fruits such as strawberries, cantaloupes, and bananas, and fresh vegetables such as cabbage and tomatoes.

symptoms The symptoms of infants with scurvy include loss of appetite, weakness, pallid skin, irritability, and lack of weight gain. When the baby teeth erupt, there is often bleeding of the gums. When the infant moves, there is pain in the legs caused by hemorrhage in the joints, and there are painful swellings about the joints. Blood spots appear on the skin. The patient has low-grade fever. There may be blood in his urine. Adults with scurvy lose weight, become weak, and develop pale skin. Their gums become tender and spongy, and eventually ulcerate. Large black and blue areas appear on the extremities, and there are frequently painful spots over the shinbones. There can be hemorrhage into the muscles of the calves, nosebleeds, and bloody vomiting. The teeth loosen and fall out.

Scurvy which involves the mouth must be distinguished from trench mouth or other local gum infections.

complications As a rule serious complications are rare. In advanced cases there can be hemorrhage and secondary infections. The loss of teeth is an important cosmetic problem.

prevention (or lessening of impact) Scurvy can be prevented by eating a balanced diet that includes adequate amounts of the foods mentioned as sources of vitamin C. Vitamin C in commercial form is easily available and should be taken by anyone who, for reasons of health, has to be on a rigid diet that eliminates foods high in this vitamin.

Scurvy

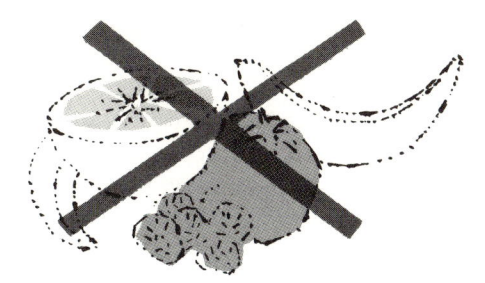

Lack of Vitamin C in diet causes Scurvy

Among best sources of Vitamin C are orange and lemon juice, tomatoes, cabbage, strawberries, cantaloupe, bananas

Signs of Scurvy

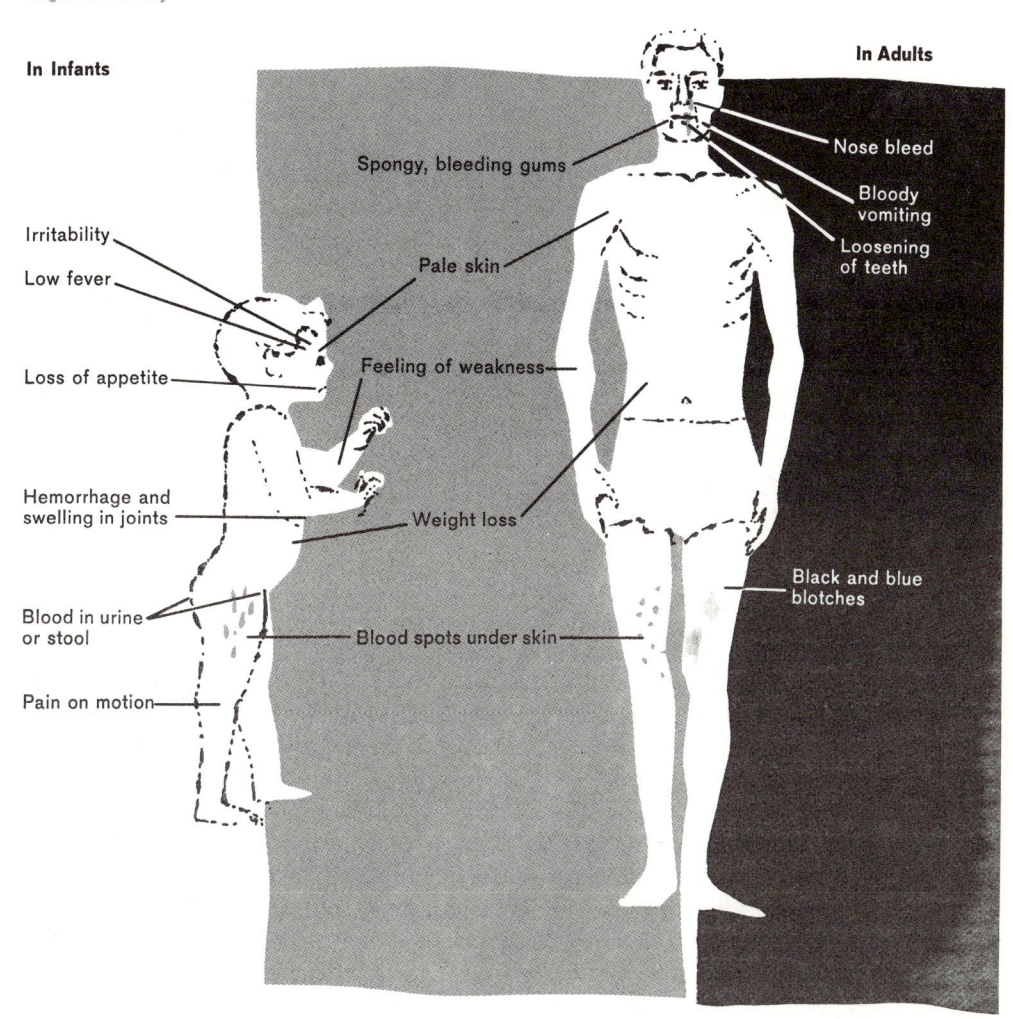

In Infants

- Irritability
- Low fever
- Loss of appetite
- Hemorrhage and swelling in joints
- Blood in urine or stool
- Pain on motion
- Spongy, bleeding gums
- Pale skin
- Feeling of weakness
- Weight loss
- Blood spots under skin

In Adults

- Nose bleed
- Bloody vomiting
- Loosening of teeth
- Black and blue blotches

weakness, spongy gums, and a tendency to develop bleeding under the skin and from the mucous membranes and bone coverings. It was once common among sailors subsisting on a diet of salted meat with few or no vegetables. Scurvy can be controlled by taking plenty of vitamin C which is now available in several medicinal forms. The material need not be injected into the blood but can be taken by mouth, after which the condition usually clears up promptly. Much better is the prevention of scurvy by the daily taking of some citrus fruit juice, tomato juice, or by eating leafy green vegetables, which add other important factors to the diet. See also NUTRITION; VITAMINS. See MEDIGRAPH page 1167.

SEASICKNESS. See MOTION SICKNESS.

SEBACEOUS CYST. See WEN.

SEBACEOUS GLANDS, the oil-producing glands of the skin. See also SKIN; SEBORRHEA.

SEBORRHEA, a functional disease caused by excessive secretion of the *sebaceous glands* in the skin. The condition may vary widely, from nothing more than *dandruff,* the commonest form, to *seborrheic dermatitis,* in which the whole scalp and sometimes the face and other parts of the body develop a greasy kind of crusting and scaling, accompanied by red irritated areas.

In some cases, dandruff begins in childhood as a simple scaling of small white bits of skin from the scalp and then continues as a mild annoyance for many years. Often, however, the process gradually becomes more and more involved with greasy discharges from the scalp and skin of the face, and "oily" seborrhea may develop, sometimes with so much discharge that drops of oil actually collect on the skin.

Physicians attribute these symptoms to a variety of causes. Some feel that these phenomena are the result of a constitutional predisposition to a kind of skin which is subject to excessive growth of oil-producing glands and enlargement of pores. Others believe that actual infection by some microorganism is involved. Changes in behavior of various internal glands of the body and such factors as faulty diet and chronic intestinal disorder are also blamed. Many feel that in all likelihood more than one of these factors, and possibly all of them, may be involved.

Treatment of troublesome dandruff should be under a doctor's direction, but the person who has seborrhea will find that more than the usual participation by the patient is required. Success depends largely on his willingness to take frequent shampoos, massage the scalp with prescribed lotions and ointments, and brush the hair daily.

The doctor has other measures which he uses to shorten the treatment time. A new preparation, derived from *selenium,* has proved effective against many of the annoying symptoms but should not be used without a doctor's advice.

The patient's general health is significant, and rest, exercise, and proper hygiene are essential. Excessive fatigue, lack of sleep, anxiety and emotional strain may be involved in inducing the state which is conducive to the development of seborrhea. If necessary, the blood should be brought to normal by dietary supplements such as vitamins and iron.

In cases in which nothing more serious than some scaling of the scalp is involved, a direct attack on the dandruff alone may be all that is required. The dandruff-prone person should shampoo his hair and scalp thoroughly at least once a week, bathe daily, and avoid wearing clothing that overheats and softens the skin.

If the oily condition becomes severe, the doctor may require special shampoos of *olive or similar oils* and *glycerin* to remove the fatty covering of the scalp and make it accessible to treatment. Following this, alkaline rinses of diluted *borax* and *ammonia* may be applied to reduce the oiliness, although these rinses must be followed by an oily application to prevent irritation of the scalp.

Seborrheic dermatitis, the most severe form of seborrhea, is ordinarily a sequel to oily dandruff and skin. Treatment is difficult and must be varied to meet the particular condition encountered. A good daily hygienic routine is essential, with ample sleep, bathing, and a diet rich in protein. *Vitamin B complex* or *vitamin B$_{12}$* may also prove beneficial. The doctor may use various special ointments, and antibiotics will help control infection if it occurs. See also SKIN; ACNE. See MEDIGRAPHS pages 31, 1171.

SECONDARY POLYCYTHEMIA. See RED BLOOD CELLS, DISEASES OF.

SEMEN, the sticky viscous white substance ejaculated from the penis during orgasm, containing the *spermatozoa,* and consisting otherwise of the secretions of the *epididymides, seminal vesicles,* and *prostate gland.* These various secretions, which provide an environment in which the sperm cells can live and move, are collectively called the *seminal plasma.* This is composed of water, proteins, sugars, salts, vitamins and other chemicals. See also REPRODUCTION SYSTEM; TESTICLES; SEMINAL VESICLES; PROSTATE; SEMINAL DUCTS; PENIS; EPIDIDYMIS; VAS DEFERENS; ORGASM.

SEMINAL DUCTS, the two efferent ducts leading from the *testicles* to the *urethra.* They consist of the *epididymides, vasa deferentia,* and *ejaculatory ducts.* They are connected with the *seminal vesicles* and receive their secretions. Their purpose is to transport sperm cells from the testicles to the seminal vesicles, and, during sexual intercourse, to the urethra. See also SEMINAL VESICLES; VAS DEFERENS; EPIDIDYMIS; TESTICLES; SPERMATIC CORDS; URETHRA; PROSTATE; PENIS; SCROTUM; REPRODUCTION SYSTEM; SEMEN; ORGASM.

the disease and its causes This is a common type of skin disorder involving the scalp, eyebrows, cheeks, and the front of the chest. It occurs in adults and is common in both males and females. The cause is unknown, but several known factors play a part: It is frequently related to acne; it is thought to be involved with hormone action; it seems to be aggravated by foods such as chocolate, fatty or fried dishes, and seafood; it is not unusual to see it before or in association with the development of psoriasis.

symptoms There is a widespread eruption involving the entire skin of the scalp, and frequently breaking out behind the ears, too. The skin is red and covered with irregular patches on which there are greasy scales. These tend to flake and occasionally take on a yellowish color. The patches vary in size and shape, and are usually dry except for the area behind the ears, where oozing is common.

The eruption spreads slowly and may also be seen in the armpit, groin, and between the buttocks.

As a rule there is no itching and the patient is more disturbed by how this disease looks than how it feels.

complications There are no serious complications.

prevention (or lessening of impact) Seborrheic dermatitis tends to resist treatment and be chronic. However, there are specific medications a doctor will prescribe. Vitamins may be recommended. Good skin hygiene will certainly do much to prevent secondary infections and minimize unsightly appearance. The patient should most conscientiously omit from his diet any foods known to aggravate this disorder.

Seborrheic Dermatitis

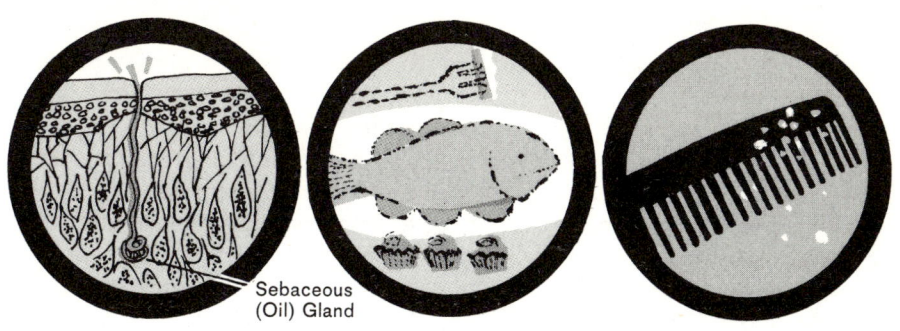

Sebaceous (Oil) Gland

1. Caused by too much production of oil by glands of skin

2. Chocolate, seafood, fatty and fried foods may stimulate overproduction of oil

3. Milder forms range from dandruff to acne — but they are not necessarily preliminary to development of seborrheic dermatitis

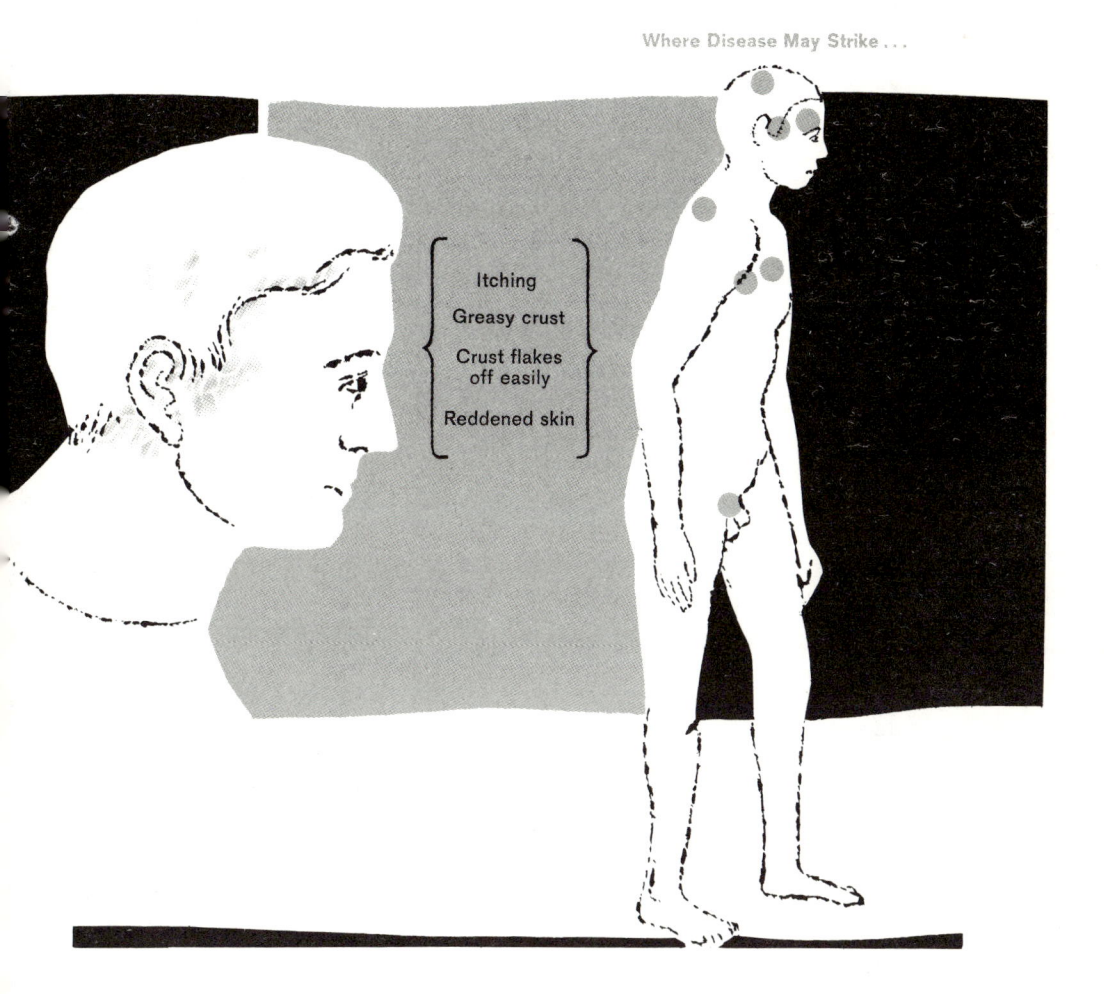

Where Disease May Strike...

{ Itching
Greasy crust
Crust flakes off easily
Reddened skin }

SEMINAL VESICLES, the convoluted pouches between the bladder and rectum (but not connected to either) which are connected with the *vasa deferentia* and the *ejaculatory ducts,* serve as storage spaces for sperm cells until ejaculation is induced by sexual activity, and secrete a viscous fluid constituting a major component of *semen* and facilitating the further passage of the sperm cells to the *urethra. See also* SEMINAL DUCTS; VAS DEFERENS; PROSTATE; SEMEN; URETHRA; TESTICLES; EPIDIDYMIS; PENIS; SCROTUM; REPRODUCTION SYSTEM.

SENESCENCE, the process of aging. As people grow older, their bodies are subject to physiological degeneration. The cells of the body begin to lose their power of repair, and the glands tend to function less efficiently. Digestion becomes disturbed, and the senses of taste, smell, sight, and hearing often weaken or begin to fail. In the aging process of the human body, the condition of the blood vessels is the most significant single factor. Hardening of the arteries, the wearing out of the muscular tissues of the blood vessels, and heart failure are the result of degenerative changes in the tissues. As the consequence of these changes, the body may either lose bulk or become corpulent. The bones are harder and more brittle, the hair grays and often falls out, the capacity for muscular and frequently mental effort decreases, and diseases affecting the circulatory system, heart, kidneys, lungs, and other organs begin to manifest themselves.

Within the limits imposed by aging, medical science can do much for these disorders, and older persons should be examined by a doctor at frequent intervals.

Many of the changes in the vision of older persons are due to changes in circulation, including hardening of the arteries. The pupil of the eye becomes smaller and less movable, and the color of the eyes becomes lighter. The lens of the eye grows and increases in weight throughout life, and a reduction in elasticity promotes the condition known as *presbyopia,* which is due to a loss of accommodation in the lens. Sometimes a *cataract,* typical of old age, forms. The exact cause is not known, and the decision whether or not to remove a cataract depends on many factors related to the person's mental and physical condition, as well as the actual condition of the eye.

The eyelids of an older person develop wrinkles, and he seems to cry more easily, sometimes suffering from an excess of tears. This is often due to relaxation of the tissues of the eye, which do not hold the material as well as do the tissues of younger persons. With surgical advances, techniques have been developed for maintaining the normal relationship between the tissues and overcoming the excess of tears.

Like the rest of the body, the teeth and jaws are subject to change in old age. The jaws change shape and the teeth tend either to fall out or require extraction. Artificial dentures often replace the loss of teeth.

The functioning of the digestive system becomes less efficient as a person grows older, and frequently a simpler, more easily digested diet is preferred. Three meals a day should still be eaten, but they can be smaller. The diet, of course, should continue to be balanced, and vitamin or mineral supplements taken if necessary. Less protein is required for tissue repair, although foods which supply energy are still essential in sizable amounts.

During late maturity, a thorough physical checkup is a wise precaution against disease in old age. Although aches and pains may multiply as one grows older, there are no diseases specifically caused by old age, and many maladies to which older persons are subject result from chronic diseases which occurred years before. The diseases that take the greatest toll of life among the aged are *heart diseases, cancer,* and *cerebral hemorrhage.* Other afflictions are *arthritis, rheumatism, diabetes, prostatic enlargement, kidney diseases, hardening of the arteries, high blood pressure,* and *nervous and mental disorders.*

With the general advance in medical science, more people are living longer. Thus older persons are coming to constitute an increasingly larger percentage of the population, and their particular problems are becoming of concern to more and more people. See also GERIATRICS; SENILITY; MENOPAUSE; MIDDLE AGE CHANGE, IN MEN. See MEDIGRAPHS pages 127, 129, 1081.

SENILITY, the extreme stage of *cerebral arteriosclerosis,* which produces in the aged symptoms approaching *dementia.* The mind of the senile person becomes feeble and he may be so confused that he requires constant care and attention, and cannot be left alone. This condition is also marked by extreme forgetfulness. In such moments, he may begin to do something in one part of the house and then suddenly go off to another room, forgetting what he had started out to do. In other instances, the senile person may wander away from his home and walk confusedly about, not even having presence of mind to ask directions.

Often the rest cycle is reversed, and the senile person sleeps during the day instead of at night. He will be active all night, moving about from room to room while the rest of the household sleeps. At daybreak, drowsiness sets in and he may sleep and doze the rest of the day.

In the most advanced stages of senility, all touch with reality may be lost and symptoms of dementia manifested. Coherent communication with others becomes impossible and helplessness, incontinence, and loss of brain function are noted. At this stage, hospitalization is often the best solution, and a large percentage of beds in mental institutions are devoted to senile persons.

In treating senility, the doctor will check and prescribe accordingly for high blood pressure, overweight, and diabetes. Any correctable illness or condition will also be treated, including diet deficiencies and anemia, both fairly common among senile persons. In most cases, the teeth and digestion of the aged will be in such poor condition that a bland diet of chopped meats and strained and puréed vegetables will be advised. An effort should be made to cater to the special tastes and preferences of the individual, who may be "cranky" about his food. In treating the reversed sleep cycle, a combination of a mild stimulant in the morning and a moderate sedative at night is effected in most cases, although the situation may be fairly difficult to control. Tranquilizing drugs, among other measures, have been found effective in treatment of the extremely confused. Much remains to be learned and done in the care and treatment of senility. *See also* GERIATRICS; SENESCENCE; PARANOIA; SCHIZOPHRENIA; MANIC-DEPRESSIVE PSYCHOSIS. *See* MEDIGRAPHS pages 127, 129, 1081.

SEPTICEMIA, another term for *bacteremia* or blood poisoning. *See* BACTEREMIA.

SEPTIC SORE THROAT, an acute infection of the throat caused by an organism, *streptococcus hemolyticus*. It is the most severe of all sore throats, and serious complications may ensue if treatment is not prompt.

Ordinarily the condition develops rapidly, starting with chill and fever that may go as high as 105° F. Swelling and soreness in and around the throat make it painful to swallow or even to move the head. As the infection spreads downward, the voice becomes hoarse, the breath short, and coughing begins.

The most immediate danger is ulceration within the throat at the point of infection, or the formation of abscesses in the neck glands where the disease causes inflammation and swelling. Not infrequently the infection may go considerably further, invading the heart or abdomen and causing acute specific illness in those areas, or in other parts of the body.

The disease is sometimes called *epidemic septic sore throat,* because it may be spread by sources of infection, such as contaminated milk, which affect large numbers of people in a community. Adequate pasteurization will prevent this, but any defect in the pasteurization process may let through a batch of milk infected with microorganisms which cause septic sore throat, as well as other diseases. This particular streptococcus infects cows and when it does is found on their udders. An infected milker may spread the disease, and milkers should always wash their hands before going to work and preferably also during the process. Infected ice cream has been found to be the source of at least one epidemic. When a number of cases of septic sore throat are reported in a community, health authorities suspect a common source of infection and often are able to trace it to one milk route and even to a particular herd of cattle.

Antibiotics, such as *penicillin* or *aureomycin,* are effective against the infection. Immediate bed rest for the duration of the illness is advised. Hot wet packs on the neck may help to combat the infection. Sprays, gargles, and other preparations applied directly to the throat are of little help.

SEVEN-YEAR ITCH. If swelling of the throat begins to interfere to any considerable extent with breathing, oxygen may be given. Despite its severity, fatalities from septic sore throat are infrequent because of the accessibility of the infection to medical care. *See* MEDIGRAPHS pages 515, 1269.

SEVEN-YEAR ITCH. *See* SCABIES.

SEX. *See* ACCESSORY SEX ORGANS; ADOLESCENCE; CASTRATION; CONCEPTION; CONTRACEPTION; EXHIBITIONISM; FEMININE HYGIENE; FERTILITY; HETEROSEXUALITY; HOMOSEXUALITY; IMPOTENCE; MASTURBATION; MENSTRUATION; MENOPAUSE; NARCISSISM; NOCTURNAL EMISSION; NYMPHOMANIA; ONANISM; ORGASM; OVARIES; OVULATION; PENIS; PITUITARY; CHILDBIRTH AND PRENATAL CARE; PREGNANCY, SIGNS OF; PROSTATE; PUBERTY; REPRODUCTION SYSTEM; RHYTHM METHOD; SADISM; SATYRIASIS; SCROTUM; SEX EDUCATION; SEXUAL INTERCOURSE; STERILITY; TESTICLES; URETHRA; UTERUS; VAGINA; VAS DEFERENS; VENEREAL DISEASE; VULVA.

SEX EDUCATION. A child shows curiosity about his body and about sex at an early age, although in a different way and on a different level than an adult. Beginning about the age of three or four, the child will start asking questions, about himself and where he came from, which he has a right to do without fear or shame. The questions should be answered truthfully and straightforwardly, giving enough information to satisfy the child's immediate curiosity. In these early stages a generalized sentence or two is often adequate.

Sex is fundamental in nature; it is perfectly normal for a child to wonder about it. The attitude toward sex which a child develops in his first five or six years is considered by many psychologists as one of the major factors in shaping his entire life and development. This attitude begins to be formed with the act of living, everything happening to the child and taking place about him leaving a subtle imprint. In this sense, many authorities say, sex education begins at home and at birth.

How the parents feel toward sex and how they act toward each other is reflected in the child. If the mother associates sex with disgust or danger, if she feels "woman's lot" is a burden and giving birth a sacrifice, she may be laying the seeds of problems that will trouble the child in later life. Similarly, the father who treats his wife as inferior may instill in the child an attitude toward sex which can cause inner conflicts that lie hidden for years.

The child early notices differences between men and women—in voice, in figure and dress, in a man's possession of a beard, in the household functions which the father and mother perform. In a home in which there is warmth and love and truthfulness, the child will feel free to ask questions about these differences and about himself. If the parent is embarrassed or evasive, or if the entire subject of sex is considered taboo, the child, too, may come to regard sex or parts of his body with disgust or shame. In time the child may think of sex as "dirty," instead of as a natural process.

One of the main difficulties parents find in answering a child's questions is lack of an accurate vocabulary. The child who learns about sex from other children generally learns words that are vulgar and uncouth. The parent wants to avoid this but often is blocked by not knowing the right words or the right approach. Knowing accurate terms will enable the parent to answer questions casually and simply, with neither innuendo nor embarrassment. Sex is everywhere in nature, in plant as well as in bird and animal life, and knowing the fundamentals of biology can provide the parent not only with a vocabulary but an approach.

The teaching of sex may use the vocabulary of science, but it is, especially in the early years, an art. The child should not be told until he asks; and, though he should be told the truth, he need not be told the *whole* truth. The child of four or five often does not want, nor can he comprehend, detailed information. A few words may be all he needs until they are absorbed and he comes up, perhaps many months later, with the next question. *The truth that he is told is the truth as he can understand it.* Thus, to a child of five who asks how his body was in his mother's body it is usually enough to explain that this came about because of the love his father had for his mother.

What is told to the child—in generalities or by illustration in the early years, with greater detail in adolescence—should be told casually. Sex is a part of living, and to the impressionable child the teaching of it should not be shown undue emphasis.

If the child is given truthful—if simple—answers in his early years, he will be better prepared for the problems that arise in puberty. Changes crowd in at this time on the growing boy and girl, bringing with the concatenation of physical transformations a host of fresh questions, stirrings, and often fears. The child now needs straightforward explanations of the physical changes, and needs, further, to understand that the sex urge is natural, that it appears in everyone and is necessary for the continuation of the species.

The child thus prepared will accept the changes without fear or shame or shock. Girls, maturing earlier than boys, will need to be prepared earlier since *menstruation* without preparation can be a shocking experience. Similarly, the boy who does not understand why it is taking place may experience fear or disgust at the onset of the *nocturnal emission*.

For parents who want to provide the child with sex education from the outset, but are doubtful about the proper way to do it, books are available on the subject. But the best teaching is by example. A sound basic attitude toward sex and life, a proper fulfilling of the role of father and mother, are more important to the development of the child than just scientific fact or finding. See also ADOLESCENCE; CONCEPTION; CONDOM; CONTRACEPTION; FALLOPIAN TUBES; FERTILITY; HOMOSEXUALITY; HYMEN; HYSTERECTOMY; IMPOTENCE; MARRIAGE; MASTURBATION; MENOPAUSE; MENSTRUATION; NOCTURNAL EMISSION; ORGASM; OVARIES; OVULATION; PENIS; PROSTATE; SCROTUM; SEMEN; SEMINAL VESICLES; SEMINAL DUCTS; STERILITY; TESTICLES; UTERUS; VAGINA; VENEREAL DISEASE; VULVA.

SEXUAL INTERCOURSE, in normal heterosexual relations, the intromission of the *penis* of the male into the *vagina* of the female, resulting by rhythmic spasmodic interaction in the ejaculation of *semen* from the penis into the female reproductive system. Under ideal psychological conditions, *mutual orgasm* is achieved. (Orgasm always occurs in the male if the act is completed.) Sexual intercourse may or may not result in *fertilization,* depending upon the availability of an *ovum* in the female tract at the time of the act. The term *coitus* is also used to indicate sexual intercourse. See also MARRIAGE; CONCEPTION; CONTRACEPTION; ORGASM; REPRODUCTION SYSTEM; HOMOSEXUALITY; MASTURBATION.

SHAKING PALSY. *See* PARALYSIS AGITANS.

SHINGLES. *See* HERPES ZOSTER.

SHOCK, the condition caused by acute failure of the peripheral circulation, the circulation of the blood in the veins and in the capillaries farthest from the heart. The essential functions of the body are diminished. Shock may occur during times of great emotional stress, injury, pain, sudden illness and accident, such as burns, and has been one of the most difficult emergencies to confront physicians.

It is believed by many doctors that *loss of blood* is the cause of shock in most cases, and therefore treatment of shock emphasizes maintaining the blood supply through use of *blood plasma* by transfusion.

The first change that occurs in shock is *dilation of the blood vessels* on the surface. When this happens, the person begins to sweat, while his skin is relatively warm. His blood pressure falls and his pulse becomes slow and feeble.

The victim of shock should first of all be placed with his head low, since a loss of blood from the brain may result in failure of the brain to function. If the state of shock continues over a period of even a few hours, it may be fatal or cause permanent impairment of the brain. He must be kept comfortably warm. Pain, which may be a contributing factor to the intensity of shock, is relieved by sedative drugs.

A *secondary shock* due to damage of the tissues follows the initial shock from a wound or injury, and may be apparent an hour or more after an injury. A person in secondary shock is pale, weak, exhausted, and, if conscious, may complain of thirst. His perspiration is cold and clammy, pulse rapid and thready and breathing rapid and shallow,

1177

the disease and its causes The anterior, or forward part, of the pituitary gland affects the working of a variety of other glands such as the thyroid, ovary and testicle, adrenal, breast, and pancreas. In addition, the anterior pituitary hormone is responsible for body growth.

When any condition prevents the pituitary gland from functioning properly, the body is profoundly affected and suffers from a variety of disorders grouped under the heading of hypopituitarism, which means underactivity of the pituitary gland. Most often this interference with the pituitary gland is the result of the destructive effects of a tumor, or some inflammatory disease, or a vascular disturbance. The age at which the disease develops determines to some extent the symptoms and end result.

symptoms When there is destruction or change in the pituitary gland *before* the onset of puberty (the age at which boys and girls mature sexually—usually in the early or middle teens), the disease is marked by dwarfism and subnormal sexual development. There is little change in other glandular functions. The patient's mentality is unaffected. He is a well-proportioned dwarf who remains sexually immature. Such cases are quite rare and are usually caused by the destructive effects of a tumor upon the anterior pituitary gland.

In cases of hypopituitarism which occur *after* the onset of puberty, there are deficiencies in most of the glands affected by the pituitary. These glands may become inactive at various times, but it may take years for the negative effects to become clear.

Symptoms of hypogonadism and Simmonds' disease—two disorders resulting from underactivity of the pituitary gland—are detailed in the accompanying Medi-Graph.

complications These depend on the cause. When a malignant tumor is responsible, one complication, of course, can be a spread of the malignancy. If it attacks the nearby optic nerves, the patient can become blind. Eventually, since there is interference with all glandular functions, the patient can die from secondary infections as well as from general loss of strength.

prevention (or lessening of impact) Nothing can be done to prevent this disease, but early recognition can help to stop its progression before secondary effects seriously affect body functions.

X ray or surgery may be effective in removing tumors. If the body metabolism is not thrown off balance too severely, treatment to replace lost hormones can be effective and give the patient a remarkable degree of recovery of lost functions.

The subject of glandular malfunction is a complicated one. This form, as well as most others, requires expert care and evaluation.

Hypogonadism and Simmonds' Disease
(Underactive Pituitary Gland Disorders)

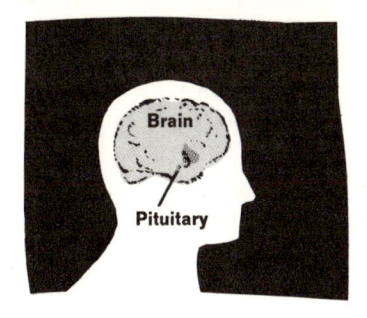

Front part of pituitary gland is attacked by tumor, impairment of blood supply or inflammation. Result may be underproduction of sex—and other—hormones.

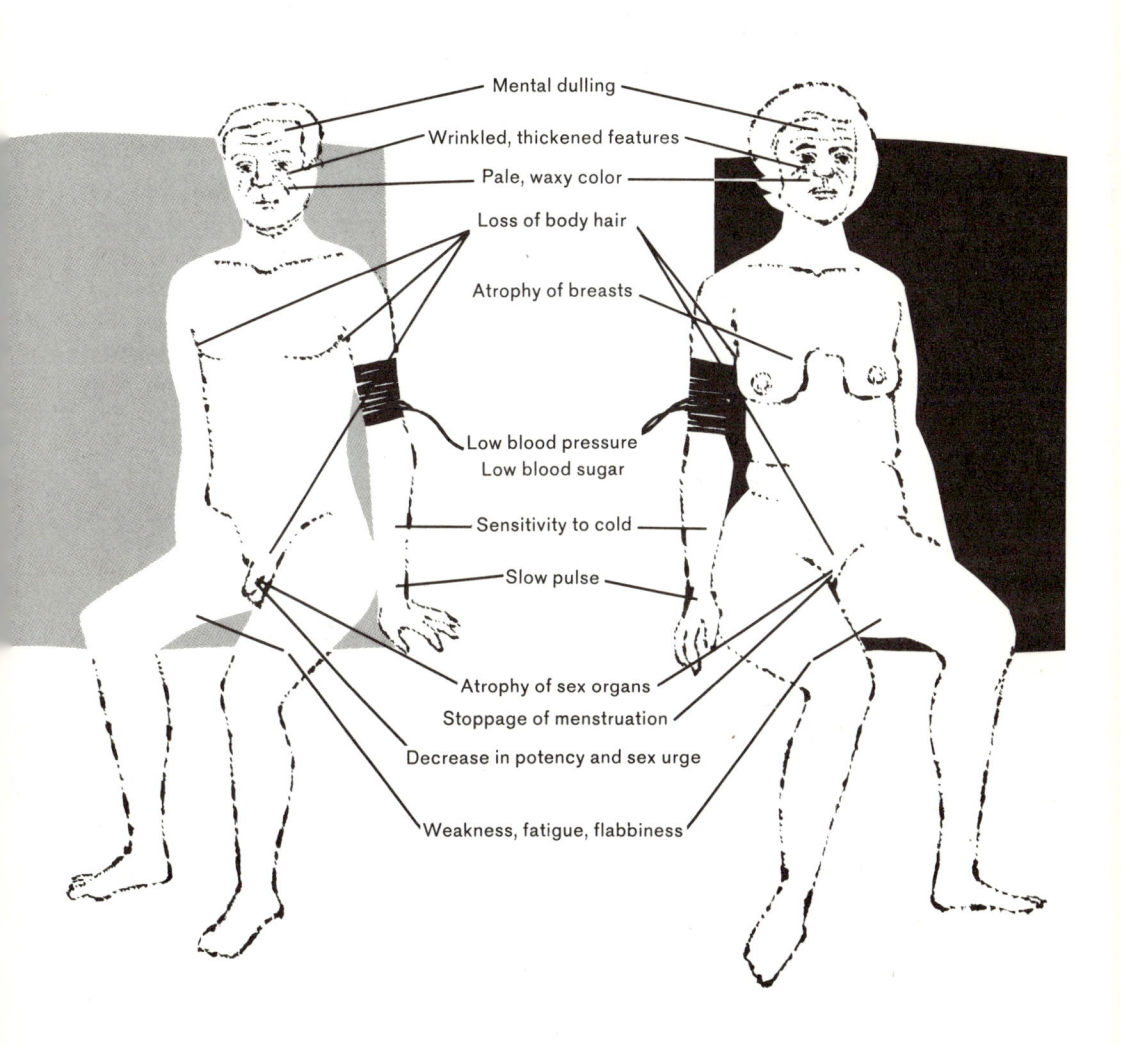

- Mental dulling
- Wrinkled, thickened features
- Pale, waxy color
- Loss of body hair
- Atrophy of breasts
- Low blood pressure
- Low blood sugar
- Sensitivity to cold
- Slow pulse
- Atrophy of sex organs
- Stoppage of menstruation
- Decrease in potency and sex urge
- Weakness, fatigue, flabbiness

1179

SHOCK TREATMENT

blood pressure low and the superficial blood vessels collapsed. Secondary shock is seen mainly after severe burns or as a late manifestation of a surgical operation.

In shock following burns, the patient, if conscious, should be given salt and soda in water (1 quart of cold water, 1 teaspoon of salt, and ½ teaspoon of baking soda) to replace the salty fluids lost from the tissues. This is only a first-aid measure to be taken until the doctor arrives.

Patients suffering from *diabetic* or *insulin shock* require special treatment which only a doctor can administer.

In surgery, continuous transfusion of blood or plasma is sometimes a part of the operative procedure. It greatly lessens the incidence of shock. See also INSULIN SHOCK THERAPY; APOPLEXY; POISONING.

SHOCK TREATMENT. See ELECTRIC SHOCK TREATMENT; INSULIN SHOCK THERAPY.

SHOULDER, a joint of the ball-and-socket type, constructed of bones held in position by powerful muscles, tendons, and ligaments. Because of its unique structure, it has a greater range of movement than any other joint in the body. However, the shoulder is unsupported from beneath and is therefore subject to dislocation in this direction.

The shoulder joint is easily injured and may become stiff and painful from a number of causes. When this occurs, the person usually must cease all activity for a time, as further movement will intensify the injury. Frequently a torn tendon may cause pain and stiffness. The tendon may be torn as a result of dislocation, fall, or strain. Infection of the *bursa* (sac) in the shoulder region may produce inflammation which inhibits movement of the shoulder.

Fractures of any of the bones in the shoulder require surgical treatment. *Dislocation* demands setting of the bones and immobilization by means of bandaging or placing the shoulder in a cast. Immobilization is also essential in case of intense pain due to *sprain, severe infection,* or *torn ligament,* and usually it is expedient to place the arm in a sling which will enable it to be supported close to the side. In most cases, this is all the treatment required. A *splint and plaster cast* to hold the arm raised and away from the body—the *abductor position*—may be desirable in other cases. After removal of splints and casts, heat, massage, and exercise will help prevent loss of function and restore mobility. Recurrent dislocation of the shoulder is fairly common, especially among athletes, and surgery is practically the only conclusive treatment for this condition. Subsequently the shoulder must be placed in a cast and after its removal appropriate exercise is required to restore normal function.

Frozen shoulder is a disorder involving the bursae and tendonous tissue, and it produces extreme pain and stiffness. Rest is of utmost significance and application of heat is often helpful. When calcium is de-

1180

SICKLE CELL ANEMIA

posited in the area, *hydrocortisone* or similar drugs may be injected. Gentle exercise and heat help to restore normal function, and in some cases such treatment is required for a long time. *See also* ARTHRITIS; BURSITIS; DISLOCATION; JOINTS AND JOINT DISEASES.

SICKLE CELL ANEMIA. *See* RED BLOOD CELLS, DISEASES OF.

SIMMONDS' DISEASE, a disorder caused by underdevelopment of the anterior lobe of the pituitary gland and characterized by deficiencies in the functioning of the endocrine glands. *See also* PITUITARY. *See* MEDIGRAPH page 1179.

SINUSES, cavities or channels within bones. Those in the head which connect with the inside of the

Sinuses—The sinuses, which surround the nose include the *frontal sinuses,* the *maxillary sinuses* on each side, and the *ethmoid sinus* in back of the nose. They help the physiology of the body in various ways. The mucous membrane that lines the sinuses is much thinner than that of the nasal cavity. In this mucous membrane, there are cells called *goblet cells* which pour out a substance called *mucus.* This mucus is ordinarily eliminated from the sinuses by the movement of the tiny hairs and line its walls. If the openings of the sinuses are not blocked by inflammation or swelling, drainage of mucus goes on constantly and with it foreign material such as germs passes into the nasal cavity and the throat. The functions of the sinuses shown symbolically in the three drawings are the provision of moisture and warmth to air that is taken into the body (*top*); drainage of material from these open areas in the skull cavity which help to lessen the weight of the skull and maintain balance on the neck (*center*); and the resonance that is given by the sinuses to the voice exactly as a resonant chamber may be used to heighten and broaden the tone for radio amplification (*bottom*).

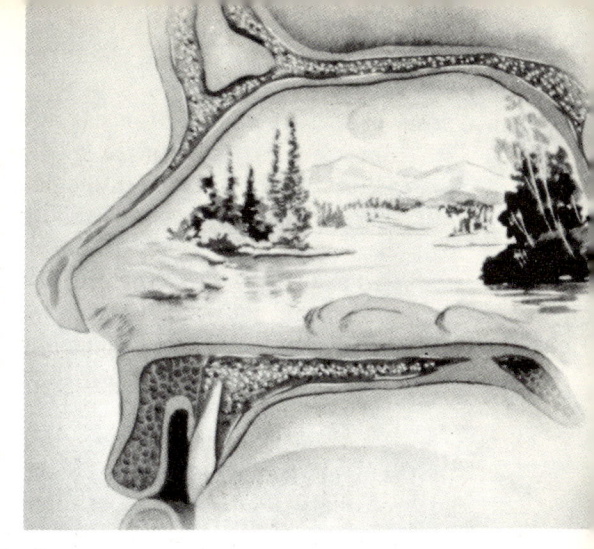

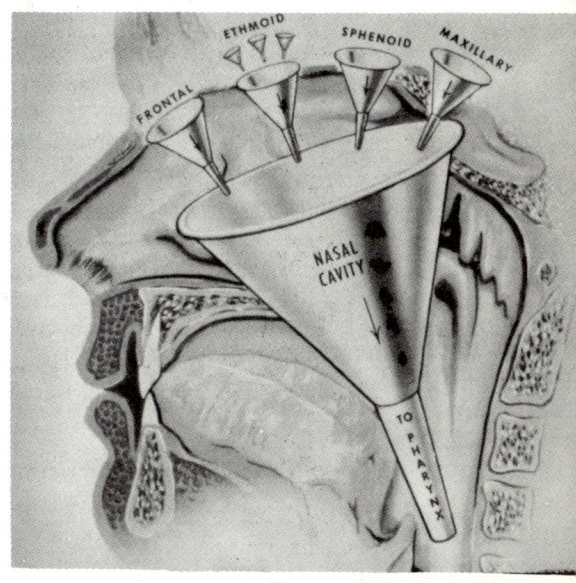

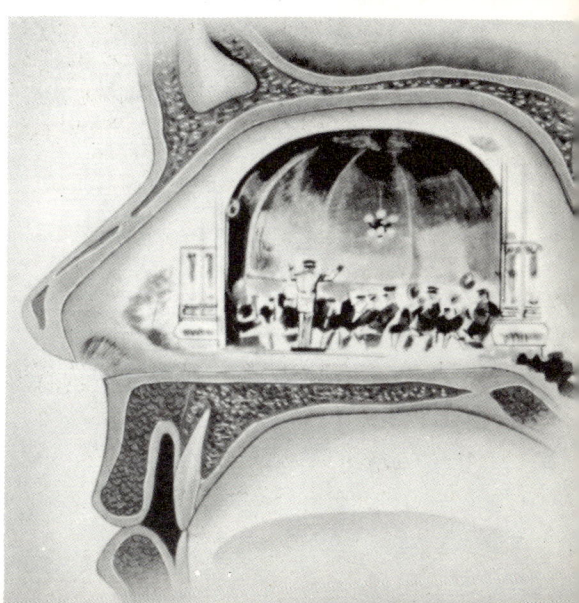

the disease and its causes Sinusitis is an infection of the membranes lining the sinus cavities. It is caused by a variety of bacteria which live and grow there. Any obstruction in the nose, such as polyps, large adenoids, or a deviated septum, may interfere with normal sinus drainage and open the way for infection. Nasal allergies are often responsible because they frequently lead to secondary infections. Sinusitis may follow a simple cold or an abscessed upper molar rupturing into the maxillary sinus. Swimming and diving frequently cause it. It is a common disease, especially along the seaboard where there are sudden changes of temperature and humidity.

A patient is susceptible to repeated attacks once he is infected. Any sinus or combination of sinuses may be involved, but the frontal and maxillary sinuses are most often affected. Infection of the sphenoid sinus occurs less often but can be more serious.

symptoms Sinusitis begins with low-grade fever, weakness, and pain over the particular sinus involved. The directions in which this pain radiates are shown on the accompanying diagram of sinuses. As a rule, there is a thick yellow or green discharge which increases and decreases as the position of the head changes. If the drainage is blocked, the infection may last beyond the few days it runs normally, and there is pain and a rise in temperature. Also, at this stage there may be swelling about the eyes and cheeks. Toothache may be the first sign of maxillary sinusitis.

complications Without drainage an infection can become severe enough to involve the bone (osteomyelitis). Another complication is meningitis which is caused by direct invasion of the brain. This happens less often now with the proper use of antibiotics. The infection can also spread to the eye, throat, ear, and lungs.

prevention (or lessening of impact) Since nasal obstructions are often specific causes of sinusitis, it is well to repair septal deviation, remove polyps and enlarged adenoid tissue, and make any other corrections necessary to permit discharge to drain freely from the nose. If a patient has an existing allergy, it should be treated. Nose clamps during swimming and diving are of help. Packaged cold vaccines relieve some people, while others benefit from a vaccine prepared from their own infected discharge.

Sinusitis

A. The Sinuses—and Where Pain from Them Strikes

1. Frontal Sinus — Directly outward to forehead.

2. Ethmoid Sinus — Back of the eyes and nose.

3. Sphenoid Sinus — Back of the head and neck.

4. Maxillary Sinus — Beneath eyes and up to forehead.

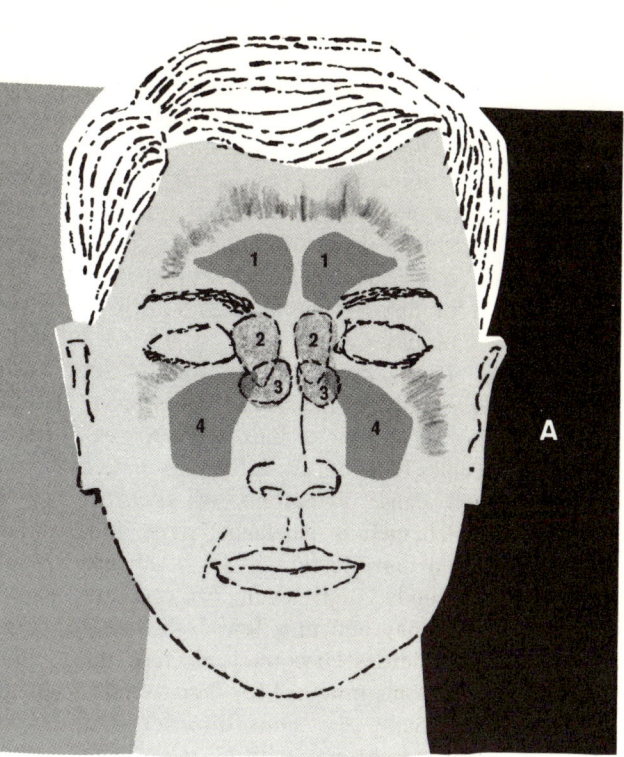

B. Cross-section View of Acute Sinusitis

1. Infection creates pus in sinus.

2. Thick yellow or green discharge seeps down into nose and throat.

3. Infection blocks normal air passage through sinus, congests nasal lining, creates feeling of pressure, tenderness, pain in surrounding area.

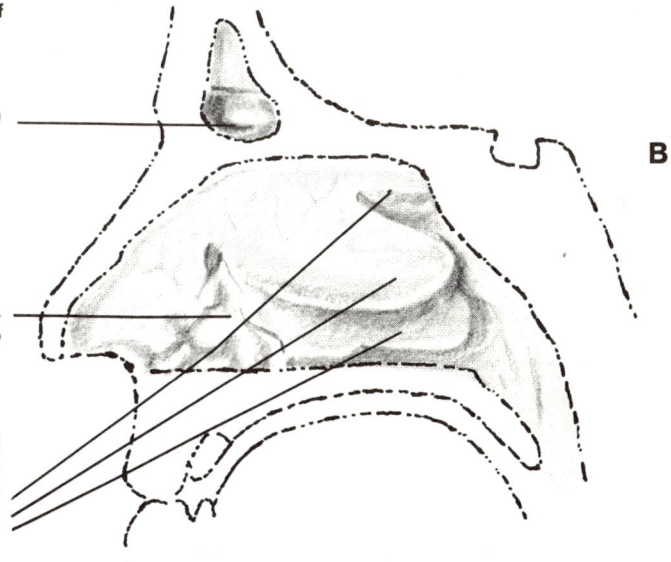

nose by narrow passageways sometimes cause trouble. The sinus in the cheekbone is called the *antrum,* the one above the eyes is the *frontal sinus,* and deeper behind the nose is the *ethmoid sinus,* which is actually a series of small sinuses, varying from three to more than fifteen in some cases.

The membranes of the sinuses are susceptible to infection. If the opening of the sinus into the nose becomes blocked, the infectious matter will cause symptoms of *sinusitis,* which include headache, pain, and, when the infection is absorbed into the body, high fever. An ordinary cold may end in a few days, but if the sinuses become infected the symptoms may last for many weeks. Eventually the sinus disorder may become chronic, with an increase in the intensity of the original infection.

The doctor usually treats an infection of the sinuses by cleansing the nose and shrinking the membranes by applying *vasoconstrictors* such as *epinephrine.* He then determines whether or not the infectious material is draining from the sinuses into the nose. X-rays will indicate whether there is any *blocking* or *polyps* or *tumorous growth.* Infection may be controlled with drops, sprays, or application of medicinal packs. Drugs may be given orally, or applied directly to the nose by washing out the sinuses. Occasionally surgical procedures are advisable. While current treatment with drugs—such as the *sulfonamides, penicillin,* and other *antibiotics*—has practically eliminated surgery, certain complications may necessitate operation to improve drainage or destroy an abscess. When polyps are growing in the sinuses, *ACTH, cortisone,* and similar hormone products have been successfully used.

Allergenic substances are sometimes responsible for sinus disorders, and the doctor may prescribe *antihistaminic drugs.* (There are several excellent antihistaminic preparations on the market obtainable without a prescription, including TRIAMINICIN® and SINUTAB®.) In chronic sinus infections, *vaccines* have been helpful once the germ responsible has been determined. In time, resistance to the infection will develop.

Persons with acute or chronic infections of the sinuses should avoid swimming, diving, and strenuous outdoor exercise. Particularly obstinate cases of sinus infection may improve in a hot dry climate. *See also* HEADACHE; MIGRAINE; ALLERGY; ASTHMA; HAY FEVER.

SINUSITIS. *See* SINUSES.

SKELETON, the bony framework which supports the soft tissue and protects the internal organs. The skeleton consists of *axial* and *appendicular* sets of bones. The *skull,* the *ribs* and *breastbone,* and the *spine* form the axial part, and the *arms* and *legs* are the appendages. Two bony girdles—the *shoulder* and the *pelvis*—connect the axis and the appendages.

The two *innominate bones* form the pelvic girdle, which is actually made into a rigid girdle by the *sacrum.* The shoulder girdle—which is formed by the *scapula* and the *clavicle*—is incomplete in front and behind, but supported in front by the uppermost part of the *sternum* (the breastbone).

The arm is attached to the axial skeleton by the *clavicle* and *scapula*. The leg is attached by the *innominate bones,* which are jointed in front to each other and at the back to the *sacrum* (the lower end of the spine).

Altogether, 206 bones comprise the human skeleton, including the tiny bones of the middle ear. The skeleton is a complex structure of bones and joints, and its movements are made possible by the *skeletal muscles* which are attached to their respective bones by *tendons.* Tendons anchor muscles to bone by means of connective tissue fibers which enter the bone structure. Together the skeleton and muscles have a great part in body function, since every body movement, voluntary and involuntary, depends on the skeletal and muscular systems.

Disorders of the skeleton embrace the various infections, inflammations, and diseases—including *cancer*—that may attack the bones. *Sprains* of the ligaments binding bones together may occur, *debility* as in foot strain or flat feet, or *dislocations* and *fractures* of bones or joints. *Arthritis* and *rheumatism* may attack the bones and joints. Various mechanical defects, such as *curvature of the spine,* can develop, or congenital deficiencies may present difficulty later in life. *See also* ARTHRITIS; BONES; DISLOCATION; FRACTURES; JOINTS AND JOINT DISORDERS; SPINE; VERTEBRA. *See* MEDIGRAPHS pages 659, 989.

SKENE'S GLANDS. *See* VULVA.

SKIN, the largest single organ in the body, forming a protective covering over it. The skin of an adult person weighs about six pounds and if spread flat would cover an area of about 16 to 20 square feet.

The skin consists of specialized cells called *epithelial cells,* of *elastic fibers,* and of numerous blood vessels called *capillaries, nerves* and *nerve endings, sweat* and *sebaceous glands,* and *hair follicles.* There are three generalized layers of the skin: the *epidermis,* the *dermis,* and the *subdermis.*

The *epidermis* (or *cuticle*) is the outer visible layer of the skin. It contains no blood vessels or nerves. Its nourishment is obtained from *lymph,* a clear fluid obtained from the blood vessels lying below in the *dermis* by a process of filtration through the cells. This explains why superficial wounds do not necessarily result in bleeding but often only in the exudation of a clear liquid. The liquid is lymph.

The epidermis itself consists of three layers. The innermost of these —called the *stratum mucosum*—is comprised of the actual living epithelial cells. These cells contain the *melanin pigments* which determine, by their relative abundance or development, the *pigmentation* (skin color) of the given individual. The more abundant or highly developed

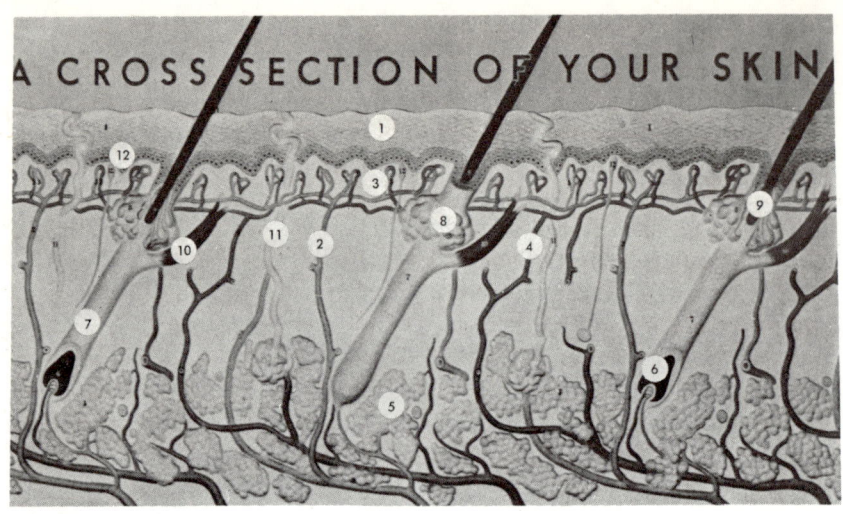

Skin—(1) outer layer, (2) arteries, (3) capillaries, (4) veins, (5) fat tissue, (6) hair root, (7) hair shaft, (8) oil gland, (9) hair, (10) hair muscle, (11) sweat gland, and (12) touch nerve.

the melanin pigments are, the darker the complexion. (*See discussion at* PIGMENTATION.)

These epithelial cells are continuously growing and multiplying. As newer cells arise, they push the older worn-out cells toward the outer layers. The older cells gradually lose their melanin pigments, become tougher in consistency, and finally die. The dead cells are eventually pushed into the outermost layer of the epidermis—called the *stratum corneum* or *cornified layer*—from which they are finally sloughed off. The cornified layer also contains *fatty material* and *keratin,* a horn-like substance which is also the principal constituent of the nails.

A thin middle layer—called the *stratum lucidum*—lies between the *stratum mucosum* and the *stratum corneum*. It consists mainly of cells in a transitional stage.

Underneath the epidermis lies the *dermis* (also called the *corium*). The dermis interlocks with the epidermis by numerous small *projections* or *ridges,* which are most clearly noticeable on the fingertips, palms and soles. These ridges are permanent, and are not affected by the growth or sloughing off of the epidermal tissue, since they are actually part of the dermis, not the epidermis.

The *dermis* consists of a complex network of elastic fibers which produces the elasticity of the skin, and of nerves, glands, hair follicles, and capillaries.

There are principal nerves—called *cutaneous nerves*—running through the dermis, and their numerous branches all terminate in *specialized nerve endings*. Each of these various types of nerve endings is concerned with a particular sensation.

Thus, *Krause's end bulb* is a nerve ending dealing with sensations of *cold; Ruffini's end organs* deal with sensations of *warmth; Meissner's corpuscle* deals with the sensation of *touch;* and the *bare nerve endings* deal with the sensation of *pain.* The first three of these *abut* the epithelial cells of the epidermis; the *bare nerve endings* actually penetrate the epidermis.

Another nerve ending—the *Pacinian corpuscle*—deals with the sensation of *deep pressure,* and lies much deeper in the dermis, or actually penetrates the *subdermis.*

There are two major types of glands in the dermis: *sweat glands* and *sebaceous glands.* The *sweat glands* are of two kinds: *eccrine* and *apocrine.* The eccrine glands are distributed over the entire surface of the body. The apocrine glands develop at puberty and occur in the underarms, nipples, navel, and genital-anal region. These two types of sweat glands differ primarily in the nature of their secretions. The secretions of the apocrine glands have a much more pungent odor—in fact, frequently offensive!

The secretions of the sweat glands are known, of course, as *sweat* (or *perspiration*). The sweat is secreted through tiny ducts called *pores* leading to the exterior. The sweat consists of water, salts, vitamins, amino acids, fatty acids, antibacterial chemicals, and some waste products.

The primary function of the sweat glands is to cool the body. The cells of the body generate great heat during their normal operations. By having some of its constituent water evaporated through the pores, the blood in the capillaries of the dermis is cooled. This cooled blood then flows back to other areas of the body, cooling them in turn. The total body temperature is thus maintained at equilibrium.

In addition to these cooling functions, the sweat glands serve to combat infection by manufacturing antibacterial substances. Individuals with excessively dry skin—viz., with inadequately functioning sweat glands—are thus often more susceptible to certain types of infection than those individuals with the good fortune to have normally functioning sweat glands.

The *mammary glands* in the female are modifications of apocrine glands. Women have twice as many apocrine glands as men.

The *sebaceous glands* are connected with the *hair follicles* which occur all over the body. Most of these hair follicles are too small to be noticeable, except in certain areas of the body such as the scalp, underarms, genital-anal region, and in men the face and chest. The sebaceous glands secrete an oily chemical called *sebum* which serves to lubricate the skin. Individuals with excessively oily skin are afflicted with overactive sebaceous glands.

The hair follicle arises in the dermis and consists of a *root* or *bulb,* and a *shaft* which penetrates the epidermis to the exterior, and to which the sebaceous gland is attached. A specialized muscle called the *arrector muscle* is attached to the root of the hair and controls its movements.

The *subdermis* (or *subcutaneous tissue*) lies below the dermis and consists primarily of fatty tissue and fibrous supporting structures. Its

1187

the disease and its causes Skin cancer is probably the most common form of cancer a doctor sees. As a rule, it responds to treatment and is the form of cancer most often cured. The exact cause is unknown. Occurring slightly more often in males than in females, it strikes hardest in the older age group.

There may be some relationship to skin cancer among people with light complexions or those heavily exposed to the sun. Exposure to X ray radiation and chronic exposure to certain chemicals are also considered to be factors in skin cancer.

The most common area for skin cancer is the face, extending over the cheeks from the nose to the ears.

symptoms There are two types of skin cancer: one, basal cell carcinoma, appears in its early form as small, hard nodules of waxy appearance. They grow very slowly and are often present for years before their presence is questioned. Although the nodules are small, they can be identified readily by a trained person.

A more serious form of this type of skin cancer, known as rodent cancer, is characterized by ulceration of the immediate area. It is rapidly destructive, penetrating the skin and involving the local area.

As with most skin tumors, basal cell cancer frequently arises from areas of thickened skin.

Another type of skin cancer is called epidermoid cancer. This form attacks principally the cheeks, ears, and back of the hands. It begins as a warty growth which bleeds easily when the surface is removed. Usually it ulcerates and is often hidden by a secondary infection. Sometimes there is local pain as it penetrates the skin. Depending upon where the malignancy is, the neighboring lymph glands may be involved.

complications There are few complications in skin cancer, provided treatment is rapid and adequate. Of course, as with any malignant disease, there is a possibility that it can spread widely. Ulceration with secondary infection is a possible complication. However, this is not nearly as important as the skin cancer itself.

prevention (or lessening of impact) There is no known way of preventing the development of skin cancer. Once the nodules are observed, investigation should follow promptly. The diagnosis can be established easily by biopsy or complete removal of the section. The doctor will urge the removal of any suspicious area. When it is indicated, X ray can be used most effectively.

Pre-cancerous moles, or areas of skin which have become thickened and are known to be pre-malignant, should be removed before the change occurs.

Skin cancer does not have to be a matter of concern and worry for the patient, provided it is not neglected.

Skin Cancer

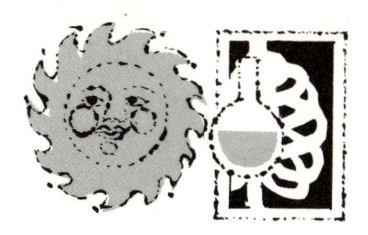

Contributing Factors
X-ray radiation, contact with industrial chemicals, chronic irritation; too much sunlight

Two Types of Skin Cancer

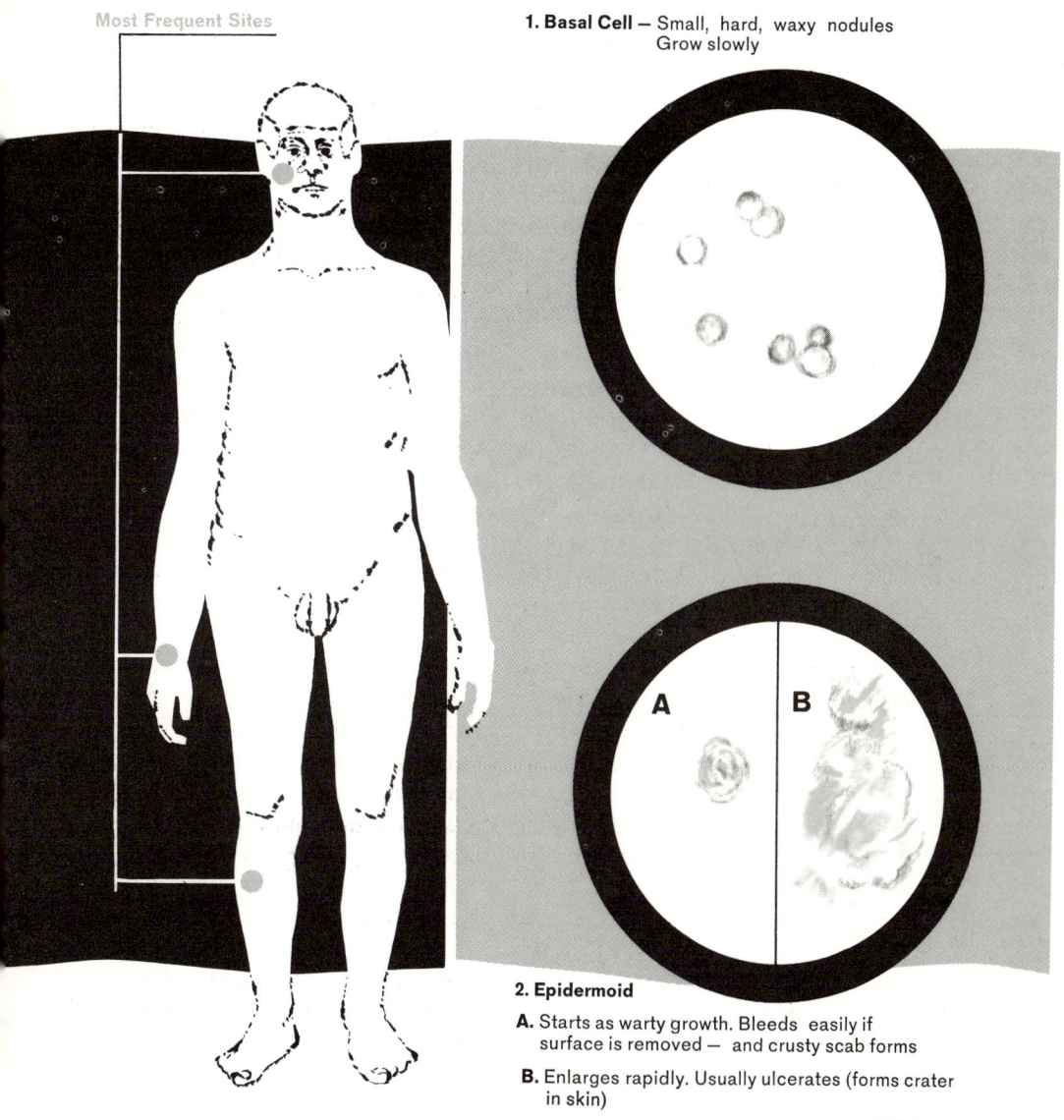

1. Basal Cell — Small, hard, waxy nodules Grow slowly

Most Frequent Sites

2. Epidermoid

A. Starts as warty growth. Bleeds easily if surface is removed — and crusty scab forms

B. Enlarges rapidly. Usually ulcerates (forms crater in skin)

purpose is to insulate the body from outside cold. This layer is missing from certain areas of the body, such as the eyelids.

The skin is an organ of the body as much as the liver, heart, or lungs. When the flow of blood to the skin is hindered for any reason, the skin becomes harder, thicker, and loses its elasticity. In old age, when blood circulation to the skin decreases, the skin loses its youthful appearance, wrinkles form, and the color changes.

Fingernails and toenails are actually modifications of skin consisting of keratin, and the mucous membranes found in body cavities such as the mouth, nose, digestive tract, and eyes are similar to skin, consisting of specialized epithelial tissue. Mucous membrane differs from outer skin in many ways, principally in the secretion of mucus and in lacking keratin, sweat glands, and hair.

Any inflammation of the skin is called *dermatitis*. Although some forms of dermatitis are due to serious internal causes, 95 per cent of the cases of disturbed skin are simple irritations due to infection or some external cause.

A change in the skin is a characteristic of many *deficiency diseases*. Vitamins have a definite relationship to the skin and at least six skin conditions are connected to vitamin deficiencies. For example, a *vitamin B_2 (riboflavin) deficiency* will cause blisters and cracking at the corners of the mouth. A *deficiency of vitamin C* leads to *scurvy* with hemorrhages in the gums and skin. A *vitamin A deficiency* results in dryness of the skin and hair, although most people who have dry skin and hair do not necessarily have this deficiency. A *vitamin B_6 (pyridoxine) deficiency* may be the cause of excessively oily skin in some cases. A deficiency of *niacin* results in *pellagra*.

Practically every skin disease has at one time or another been treated by some kind of diet. *Psoriasis*, for example, has been treated with doses of vitamin D, but it is a stubborn ailment and its cause is not yet known. *Urticaria* and various forms of *eczema* which are allergies to certain proteins are related to diet.

Many different diets have been tried in treatment of blackheads, pimples, and *acne*—for instance, diets without meat, without sugar, or without fats. At present most skin specialists agree that a low-fat diet is beneficial, since in many cases of acne an overactivity of the oil glands of the skin is present. Most would also advocate avoidance of excessive sugar consumption.

Particular foods seem to aggravate some acne, most frequently *chocolate, nuts, shellfish, peanuts, pork* and *pork products, tunafish, milk, milk products* and *cheese*. The only conclusion that may be drawn is that acne cannot be controlled by diet alone, but that a well-balanced diet is certainly an important part of maintaining healthy attractive skin.

Certain illnesses induce various abnormalities of skin structure known as *primary* or *secondary lesions*. The primary lesions include *papules, vesicles, pustules, bullae,* and *scales,* The secondary lesions, which result from a primary condition, include *atrophy, pigmentation, sclerosis* or *hardening, ulceration, crusts,* and *lichens.*

Normal skin will thrive well with nothing more than a reasonable amount of cleanliness. The skin of a baby requires more care than that of an adult, since it is more easily irritated. Women, especially, are concerned with the appearance of their skin and are often susceptible to the advertising claims of various products for the skin. However, no substance applied to the skin can "feed it," and any benefit derived is only superficial and temporary. A substance powerful enough to actually alter the skin would be completely unsafe to use. *See also* ACNE; ACNE ROSACEA; ALBINO; ALLERGY; BARBER'S ITCH; CANCER; COSMETICS; ECZEMA; ERYSIPELAS; HAIR; HERPES ZOSTER; HIVES; IMPETIGO; MELANOSIS; NAILS; PIGMENTATION; PSORIASIS; RINGWORM; SCABIES; SPOROTRICHOSIS; SYPHILIS; TATTOOING; TULAREMIA; VITILIGO. *See* MEDIGRAPHS pages 31, 441, 759, 763, 1043, 1087, 1171, 1189, 1331.

SKULL, the entire bony framework of the head, consisting of the *cranium* and the *face.* The *cranium* is made up of the *frontal bone*—the front part of the cranium—the *occipital* which lies behind, and the *sphenoid, temporal,* and *parietal bones* at the side. The *roof* or *vault* is formed by the *frontal* and *parietal bones,* and the *base* of the skull by the *occipital, temporal, sphenoid,* and *ethmoid bones.*

The *occipital bone* has a large opening through which the *brain* is connected with the *spinal cord;* in addition, other openings provide for the passage of numerous *nerves* and *blood vessels.*

The bones of the face fit closely beneath the *orbits* of the eyes, around the *nasal cavities* and *mouth,* and in the *cheek.*

The skull of a baby is thin and soft. The bones that form the vault of the newborn baby's skull are separated and the membranous space between is called *fontanelle.* The movement of these bones affects the shape of the head, which may be temporarily altered by molding during birth.

Various diseases may provoke changes in the shape of the head, such as *rickets, hydrocephalus, acromegaly,* and *osteitis deformans,* and some birth injuries and congenital deformities also affect the shape.

The skull is subject to *fractures* of two types: the *closed* or *simple fracture,* and the *open* or *compound fracture.* Simple fractures vary from a small fracture line to extensive cracking of the bones throughout the skull. Simple fractures may be complicated if one of the pieces of bone presses on the brain. Other complications occur when the fracture crosses a major artery or vein or involves a *cranial nerve.* In most simple fractures, healing progresses without much treatment, but special surgery is usually imperative in cases of fracture across a major artery. Compound fractures of the skull are more serious and care must be taken to guard against *meningitis. Sulfa*

1191

drugs and *antibiotics* have been helpful in reducing the incidence of this infection in skull fractures. *See also* BRAIN; CONCUSSION; HEAD INJURIES. *See* MEDIGRAPHS pages 659, 1221.

SLEEP, the periodic state of rest during which there is a noticeable decrease of consciousness and activity. The average person requires sleep just as he does food, and the demand for sleep is as regular as that for food. During sleep, the body—and in particular, the brain—has an opportunity to repair itself, to get rid of *wastes* that have accumulated in the tissues during the day. The rate of metabolism during sleep is at its lowest point, being sufficient only to keep the vital parts of the body in operation. Blood pressure drops, the pulse rate slows down, breathing is irregular and slackened. The body is less sensitive to pain, light, and sound. Even the temperature is somewhat lower than during waking hours.

An infant sleeps almost all of the time, awakening usually only for feeding. A child of two or three years of age should sleep twelve or thirteen hours a day. Seven or eight hours of sleep is normally adequate for an adult. More hours of sleep are required in the early years of life, since the body tissues build reserves of energy during sleep necessary to meet the greater demands of the growing body. The aged person usually sleeps only about six hours at night; occasionally four hours' sleep seems to be adequate. The amount of sleep needed varies among people, but everyone should have enough to awaken rested and refreshed. *See also* BRAIN; CEREBRUM; NARCOLEPSY; SENILITY; SNORING; SOMNAMBULISM.

SLEEPING SICKNESS. *See* ENCEPHALITIS.

SLEEPLESSNESS. *See* INSOMNIA.

SLIPPED DISC. The *backbone* as an integrated system is so designed and put together that it breaks only under the most extraordinary and violent shocks. It can support a weight far larger than that of the body of which it is a part, and can move this body in practically any direction. In addition, the backbone is capable of a range of movements extending from a stevedore's lift to an acrobat's contortions and a ballet dancer's delicacy and discipline.

The *intervertebral disc,* a little cushion of *cartilage* that lies between every second *vertebra* of the *spinal column,* makes all this possible. The center of each disc is composed of a special material called *nucleus pulposus,* which tends to move about slightly in correspondence to movements of the body. These discs cushion the body and especially the head against direct impact of the shock of walking which a solid bone would transmit. They also permit an ease and degree of rotation of the vertebrae which would otherwise be impossible.

The functions and changes in these discs have only recently been comprehended. The *jeep disease* of World War II—severe and persistent back pain associated with constant riding in a jeep over rough roads—led to medical investigation which proved that the pain was caused by dislocation of one of the intervertebral discs which had been squeezed or bumped out of position by violent movement. Sometimes the *nucleus pulposus* ruptures, loses liquid, and contributes to the squeezing that displaces the disc.

Occasionally a disc is displaced during common experiences of everyday life. An automobile accident may throw a sudden and excessive shock on the spine and cause an injury at first not apparent. A bumpy airplane landing may have the same effect. Many forms of athletic exercise involve some risk of injuring a disc. Activities, such as football, baseball, and gymnastic work which subject the spine to frequent sharp heavy shocks while the back is in an unusual position tend to do this most frequently.

The detection of a dislocated disc is not a simple matter and may require prolonged study. The injury is not apparent through simple exploration with the fingers. X-ray and careful review of the symptoms will help the doctor make a diagnosis.

Rest, wearing braces, and surgery are all alternative remedies for the condition. The doctor's judgment alone can determine the best treatment. *See also* SPINE; SPINAL CORD; SPINAL CURVATURE; SPINAL FRACTURE; SPONDYLOLISTHESIS. *See* MEDIGRAPHS pages 947, 1211.

SMALLPOX, or *variola,* a contagious infectious disease, often fatal, with fever followed by a papular

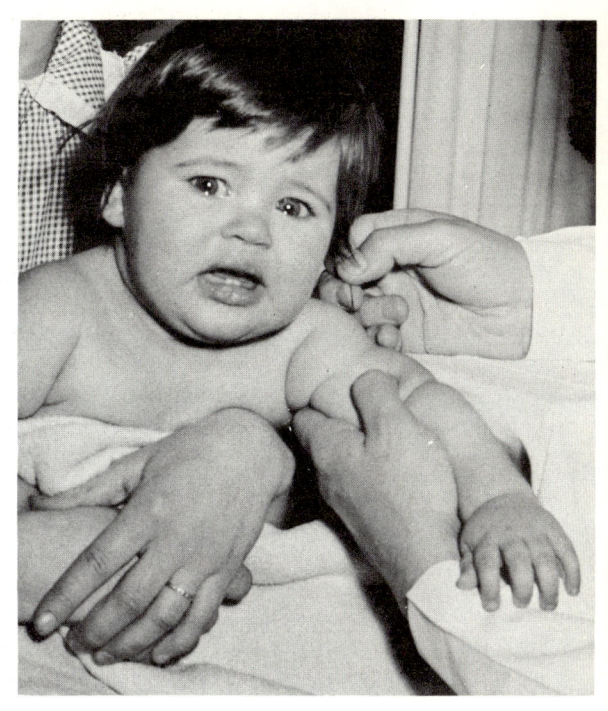

Smallpox—Child being vaccinated against smallpox. Since immunity to smallpox is not permanent, vaccinations should be repeated.

eruption which results in pitted scars. The introduction of *vaccination,* developed by the English physician Edward Jenner in 1796, and the more recently improved techniques for *quarantine* and *isolation* have brought smallpox almost completely under control and it is now comparatively rare.

The virus of smallpox is present in the discharge from the nose and throat, in blisters on the skin, in the scabs that eventually fall off, and in the excretions from the body. The disease may spread from any of these sources, which accounts for the ease and rapidity with which the disease infects anyone who is not immune.

1193

the disease and its causes Smallpox is a highly contagious virus disease which can be very serious in unvaccinated people. It is spread by direct contact with an infected person or any article he has handled, or by a carrier. The virus is present in discharges from nose and throat, in skin blisters, in the scabs which later fall off, and in body excretions. There are no recognizable symptoms during the incubation period, which lasts from 10 to 14 days. A patient becomes permanently immune to smallpox after an attack.

symptoms The disease begins suddenly, with high fever accompanied by a rash. There may be vomiting, diarrhea, aches and pains. Convulsions and delirium may occur if the temperature climbs high enough.

In its early stages the rash may resemble measles. It starts on the face and forearms and spreads to the upper arms and body. By the third day the lower extremities are covered. About the fourth day it comes to look like a series of water blisters, as illustrated. These take on the appearance of pus blisters as the illness progresses. All of the rash on a person's body looks alike at any one time. This is different from the rash of chickenpox, where all the different stages of the rash may appear at one time. Throughout the development of the smallpox rash there is likely to be high fever.

A mild form of smallpox called variloid may occur in people who are *partially* protected by a vaccination they may have received years before.

complications In more severe forms of smallpox, bleeding occurs from the mouth and the rash may resemble blood blisters. In confluent smallpox, which is a severe form of the disease, the rash is so dense it appears to run together. Such cases are often fatal.

Complications include secondary infections of the skin, such as boils, abscesses, and erysipelas. Ear infections, pneumonia, and heart failure are also complicating features.

prevention (or lessening of impact) Everyone should be vaccinated because it is almost a guarantee that one will not get smallpox. This should be repeated every three years to maintain immunity. Anyone planning to spend time in a foreign country where smallpox is known to exist should be certain to get a revaccination.

Isolate the patient with this disease, and sterilize or destroy anything with which he has come in contact. Good care includes keeping the patient in bed, keeping him clean and comfortable, and seeing to it that he gets plenty of liquids.

Smallpox

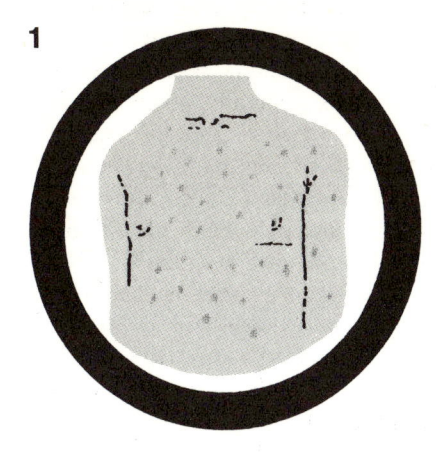

1. Rash
Sudden outbreak of fever is accompanied by rash. It starts on face and forearms, spreads to upper arms and rest of body by 3rd day. Rash turns from red spots to pimples.

2. Blisters
Around 4th day, blisters with gray pinpoint centers form over pimples

3. Pus Globules
Blisters keep enlarging, and around 7th day fill with yellow pus.

4. Pockmarks
Around 10th day pus globules begin to dry up and form scabs. In more severe cases of smallpox, permanent pockmarks are left after scabs disappear.

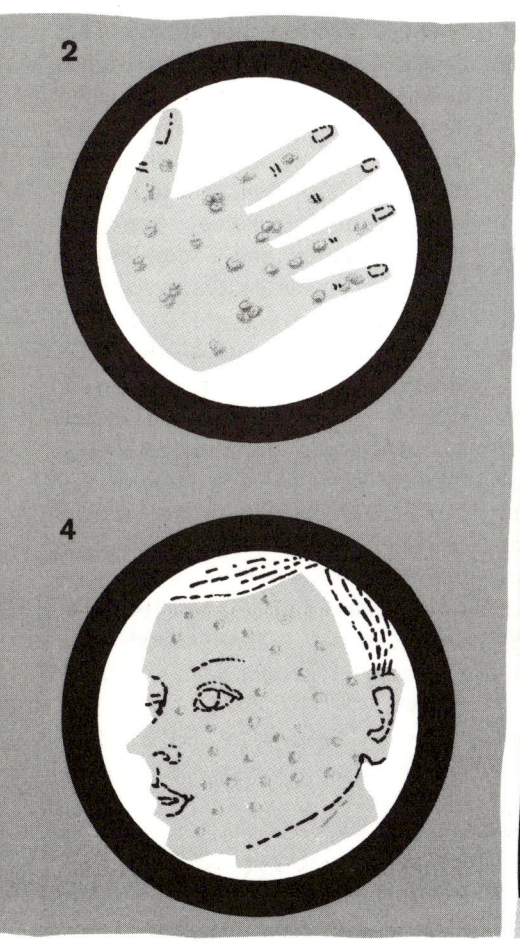

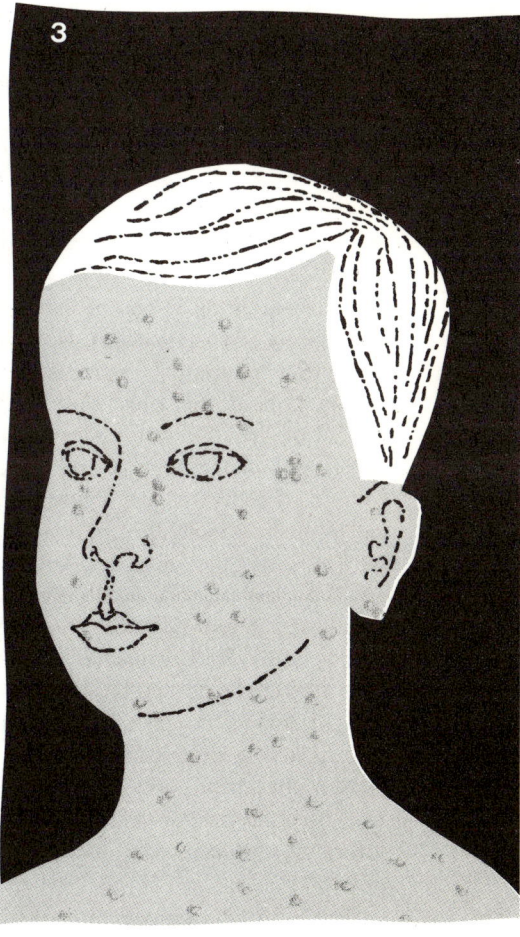

The incubation period is generally eight to twelve days. Smallpox begins with violent headache, chill, pain in the back and limbs and a high fever, and, in children, convulsions and vomiting. Within three or four days small reddened pimples appear over the face and wrists and spread rapidly to the arms and chest. These form blisters in a day or two and in about eight or nine days begin to dry, leaving a blackish crust. The face swells and feels irritated and the rash, particularly on the face, can be agonizing. The eyelids may be swollen shut. After three or four weeks the crusts fall off and the characteristic pitting scars or pockmarks of smallpox remain.

Complications caused by bacterial infection result in *bronchopneumonia, conjunctivitis,* or more serious damage to the eyes or middle ear.

Since smallpox is one of the most contagious diseases known, isolation and strict quarantine are essential. It can spread not only during the course of the illness but also during the long convalescent period which follows. Clothing, bed linens, and any object which the patient has handled carry the infection. Any person who has been in contact with a smallpox patient should be vaccinated, unless he has had a vaccination during the preceding five years. Vaccination may even protect the patient if it is done during the early incubation period, and may, if effective, result in milder symptoms. One attack of smallpox gives lifelong immunity.

The immunity gained by vaccination is temporary and vaccinations must therefore be repeated at five- to seven-year intervals. The first vaccination is generally given between the ages of three months and one year and is repeated between the ages of seven and eleven years, especially if an epidemic is present or if travel is planned to areas where the disease is more common than in the United States. *See also* IMMUNITY; IMMUNIZATION; INFECTION; INFECTIOUS DISEASES; VACCINATION. *See* MEDIGRAPH page 1195.

SMELL, the perception of odor. The degree of perceptiveness varies among persons, some having a highly developed sense of smell and others having very little. Sense of smell appears to be less significant to human beings than, for example, sense of sight or hearing, and a total loss of the *olfactory sense* usually requires little adjustment.

To test olfactory sensitivity, well-defined odors are used. A person with a high sensitivity can detect *camphor* in a solution of 1:30,000,000 and *vanilla* in a solution of 1:10,000,000. Apparently the strongest odor is that of *mercaptan,* a derivative of *alcohol* in which *oxygen* is replaced by *sulphur*. It can be detected when 1/23,000,000th of a milligram is present in a quart of water.

Loss of the sense of smell is called *anosmia. See also* ANOSMIA; NOSE; OZENA.

SMOKING AND LUNG CANCER. Statisticians have noted an increasing incidence of deaths attributable to lung cancer. *Statistical evidence* definitely establishes a relationship between this increased incidence of lung cancer and *smoking*—in particular, the smoking of *cigarettes*. Chemical or *physiological evidence* of a *direct cause-effect relationship* between these two phenomena remains somewhat inconclusive. Some of the increased incidence of lung cancer can undoubtedly be ascribed to the dangerous pollution of the atmosphere over many of our great cities. However, all available evidence at our disposal does indicate that habitual cigarette smokers are far more likely to contract the disease than those who smoke few or no cigarettes. (Statistical—and possibly also chemical—evidence indicates there is less hazard in *pipe* smoking, and the least hazard of all in *cigar* smoking—except, of course, in not smoking at all!) The United States government now requires that all packages of cigarettes carry a printed warning to the effect that cigarette smoking may be injurious to health. *See also* CANCER; BUERGER'S DISEASE; TOBACCO. *See* MEDIGRAPHS pages 283, 849, 865.

SNAKEBITE. Several types of snakes are poisonous—that is, capable of injecting a poisonous venom into their victims by biting. These include the *cobra, viper, rattlesnake, water moccasin (cottonmouth), copperhead,* and *coral snake*. All of these snakes are extremely dangerous and should be avoided. The bite of the cobra and the coral snake is usually fatal, as their toxin is exceedingly virulent and acts quickly to paralyze the entire nervous system, including the brain. The bites of the other snakes need not necessarily be fatal if treated properly at once, but fatality almost inevitably ensues if such treatment is not immediately administered.

Emergency treatment consists of making a crosswise incision through the fang punctures with a knife previously sterilized by flame or cleaned with iodine or alcohol. Extreme care should be taken not to sever any arteries. Suction—by mouth or suction cup—should then be applied until all the blood in the vicinity of the wound has been removed. (If suction is not feasible, the wound can be squeezed to remove the blood, but suction is always preferable because of its greater efficiency.) No great danger is presented by sucking the venom by mouth, provided there are no open sores present in the mouth or gums.

A tourniquet should be placed above the bite and the victim carried by stretcher to a physician. If at all possible, the snake should be killed and taken to the physician for identification. The physician will administer the proper type of *antivenom serum*, which serves to neutralize the remaining toxin. Under no circumstances should alcohol or stimulants be administered, as they accelerate the circulation of the blood and thus promote the further absorption of the toxin.

The bite of the *Gila monster* and of poisonous *scorpions* should be treated in the same manner as snakebite. *See also* INSECT BITES; BEE STINGS; BLACK WIDOW SPIDER.

SNEEZING

SNEEZING, or *sternutation,* a natural reflex action involving a deep intake of breath followed by closure of the *glottis*; the mechanism is similar to that of a cough. A violent expiration effort ensues, the glottis opens, a blast of air is sent out through the nose, taking with it *mucus* and other material. Frequently the eyes water immediately following a sneeze.

Paroxysms of sneezing and watering eyes are characteristic of *hay fever* and other allergic conditions. A sneeze may occur without an irritant, such as when a person stares at a bright sky or stands barefoot on a cold floor. Sneezes can often be suppressed by placing a steady pressure between the nose and lip with one or two fingers.

Sneezing can be a symptom of a *common cold* or of some respiratory disease such as *influenza*. Since a sneeze disseminates virus or bacteria, it should always be covered with a handkerchief or tissue.

In cases of persistent sneezing the nose should be examined by a doctor, since a disordered *septum* or other source of irritation may exist which requires special attention. Treatment of sneezing always involves treating the underlying condition.

SNORING, the rough audible sound made by breathing through the nose in such a way as to cause a vibration of the *soft palate*. The noise made by snoring is due to the intermittent passage of air at places in the mouth where there may be partial obstruction. *Adenoids* sometimes cause snoring, especially in children.

Snoring can occur in several ways. During sleep a partial relaxation of the muscles holding the vocal cords may occur so that they fall closely together and interfere with the passage of air. Or, when a person is sleeping deeply or is unconscious, and lying on his back, the tongue may fall back and partially close the opening through which air passes. This is what causes the noisy breathing called *stertor* which occurs in *concussions* and *apoplexy*.

Sometimes, because of irritation or inflammation, mucus may collect in the nose or in the passages behind the nose, or the muscles associated with the nose and throat may be abnormally tense and interfere with passage of air. If the nose is blocked and the lips are held tightly together, a whistling sound occurs as the air passes out.

Snoring sounds seldom disturb the person snoring. Often he will stop snoring if, when he is lying on his back, he is turned to the side. Closing his mouth, or pushing the lower jaw forward and with it the base of the tongue, is sometimes effective.

SODIUM BICARBONATE, also known as *baking soda,* a white crystalline powder. Given as an antacid, it overcomes excess acidity of the juices of the stomach and excess acidity of the body generally. In cases of *acidosis,* which may be due to *diabetes* or another condition, large doses of baking soda may be taken orally. Because it can liquefy mucus, a sodium bicarbonate-water solution is sometimes used to cleanse the nose and other mucous surfaces. A lotion made of a teaspoon of baking powder to a pint of water helps to relieve itching, and a baking soda bath may be beneficial in helping similar conditions.

SODOMY, a legal term denoting either *pederasty* (intromission of the penis into the anus of another person, whether male or female) or *bestiality* (sexual intercourse with animals) or both. In some jurisdictions, sodomy also denotes any sexually deviant act performed by a male with a female or between two males, including *irrumation* (penis-mouth copulation), *fellation* (mouth-penis copulation), *mutual masturbation,* or *simple molestation.* A person engaging in *bestiality* is considered psychotic.

SOMNAMBULISM refers to a sleep or sleeplike state during which walking or other activities are performed. It is fairly common in children. In adults it is rarer and of more serious significance. Usually sleepwalking stems from some conflict in the mind which is unresolved and continues to stimulate the person even during the period of sleep. Usually when the person's doubt or fear is removed—which, in serious cases, may require psychiatric help—the sleepwalking ceases. A person awakened during sleepwalking is usually perplexed and distressed. He should not be criticized or scolded, but consoled and returned to bed.

SORE THROAT refers to inflammation of the *pharynx,* called *pharyngitis,* or of the *tonsils,* called *tonsillitis.* In a *common cold,* the soreness is usually in the back wall of the upper throat and affects the *nasopharynx* and the *palate. See also* COMMON COLD; HOARSENESS; LARYNGITIS; PHARYNX; QUINSY; SEPTIC SORE THROAT. *See* MEDIGRAPHS pages 515, 1269.

SPACE MEDICINE. Man's venture into outer space has opened up an entire new field of medicine commonly referred to as *space medicine.* Space medicine has evolved from the earlier aviation medicine designed to protect aviators from possible harmful effects of flying such as *altitude sickness* and *motion sickness.* However, the problems in space medicine are infinitely more complex and present a unique challenge to modern medical science.

The scientist engaged in space medicine is concerned with the protection, health, and safety of the astronaut. He works directly with the astronaut in his training program, devises workable methods of adjustment to the conditions of outer space, and is involved directly or indirectly with the preparations for all the varied phases of space flight. He is consulted by the engineers and physicists concerning the engineering of the space vehicle and the design of astronautical equipment.

The space vehicle includes all the necessities required to maintain the life, safety, and comfort of its occupants. As there is no air in space, an

1199

artificial atmosphere of oxygen is created inside the vehicle. Chemical means are used to remove the carbon dioxide breathed out by the astronauts and to preclude any other contamination of the oxygen. Temperature and pressure settings inside the vehicle are maintained at comfortable levels prescribed by the space physician. Although the space capsule itself is airtight, the astronauts are provided with a specially constructed space suit as protection against conceivable leaks in the capsule.

Urine is voided by means of a container built into the space suit. Defecation is managed in the same manner. (The necessity for defecation is minimized on shorter space flights by a low-residue diet preceding the flight.)

Food and liquids are consumed by means of plastic containers which can be squeezed to eject their contents directly into the mouth. The tolerance of the astronauts to the high-gravity forces generated by the launching and reentry processes is maximized by favorable positioning within the capsule. Shielding substances are employed to protect them from heat and sunburn.

The physical condition of the astronauts in flight is studied continuously by the space physician stationed on earth. Such measurements as blood pressure, body temperature, respiratory rate, and electrocardiograms are recorded on the spacecraft and radioed to earth. Significant abnormalities have not been noted in early space flights involving the orbiting of the earth itself. What possible future flights to the moon and planets may entail remains to be seen.

The psychological well-being of the astronauts is as important as their physical health. Future extended space travel will subject them to lengthy periods of isolation from society, and their ability to perform efficiently within the confined artificial world of the spacecraft will depend to a large extent on their emotional equanimity.

Weightlessness—the state of zero gravity—which astronauts experience in space is a peculiar phenomenon which still requires much study and observation. During weightlessness, the astronauts experience a situation devoid of normal directions, such as "up" and "down," and in which normal orientation is rendered difficult or impossible. Space physicians have ascertained that under these conditions the eye assumes the crucial role in the process of orientation. Great emphasis is placed on protection of the eye; coated glasses and ports have been designed to obviate possible retinal burns from sunlight or other sources.

Despite the disadvantages of weightlessness, the performance of astronauts under this state has been remarkably good. It is possible, however, that on longer flights weightlessness may alter the normal terrestrial cycle of sleep and wakefulness. In such a contingency, drugs, exercise, and other means may help to restore the normal cycle.

Space medicine is intimately con-

The field of space medicine, still in its infancy, is assuming an increasingly commanding role in society, as more and more astronauts are sent on space exploration missions. The space physician is concerned with the health of the astronauts before, during, and after the space flight. Some of the techniques which have been developed in this specialized field have been adapted successfully to other areas of medicine as well. The astronaut's ability to adapt to conditions alien to his normal environment is the crux of the problems involved in space medicine. Physiological research under simulated conditions here on earth has revealed much information about human adaptation to space conditions and greatly minimized the dangers entailed.

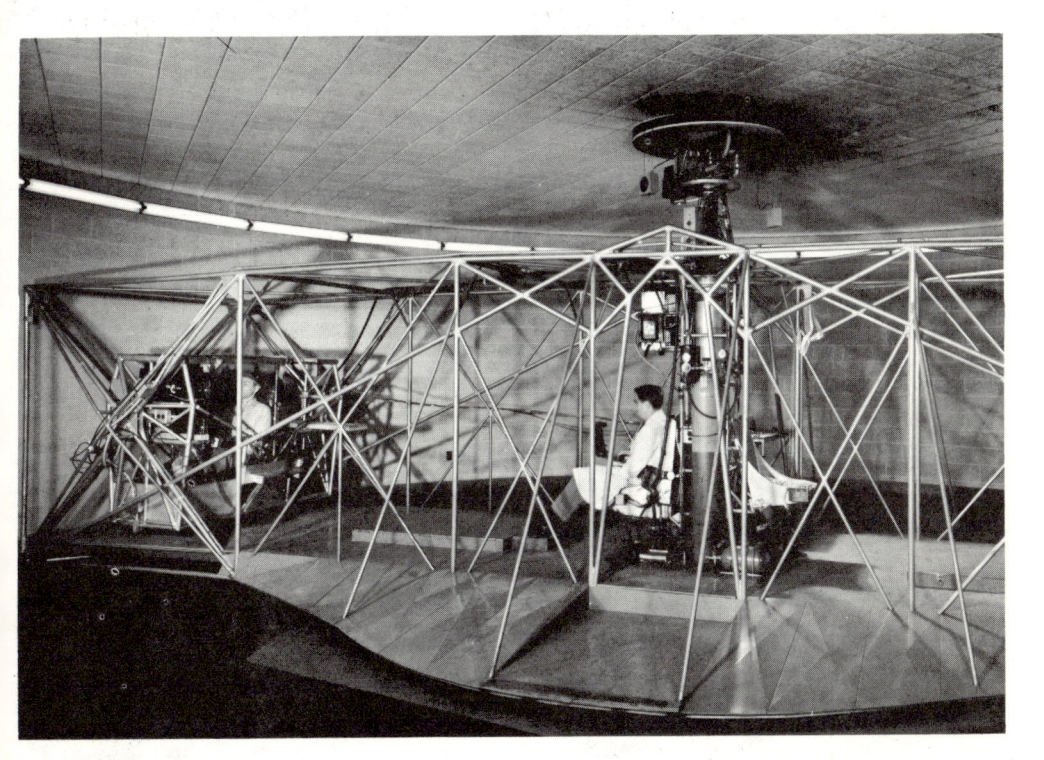

This centrifuge for human physiologic research has produced important information about the effects of gravitational forces upon the various systems of the human body. Although designed primarily for airplane pilots, it has been useful in the testing of astronauts as well. At left is the pilot in a simulated pilot's compartment. At center is an observer. The entire apparatus is made to revolve at great speed about the axis in the center, thus exerting great centrifugal forces upon the pilot.

Below: The medically tailored cuff on the astronaut's left arm monitors his blood pressure during his space flight. The astronaut presses a button on his instrument panel to inflate the cuff for a blood pressure reading.

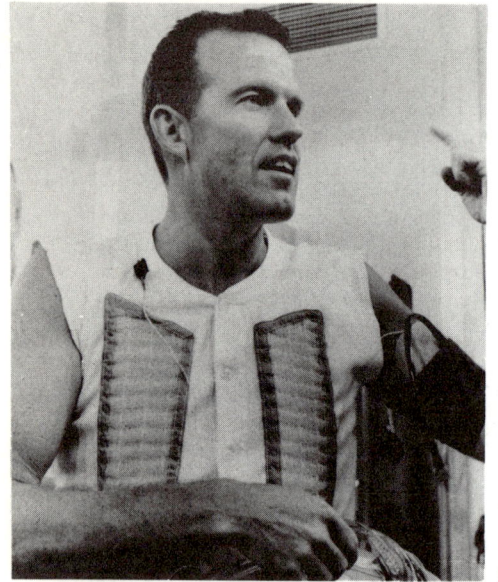

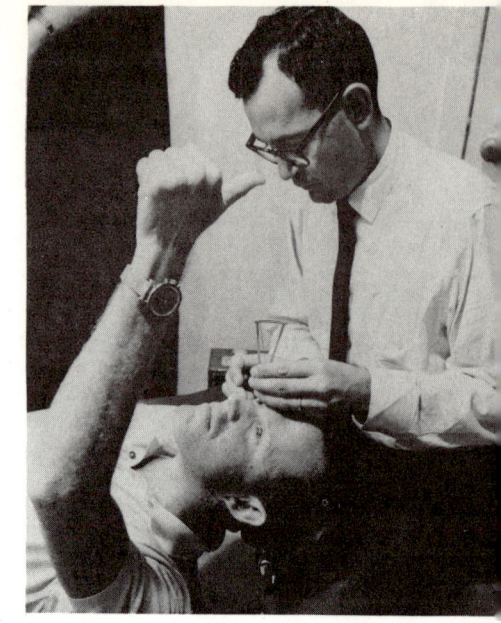

Above: The astronaut is given an eye examination prior to the space flight. The eyes are vital in space orientation. Below: John Glenn, the first American to orbit the earth, undergoes an examination following his return to earth.

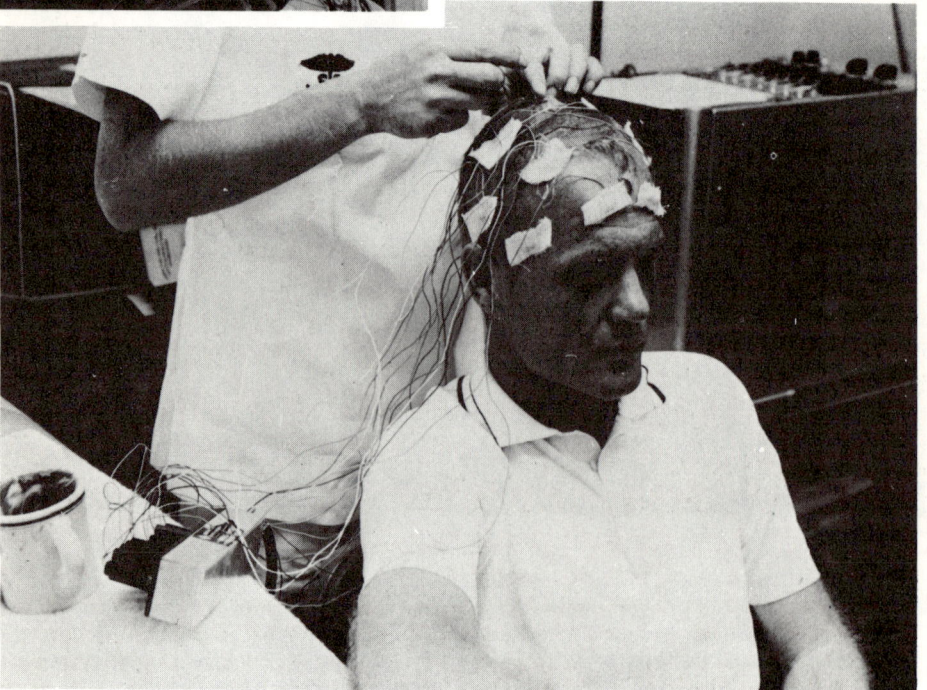

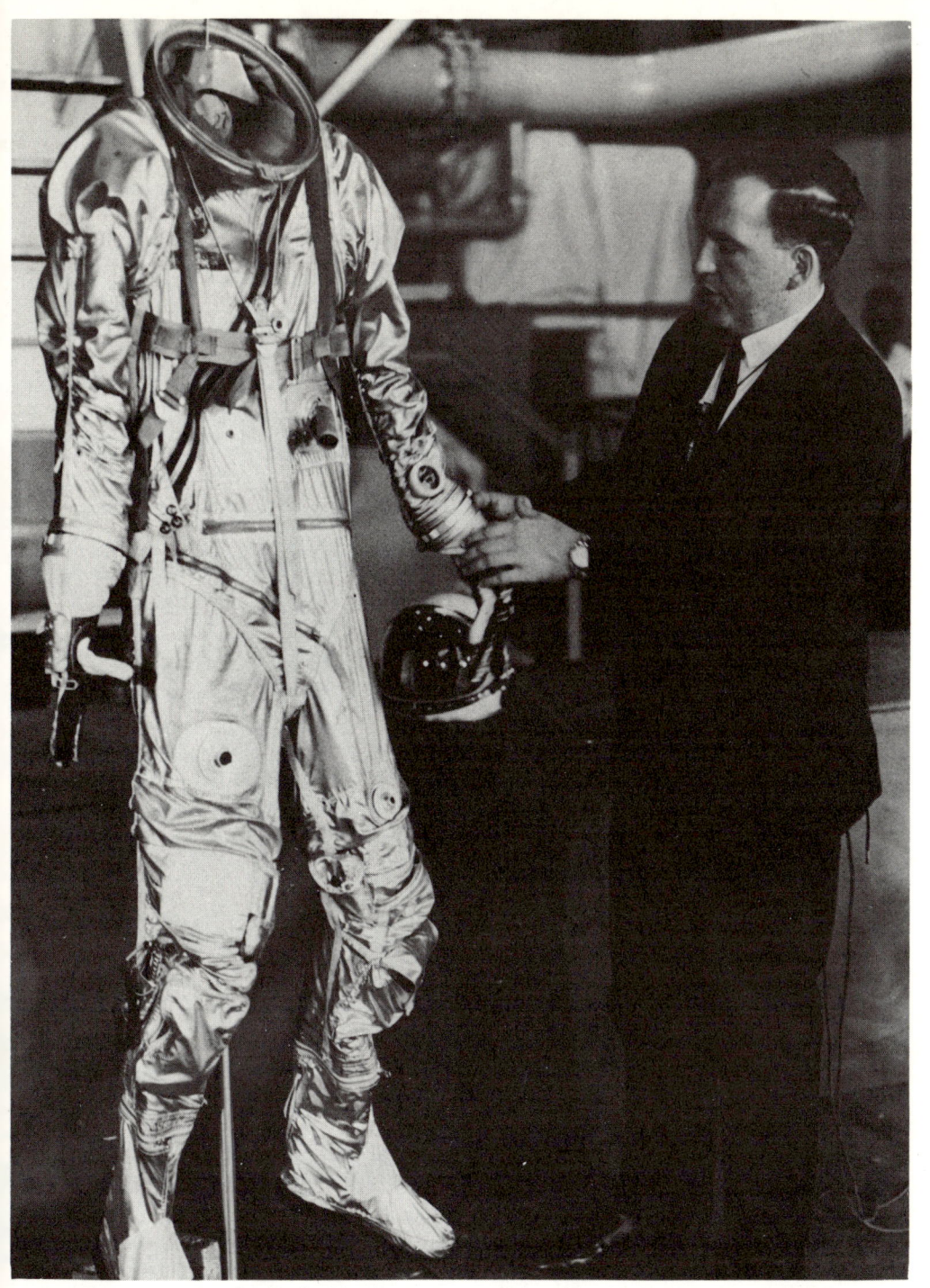

The space suit worn by the first American astronauts. The suit was specially constructed to protect the astronaut against sudden unforeseen leaks in the spacecraft. It is constantly being modified and improved by trial and error.

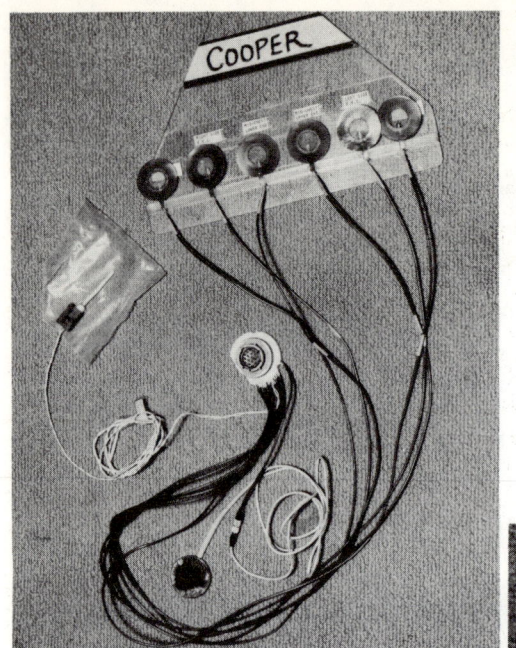

A variety of medical instruments, specially designed by space scientists and physicians, is employed to monitor the metabolism of the astronauts while in space. The instruments shown at left are *biosensors*, designed to monitor the heartbeat and respiration rate of the astronaut while in orbit.

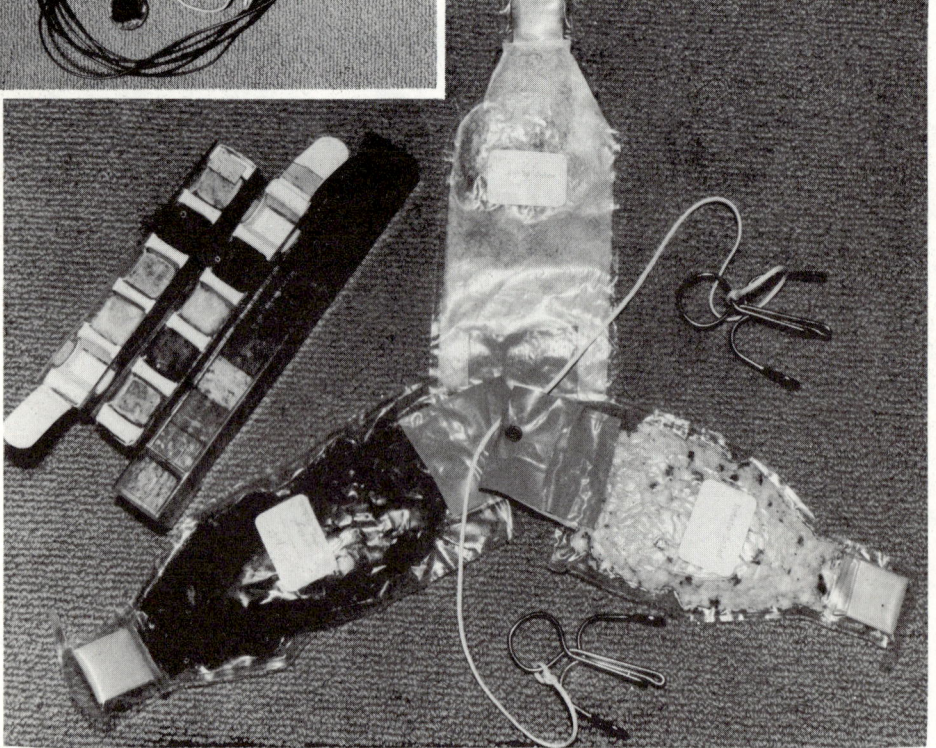

The state of weightlessness in which the astronaut must function while in space and the absence of gravity require the preparation of specially packaged foods that can be consumed without difficulty: On the earliest American space flights, astronauts consumed bite-sized portions of ready-to-eat food. Later, experiments were made with hydrated food in plastic bags and with liquid "squeeze-bottle" food.

nected with the study of astronomy and with speculation or deductions concerning the probable nature of the environmental situations on other celestial bodies likely to be visited at some future time by astronauts. Particularly intriguing is the possibility of vegetation or other forms of life on other planets—a very definite possibility in the case of Mars, at least. Also important is the study of the deadly radiation known to exist in outer space and, indeed, to encircle the earth itself. Much still remains to be learned about the hazards of radioactivity.

Progress in space medicine has been substantial and has produced important medical results in other areas of medicine as well, notably the development of *micro-instrumentation* and *biotelemetry*. See also ALTITUDE SICKNESS; MOTION SICKNESS.

SPANISH FLY. See CANTHARIDES.

SPASM, an involuntary sudden contraction of a muscle. The usual cause is irritation of the nerve cells or nerves which supply the muscle. A sustained contraction is called *tonic*. If contraction and relaxation rapidly alternate, it is a *clonic spasm*. A general spasm over the body is a *convulsion* or *fit*. Massive spasms are characterized by sudden movements which involve most of the body musculature and last from a fraction of a second to several seconds. They may affect infants and young children. The commonest form of spasm is one in which the limbs and trunk are suddenly flexed, followed by relaxation. Similar attacks may occur in series.

Almost anyone can at some time have a muscle spasm. Sudden chilling of the body during swimming may cause a muscle spasm, or whenever the circulation of the blood in any part of the body is greatly diminished sudden involuntary contractions may occur. Disorders in the nervous system—for example, the death of a nerve cell in the interior portion of the spinal cord—may result in paralysis of the muscles with spasm of the opposing muscles.

Sometimes children develop *habit spasms*—not to be confused with *chorea* or *St Vitus' dance*. The movements of habit spasm are quicker and always repeated in the same way, whereas the movements of chorea are irregular and variable. Spasms in children may sometimes occur as a result of distress, such as fear of punishment.

Whenever a spasm of the muscle occurs, examination by a doctor is necessary to determine the source. If it is a condition affecting the nerves, medical or surgical management may be required. In some instances, injection of one of various substances around the nerves of the area involved is the only treatment to stop a spasm. See also CHOREA; CONVULSION; HABIT SPASM; ORGASM; TIC DOULOUREUX.

SPEECH, the process of uttering articulate sounds representing ideas or feelings. The centers of the brain involving the capacity for speech are in the *cortex*. An injury or disease that interferes with cells of the cortex or with fibers that link them, as in *aphasia,* hinders the thought processes of speech.

Sound is produced by vibrations of the vocal cords as air rushes through the *larynx*. In *laryngitis,* the vocal cords are affected and the voice becomes a whisper. Paralysis of the cords causes complete loss of voice, or *aphonia*. The voice may be suddenly lost in *hysteria*. Here the cords remain normal and the cause is emotional.

Sound produced by the larynx is modified by *articulation,* which involves alterations in the shape of the *mouth* and *pharynx* and movements of the *teeth, tongue,* and *palate*. The nerve centers which control articulation are in the *medulla* and are connected with the speech centers in the cortex. Articulation may be affected wholly or partially by damage in these areas.

Lisping, stammering, and *stuttering* are speech defects which can be corrected by training and various exercises. Speech defects caused by *harelip* or *cleft palate* may be corrected by surgical treatment, or *prosthesis*. Surgeons, psychologists, otolaryngologists, speech therapists— all can help in the correction of faulty speech.

Learning to talk is a sign of a child's mental development, but delayed speech should be no cause for alarm unless it is due to mental defect or deafness. If a child still does not speak by the age of one year, he should be taken to a doctor so that his hearing and general intelligence may be tested. Children learn to speak by imitation and will adopt the accents, inflections, and mannerisms of those around them. The best way to encourage correct speech in a child is to listen with interest to what he has to say, making as few corrections in his speech as possible, and speak to him in a correct, modulated and articulate way.

Here are seven rules which parents should follow in developing habits of good speech in their children:

1. Do not correct the child's pronunciation or enunciation. Praise that which is correct, but do not stress that which is wrong.

2. Do not imitate the child's baby talk. By doing this, you simply confirm him in his error. If you speak good English, he will imitate it as soon as he can.

3. Never "talk down" to babies and little children.

4. Do not nag, coax, or raise your voice in an effort to get the baby to talk. Speech will come naturally.

5. If any of the baby's relatives or playmates or you stammer, give the baby an opportunity to learn to talk from someone else. Children imitate what they hear.

6. Give the child a chance to learn to talk and listen to him when he talks. This will encourage him.

7. Tell the child to listen. However, do not ignore him but include him whenever possible in the conversation.

See also APHASIA; STUTTERING AND STAMMERING.

SPERMATIC CORDS, the cords by which the *testicles* are suspended in the *scrotum* from the body, and through which the *vasa deferentia* pass from the *epididymides* to the *inguinal canals* and the *seminal vesicles* in the *pelvis*. The spermatic cords consist of veins, arteries, lymphatics, and nerves, as well as the vasa deferentia. Their movements—which move the testicles toward or away from the body as external temperature conditions warrant—are controlled by the *cremasteric muscles*. See also SCROTUM; SEMINAL DUCTS; REPRODUCTION SYSTEM; TESTICLES; VAS DEFERENS.

SPHINCTER. See URINATION.

SPIDER BITES. See BLACK WIDOW SPIDER.

SPINA BIFIDA. An essential step in the development of the human embryo before birth is the growing together of two sides of the original channel in the back, thus forming the space where the spinal cord will lie. Failure of these to grow together results in a structural condition known as *spina bifida,* meaning literally a *split spine*.

This condition occurs in approximately one in every 1,000 births, but the specific form of the defect always varies. Ordinarily *spina bifida* will be only a gap in the coverings which should enclose the spinal cord. In other instances, however, one or more vertebrae may be absent. This deformity may be accompanied by a bulge in the sheathing of the spinal cord projecting to the exterior, as in a *hernia*. This creates in the back a bulbous body filled with liquid.

Some cases of *spina bifida* are accompanied by what is called *hydrocephaly,* derived from words meaning *water* and *head*. In this condition the fluid which is normally required within the membrane containing the brain increases inordinately in quantity and the skull bones expand to compensate. The size of the head becomes grossly disproportionate to that of the body.

Immediate medical attention should be given to every such case. Exposure of any part of the nervous system, as occurs in *spina bifida,* is extremely serious. Surgical repair will benefit at least half the children affected by the condition but must be undertaken as early as possible to obtain the greatest benefit. The elimination of the bulge in the back often will accomplish much for the patient.

If the condition is left unattended, the distortion of the spinal nerves and the strain to which they are subjected will disturb their function. When the abnormality occurs in the lower spine, the defect may cause paralysis of the legs and loss of normal control over bladder and bowel action. If the nerve supply of the skin is inadequate, ulcers may develop. See also HYDROCEPHALUS.

SPINAL CORD, the relatively large branch of nervous tissue that extends from the *brain* down through the *vertebrae*. The brain and the spinal cord together constitute the *central nervous system*.

The spinal cord is the medium for communication between the brain and many other parts of the body, and also effects numerous *reflex actions*. Some of these are: reflexes controlling many essential muscular movements, such as those jerking the body away from sources of pain; reflexes partly controlling the bowel and urinary bladder; erection of the penis; and movements in the digestive and circulatory systems and other organs. The spinal cord transmits sensations of touch to the brain.

The cord is about eighteen inches long and approximately the thickness of the little finger. Branching from it to the left and right, into the body itself, are thirty-one pairs of nerves. The *vertebral column* — or *backbone* — is much longer than the eighteen inches of the spinal cord. Consequently many of the projecting branches which serve lower parts of the body, and so leave the vertebral column lower, must extend through the rest of the column down to the point where they branch out of it.

The spinal cord may be disordered in a number of ways. In *myelitis*—such as *poliomyelitis*—it is inflamed.

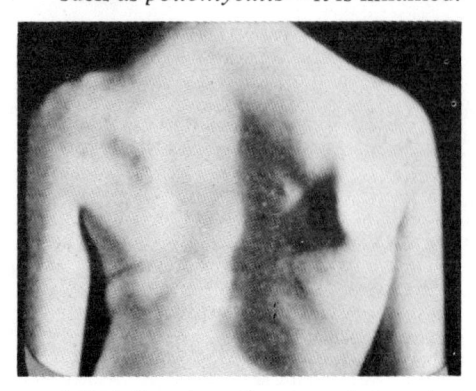

Spinal Curvature—Curvature of the spinal column of unknown causation. Curvatures may result from faulty development of the spine or from diseases of the spinal column.

Sclerosis, in which tissue associated with nerves hardens and damages them, may affect the spinal cord. *Meningitis* is inflammation of the membranes which encase both the brain and the spinal cord. The cord may be affected by *concussion,* inducing temporary paralysis, or it may be directly injured, as when the vertebral column itself breaks. See also BRAIN. See MEDIGRAPHS pages 1063, 1211, 1221.

SPINAL CURVATURE. The spine is one of the most fundamental structural elements of the body and forms a basis around which other essential parts are arranged. Seen from the side, the spine has a modified S shape, giving it a springiness and elasticity that protect the delicate organs in the head and elsewhere from constant bumps and shocks. Seen from the front, it is a straight line. When this line loses its straightness and becomes a looplike curve, either to the right or to the left, the resulting condition is *scoliosis,* or curvature of the spine.

This curvature frequently is a symptom or a sequel of another disorder rather than a disorder itself. Usually the backbone is extraordinarily protected by the system of muscles and ligaments that combine with the spine to give the body its normal erectness. However, an inadequacy may occur in these muscles which permits the spine to curve toward either side. One or more bones, rather than the muscles, may suffer breakdown, and thus throw other bones and tissues out of place.

Scoliosis may occur from habitual

bad posture. At first, only the positions of the parts are abnormal and the tissues remain unaffected. Later, however, if the fault is not corrected, tissue changes do occur and the curvature will become more or less permanent.

Correct posture is especially essential for children, and parents should keep careful watch to insure the child's correct posture and eliminate any postural defects promptly to avoid any permanent deformity. Often special exercises aid in developing muscular strength, which may be lacking, to hold the spine in its natural erect position.

The structural significance of the spine makes almost inevitable the displacement of other parts of the body when spinal deformity occurs. The lung of the side opposite the curvature may become overcompressed; one or more nerves may suffer undue pressure. Frequently the lower rib or ribs will be thrown down against the thigh with no apparent spinal displacement.

Such disorders should be examined by the doctor to determine whether or not the displacement observed is originating with a curvature in the spine which has hitherto escaped notice and diagnosis. The patient is observed standing in his habitual relaxed position and then attempting to straighten his back as fully as possible. The doctor may check the form of the spine against a straight vertical standard such as a plumb line.

Orthopedists, who specialize in correcting deformities, can correct bad posture and support weak bodily structures with external mechanical means such as braces and casts. Ordinarily, however, this is a last resort and emphasis is first placed on training by exercises. *See* MEDIGRAPH page 1211.

SPINAL FRACTURE, any break of the bones of the spine. It is a grave injury since the spine is the structural foundation for most of the body and is the intermediary for communication between the brain and the body. Before the advent of x-ray, the only positive sign that a back was broken was usually paralysis in one or more parts of the body. X-ray permits a much more thorough and certain diagnosis. Treatment of such fractures has also improved.

Serious injury to the spine results from a violent shock or blow. Since the spine is well protected by its structure and surrounding tissues, it must be struck or strained with unusual force to break. Spinal injury can occur in automobile accidents, falls, in excessive efforts to move or lift a heavy load, or from a sudden violent jerk. The most severe breaks in the back occur in the region of the neck, where there are a greater number of nerves affecting other parts of the body than at a lower point of the back. The most serious consequences come from a fracture which invades or tears the spinal cord or causes a hemorrhage into it. Occasionally the cord may be injured as seriously as from a break when two or more vertebrae, the bones which make up the spine, are forced apart without actual fracture to the bones themselves.

the injury and its causes Between the vertebrae of the spine there are spinal discs made of cartilage which serve as shock absorbers. Acute injuries, congenital weakness, or chronic injuries which may have occurred years before the onset of pain, can cause weakening of the ligaments which bind the spine. At the weakest point these ligaments may tear, permitting the spinal disc to protrude, or herniate. Protrusion of the disc, with pressure on the nerve roots, is one of the commonest causes of low back pain, causing the kind of low back disorder which used to be described as lumbago, sciatica, sacro-iliac sprains, and low back sprains.

symptoms Low back pain or irritation of the involved nerve root is one of the earliest symptoms of a slipped disc. At this stage, rest will generally result in less pain because the disc works back to its more normal position. However, if it does not slip back completely, the nerve root irritation continues and causes pain down the back of the leg, sometimes numbness, and the kind of discomfort commonly called "sciatica." The continued pressure on the sciatic nerve causes intense pain which is aggravated by any back movements, sneezing, coughing, or other abrupt motion. The outer surface of the foot and toes may tingle or become numb. When the patient stands he tilts his back. When he raises his leg straight up, he gets a definite pain in the back. Continued nerve pressure causes weakness and atrophy of the muscles, and definite loss of sensation. Paralysis can result from this chronic pressure on the nerve, and the patient cannot use his bladder and bowel.
The sciatic pain from the buttock down the length of the affected leg can become so excruciating that motion becomes severely limited, if not impossible, and the patient is bedridden.

complications These depend on the extent of nerve damage caused by the pressure of the displaced disc. The paralysis and interference with bladder and bowel functions are serious problems. In addition to the further complications they may bring, they can prevent the patient from working or from carrying on other normal activities.

prevention (or lessening of impact) Any case of low back pain or sciatica should be thoroughly investigated to rule out the possibility of a herniated spinal disc. The diagnosis can generally be made from just a physical examination, but sometimes X ray or spinal canal studies are necessary. Bed rest and heat may prevent the development of the more serious effects of a slipped disc if they are used early enough. Many patients find orthopedic supports such as corsets or low back braces helpful. Heavy lifting, bending, pushing, and pulling should be avoided.
When there is no improvement after the simpler recommendations have been followed, back traction or surgery may be necessary.

Slipped Disc

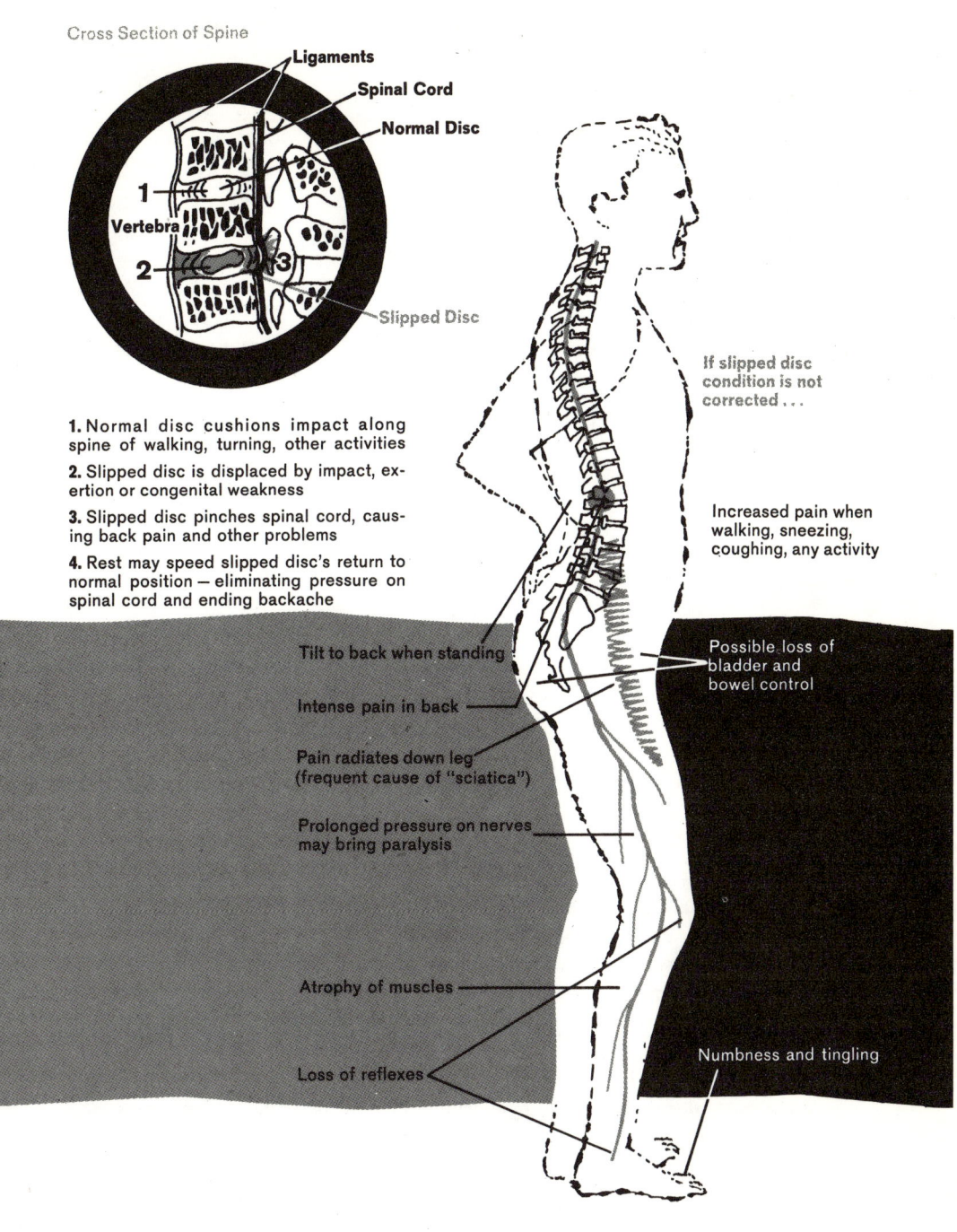

Cross Section of Spine

- Ligaments
- Spinal Cord
- Normal Disc
- 1 Vertebra
- 2
- 3
- Slipped Disc

1. Normal disc cushions impact along spine of walking, turning, other activities
2. Slipped disc is displaced by impact, exertion or congenital weakness
3. Slipped disc pinches spinal cord, causing back pain and other problems
4. Rest may speed slipped disc's return to normal position — eliminating pressure on spinal cord and ending backache

If slipped disc condition is not corrected...

Increased pain when walking, sneezing, coughing, any activity

Tilt to back when standing

Intense pain in back

Pain radiates down leg (frequent cause of "sciatica")

Prolonged pressure on nerves may bring paralysis

Possible loss of bladder and bowel control

Atrophy of muscles

Loss of reflexes

Numbness and tingling

SPINE

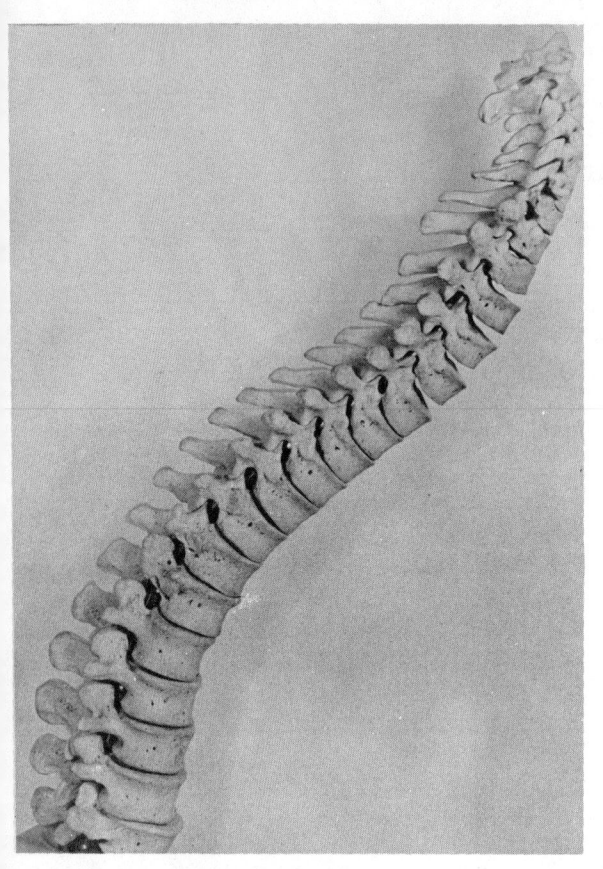

Spine—Model showing the position of the backbone when a person is bent forward with the head held erect. The spine is viewed from the right side. The bones of the spinal column increase in size downward. The cervical at the top is the smallest bone and the lumbar toward the bottom is the largest.

Spinal fracture, or any injury to the spinal cord or back or spine that seems to involve the nervous system, requires the immediate attention of a *neurologist*. X-ray study of all bones involved is essential.

Restoring the bones affected to their normal position is a primary expedient, usually done by a *surgeon* or *orthopedist,* a specialist in correction of deformities of the back and limbs. Supports to hold the bones in place while they are healing will then be applied. In some instances when nerves associated with the excretory functions have been damaged, the patient will need assistance with bladder and bowel action.

When there is any possibility that a person has a broken back, the person should be moved as little as possible and a doctor called immediately. Under the supervision of the doctor, the injured person will be placed, with a minimum of movement, onto a board for transport to the hospital. If the neck is broken, it is essential that the head be kept motionless. Deadening of sensation in parts of the body below the point of injury and loss of bowel and bladder control are signs of serious damage. Serious spinal injury will probably produce shock and the victim must be kept warm and, if it can be done without moving him, the head placed lower than the rest of the body. *See* MEDIGRAPHS pages 659, 1221.

SPINE, the column of small bones, called *vertebrae,* and associated tissues which maintains the body in its erect posture. The spine or backbone is a kind of natural spring, elastic in character and shaped like an S, which prevents the body from suffering the incessant shocks it would get if the spine were a single solid bone. Between the vertebrae are *cartilaginous discs,* which have further shock-absorbing action and which permit turning and twisting motion without friction among the vertebrae.

The spine also carries the spinal cord and its extensions, which provide not only intercommunication between the brain and much of the body but regulate many reflex functions.

The spine, made up of such heavy bones and so well protected by associated muscles, is one of the most secure parts of the body. *See also* BACKACHE; CHIROPRACTIC; SLIPPED DISC; SPINAL CORD. *See* MEDIGRAPHS pages 1211, 1221.

SPLEEN, a large, ductless, gland-like organ which lies in the upper left part of the abdomen, just below the diaphragm and toward the rear of the body.

Although the functions of the spleen are known to have significant relationships to the character and circulation of the blood, they are not fully understood. One unanswered problem concerns the dissolution and disposal of red cells of the blood which have exhausted their usefulness, and another surrounds the production of new blood cells. Since such cells are intimately concerned with combatting infection, the spleen is further implicated in the *control of disease.*

At times the spleen contracts, discharging a quantity of blood into the general circulation. Therefore, when an animal or human being exercises intensively, the spleen is believed to *maintain the proper volume of blood circulating in the blood vessels.*

Animal experiments have provided some interesting information regarding the spleen. The organ it-

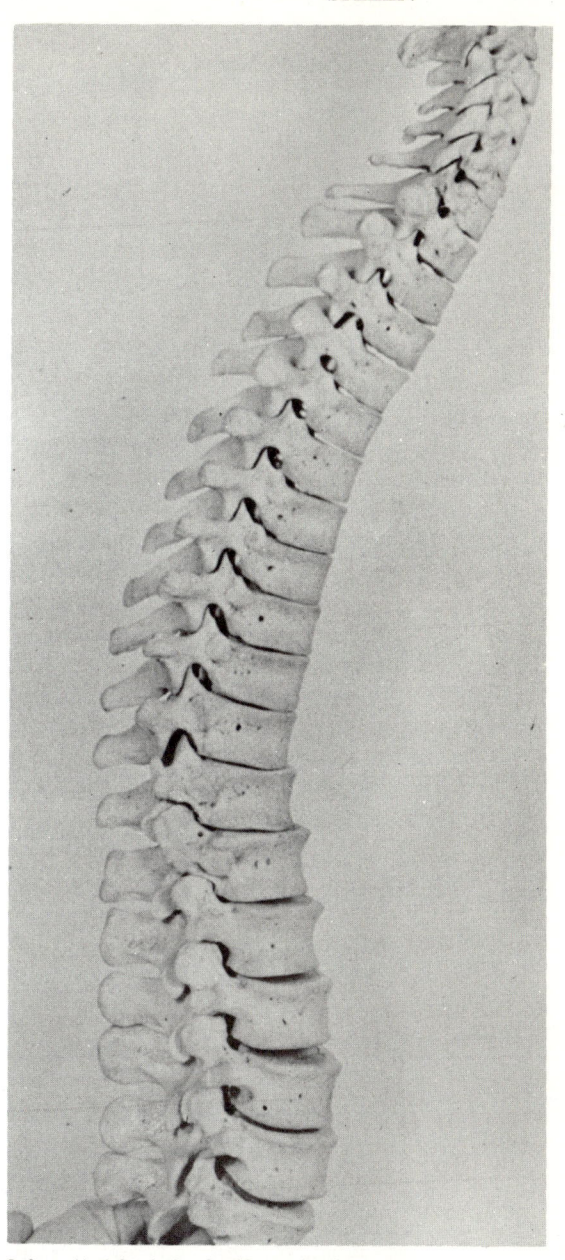

Spine—Model of the backbone in the erect position as seen from the right side. The spine is made up of 33 vertebrae, 24 of which are movable. The pattern of the spine permits flexibility in bending. When in the erect position, the spine forms a normal shallow S curvature.

self evidently does not experience pain. Thus, by operation, a celluloid window can be inserted in an animal's abdominal wall and the behavior of the spleen can be watched directly. The spleen can also be transplanted to a location outside the abdomen. When this is done, skin rapidly grows over the spleen, and its expansion and contraction can be observed directly.

An ancient idea, that the spleen is related to emotions, is expressed in the phrase *venting your spleen.* Experiments on dogs tend to justify this. A dog which was a confirmed cat chaser was trained to lie motionless on a table. Then the doctor would put before the dog's nose, alternately, first a duster which had not touched a cat, then a duster which had been in a basket with a cat. Although the dog continued to lie motionless when it smelled the second duster, its spleen could be observed to contract. Smelling the other duster left the dog's spleen unaffected.

Other animal experiments have revealed the contraction and discharge of blood under the influence of exercise. When the exertion is intensive enough, the kidney may become so depleted of blood that it suffers actual damage. Evidently, then, the activity of the spleen in maintaining evenness of blood circulation helps to protect other organs which might be adversely affected without this supplement.

Enlargement of the spleen is a disorder of variable sources. Sometimes enlargement is due to splenic destructive activity against worn-out blood cells and disease-creating organisms which are retained within the spleen. Sometimes a fatty material enlarges the spleen. Enlargement of the spleen appears in several major infectious diseases, among them malaria.

Other conditions which tend to chronic splenic enlargement are *Hodgkin's disease, splenic anemia, pernicious anemia, leukemia,* and *hydatid* and *amyloid diseases.* Furthermore, acute enlargement may accompany *enteric fever, anthrax, pyemia, septicemia,* and other infections.

Rupture may occur either because of external injury, as in an automobile accident, or spontaneously in connection with a massive enlargement. *Hemorrhage* is then intense, because the extensive blood supply which normally passes through or is bound in the spleen pours into the abdomen. If delay is not protracted, the condition can be treated surgically.

Splenic enlargement may accompany *leukemia* or a condition known as *Banti's disease,* in which severe anemia occurs.

An enlarged spleen is not always explicable, and if an adequate cause is not ascertained the organ must be removed. In such cases a *lymphoma* or tumor of lymphoid tissue may be responsible. In certain specific diseases—such as *purpura hemorrhagica* or *thrombocytopenia,* a clotting disorder of the blood—removal of the spleen is considered beneficial. In the case of *Banti's disease,* splenectomy is not generally recommended. The spleen is not essential to life—as is, for example, the liver—and its removal rarely produces adverse effects. *See also* THROMBOCYTOPENIA.

SPLENIC DISEASE. Primary disorders of the spleen are so rare that the spleen has been considered an anticancerous organ, although secondary cancer of the spleen does occur. However, like other tissues of the body the spleen is liable to injuries from falls, wounds, and accidents. In some disorders the spleen fills the entire left side of the abdomen and weighs many pounds. Disturbance of circulation of the blood in the spleen is characterized by acute abdominal pain and a sudden increase in the size of the organ.

Among unusual conditions affecting the spleen are the appearance of *accessory spleens* scattered through the abdomen; and *floating* or *wandering spleen,* in which the tissues which hold it in place become relaxed and the organ moves from position, a condition far more frequent in women than men.

Often the spleen is enlarged in *malaria, leukemia* and other blood diseases, and can be a symptom of many generalized diseases. In *Banti's syndrome,* extreme enlargement of the spleen is associated with severe *anemia.*

Sometimes surgical removal of the spleen is considered helpful—for instance, in severe cases of *purpura hemorrhagica* or *thrombocytopenia,* a condition in which the blood does not clot easily. The spleen may also be removed when *tumors* are present.

Steroid hormones, ACTH, and *cortisone* are valuable in splenic disease to lessen the destruction of red blood cells. ACTH and cortisone may be employed before an operation for removal of the spleen, often in connection with transfusions of whole fresh blood. *See also* SPLEEN.

SPONDYLOLISTHESIS, or *slipped vertebra,* a condition in which an exaggerated lumbar curve is formed when the fifth vertebra is so affected as to slip forward toward the front of the body. This abnormality is caused by defective growth of bone in the neural arch. Because support is lacking, the condition causes backache, which disappears when the person rests. The pain reappears on exertion and is felt down the thigh and leg. *See also* SLIPPED DISC. *See* MEDIGRAPH page 1211.

SPOROTRICHOSIS, an infection of the skin and mucous membranes, caused by a fungus, the *Sporotrichum schenckii,* which grows on plants and brush. Persons exposed to vegetation, such as gardeners or farmers, are most apt to become infected, usually by acquiring the fungus on the skin or a break in the skin. Sporotrichosis has also been found in horses, dogs, and cats.

About twenty days to three months after contact with the fungus, a hard rubbery growth appears at the site of injury. The growth hardens, becomes inflamed, and gradually breaks through the skin, discharging a small amount of thin pus. The surrounding skin becomes discolored and finally turns black. The infec-

the injury and its causes SPRAIN A sprain occurs when there is rupture of individual fibers or small groups of fibers of the *ligament* which holds a joint together. It is caused by the stretching of these ligaments in an injury. All joints can be involved in sprains. In areas where the ligaments surrounding a joint are very extensive, the involvement can extend over a considerable area. An example of this is the ankle, where discomfort from a sprain may extend to the top of the foot.

STRAIN A strain is the parting or rupture of certain strands or fibers of a *muscle*. It is usually brought on by extreme muscle activity, particularly by heavy activity to which the muscle is not accustomed. Strains occur most commonly in the muscles of the back. However, the arms and legs are also subject to strains, especially in people involved in athletics or any activity in which these parts are used extensively.

symptoms As shown in the Medi-Graph, the symptoms are pain and swelling which limit the use and motion of the joint or muscle involved. Pain increases when there is tension on the injured part, and decreases when the part is in a relaxed position. Black and blue marks discolor the skin, marking the spread of blood surrounding the injured area.

complications SPRAIN There are no serious complications involved in sprains except the disability they cause.
STRAIN Occasionally a complication of strain is the development of adhesions (an abnormal sticking together) between the torn muscle fibers. This results in prolonged pain and disability.

prevention (or lessening of impact) SPRAIN Once it is established that there is no broken bone, the sprained area should be rested. For the first 24 hours cold should be applied to reduce the swelling. Follow with heat and general massage. In cases of severe swelling, it is best to strap the joint firmly so that the injured part is rested as much as possible. The physician will generally allow the patient to undertake modified activity, and suggest that the patient make progressive use of the injured part as he finds he can do so.
STRAIN If the pain is very severe, the patient should be put to bed with the injured part raised up and at rest. Heat is usually very helpful, and gentle massage hastens recovery. It is advisable that the patient exercise the part in gradually increasing amounts as soon as he is able. If necessary, the part can be bandaged for support with a light splint or elastic type bandage.

Sprains and Strains

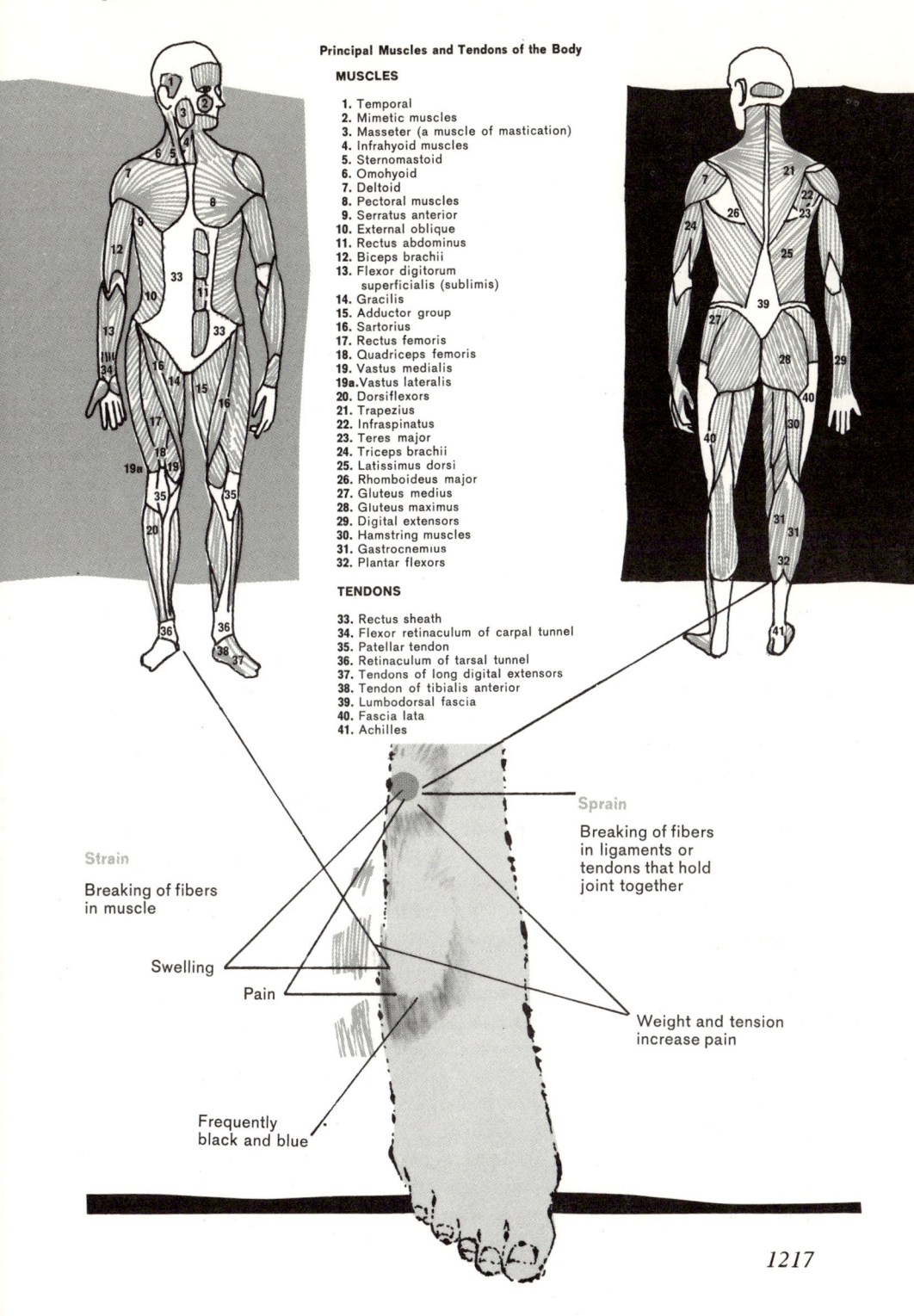

Principal Muscles and Tendons of the Body

MUSCLES

1. Temporal
2. Mimetic muscles
3. Masseter (a muscle of mastication)
4. Infrahyoid muscles
5. Sternomastoid
6. Omohyoid
7. Deltoid
8. Pectoral muscles
9. Serratus anterior
10. External oblique
11. Rectus abdominus
12. Biceps brachii
13. Flexor digitorum superficialis (sublimis)
14. Gracilis
15. Adductor group
16. Sartorius
17. Rectus femoris
18. Quadriceps femoris
19. Vastus medialis
19a. Vastus lateralis
20. Dorsiflexors
21. Trapezius
22. Infraspinatus
23. Teres major
24. Triceps brachii
25. Latissimus dorsi
26. Rhomboideus major
27. Gluteus medius
28. Gluteus maximus
29. Digital extensors
30. Hamstring muscles
31. Gastrocnemius
32. Plantar flexors

TENDONS

33. Rectus sheath
34. Flexor retinaculum of carpal tunnel
35. Patellar tendon
36. Retinaculum of tarsal tunnel
37. Tendons of long digital extensors
38. Tendon of tibialis anterior
39. Lumbodorsal fascia
40. Fascia lata
41. Achilles

Strain
Breaking of fibers in muscle

Sprain
Breaking of fibers in ligaments or tendons that hold joint together

Swelling

Pain

Weight and tension increase pain

Frequently black and blue

1217

tion may spread to other skin areas, but rarely affects any internal organs.

Potassium iodide has been used successfully to treat sporotrichosis and is often continued for at least a month after apparent recovery as a safety measure. Abscesses which are slow in healing may be drained to hasten recovery and then treated with the iodide. *See* MEDIGRAPH page 665.

SPRAINS, injuries in the area of a joint, in which a sudden movement or a fall will stretch or overstrain connective tissue fibers belonging to the *ligaments, muscles,* or *tendons* so that they are torn or ruptured. Fluid or blood then gets into the joint. Sometimes a sprain is so severe that a bone is broken. For this reason every severe sprain should be x-rayed. The opening of the football season and the onset of winter produce a sudden increase in the number of sprains, particularly of the ankle.

It is advisable to treat the injury as soon as possible. A firm bandage should be applied evenly and smoothly over the joint in order to limit internal bleeding. If materials are available, the sprain may be treated by putting a layer of cotton wool about an inch thick over the joint, and for an inch or two beyond it on either side, and bandaging as firmly as possible without causing discomfort.

First-aid measures are helpful, but most sprains require medical attention. Ordinarily a simple sprain is treated by rest, elevation of the leg and ankle, and the application of an ice bag. The doctor will immobilize the joint by strapping or he may use adhesive materials or even apply a plaster cast. Current treatment, however, recommends movement of the joint as soon as possible. In order to control accompanying pain, the physician may inject an anesthetic substance into the injured area, thus permitting the patient to use the foot or hand.

Movement is difficult in a joint which has been fixed in one position for a long time, particularly if inflammation and swelling are pronounced. In such cases movement is not attempted immediately, but gradually. The bandage may be removed for a short time, and the joint gently massaged to aid softening of the tissues and relaxation of the stiffness. Heat should not be applied to a sprained ankle until the danger of congestion and hemorrhage has been controlled. The value of heat is greatest in the final stages, when repair has begun, in order to encourage circulation and absorption of excess fluid. *See also* JOINTS AND JOINT DISORDERS. *See* MEDI-GRAPHS pages 659, 1217.

SPRUE, a feverless chronic disease. *Sprue* comes from the Dutch word that describes an *inflammation of the mouth.* The disease, known for more than two thousand years, is generally considered to be a tropical ailment, although it will occur in persons who do not live in the tropics. Both *tropical* and *nontropical sprue* are probably *nutritional deficiency disorders of the small intestine,* marked by impaired absorption of food elements, particularly fats. However, the exact cause is unknown.

Symptoms of sprue are *diarrhea, cramps,* and *distended stomach* due to gas. The material from the bowels is pale, greasy, unformed and foul, and occasionally watery. The person with sprue becomes emaciated, muscles and fat waste away, and, in advanced cases, recovery is difficult. Clubbed fingers and spotted skin may develop. When the person also suffers from a vitamin B complex deficiency, fissures develop at the corners of the mouth and the tongue is smooth and fiery red.

In the past, many different kinds of diets were tried in treating sprue. Currently *liver preparations* and *folic acid* have produced favorable results. In sprue, treatment also involves a careful control of the diet, which should be moderately bland, low in fat, and high in proteins. Calcium intake can be increased with *skim milk* and *calcium lactate tablets,* and *ripe bananas, vitamin* B_{12}, and *iron supplements* have been found beneficial. Occasionally *antibiotics* and *cortisone* have been temporarily successful, but their prolonged use presents certain problems. Sometimes small and repeated *blood transfusions* have been helpful, even life-saving, in critical cases of sprue.

SQUINT, or *strabismus,* failure to focus both eyes on the same point. In the most common form, one eye looks toward the object while the other is turned from it.

There are many kinds of squints, caused by a large number of disorders and diseases in the eye, the muscles that move it, the nerves supplying them, and the brain which controls and coordinates the nerve impulses.

An eye specialist (*ophthalmologist*) can determine the exact type of squint a person has and then prescribe treatment. Frequently a squint may be cured by wearing special glasses. Sometimes the squinting eye must be trained and special exercises with certain instruments are prescribed. In some cases surgery on the muscles of the eyeball may be advisable.

Treatment is generally effective, but requires the cooperation of the patient. When a child has a squint, sympathetic attitudes on the part of his family and persons around him can be of great help. *See also* EYE.

STAMMERING. *See* STUTTERING AND STAMMERING.

STANFORD-BINET TEST. The Stanford-Binet "I.Q." or Intelligence Quotient test is a revision of the Binet-Simon tests which were originally conducted in France by two French psychologists, Binet and Simon, who had been commissioned by the French government to study the conditions of mentally defective persons. They did extensive research to determine what the normal child should be expected to do at any particular age.

No test has yet been developed which can conclusively measure someone's intelligence, but many different methods have been tried, with

1219

the injury and its causes Whiplash is seen more and more and has become a distressing medical and legal problem. It is generally the result of an automobile accident in which a car that is slowing down or completely stopped is hit forcibly from the rear. Studies show that in such cases the patient's head is first snapped back and then forward, with considerable force. A head-on collision with any object can also cause whiplash. The damage that results is something like a severe sprain that might be found about any joint. Damage is usually done to the ligaments supporting the vertebrae of the neck. There is stretching, some tearing, and sometimes internal bleeding around the injured area. The injury can take a very long time to heal, and during the recovery period the patient cannot do anything that would put strain on his arms, shoulders, and neck.

symptoms At the time of the accident there may be only a few symptoms or none at all. The patient may complain of a slight neck pain or inability to move his head freely. After 24 hours the neck pain increases and the victim cannot move his head in any direction, particularly forward and backward, without pain. Muscles over the front or back of the neck can become very tight and tender to touch. The pain radiates into the shoulders or down to the fingertips. Weakness, numbness, or tingling in one or both arms is not unusual. Occasionally the patient complains that he has a headache and feels dizzy and nauseated when he changes his position.

complications The accident causing whiplash can also cause a fracture or dislocation of a vertebra of the neck. Sometimes herniation of a cervical disc occurs. This means that one of the discs located between the neck's vertebrae has been pushed out of position. It may then press on the nerves emerging from the spinal column and cause severe pain.
This herniated disc or other severe nerve injury resulting from the whiplash can interfere with full use of the upper extremities and be a serious handicap to a working man or woman.

prevention (or lessening of impact) The most logical preventive step is to drive carefully. Cars should be equipped with such safety equipment as seat belts and head rests and these should be used whenever the car is in use. Drug therapy, neck supports, and physiotherapy are available for the patient with a whiplash injury to the neck. Orthopedic and medical care can make him more comfortable and minimize his disability.

Whiplash Injury of the Neck

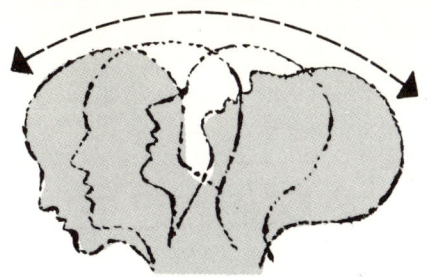

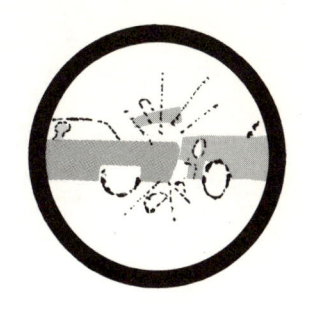

1. Accident As result of sharp impact, head snaps back and forth with great force

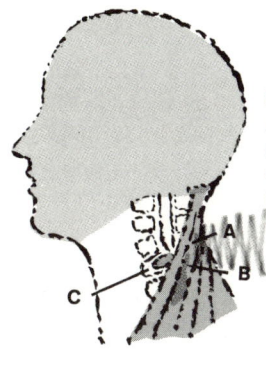

2. Damage
A. Stretching and tearing of ligaments
B. Bleeding around injured area
C. Occasionally goes on to severe nerve injury. Herniation of cervical disc, fracture or dislocation may be accompanying injuries

3. Initial Reaction
May be slight neck pain and limitation of head movement—or little noticeable pain

4. After 24 Hours
Weakness
Headache
Dizziness
Nausea
Front and back neck muscles tender to touch
Pain may radiate on position change
Increased pain—especially when moving head forward or backward
Numbness
Tingling

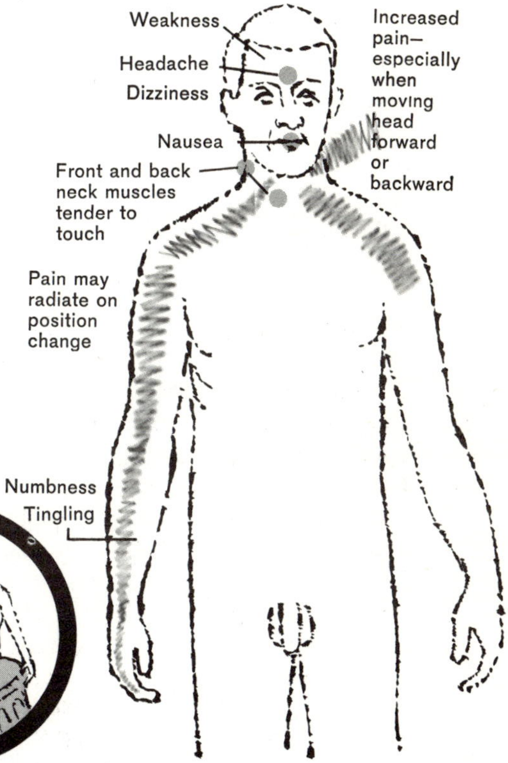

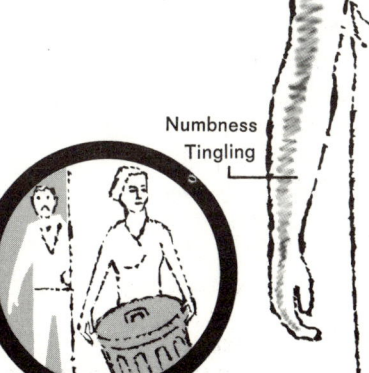

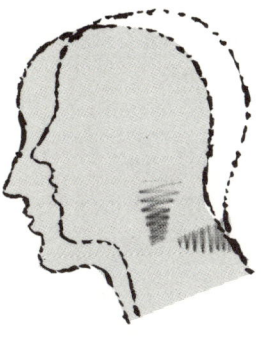

5. Next Several Weeks
Pain and weakness in neck, shoulders, arms during lifting or other strain producing activities

1221

varying degrees of success. The Stanford revision of the Binet-Simon test is one of the most widely used at present. The "I.Q.", a numerical rating, is determined by dividing the chronological age of the child tested into the age level the child achieves on the test and multiplying the result by 100. For example, a ten-year-old child who has the capacity of a twelve-year-old child, according to the standard of achievement for each age group, has an I.Q. rating of 120. The average child is therefore rated at 100. Only one quality is tested, the reasoning intelligence. According to this scale, a person scoring below 70 is a moron; below 50, an imbecile; and below 20, an idiot. Out of a total of 500,000 mentally deficient persons in the United States, 30,000 are classified as idiots, 100,000 as imbeciles, and the rest as morons. See also INTELLIGENCE; GENIUS; FEEBLE-MINDEDNESS.

ST. ANTHONY'S FIRE. See ERYSIPELAS.

STERILITY, the incapacity to produce children, a complex phenomenon involving a variety of factors. Chief responsibility may be borne by the woman, the man, or both. Even when one or the other is specifically accountable, sterility may apply only to a given set of circumstances; in another situation the same person might not be sterile. Because of its variability, sterility may properly be regarded as characteristic of a particular union of two persons, rather than of either the man or the woman separately. Scientists have determined that circumstances pertaining to the marriage relationship may cause sterility.

Some marriages are deliberately childless, the husband and wife having decided to take measures to assure this. Other marriages, childless for other reasons, constitute 10 per cent of all marriages in the United States and Great Britain, according to investigators.

In the past, a childless marriage was often assumed to be solely the responsibility of the wife. However, medical statistics indicate that men are responsible for 30 to 40 per cent of all instances of childlessness. Diagnosis of the condition and endeavors to correct it demand first an examination of the husband. If the results indicate that he is responsible, the general physical condition of the wife is determined. A frequent cause of sterility in men is some disorder associated with the male reproductive cell, the *sperm,* one of which must fertilize an *ovum,* or female egg cell to produce conception. These male cells are produced in the *testicles,* the two male sex glands, and stored in the *seminal vesicles,* higher in the body.

Such disorders may involve various organs or tissues. The glands may not produce sperm cells even though otherwise the man appears to be sexually normal. The sperm cells produced may be weak or malformed, so that they cannot function properly and carry the fertilization process to the final stage. Furthermore, there may be insufficient numbers of them; although only one sperm can fertilize a given egg cell, a normal male provides as many as several hundred million of them on each ejaculation. Any of these conditions may be responsible for the woman's failure to conceive, and the doctor has means for testing to find out whether or not such a condition is present.

Conditions in the woman which prevent conception are even more varied than in the man. Among the simplest are *infection, inflammation,* or *injury* of the parts of the body involved. Sometimes the cause is blockage of a passage through which the sperm cells should travel. Occasionally congenital deformities of the sexual organs may cause such *occlusion* or otherwise render conception impossible. In a few instances the uterus may be undeveloped or missing entirely.

A frequent cause of sterility in women is some irregularity in the system of glands of internal secretion, the *endocrine glands,* or of their products, the *hormones.* The sex glands are a significant part of the whole glandular network, and a mishap in the latter can affect the female sexual cycle at one of several points, making conception difficult or impossible.

Other conditions which can induce sterility include *faulty diet,* a subject not yet thoroughly understood, and *emotional or mental disturbances* which can react upon physical factors.

That a woman has not attempted to prevent conception and still has not conceived does not necessarily mean that pregnancy is impossible for her. The condition may continue for years and then terminate in a normal pregnancy and delivery.

Complete physical examination of both husband and wife by a doctor is essential for the couple who seem sterile and wish to correct it. Such an examination will include studies of sperm cells of the husband and examination of the wife's sexual organs to determine their condition and whether or not the necessary tubes are open and functioning properly. A complete record of the sex experiences of both husband and wife is also imperative. The cause or causes that the physician finds operative will determine the recommendations. Often a previously sterile couple can achieve conception by careful use of knowledge of the alternating periods of fertility and infertility in the female, regulated by the *menstrual cycle.* When a disease has closed one or both of the Fallopian tubes within the woman, attempts to free them by surgery or forcing a passage of air through them are only rarely successful. *See* MEDIGRAPHS pages 469, 923, 995, 1179, 1307.

STERILIZATION, an operation which renders the male incapable of fertilizing the female by severing the *vasa deferentia,* making it impossible for sperm cells from the testicles to reach the outside. The operation is not necessarily irreversible, but probably is so in the majority of cases. Sterilized males can still enjoy sexual intercourse, ejaculating the secretions of the accessory sex glands. It is to be distinguished from *castration,* which involves excision of the

1223

testicles. A sterilized male does not lose any of his secondary sexual characteristics; the male hormones produced by the testicles continue to circulate in the blood stream. See also STERILITY; FERTILITY; CASTRATION; IMPOTENCE; VAS DEFERENS; REPRODUCTION SYSTEM; SEXUAL INTERCOURSE; CYSTIC FIBROSIS.

STOMACH, the portion of the *alimentary tract*—the digestive tube—which extends from the lower end of the *esophagus* or *gullet*—the canal extending from the *pharynx*—to the beginning of the *duodenum* or first part of the small intestine. The normal stomach is J-shaped with a bulge above and to the left of the junction with the esophagus. The shape varies according to its fullness or emptiness and the position of the person.

The stomach narrows to join the small intestine, forming the *pyloric canal* which has a thick muscular valve called the *pyloric sphincter*. Three muscular coats in the wall of the stomach are covered inside by a layer of mucus and a submucous lining containing blood vessels, lymphatics, and nerves. The internal surface of the stomach contains the minute gastric glands which manufacture *hydrochloric acid* and certain ferments which digest food into simpler substances. The muscular walls grind and mix the food with the gastric juices. About every twenty seconds, a wave of contraction passes along the stomach from the upper part to the pylorus. During digestion, the contractions also cause partially digested food to pass into the duodenum in the form of *chyme,* a thick fluid.

Various congenital deformities may affect the stomach, such as *enlargement of the muscle of the pyloric valve. Gastroptosis* (dropped stomach) may occur later in life. Surgery is generally successful in correcting congenital abnormalities when they are known.

Inflammation of the lining of the stomach is a common disorder, occurring in various forms and at any time throughout life. *Peptic ulcers* are another common stomach disorder, resulting from action of the gastric juices on the stomach wall. An increase in the amount or concentration of gastric juice causes acidity.

Cancer of the stomach is responsible for a great number of deaths each year in the United States. It usually occurs in late middle age and more often in men than women, men past forty-five being the most frequent victims. Cancer of the stomach is of several types. including *ulcerating cancer, tumor* growing in the stomach cavity, and a *diffuse thickening* of the stomach wall. Loss of weight, appetite, and general normal health are symptoms of stomach cancer, but unfortunately the cancer is often too far advanced before it is detected to be effectively treated and may have spread to regional lymph nodes and other organs. Because of the danger of stomach cancer, any form of stomach "upset" after middle age should receive immediate medical attention. If the cancer is discovered soon enough, an operation to remove the cancer with a portion or even all of the stomach can be successful in curing the condition, and so it is imperative that it be diagnosed at the earliest possible time. Cancer of the stomach is too often a hopelessly fatal disease because of a late diagnosis. See also DIGESTION; FISTULA; FOOD POISONING; GASTRITIS; INDIGESTION; PEPTIC ULCER. See MEDIGRAPHS pages 297, 1297.

STOMACH ACHE. See ABDOMINAL PAIN.

STOMACH ULCER. See PEPTIC ULCER.

STOMATITIS, an inflammation of the mucous membranes of the mouth, sometimes attributable to a riboflavin deficiency. See also DEFICIENCY DISEASES.

STREPTOCOCCUS, a genus of *bacteria* which grows in chains, resembling tiny strings of beads when viewed under the microscope. *Streptococcus* germs are present in infections such as *erysipelas, scarlet fever, subacute bacterial endocarditis, puerperal fever, septic sore throat,* and certain forms of *enteritis* and *rheumatic fever.*

STREPTOMYCIN, an *antibiotic* drug obtained from the moldlike microscopic plant, *Streptomyces griseus.* It is similar to *penicillin* in its antibacterial action and method of manufacture, and has been found particularly effective against many disease-producing germs that penicillin also attacks. In addition it is a powerful agent against some diseases that are not affected by penicillin, such as *tularemia,* a severe infectious disease acquired in handling infected rabbits.

Streptomycin is also effective in treating certain types of *blood* and *urinary infections* which are not helped by other drugs. Reports indicate that it may cure *tuberculous meningitis,* and it has been successfully used in diseases produced by the *common colon bacillus. Pneumonia, streptococcus infections, staphylococcal pneumonia,* and *staphylococcal meningitis* are among the many diseases in which streptomycin has been effectively used.

Streptomycin is taken orally or injected directly into the blood stream, as the condition dictates. In cases of meningitis, it is injected into the spinal fluid. See also ANTIBIOTICS.

STRESS, a state of tension or pressure which may be physical, such as results from accident or injury; or emotional, such as stress caused by an impending threat or other difficult situation. It is in the latter, the psychological sense that the word stress is generally used in medicine today.

People have been aware that emotions affect the body long before science proved it experimentally. Expressions such as "became paralyzed with fear," "sick with disgust," "trembling with anger," are commonly heard in everyday life. Emotions are, however, more far-reaching than such visible evidence indicates. Any emotion, mild or severe, registers in every cell and tissue of the body. With a strong emotion, such as fear, the entire body tone changes: blood pressure rises, heart and breathing are faster, the adrenal glands become more active, and changes in the gastrointestinal tract and shifting of blood supply take place.

The stress may be situational, that is, it may be caused by a specific difficult situation or danger; or the stress may be present without an actual threat but because of underlying emotional problems. Moreover, the physiological changes of a stress situation may sometimes be brought about by merely discussing the threat, as illustrated, for example, by a girl who repressed feelings of hostility toward her family but brought them into the open in the doctor's office.

Stress, it is thus evident, can build up. If the stress resulting from underlying emotional problems continues for a long time, various physical symptoms may be produced. The patient may develop high blood pressure, stomach ulcers, diarrhea, constipation or other conditions. Some authorities estimate that at least one half of general medical practice is for such stress-induced diseases.

These diseases are considered by some to be protective measures taken by the individual against threats or symbols of danger which the early experience of the individual unconsciously interprets as actual fearful dangers. Why some people react to life stresses with peptic ulcer, others with high blood pressure or diarrhea or headache or no disease at all, depends on many factors, on which there is no general agreement. Most theories, however, take into account early infantile and childhood experiences, or a total life experience together with physiological factors.

There are people in whom life stresses build up to a degree in which the "mental load" is too burdensome. In such cases what is commonly called a *nervous breakdown* may result, the duration and severity of which depend also on a complex of factors. Relatively minor stresses may find expression in a variety of ways. A common outlet for repressed hostility, for example, may be seen in the individual who drives recklessly and violently, almost obviously in pursuit of an accident.

Apart from the repressed and unresolved mental conflicts of the individual, social attitudes add their own stresses. These social attitudes vary with different cultures and they vary also in different times. However, basic in treating certain diseases, many believe, is the uncovering of hidden emotional conflicts that find expression in those diseases and in personality disorders. The stresses of life, they feel, can be managed if the personality has not been impaired by early life experiences. *See also* ANXIETY; EMOTIONAL HEALTH; FEAR; PSYCHOSOMATIC DISORDERS.

STROKE, a sudden and severe seizure or fit of disease. The term is generally used for *apoplexy,* and in connection with sunstroke and heatstroke. *See also* APOPLEXY; HEAT SICKNESS. *See* MEDIGRAPH page 1229.

STUTTERING AND STAMMERING may be described as spasmodic speech defects, resulting in a sudden check in the flow of words, or a rapid repetition of a consonant or consonants with which the person has difficulty. Usually the difficulty is with the sounds *p, b, m,* and *w,* which are sounds made by the lips. The stutterer or stammerer does not, however, always have difficulty with the same sounds. His emotional state at the time of speaking may be a factor in how he speaks.

Stuttering or stammering are almost never due to any organic weakness, either in the organs used in speaking or in the nerves and nerve centers which control them. Physical factors may, however, sometimes aggravate it. The doctor will first make sure that inflammation of *adenoids,* abnormal length of *uvula,* abnormal size of the *tongue,* and improper development of the *mouth* are not involved.

Often children who stutter develop behavior changes; a fear of appearing ridiculous produces a subsequent lack of confidence. Persons naturally left-handed but trained to use their right hand stammer more frequently than others, and males more often than females. Anyone acutely embarrassed or terrified is likely to stammer, until his emotion is under control. Stammering is usually an expression of self-consciousness, shyness, or fear. In an eager youngster, however, it may be nothing more than failure to keep up with his rapid flow of thought; words and thoughts are conceived faster than they can be expressed. Stammerers almost always can sing and talk to themselves quite fluently.

Because stuttering and stammering are primarily conditions which have emotional causes, treatment is directed toward the person's mental conflicts. When the conflict is resolved, the person will probably regain self-confidence and the speech defect disappears. The person with a speech defect may benefit from special speech correction classes. A class is often preferable to personal instruction since the person will be encouraged by the progress of others and the realization that he is not alone in his problem. His family and friends must be patient, tolerant, and confident; anger and impatience will only aggravate the situation. *See also* PSYCHOSOMATIC DISORDERS.

STY. *See* EYE.

SUFFOCATION. *See* ASPHYXIA.

SUICIDE. Every year about 20,000 people in the United States kill themselves. Suicide is not, therefore, an exceedingly prominent cause of death. Nevertheless, suicides are always attracting attention because of the natural drama associated with them.

Why do three and a half times as many men as women attempt suicide? Why is the tendency to commit suicide greater among older than among young people? It seems that

the disease and its causes The term stroke is a broad descriptive word used to describe the effects of any interference with circulation within the brain. Strokes are properly called cerebral vascular accidents. They occur in a number of ways, as shown in the Medi-Graph. The blood supply to the brain is blocked by a thrombosis or clot which blocks the entrance to a narrowed and roughened section of artery; an embolus, which is a clot that is carried from another part of the body, usually the heart, blocks normal blood passage; a brain artery bursts and is unable to furnish brain cells with essential, nourishing blood; and, in rare instances, brain tumors or abscesses press on an artery and close it off.

A doctor cannot always be sure of the precise cause of a stroke, but he makes his diagnosis on the basis of the manner in which the attack occurred, the age of the patient, X ray studies, and the presence of possible contributing factors such as arteriosclerosis, high blood pressure, rheumatic or coronary heart disease, and diabetes. While the patient's condition seems to be the same regardless of the cause of the attack, the outlook and treatment differ.

Both men and women are affected, usually in the older age group.

symptoms A stroke can occur without any warning and without any seeming relation to any event in the life of the patient or his physical condition. He can awake from sleep and show signs of paralysis affecting his extremities or his face. However, frequently there is warning—usually a period of numbness on one side, perhaps some headache, and often weakness of the face or an extremity which disappears after a time.

When the attack comes full force, there is paralysis of one side of the body, with all the symptoms noted in the Medi-Graph. Generally, strokes caused by a cerebral thrombosis are slower to develop than those caused by hemorrhage or emboli. In the case of emboli, there is immediate collapse and sometimes shock. Hemorrhage may cause severe headache and stiffness of the neck before the paralysis develops.

The areas of weakness or paralysis depend upon just where the accident occurs in the brain. Small blood vessel damage causes local areas of weakness or numbness; larger cerebral blood vessel damage causes larger areas of paralysis and weakness.

complications These depend upon the severity of the attack. Severe brain destruction can cause death. Specific areas of brain damage can cause respiratory and cardiac failure. Patients who become paralyzed are subject to the complications of bed rest—pneumonia, kidney infections, bed sores, and blood clots.

prevention (or lessening of impact) Anti-coagulants help patients with heart disease capable of forming emboli. Surgery is effective in cases with early signs of thrombosis in the neck arteries. Severe high blood pressure must be treated by a physician. When paralysis has occurred, the patient must be protected against secondary infection and started on physical therapy as soon as possible.

Stroke (Apoplexy)

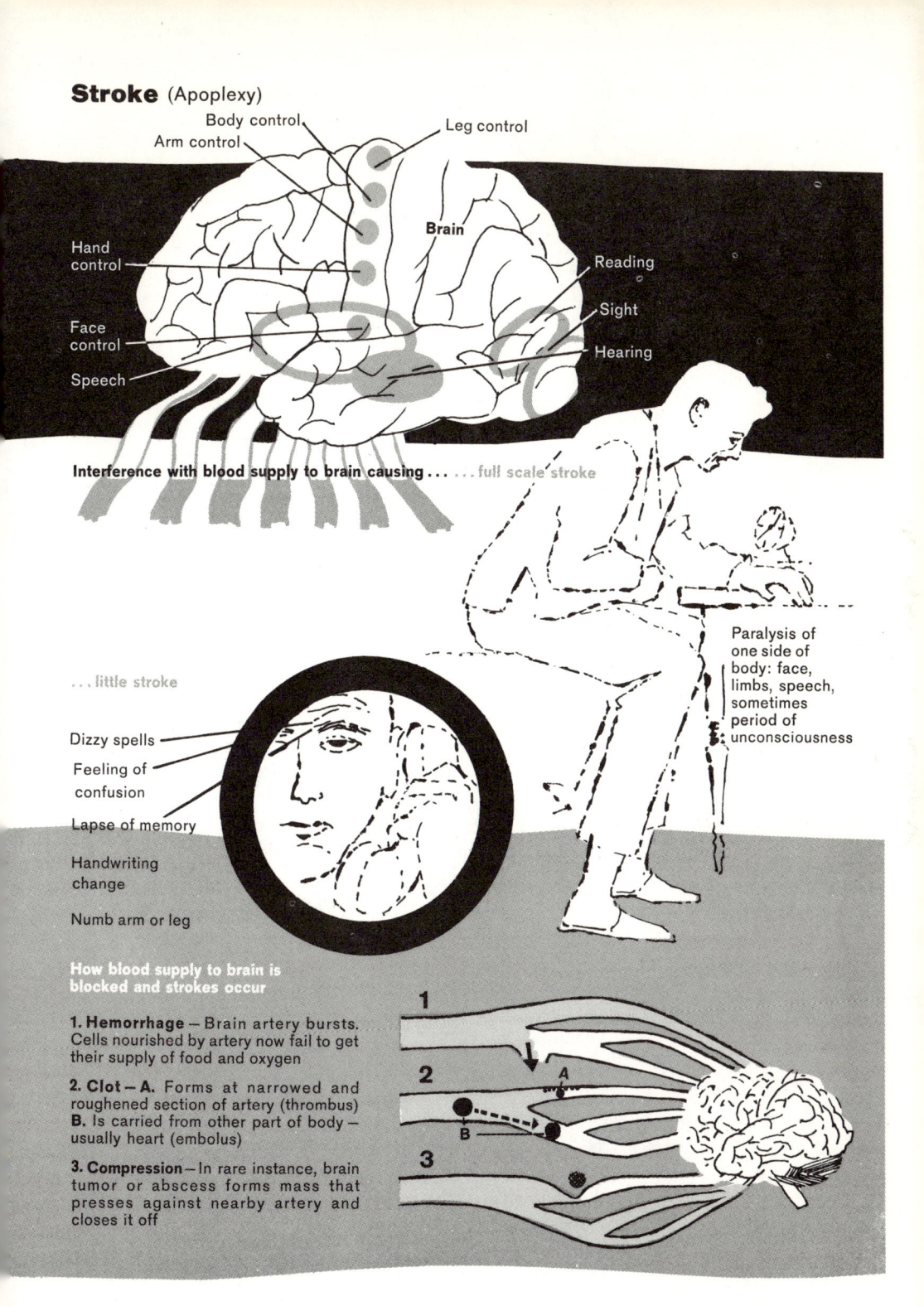

Body control
Arm control
Leg control
Hand control
Brain
Reading
Sight
Hearing
Face control
Speech

Interference with blood supply to brain causing ..... full scale stroke

Paralysis of one side of body: face, limbs, speech, sometimes period of unconsciousness

... little stroke

Dizzy spells
Feeling of confusion
Lapse of memory
Handwriting change
Numb arm or leg

How blood supply to brain is blocked and strokes occur

1. Hemorrhage — Brain artery bursts. Cells nourished by artery now fail to get their supply of food and oxygen

2. Clot — **A.** Forms at narrowed and roughened section of artery (thrombus) **B.** Is carried from other part of body — usually heart (embolus)

3. Compression — In rare instance, brain tumor or abscess forms mass that presses against nearby artery and closes it off

1229

suicide results chiefly from the discouragement and hopelessness of later years of life. During war the suicide rate always drops.

People differ as to the methods by which they commit suicide. The agents most frequently used are firearms and poisons, which account altogether for about one half of all suicides. Then there are asphyxiation and hanging. These four techniques account for 83 per cent of all suicides.

People who commit suicide represent a group who are easily upset emotionally. They break down under strains which other people manage to surmount. Sometimes the strain arises from economic conditions, sometimes because of trouble with friends and relatives.

The psychologists are convinced that there is a steady progression of the tendency to self-destruction long before the self-destruction is finally consummated. Obviously, therefore, there is time when such a tendency is discovered to undertake corrective action with a view to overcoming the desire.

The ability to adjust oneself emotionally to one's surroundings is perhaps most important to the prevention of suicides. The conditions that influence people, such as poverty, unemployment, ill-health, mental abnormality, physical suffering or handicaps, may lead people to thoughts of self-destruction. Loss of honor and prestige, disappointment in love, failure in achieving one's ambitions, or any other failure in adequacy may result in thought of suicide.

Obviously the way to prevent suicide is to develop a proper attitude toward life in the young. This is the responsibility of the entire community as well as of the home. Young people must be given a proper mental and emotional outlook. They must learn to act properly toward the difficult situations that invariably arise in the human life. *See also* MANIC-DEPRESSIVE PSYCHOSIS; PARANOIA.

SULFONAMIDE DRUGS, or *sulfa drugs,* are derived from or are compounds of *sulfonamide,* and their introduction into medicine marked a turning point in the treatment of disease. Among the sulfonamide drugs are *sulfadiazine, sulfapyridine, Gantrisin, Kynex,* and others. These drugs act effectively on diseases caused by *staphylococcus, meningococcus, streptococcus,* and *organisms* of the *dysentery group.*

Before sulfa drugs, treatment of such diseases as *lobar pneumonia* and *spinal meningitis* depended on serums, which were only moderately successful. Management of infections of the middle ear was so ineffective that loss of hearing and *mastoiditis* often followed. Treatment of *gonorrhea* depended on repeated and frequently unsuccessful urethral injections. The use of sulfa drugs virtually revolutionized treatment of these and other conditions.

The sulfonamides differ in degree of activity, rate of absorption or metabolic and toxic effects, and should only be taken under the supervision and recommendation of a doctor. In some persons they cause undesirable side effects, such as rash, fever, and a lowering of the number of white cells in the blood. While these complications are infrequent, care must still be exercised in use of the drugs.

Penicillin and other *antibiotics* have superseded sulfa drugs in many cases, or the sulfa drugs are used in combination with antibiotics as anti-infective systemic drugs to combat bacterial infection.

SUNBURN, known medically as *erythema solare,* discoloration or inflammation of the skin, developing from overexposure to the sun. It may be as simple as a slight reddening of the skin or severe enough to cause blistering, fever, and nausea. Ointments, lotions, or creams help to relieve the discomfort, which results from exposure of the nerve endings.

More severe sunburns, involving blisters, dizziness, headache, fever, vomiting, and other symptoms of constitutional disturbance due to the secondary toxic effects of the burn, should be treated as if the burn had resulted from other causes, such as fire or hot water. A burn from the sun is a burn fully as much as any other, and the victim should consult a physician.

Danger from sunlight is chiefly due to the effects of *ultraviolet rays,* the short heat rays. More ultraviolet light penetrates near the water than inland, and a cool day with brilliant sunshine may be more scorching than a hot but hazy day. The burning effect of bright sunlight reflected from snow is well known.

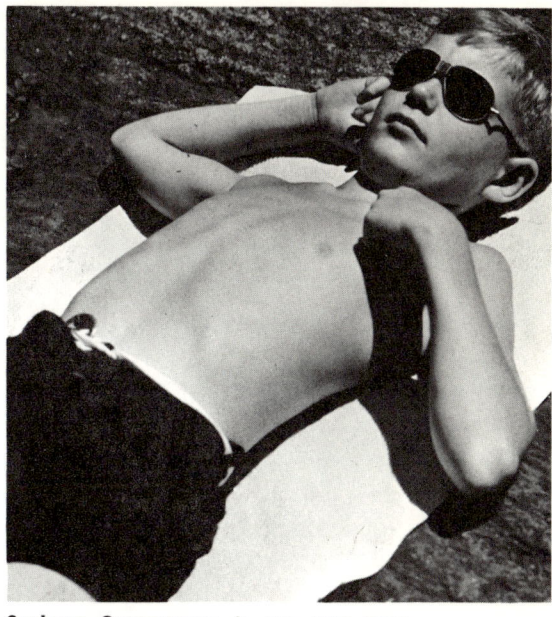

Sunburn—Overexposure to sun may cause severe sunburn, sunstroke or heat exhaustion. Suntanning should be done gradually. Exposure times can be increased by ten to fifteen minutes each day. Persons with fair complexions should be extremely careful because their skin absorbs more of the sun's rays than does that of darker persons.

The skin of an infant is much more delicate than that of adults and will burn and become inflamed more promptly. Special care should therefore be taken to avoid overexposure of an infant to the sun. Blond or red-haired persons with fair skin are particularly susceptible to burning, but everyone should acquire resistance to sunburn by gradual exposure, beginning with perhaps only five or ten minutes in the direct sun. *See also* SKIN; PIGMENTATION.

SUNSTROKE. *See* HEAT SICKNESS.

SUPPURATION refers to the formation of pus.

1231

SURGEON, a doctor who specializes in operative techniques. Formerly, a surgeon undertook anything that was to be done which involved the use of the knife on the human body. Now operations are so technical and the associated care of the patients so involved and intricate that surgery has broken up into a great number of specialties. These include surgery of the brain and nervous system, surgery of the heart and the associated blood vessels, surgery of the stomach and the intestines, surgery of the lung and chest, orthopedic surgery, genitalurinary surgery, gynecological surgery, plastic surgery and rehabilitative surgery. In many large schools and hospitals today, there are divisions for each of these surgical specialties. Moreover, the American Board of Surgery which certifies a surgeon as to his qualifications, has recognized some of these specialty branches as sub-divisions of surgery with special examining boards. The training of the surgeon has become long and arduous in the United States requiring not only a degree in medicine but also general internship followed by a surgical residency and sometimes an assistantship of many years before the surgeon undertakes to practice alone. In the hospital or clinic the surgeon no longer functions merely with the aid of an anesthetist and a nurse but is now associated with a large group of persons known as a surgical team. Such a team might include the surgeon, the anesthetist, the surgeon's assistant, the surgical nurse and often associated personnel to take care of blood transfusion, the use of various fluids and resuscitation. *See also* SURGERY; SURGERY, HISTORY OF; SURGERY OF OLDER PEOPLE.

SURGERY, the art of treating injuries or diseases by operative techniques. The surgeon has always been an integral part of medical science. Some of the earliest medical writings known are devoted chiefly to records of surgical cases. Strangely, however, the great advances in surgery have been dependent on medical discoveries in other fields. These advances include the discovery of *anesthesia* by Morton and Long in 1847; the discovery of the principle of *antisepsis,* which prevented infection during surgery, and the *wearing of rubber gloves,* introduced by Halstead. The use of *blood transfusion,* the *control of fluid* in the body, the feeding of patients by a variety of techniques and the use of drugs for controlling various symptoms have also aided success in surgery.

It was only a comparatively short time ago when few surgeons dared to invade the interior of the body as a whole, let alone the brain. Today there is no portion of the human body that is not invaded successfully. Previously surgery was largely mutilating, involving the removal of diseased organs or tissues. The surgery of today is called *physiological surgery* and is aimed at restoring normal function of various organs and tissues when these functions have failed. Under these circumstances, the surgeon today

Surgery has undergone remarkable advances in recent years. The use of antibiotics to prevent infections and new methods of treating surgical shock have given great impetus to the development of advanced surgical techniques. Many operations performed routinely today were considered marginal risks only a few years ago. Some of the most dramatic achievements have been made in the field of heart surgery. The heart can now be operated upon directly for extensive correction of congenital defects. Patients who were previously invalids can now be liberated to lead normal lives.

These photographs were taken during actual surgery on the heart. At right, an instrument called the *aortic valvulotome* is being tested. It is inserted into the ventricle of the heart to dilate the aortic valve.

Below: Strictures of the aortic and mitral valves of the heart are being widened. The left side of the heart has been opened and the ribs are held back to expose the heart.

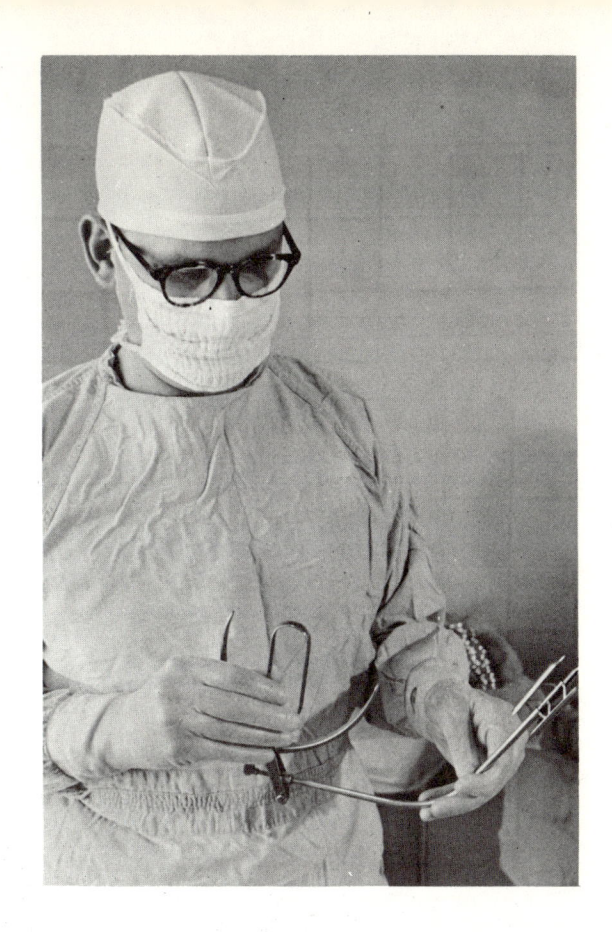

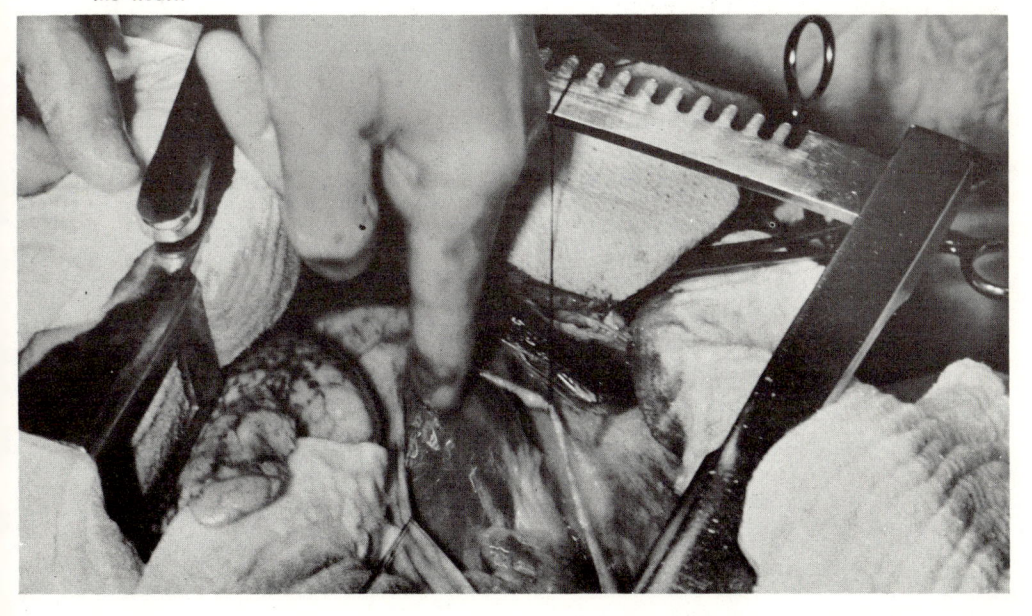

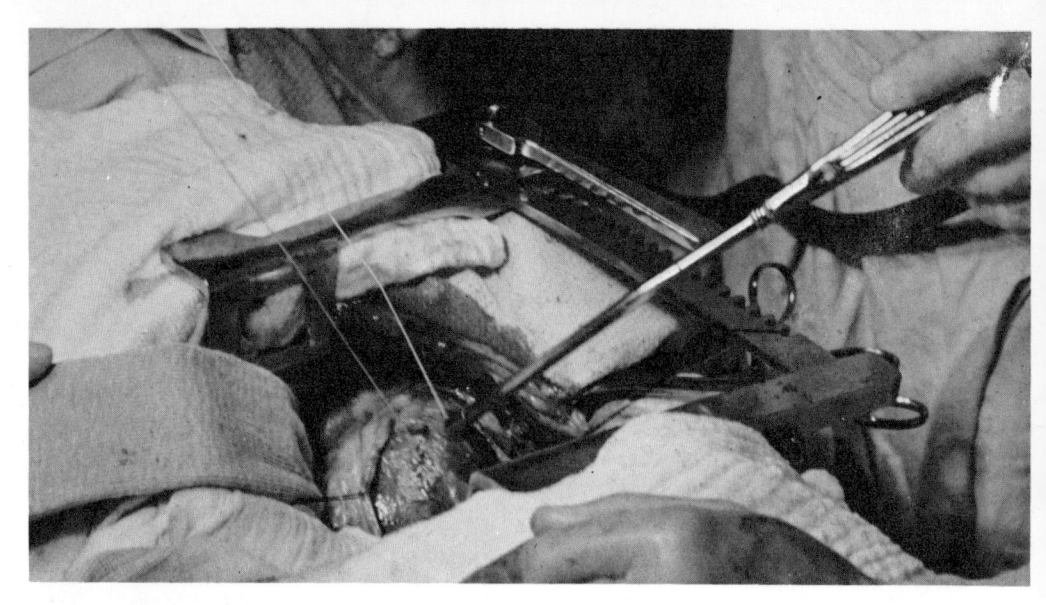

Above: a purse-string suture is being placed in the myocardium of the left ventricle. Below: the surgeon holds his left finger over the stab wound just made at the center of the purse-string suture. The valvulotome, shown on the preceding page, is here introduced into the aortic valve in a closed position. The valve will be opened.

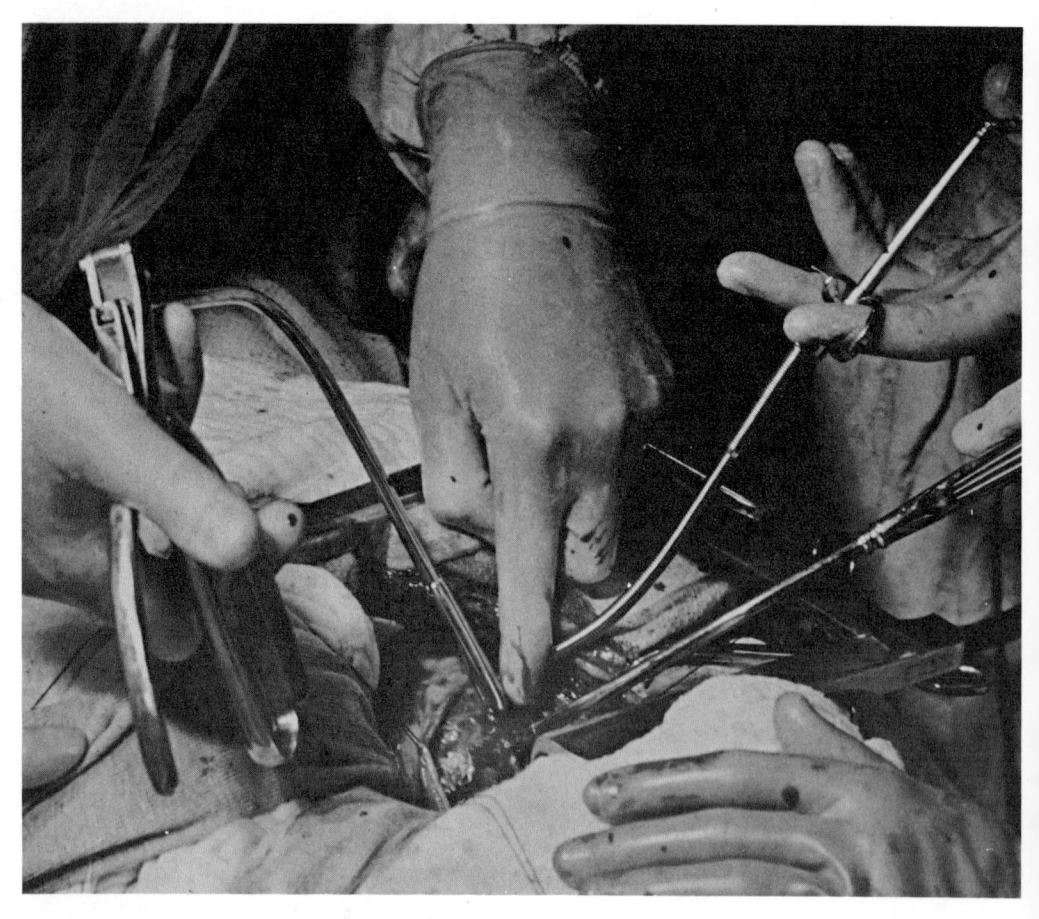

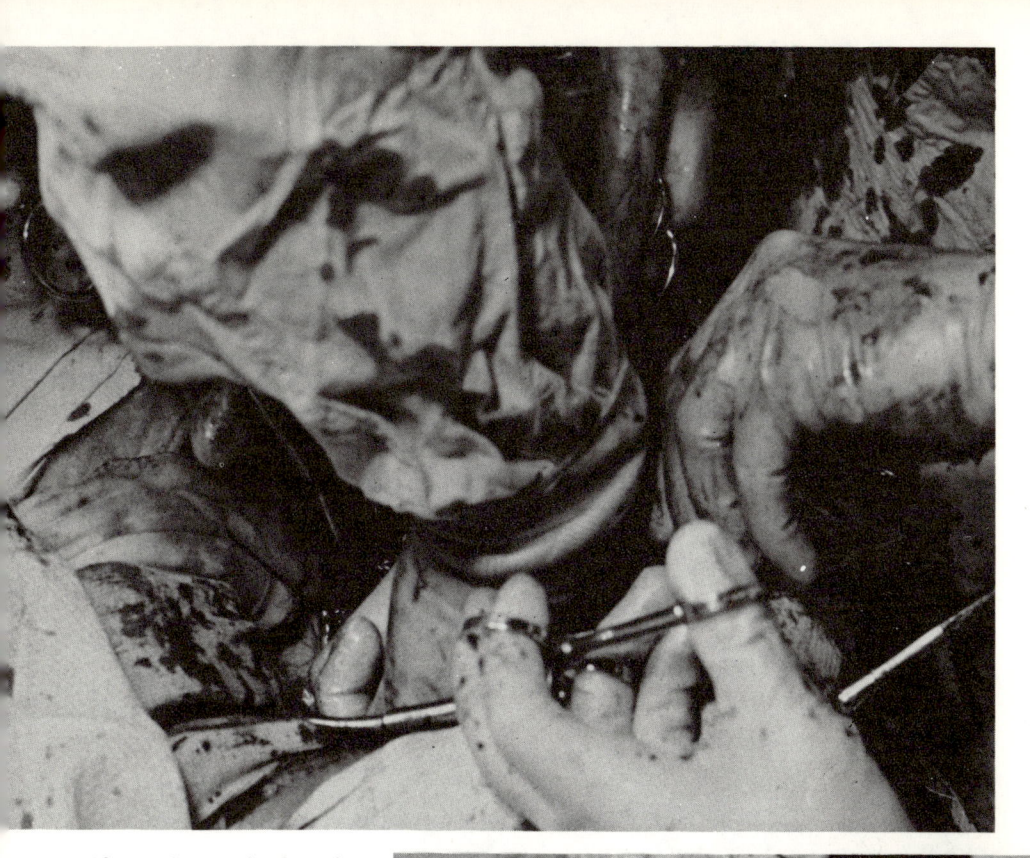

Above: the mitral valve is being opened. The finger is introduced into the valve and the sides split to widen the opening. The technique is called *finger fraction*.

Right: the surgery is completed and the chest is closed.

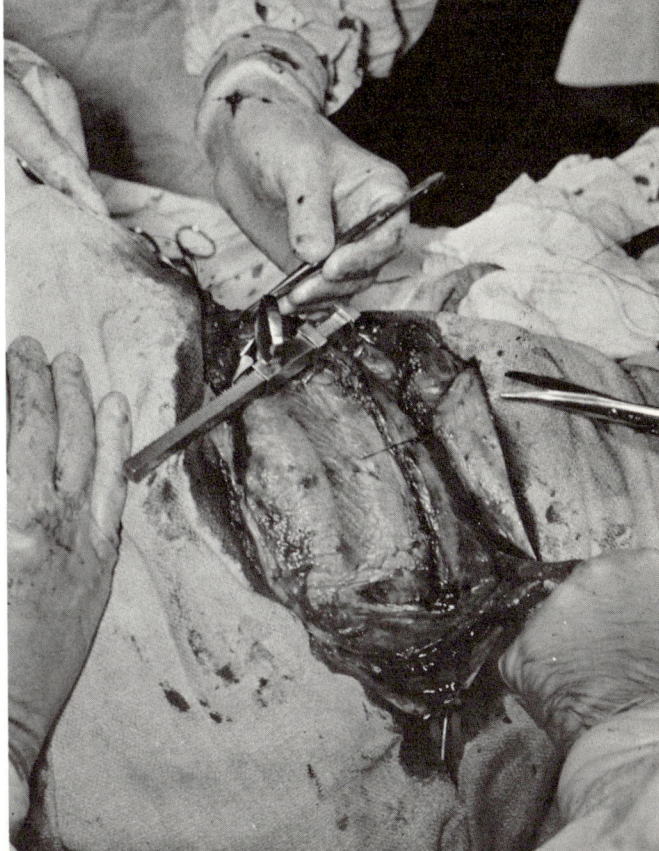

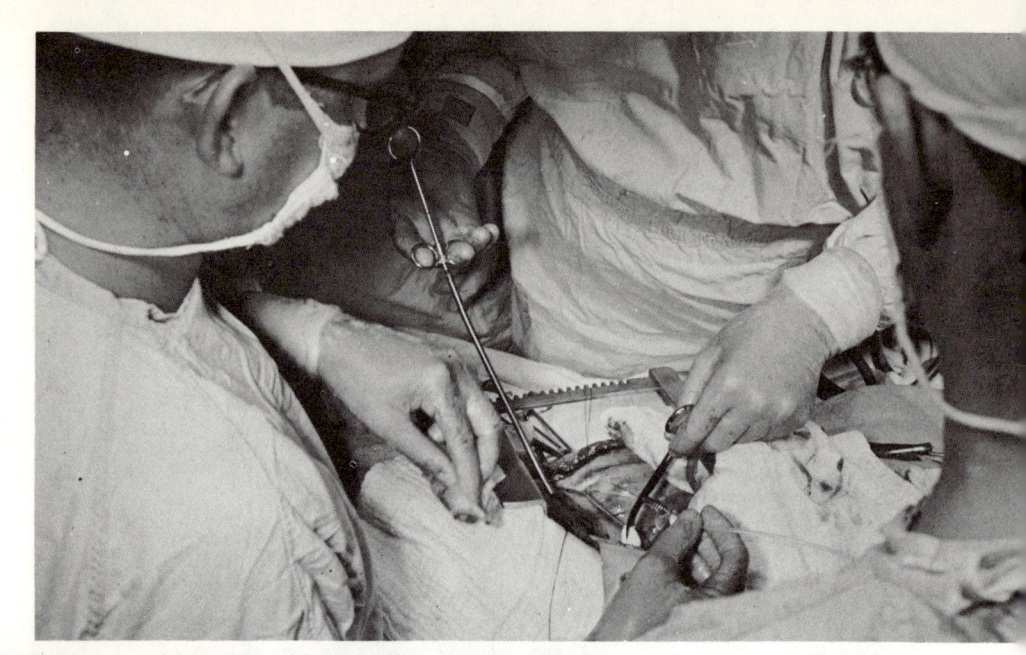

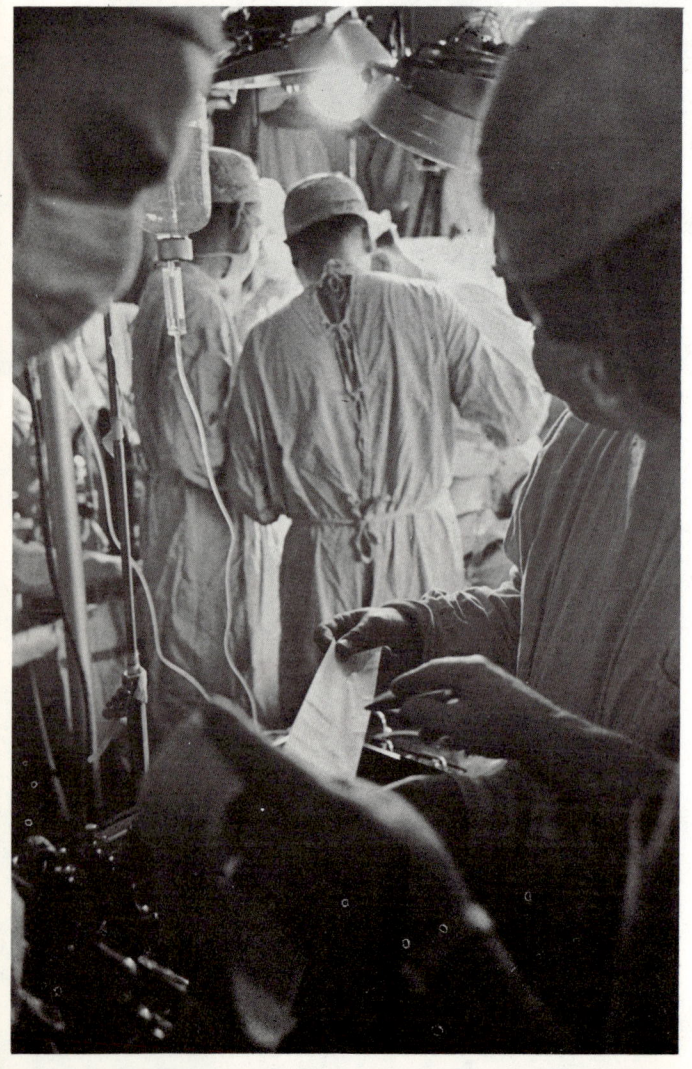

During the course of the operation, the surgeons take pressure readings by means of an instrument called a *manometer* connected to a needle which is inserted into the left heart chambers. This procedure is depicted above. At left, these pressure readings are being compared with readings taken prior to surgery. In this case, a reduced pressure reading indicates success in relieving the stenotic valves from excessive constriction—the disturbance which it was proposed to correct by the operation shown in these photographs. Many similar heart defects can now be corrected by comparable operations, thanks to the extraordinary refinement of surgical techniques in recent years.

does procedures which would have been called highly radical just a few years ago. Examples are removal of almost all of the organs of the pelvis for the treatment of cancer, the removal of the esophagus because of the presence of cancer, the complete removal of the stomach, the removal of the breast with all of its associated lymph glands, the removal of the colon because of chronic ulcerative colitis or the appearance of polyps and diverticuli which may be related to cancer. This does not include the operations that have been done on the heart or removal of the lung in whole or in part and the extensive operations on the brain and other portions of the nervous system. *See also* SURGEON; SURGERY, HISTORY OF; SURGERY OF OLDER PEOPLE.

SURGERY, HISTORY OF. The rise of surgery depended upon the knowledge of such fundamental sciences as *anatomy, physiology, pathology* and *anesthesia*. Just as the *stethoscope* is the sign of the physician, the *scalpel* or surgical knife is the token of the surgeon. The first scalpel ever seen in an illustration appears in the Temple of Esculapius on the Acropolis in Athens and dates back to 300 B.C. Scalpels continue to be modified in shape and form; the final important modifications were made with relationship to ease of sterilization. Handles with ivory and boned wood and tortoise shell went out with the coming of Lister.

Ligatures for tying off blood vessels and for stopping hemorrhage were known as far back as the time of Galen, in Rome around 150 A.D. Apparently the *saw* has been known to man since before the birth of history and is supposed to have been conceived from studying the teeth of fish and such animals as the sawfish. Saws for surgery were modified continuously until the time of the modern saw which is electrically operated. Trepanning and opening of the skull was employed by the ancient Incas of South America. The practice was freely engaged upon in the time of Hippocrates and the ancient Egyptians.

Devices for dilating various openings of the body in order to permit the entrance of instruments and hands go back also to the ancients but the modern devices are far superior both as to perfection, as to the fit and to illumination. The discovery of electric light and its adaption to surgical and medical instruments may be considered among the greatest of medical discoveries and new devices are introduced every year for such procedures.

Tapping for the release of fluid from the cavities of the body was performed by the ancient Greeks and Romans and the new devices which are known as *trocars* also are continuously modified with the introduction in more recent times of *air suction* and the use of the *x-ray* for indicating the area where a trocar is to be inserted.

Even in recent years new discoveries were made in relationship to the operating table which began with a simple board and four legs and which now has reached the

1237

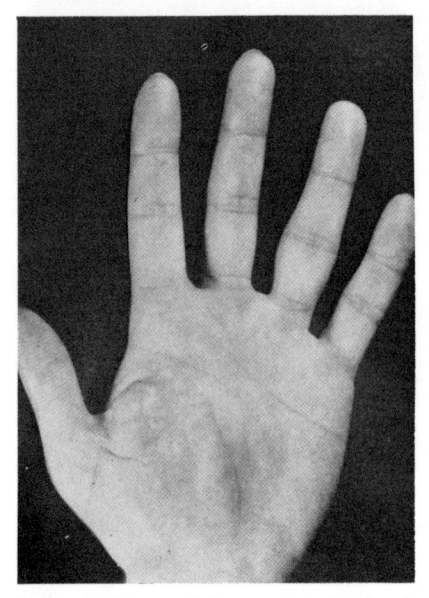

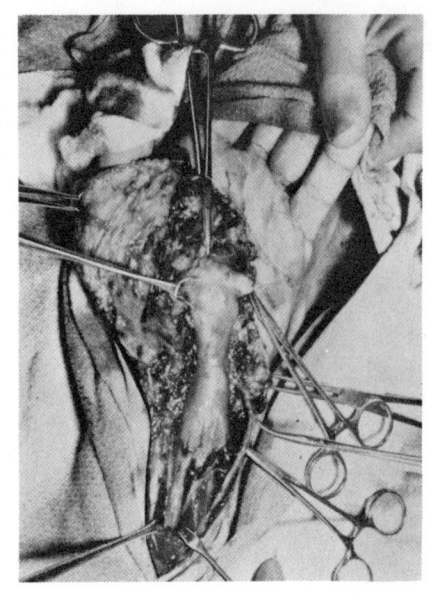

Surgery, History of—Tumor of the left hand, located just below the thumb in the palm area. In the picture (*on the right*) the tumor is being removed. Incision has been made and the interior of the palm is well exposed. Edges of the wound are held apart by retractors, and the tumor is freed from the surrounding tissues. The scissors-like instruments are hemostats which are used in clamping blood vessels to prevent hemorrhage. Hemostats have blunt points, do not cut and are self-locking. They are frequently used in surgery.

stage of tables that can be adjusted to any position, tables which provide for the anesthetist and the nurses and for holding arms and legs and various portions of the body exactly as needed. There are tables which permit the head to be dropped backward for operations on the nose and throat and indeed special devices for brain surgery. *See also* SURGEON; SURGERY; SURGERY OF OLDER PEOPLE.

SURGERY OF OLDER PEOPLE. An analysis of surgical operations done on older people have shown that, under modern conditions, surgery is performed on the aged with little risk; this is especially true when it is done as an elective operation rather than as an emergency. Much emergency surgery on older people could be avoided if chronic conditions requiring surgery were cared for before emergencies developed. Postponing an operation saps a patient's strength and increases the risk of shock and other complications. *See also* SURGEON; SURGERY, HISTORY OF.

SWEAT. SEE PERSPIRATION.

SWIMMING POOLS. The chief disorders transmitted through swimming pools are *inflammation of the eye, boils, ear infections, chronic inflammation of the nose and sinuses, sore throat,* various *skin infections*—particularly *ringworm* and *athlete's foot*

SYMPATHETIC NERVOUS SYSTEM

—*infections of the bowels* and *dysentery*. As a precaution, most public swimming pools require that all persons take a shower and walk through a footbath before entering the pool. No one with any ailment or infection should ever swim in a pool with other persons.

To keep the water in the pool clean and safe, chemicals are usually added. Ultraviolet rays are sometimes used for this purpose. Filter systems help remove sediment and infectious materials and pools are usually drained regularly.

Private pools should maintain the same strict sanitary conditions that most public pools do. Usually filters, chemicals, and purifiers are sold along with the pool, and in some places a special service will regularly clean and purify the pool.

SYMPATHETIC NERVOUS SYSTEM, or *autonomic nervous system,* supplies and exerts a regulatory activity to most of the involuntary organs of the body—glands, heart, blood vessels, for example—and involuntary muscles in the internal organs.

The system consists of a network of nerves and a series of nerve cell collections called *ganglia*. Some ganglia are connected to the *spinal cord* by *fibers*. Meshworks of fibers are sent out by the vertebral ganglia to the organs located in the abdomen and pelvis. Ganglia also arise within the brain and supply the tear and salivary glands and the pupils of the eye, and are connected with nerves that affect the ears.

Impulses through sympathetic nerve fibers cause *dilation of the pupil, sweating, quickening* and *augmentation of the heartbeat, stoppage of the flow of gastric juice, contraction of arteries,* and many other body actions. All these functions are automatic or involuntary.

In contrast, the action of the *parasympathetic nervous system*—that division between the *cranium* and the *sacrum*—is somewhat antagonistic to the sympathetic action. Thus, it *slows the heart* and *stimulates the flow of gastric juices.*

The blood supply to any part of the body can be increased by interruption of the sympathetic nerves that pass to that part. In hypertension, *sympathectomy*—cutting off the sympathetic nerves by surgery—is sometimes employed to increase the flow of blood into the abdominal area and lower limbs and thus decrease the blood pressure. Currently drugs are preferred to surgery to block the sympathetic nerves. Interruption or treatment of the sympathetic nervous system has occasionally been used in heart conditions such as *angina pectoris,* in cases of severe pain involving the urinary tract, to control serious disorders of the sweat glands, and to aid movement of the bowels.

The sympathetic nervous system is responsible for the physical sensations that accompany emotion. For example, suppressed resentment may cause overactivity of the muscles and glands of the stomach, and actual pain can result. In some psychotic or neurotic conditions, the system is involved and changes can occur in affected organs. *See also* BRAIN; SPINAL CORD.

SYNDROME, a set of *specific symptoms* which occur regularly in the same combination and constitute a *specific disease.* Dozens of disorders are known as *syndromes,* a large number of them bearing the name of the first doctor to note the syndrome, connect it with the underlying disease condition, and call attention to it. Well-known syndromes are *Cushing's syndrome,* indicating tumor in certain parts of the brain; *Korsakoff's syndrome* or *psychosis,* associated with chronic alcoholism; and *Addisonian syndrome,* a condition caused by insufficiency of the adrenal glands.

SYNOUSIOLOGY, the science and art of sexual intercourse.

SYNOVITIS, inflammation of the *synovial membranes,* those membranes which line the joints. The chief manifestation is an outpouring of fluid into the joint cavity. It may occur as a reaction to injury or as a result of infection somewhere else in the body.

Water on the knee is a typical instance of synovitis. A combination of rest and gentle pressure from bandaging will help to induce absorption of the fluid. *See also* JOINTS AND JOINT DISORDERS.

SYPHILIS, a contagious *venereal disease* which can infect any of the body tissues. It is characterized by a variety of lesions, of which the *chancre* (primary lesion), the *mucous patch,* and the *gumma* are the most distinctive. It is caused by a spirochete, *Treponema pallidum.*

The origin of syphilis is not known, but it has been claimed that Columbus's crew first introduced it into Europe after their return from the New World. A few of the crew members were with Charles VII of France when he invaded Italy in 1495, and a terrible epidemic of syphilis broke out there, rapidly spreading over all of Europe. Today syphilis is world-wide and still one of the major scourges of mankind. Figures released by the World Health Organization in 1968 indicated an alarming spread of syphilis, along with the development of new strains resistant to treatment with existing antibiotics.

The vast majority of adult cases of syphilis are acquired through *sexual contact.* Treatment usually seems to render the infected person incapable of transmitting the disease, but there is some evidence that persons presumably cured can still infect others.

A few hours after exposure, the syphilis spirochete penetrates the skin or mucous membrane and enters the blood stream and tissues. The hard chancre, the *primary stage* of the disease, does not appear until ten to ninety days later, three weeks being the average time. Usually the chancre is found on the genitals or in the mouth, but it may appear elsewhere and occasionally not at all. The fluid from the chancre is highly infectious.

Even without treatment, chancres generally disappear in ten to forty days, and the *secondary stage,* char-

1240

acterized by small raised red areas on the skin or small mucous patches in the mouth or on the reproductive organs, begins two to six months later. Generally lymph nodes throughout the body become enlarged. These lesions of secondary syphilis heal by themselves in three to twelve weeks, but may recur later.

The *tertiary stage* of syphilis sometimes develops almost immediately after the secondary symptoms have disappeared, or, in some cases, may be delayed for years. Ulcer-like draining *lesions* appear on the skin; hard nodules or *gumma* occur in the internal organs or tissue under the skin. The blood vessels and heart are often damaged and the lungs may be affected during this stage.

Neurosyphilis or syphilis of the central nervous system can accompany either the second or third stage of syphilis, although more commonly the third. When the spinal cord is involved, loss of coordination of limbs may ensue. In *general paresis,* the brain is infected and mental faculties deteriorate and the limbs become paralyzed.

Syphilis is the only venereal disease that may be acquired *congenitally* by the passing of the spirochete from the mother to the unborn child. Syphilitic infection may cause abortion or stillbirth. Infants who are born with syphilis may soon die; or, if they survive, may later develop *blindness, deafness, paralysis, deformities,* or even *mental disturbances.* Because of these terrible consequences, every prospective mother should be examined for syphilis so that, if she does have it, treatment can begin immediately. Even if treatment is delayed until the fourth or fifth month of pregnancy, the child may still be born healthy. If, however, treatment has been inadequate or absent, the newborn child should immediately be given *penicillin.* The amount given to children depends on the age the treatment begins; children over two years receive the same dose as adults.

Usually the first symptom of syphilis is a sore at the point where the germ has entered the body. The doctor makes his diagnosis by studying the material from the sore under a microscope. In the *Darkfield method,* the germs appear light and the rest of the slide dark. He will also give the patient a *Wasserman, Kahn,* or one of the other standard serological tests for syphilis.

When the syphilis germ enters the body, it multiplies quickly and gradually invades every organ and tissue, certain germs being limited to certain parts of the body. Syphilis can therefore imitate a wide variety of diseases.

Current treatment of syphilis with penicillin and other antibiotics has largely replaced former methods of treatment. These drugs can halt the spread of the disease within a few days. Penicillin is used not only for early syphilis but to alleviate the symptoms of neurosyphilis and in congenital syphilis. Because of the notable success, it was at first thought that penicillin and the antibiotics might completely wipe out syphilis, but recent figures compiled by the Venereal Disease Program showed an increase in primary and secondary syphilis in numerous states. This increase occurred among both sexes.

A person who has syphilis should lead a continent life, with proper diet and adequate sleep. He should sleep alone and not have sexual intercourse until his physician is sure he is free of contagion. Intercourse will not only interfere with the cure of the disease, but is likely to transmit the disease to the other person. In many states syphilis is a bar to marriage and a physician's certificate or affidavit is required from applicants stating that they are free from venereal disease. Other states require only that the applicants be tested for syphilis, as a mutual warning. Needless to say, anyone with syphilis should postpone marriage until free of contagion. The syphilitic person should be especially careful that others are not exposed to the disease from contact with his personal articles, such as towels, drinking glass, toothbrush, etc. Anything that touches the open sores should be disinfected or destroyed.

It cannot be too strongly urged that anyone who suspects that he has syphilis see a doctor immediately. Some people through false shame or modesty permit the disease to spread to a critical point before seeking medical aid. The fact that a person has once had syphilis should always be mentioned when he later sees a doctor or dentist for other reasons, since it may furnish a clue to treatment. *See also* CHANCRE; PARESIS; GONORRHEA; CHANCROID; LYMPHOGRANULOMA VENEREUM. *See* MEDIGRAPH page 1311.

SYRINGE, an instrument used to inject fluid beneath the skin or into a cavity. It consists of a *nozzle, barrel,* and *plunger* or *rubber bulb.* There are various special types of syringe, such as the *rectal syringe* and the *urethral syringe.*

T

TABES, a wasting or degeneration. Although there are many types of *tabes,* the term usually designates *tabes dorsalis,* also known as *locomotor ataxia. See also* LOCOMOTOR ATAXIA.

TACHYPHAGIA, the vulgar habit of rapid eating. The *tachyphage* is one who gulps his meals without stopping to sit down, or eats so fast he does not relax and enjoy his food.

The tachyphage does not improve his digestive apparatus by this mode of life. The state of his stomach is usually so troublesome that none of the normal pleasures of life, eating, drinking, or even the esthetic and intellectual joys, are ever his.

Fortunate is the tachyphage who, discovering his folly early, can take the necessary corrective measures while he is still in relatively good health. These include regular hours for meals, the use of a proper menu, the exclusion of shop talk from the table and, above all, slow eating.

TALIPES, any one of a variety of deformities of the human foot, especially those of congenital origin, such as *clubfoot. See also* CLUBFOOT.

TAPEWORM. *See* WORMS.

TATTOOING, the production of permanent coloration in designated areas of the skin by introducing foreign substances, by pricking in coloring matter, or by making scars. Tattooing dates from prehistoric times when men pigmented their skin, usually in connection with religious worship. Ritual tattooing is still practiced in Africa and in other parts of the world.

In tattooing, mineral and vegetable pigments are carried by needles directly into the true skin. Tattooing of the skin may sometimes occur accidentally, as when particles of powder are deposited in the skin and leave permanent stains. Miners occasionally have permanent discoloration due to the imbedding of coal dust in scratches. Silver and iron have an effect of tattooing when deposited in the skin.

The tattooer will sometimes use his own saliva as the moistening agent in tattooing, and various diseases, including *tuberculosis, erysipelas, bacterial infection, viral hepatitis,* and even *venereal diseases* have been transmitted in this manner. Occasionally tattooing produces reactions in the skin which result in the development of *tumors.*

One of the methods to remove a tattoo is peeling the skin with a caustic substance. This is quite dangerous and even specialists in diseases of the skin hesitate to attempt it. It is also possible to cut away the entire tattooed area, if it is not too large, and graft new skin from another portion of the body over the area. A new and successful method involves sterilizing the area with antiseptics and then sandpapering the tattooed skin off its base. Bleeding is controlled and prompt healing encouraged. Recently special *burrs* and *emery wheels* powered by motors have been used for *planing.* The skin is first made insensitive to pain by freezing it with *Freon. See also* SKIN; ACNE.

TEAR GLANDS. The little indentation at the inner end of the eye is known as the *tear gland* and serves as a kind of reservoir for tears. From this reservoir several small tubes, called *tear ducts,* carry the tears to the eyes.

Another tube, the *nasal duct,* carries a similar fluid to the nose. For this reason, whenever a person sheds tears, he will also find it necessary to blow his nose.

The tear glands, as well as the ducts, may occasionally become infected. When this occurs, a swelling is seen at the corner of the eye and a small amount of pus will form. Often a person with this condition will press out the pus and apply a commercial medication without consulting a doctor, but professional assistance is always recommended since the infection may in some cases be serious enough to require the cutting or even the removal of the gland. *See also* EYE.

TEETH, the calcified organs supported by sockets and gums of both jaws. Their chief function is to grind food into pieces small enough to be easily swallowed and digested. The teeth help to form words and also give expression. Their loss is usually associated with old age, and loss of

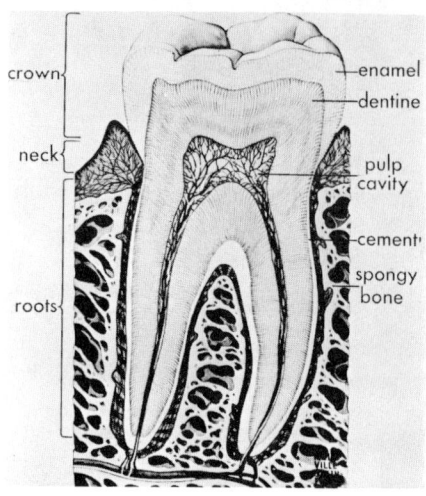

Teeth—Cross section of a tooth showing the *crown, neck* and *roots* and internal structures. Within the *pulp cavity* can be found nerves and blood vessels.

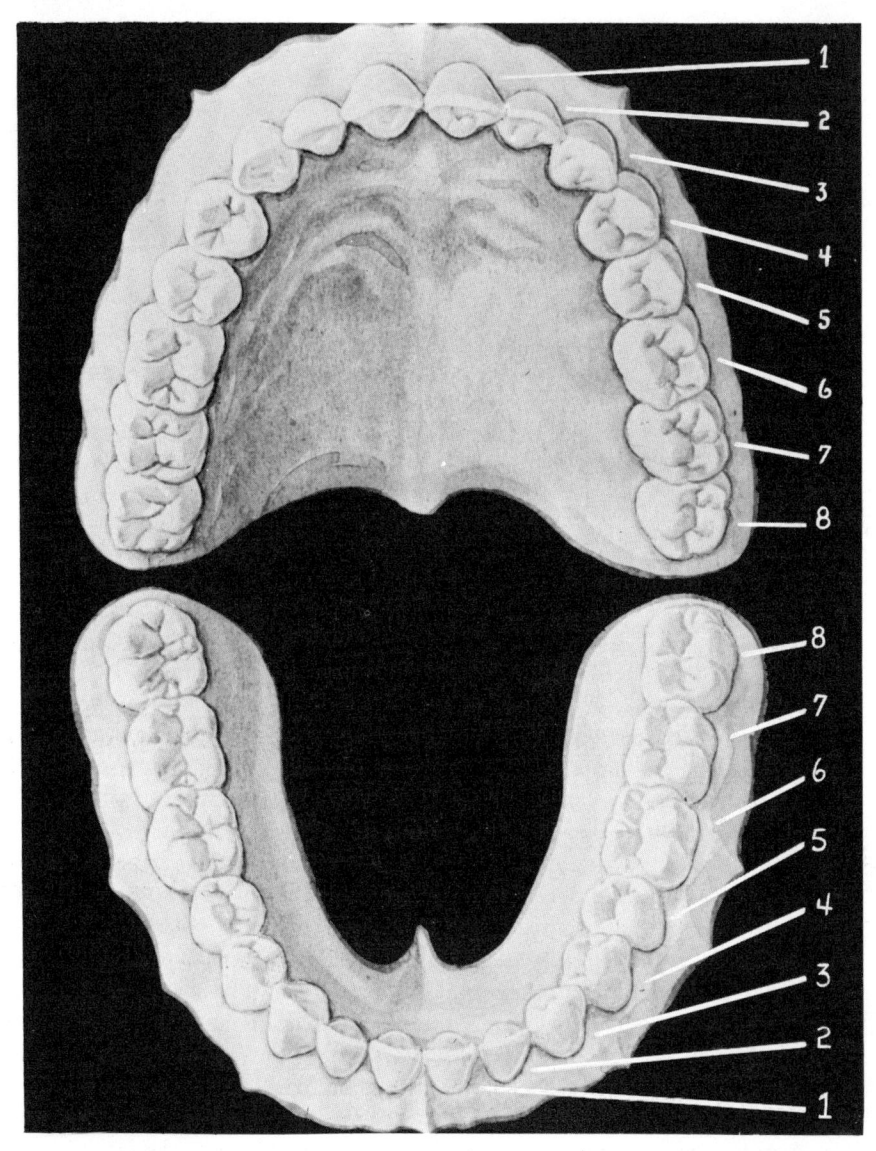

Teeth—A full set of permanent teeth, 32 in number. Upper jaw: (1) central incisor, (2) lateral incisor, (3) cuspid, (4) first bicuspid, (5) second bicuspid; (6) first molar, (7) second molar, (8) third molar. Lower jaw: (8) third molar, (7) second molar, (6) first molar, (5) second bicuspid, (4) first bicuspid, (3) cuspid, (2) lateral incisor, and (1) central incisor.

teeth in a young person may require a major emotional adjustment. Sound teeth contribute to health, while decayed teeth and diseased gums permit germs to enter the body. Thus the teeth may become focal points of infection and lead to other disorders.

Anatomy of teeth. Teeth are composed largely of mineral salts, chiefly *calcium* and *phosphorus*, and also

1245

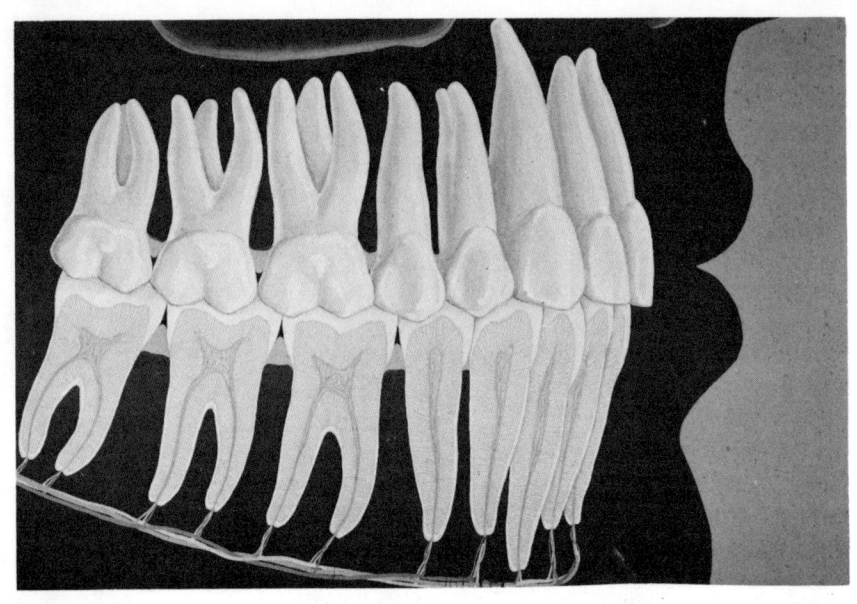

Teeth—Adult dentition, showing right side of the jaw. From left to right: third molars, second molars, first molars, second bicuspid, first bicuspid, cuspid, lateral incisor, central incisor.

magnesium, *fluorine*, and other minerals. A tooth consists of a *crown*, a *neck*, and one or more *roots*. The roots contain *dentin*, an ivory-like substance which is also found beneath the crown, surrounding a hollow, known as the *pulp cavity*, which is in the center. The pulp contains *blood vessels, nerves*, and loose *connective tissue*, including specialized *nerve cells*.

The *crown*, composed of the intensely hard *enamel* which caps the tooth, may have two or more *cusps*, or points, on its biting surface. Enamel is similar in substance to the hair and nails. If the *enamel* is damaged by accident or disease once the tooth has come into position, *natural* repair is not possible, nor can decay on the surface or in fissures in the enamel be helped by drugs, vitamins, or nourishment from the blood stream. However, this is not true for the rest of the tooth.

The root of the tooth is covered by *cement* which in its structure resembles *bone*. The *periodontal membrane* is the membrane that holds the tooth within the jawbone, and the *alveolar bone* supports the tooth and anchors it to the jaw. The alveolus also supplies calcium salts to other parts of the body and acts as a kind of reservoir. Alveolar bone is therefore easily affected by any disease that interferes with the calcium metabolism of the body.

The *gums* are the soft tissues that cover the alveolar bone, and are continuous with the mucous membranes of the mouth, lips, and cheeks.

Dentition. The process of cutting teeth is ordinarily called *teething* or *dentition*. There are two dentitions; the first produces the *primary teeth*,

TEETH

(also known as the *deciduous, temporary,* or *milk* teeth), and the second produces the *permanent teeth*.

There are *twenty* primary teeth: four *incisors,* two *canines,* and four *molars* in each jaw (upper and lower). The incisors are the front cutting teeth; the two in the middle are called *central incisors,* and those on either side are called *lateral incisors*. Outside these are the canine teeth which are sharp, pointed, and able to tear food. Beyond the canines are the molars (grinding teeth). The arrangement of teeth is the same in the upper and lower jaws and on the right and left sides.

The permanent set contains *thirty-two* teeth. Twenty of these gradually replace the primary dentition, a process which starts at about six or seven years of age and finishes at about twelve years or older. This dentition begins with the appearance of the first permanent molars, and afterward other permanent teeth are cut, including the central and lateral incisors, the first and second premolars (or bicuspids), the canines (cuspids), and the second molar. The premolars which replace milk molars have two *cusps* on the crown and for that reason are called the bicuspids. The *third* molar teeth—the *wisdom teeth*—may appear between the ages of seventeen and twenty-five or later, or not at all.

Disorders and diseases of teeth. The first teething is sometimes painful and the gums swollen, hot, and tender. The child may be generally upset, and colds, earache, and fever are not uncommon during this period. The second dentition rarely causes any trouble, with the exception of aching which may accompany eruption of the wisdom teeth.

Sometimes *malocclusion*—irregularity in placement of teeth—may be found in the deciduous and the permanent dentitions. A special branch of dentistry, *orthodontia,* has been developed to correct malocclusion, and the earlier the condition reaches the attention of the specialist the quicker and more effective the treatment will be.

Total or partial *anodontia,* or lack of teeth is rare. *Rickets* may be the cause of decayed dentition or malformation of teeth. Premature eruption of teeth has little significance, except that it may cause discomfort to a mother who is still nursing.

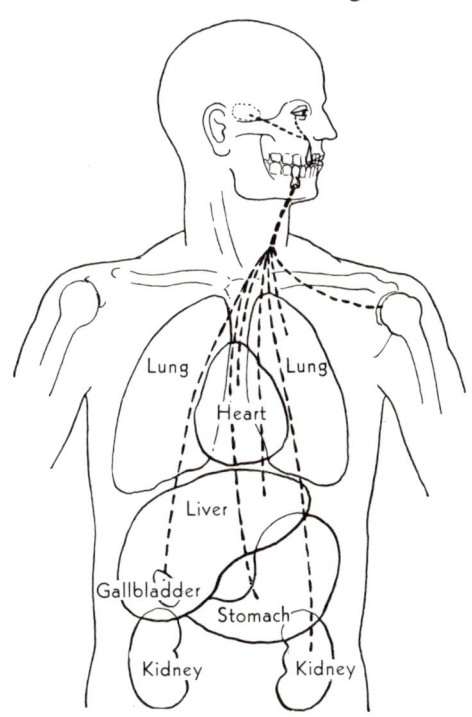

Teeth—The diagram illustrates the organs affected by abscessed teeth.

1247

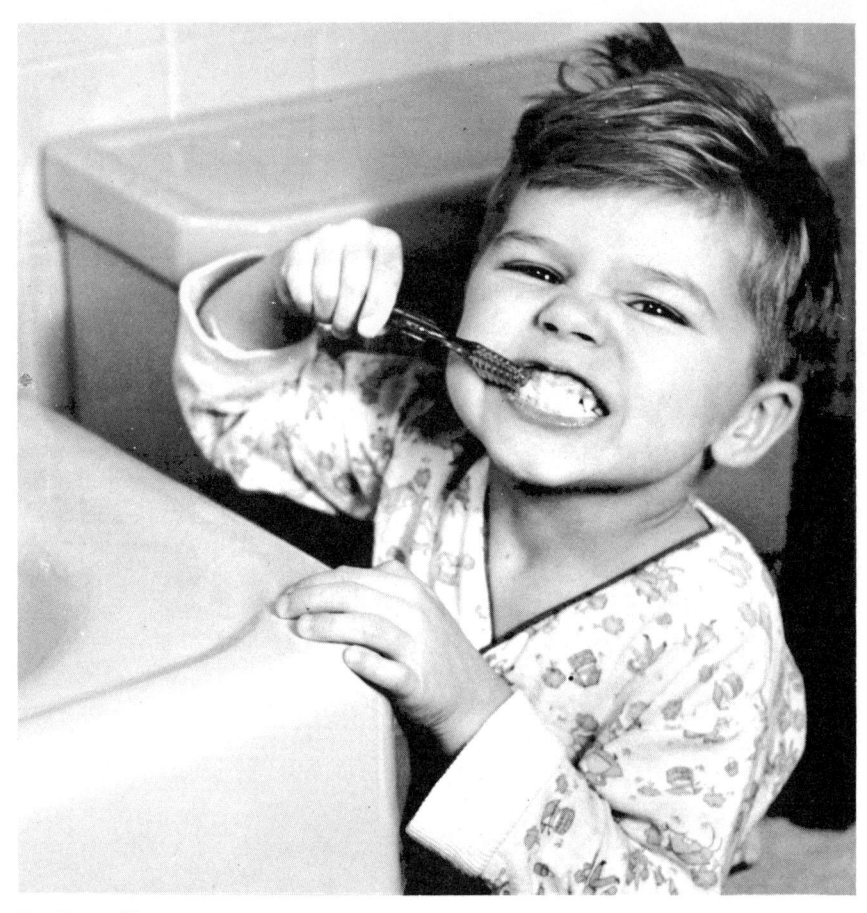

Tooth Brushing—At two years of age, most children are fascinated to see parents brushing teeth, and will want to imitate them. By example and instruction, the child can learn to brush from the gums to the edges of the teeth. Teeth should be brushed morning and night, and, whenever possible, after every meal and snack.

Mottling and *discoloration* may occur during formation of teeth, and is caused by excess *fluorine* in the drinking water or the food. Occasionally the child's teeth are malformed or incompletely calcified. These conditions should be treated by a dentist.

A small amount of fluorine in drinking water, about one part per million, has been found to help protect teeth against decay in children. Fluoridation of water has been tried successfully in many communities and is approved by leading scientific organizations in medicine and dentistry.

Unless teeth are adequately cleansed, tartar may form about the neck of the tooth and lead to infection of the gums, to *pyorrhea* and other disorders, and to diseases of the mouth. Food may adhere in spaces between the teeth and ferment, and acid substances attack the enamel and cause dental *caries* (tooth decay).

Sometimes, the pulp of the teeth becomes seriously infected or *abscessed*. An abscessed tooth is a serious disorder which may adversely affect other organs and metabolic processes. The pus caused by the abscess may spread and cause the lips, cheeks, tongue, mouth and nose to become swollen and painful. Abscessed teeth should be removed during their quiescent phase—during a period in which the swelling of surrounding tissues has receded.

Wisdom teeth which become *impacted*—viz., cannot erupt properly—may become infected and lead to metabolic disorders. Impacted wisdom teeth should be removed at the first sign of pain or infection.

Dental health. Although heredity helps determine the health of the teeth, good diet, adequate mastication, good mouth hygiene, and regular visits to the dentist for examination and cleaning are important.

There is no single diet which can insure good teeth, but a well-balanced diet, containing proper amounts of proteins, carbohydrates, fats, minerals, and vitamins, will encourage dental health just as it will general health. The teeth particularly need *phosphorus* and *calcium,* which are found abundantly in milk and milk products especially, and in leafy green vegetables, wholegrain cereal, and fish.

Dentists recommend that teeth get plenty of chewing exercise, and every diet should include enough crisp and textured foods which require vigorous chewing. Chewing benefits not only teeth but jaws, nasal and breathing passages, and the stomach as well. Chewing crisp fruits and vegetables also helps to keep the teeth clean.

Brushing the teeth should be part of everyone's daily routine. The upper teeth should be brushed down from the gum, and the lower teeth brushed up from the gum. Regular use of dental floss will help keep the areas between the teeth free of food deposits.

Small cavities which appear in the teeth will grow larger if not treated. The dentist should be consulted and the teeth examined preferably three times, and no less than twice, a year. *See also* DENTAL CARIES; DENTIFRICE; DENTAL RESEARCH, CURRENT; FLUORIDATION; ORTHODONTIA; PYORRHEA; VINCENT'S ANGINA.

TEMPERATURE, the degree of intensity of heat, especially as measured by a calibrated thermometer. The normal temperature of the human body is 98.6° F., with occasional variations during the day, amounting to no more than one degree. The temperature is generally slightly higher toward evening, when it may be 99.1° F., and in early morning it may fall to about 97.3°F.

A strict balance must be kept in the body between *heat production* and *heat loss.* To maintain a normal temperature, excess heat is expelled from the body or extra heat produced. *Heat is lost* chiefly through *perspiration* and through the air and vapor expelled from the *lungs. Heat is produced* by chemical action in the

TEMPERATURE

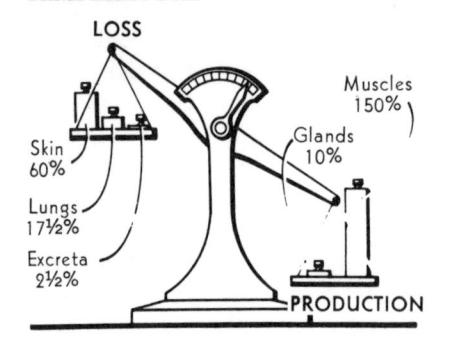

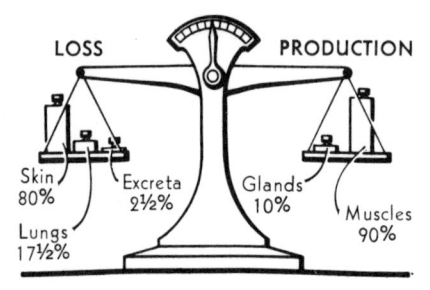

Temperature—When the body's chemistry operates normally, the heat produced by muscles and by glands is lost by way of the skin, the lungs, and the excreta. When there is fever, the loss is unable to keep up with the production.

muscles and in the *glands,* especially in the *liver.* Shivering, an involuntary muscular action, produces heat.

The sensation of heat or cold is not due to a change in body temperature but to a change in the temperature of the *skin.* When the skin feels cold or hot, a message is sent to the brain, the site of a mechanism which controls temperature. This mechanism is set into action with a corresponding drop or rise in temperature.

Disease may disturb the heat-regulating mechanism and cause the temperature to increase or decrease. The temperature of a person sick with a fever may rise to 104° F. or even higher. In severe cases, such as at the time of death, the fever may reach as high as 107° F. to 109° F. The average fever thermometer has a maximum calibration of about 110° F., above which death usually occurs. Cases have been recorded of death from heatstroke in which the persons had temperatures of over 110° F.

A temperature below 96° F. may represent collapse. In certain diseases and operative procedures, body temperature may be considerably below this figure for a period of time.

Chilling of the body ordinarily is considered harmful to health. Chilling is more serious for a person with a chronic infection of the nose and throat than for one in good health, and the response to chilling may be congestion in the nose and sinuses and the appearance of a condition

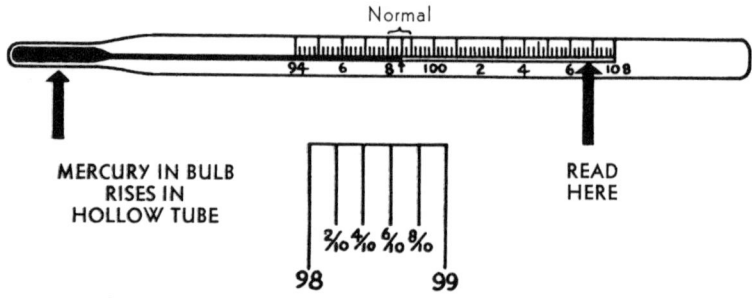

Temperature—The normal range of temperature is between 98 and 99 degrees Fahrenheit.

To read, look along the sharper edge between the numbers and the lines.

TENDON

like a cold. Some people are more susceptible to chilling than others, or are so sensitive to either heat or cold that symptoms of allergy are manifested. *See also* CHILBLAINS; FEVER; FROSTBITE; HAZARDS OF COLD; THERMOMETER.

TENDON, or *sinew,* a fibrous band of connective tisue which unites a muscle with another part of the body, and transmits the force exerted by the muscle. *See also* ACHILLES' TENDON; BURSITIS; MUSCLE.

TESTES. *See* TESTICLES.

TESTICLES, or *testes,* the two male sex glands which hang outside the body in a sac of skin called the *scrotum.* They perform two significant functions: they produce both the *male reproductive cells*—the *sperm*—and the *male sex hormone* —the internal secretion which causes the body to assume the attributes of masculinity.

Both *sperm* and the so-called *interstitial cells* originate within the testicle in tubular structures called *seminiferous tubules.* When the sperm cells mature, they migrate through the *epididymis* and the *vas deferens* to one of the two *seminal vesicles* located near the urinary bladder, where they remain until ejaculation. The interstitial cells remain in the testicle occupying the spaces between the tubules, and produce male sex hormones.

The hormone known medically as *testosterone* has been extensively studied and found to have many effects in the body. Appearing in

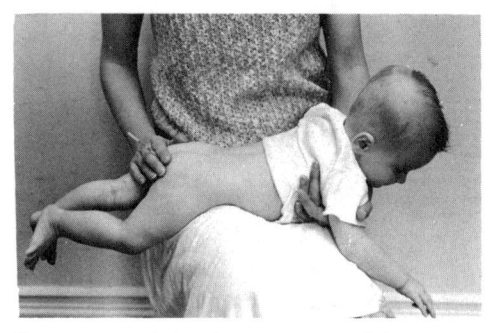

TESTICLES

Temperature—It is safest to use a rectal thermometer for children under six. Laying the child on his stomach in his mother's lap, or on a bed or table, with his legs hanging over the edge, will expose the rectum naturally and easily.

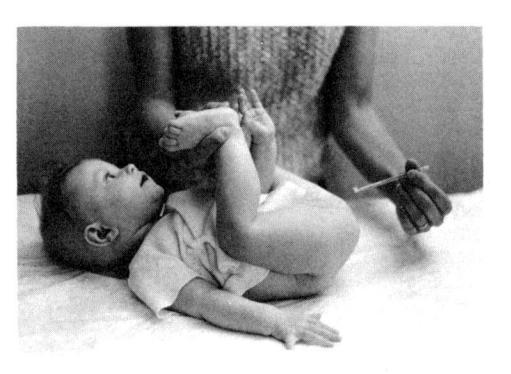

Temperature—Rectal temperature can also be taken with the baby lying on his back with his legs held up. Readings should be made only if a child shows definite signs of illness. Temperature will rise toward the end of the day.

quantity only as puberty approaches, it evokes growth of the sex organs to their adult size. Stronger and heavier male bones and muscles are dependent on the testosterone, which also causes the vocal cords in the larynx to enlarge, resulting in the characteristic pitch of the male voice, and promotes the growth of body and facial hair.

Testosterone has a definite effect on emotional and mental develop-

TEST	PURPOSE OF TEST	HOW TEST IS MADE
Schick	To determine if person tested is susceptible to diphtheria.	Minute amount (1/10 cc.) of diluted diphtheria toxin is injected into skin on front surface of forearm with hypodermic syringe and needle.
Dick	To determine if person tested is immune to scarlet fever.	By injecting 1/10 cc. of diluted scarlet-fever toxin into skin on front surface of forearm with hypodermic syringe and needle.
Widal	To determine if person tested has typhoid or paratyphoid fever.	The finger is pricked, and about 1 cc. of blood is collected. Several dilutions of the blood serum are made with salt solution; it is then added to cultures of typhoid bacilli and paratyphoid bacilli. These mixtures are placed in an incubator at about 98° F. for an hour, then are examined to determine if the germs have been clumped by the serum.
Tuberculin	To aid in determining presence of tuberculosis infection.	Diluted solution of tuberculin is injected into the skin, usually on front surface of forearm. Tuberculin is prepared from culture of tubercle bacilli. Test is examined after forty-eight hours.
Sedimentation	To aid in diagnosing tuberculosis and acute infections such as rheumatic fever.	Five to 10 cc. of blood are drawn from patient's vein and mixed with one drop of a potassium-oxalate solution. Special tube is then used to determine amount of settling of red blood cells. Speed of settling is called sedimentation rate.
Complement Fixation	To aid in diagnosing syphilis. (Also called Wassermann, Kahn test, etc.)	To blood serum or spinal fluid from patient are added various extracts and serums.
Aschheim-Zondek	To determine if pregnancy has occurred.	Specimen of urine from the patient is made slightly acid, filtered, and then injected into number of young, normal mice. (In Friedman modification, rabbits are used.)
Basal Metabolism	To aid in diagnosing thyroid and other glandular disturbances.	Patient breathes into and out of container of oxygen. His heat-production rate is determined by his rate of oxygen consumption. Percentage of variation from normal heat-production rate is called his basal-metabolic rate.
Hemoglobin Determination	To determine amount of hemoglobin in blood.	Patient's fingertip or ear lobe is punctured, and a measured amount of blood is drawn into a pipette. Prior to further laboratory test, blood is placed in tube containing hydrochloric acid.
Red Blood Cell Determination	To determine presence of anemia or polycythemia.	A drop of patient's blood is diluted in a special pipette, and after proper preparation, the red blood cells are counted.
White Blood Cell Determination	To aid in determining presence of infections or leukemia.	Blood from patient is diluted with a special fluid that destroys the red blood cells but does not injure the white cells. After proper preparation, the white cells are counted.
Urine	To determine presence of kidney disease or diabetes.	Urine specimen is examined for presence of albumin, red and white blood cells, and sugar.
Clotting Time	To test clotting ability of blood.	Skin is punctured and time estimated before bleeding stops.
Prothrombin Time	To determine vitamin-K deficiency.	Test to determine adequacy of a substance in blood necessary for clotting.
Blood Pressure	To detect high or low blood pressure.	Measured with mercury column or spring instrument by putting cuff around patient's arm and getting record at contraction (systolic) and relaxation (diastolic) of heart.

INTERPRETATION OF TEST	REMARKS
Positive reaction shown by red area at point where toxin was injected. Negative reaction indicates person is immune to diphtheria.	Schick testing of children about every two or three years is advised by many physicians; also testing of adults before inoculation during epidemics.
Positive reaction consists of red area one centimeter or more in diameter, occurring eighteen to twenty-four hours after injection. No reaction indicates immunity to scarlet fever.	Some physicians do not consider the Dick-test results comparable in dependability with those of the Schick test.
Clumping of germs brought about by this serum indicates that patient has typhoid fever.	Test is of no value if person has had typhoid fever previously, or if he has been vaccinated against the disease.
Positive reaction is a red area about the point of injection after forty-eight hours.	Tuberculin test should always be considered in conjunction with other examinations.
Speeded-up sedimentation rate is evidence of the presence of some infection.	Many factors influence sedimentation rate, such as room temperature, concentration of red blood cells, length of sedimentation tube.
Reactions are judged by degree to which destruction of red blood cells is prevented.	Some doctors now deem it advisable to report the complement-fixation reactions only as positive, doubtful, or negative.
If the mice's ovaries are enlarged, test is positive for pregnancy.	Test stated to be reliable after tenth day following first missed menstrual period. Test remains positive until seven days after the birth of a full-term baby. Other new tests involve use of frogs, rabbits, etc.
Ten percent or more above or below normal—between plus or minus seven—indicates an abnormal condition. Above is a sign of hyperthyroidism.	Useful only in conjunction with physical examination and study of patient's symptoms. For accurate results in test, patient must be completely relaxed. Test is made after patient has fasted for twelve hours and has rested thirty minutes just before test.
Decrease in hemoglobin means anemia.	Sahli's method is briefly described here. There are other methods, but none is absolutely accurate.
Decrease of red blood cells below 4,500,000 to 6,000,000 per cubic millimeter indicates anemia.	When normal care is taken in this test, results are invariably reliable.
Above normal usually indicates infection.	Same as above.
Albumin may indicate acute or chronic kidney inflammation or infection of kidney. Red blood cells may be present in acute nephritis and in tumors or stones of the kidney. Large numbers of white blood cells indicate a bladder infection or infection of the kidney pelvis. Sugar usually means diabetes.	Color and odor of urine, presence of sediment, its reaction—that is, whether alkaline or acid—its specific gravity, are all important in diagnosing kidney and related disorders.
Usual time is one to three minutes.	Used in purpura and hemophilia.
Test shows insufficient amount of substance necessary for clotting blood.	Technique used before gall-bladder operations and in liver inflammation.
Normal rate is approximately 120 plus years, over twenty to thirty.	Routine in life-insurance examination.

the disease and its causes Tetanus is an acute infection of the central nervous system caused by a specific type of bacteria and the poison they create. The bacteria are usually found in dust, dirt, and manure. The patient is infected through a puncture wound caused by anything sharp—such as a nail or splinter, or an insect or dog bite. Any skin opening is a port of entry, but deep wounds are dangerous because the tetanus germ thrives best without oxygen. It can occur in anyone . . . in any age group . . . at any time of the year. The incubation period is 3 days to 3 weeks.

symptoms This disease is characterized by pain and stiffness of the muscles of any part of the body. This is usually preceded by headache, temperature, stiff neck, and then muscle spasm. The wound of entry shows all the signs of infection. The muscles of the jaw are particularly involved, and it becomes painful and difficult to open the mouth. It is from this that the name lockjaw comes.
Swallowing may be difficult. Breathing is labored and irregular. The entire back may go into such spasm that the victim arches until he is lying on just his head and heels. Convulsions occur. In severe cases the patient dies in as few as 3 days. In less severe instances, the course of the illness is 2 to 3 weeks.

complications Secondary infections such as pneumonia are common. Heart failure can cause death. Patients who recover sometimes have deformed backs as a result of the severe muscle spasm. The disease is frequently fatal, although it need not be if properly diagnosed and treated early. When therapy is delayed, the poison or toxin invades the body disastrously.

prevention (or lessening of impact) Since the tetanus vaccine available is highly effective, immunization should be started during the first year of life. It is a series of 3 injections. Booster shots should be given for any dirty, potentially infected wound. Patients who have not been immunized and require immediate protection can be given an antitoxin, but many people react adversely to it because it is made of horse serum. Highly specialized care is needed if there is to be any hope of saving the life of a patient ill with tetanus. Specific medications are available for the muscle spasms and for complications. Hospitalization is a "must." Often the patient must be fed intravenously and may require a respirator to help him breathe.

Tetanus (Lockjaw)

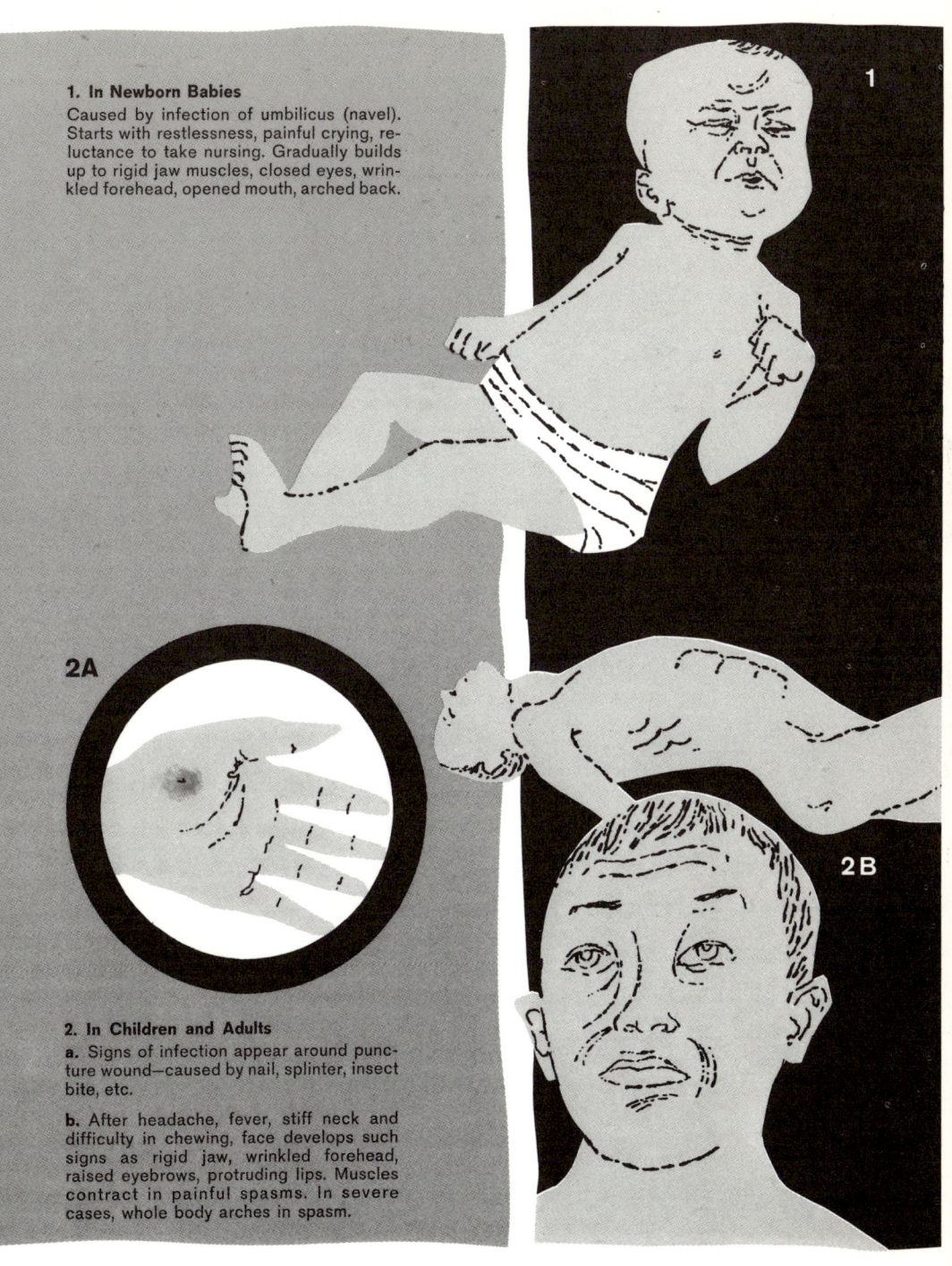

1. In Newborn Babies
Caused by infection of umbilicus (navel). Starts with restlessness, painful crying, reluctance to take nursing. Gradually builds up to rigid jaw muscles, closed eyes, wrinkled forehead, opened mouth, arched back.

2. In Children and Adults
a. Signs of infection appear around puncture wound—caused by nail, splinter, insect bite, etc.

b. After headache, fever, stiff neck and difficulty in chewing, face develops such signs as rigid jaw, wrinkled forehead, raised eyebrows, protruding lips. Muscles contract in painful spasms. In severe cases, whole body arches in spasm.

ment, catalyzing adult interest in sex, and ideas and attitudes usually identified as adult and masculine.

The body may contain at least one other male sex hormone, if not more, but this has not as yet been scientifically established.

The term *eunuch* signifies a male deprived of the testicles or of the entire external male genitalia. Such men tend to lose many or most typically male characteristics, particularly if the mutilation is performed before puberty.

Disorders of the testicles are *infection,* damage from *mumps, cancer,* or *failure to descend* normally into the scrotum. In addition, *typhoid* and *undulant fever* may affect these organs. Mumps reach the testicles in approximately one in a hundred cases, but sometimes more frequently in a major epidemic. Mumps cause testicles to swell painfully and sometimes destroy their function permanently, a complication called *orchitis. Epididymitis* is an infection of the epididymis, the hoodlike structure covering the upper end of each testicle. The sulfa and antibiotic drugs are used advantageously in testicular infections.

The testicles normally descend from within the body to the scrotum at birth. However, this does not always occur. Since the internal temperature of the body is too high to permit the organs to produce sperm cells, the glands cannot develop and function properly. Therefore, when testicles do not descend, some of the male characteristics may be latent. Treatment by hormones alone may be sufficient, but often surgery is indicated to correct this condition, called *cryptorchism.*

Cancer of the testicles is rare. The first sign is usually in the spermatic cords. Pain or other symptoms in the testicle itself occur later. *See also* ORCHITIS; REPRODUCTION SYSTEM; UNDESCENDED TESTES; SEMEN; SEMINAL DUCTS; SPERMATIC CORDS; VAS DEFERENS; EPIDIDYMIS; SCROTUM; PENIS; CASTRATION; FERTILITY; STERILITY; IMPOTENCE; STERILIZATION. *See* MEDIGRAPHS pages 923, 1179, 1307.

TESTS. The medical test is an important diagnostic tool. Tests range from the blood pressure test which the family doctor performs every day to the more complex tests that are conducted in the medical laboratory or hospital. The medical test may be used to detect the presence of a specific disease or condition; to determine susceptibility or immunity to a specific disease; to measure the rate and manner in which the body is functioning, and for various other purposes. Very often a combination of tests are used in diagnosis. The chart shows some of the more common tests (pp. 1252-1253).

TETANUS, or *lockjaw,* an infectious disease, often fatal, which especially attacks the muscles of the neck and lower jaw. This disease is caused by the *tetanus bacillus,* a germ which ordinarily infests the intestines of cattle, horses, or men, and which is also found in the earth. The germ invades human beings primarily through wounds. Since it

1256

thrives best without oxygen, it is found most abundantly in deeper wounds, especially those which contain soil or foreign refuse.

About seven days after the invasion of the germ, the person infected is likely to feel a kind of pulling pain in the wound. This is accompanied by a spasm of the muscles. He may develop chills and fever, a painful headache, and probably a general feeling of irritability. Stiffness is first evident in the muscles of the jaw and neck, and a series of violent convulsions and spasm may soon follow. Sometimes occurring as frequently as every minute, these spasms may be so extensive that every muscle in the body is involved.

The tetanus bacillus engenders an exceedingly strong poison which may be fatal. Prevention of the disease consists of injecting an *antitoxin* under the skin as soon as a wound has been inflicted. The wound is then opened wide, thoroughly cleaned of foreign matter, and cleansed with antiseptic. This preventive technique is so efficient that not one death from tetanus was recorded among the U.S. forces during World War II. *See also* IMMUNIZATION. *See* MEDIGRAPH page 1255.

TETANY. *See* PARATHYROID GLANDS.

TEXAS FEVER. *See* UNDULANT FEVER.

THALASSEMIA. *See* RED BLOOD CELLS, DISEASES OF.

THERMOMETER, in medicine, the instrument used to take the temperature of the body. In the United States, the *Fahrenheit* scale is most frequently used, usually calibrated between 94° and 110°. The normal body temperature, 98.6°, is generally indicated by an arrow. The *Centigrade* thermometer is used in Europe, Asia, and other countries.

Before taking a temperature, the mercury must be shaken down below the normal mark. This is done either by firmly grasping the stem between the thumb and forefinger and shaking the thermometer forcibly in the air, or by holding the stem in the same way and striking the inner side of the wrist on the knee.

The temperature can be taken in the mouth, armpit, groin, or rectum. Before placing a thermometer in the armpit or groin, the part should be thoroughly dried and the thermometer placed between two skin surfaces, care being taken that clothing does not come between the bulb and the skin. For rectal temperatures, the bulb of the thermometer is smeared with a little petroleum jelly and then gently manipulated into place. The thermometer should remain in the mouth or rectum for three to five minutes, and in the armpit or groin for seven to ten minutes. After use, the thermometer should be thoroughly cleansed, sterilized, and stored in a safe place.

THIAMIN DEFICIENCY. The chief symptoms of a disease called *beriberi* are due to a lack of one of the portions of the vitamin B complex called *thiamin*. Thiamin is soluble in water, damaged by heat and found chiefly in whole cereals, peas, beans, lean meats, nuts and yeast. Refined sugar, milled rice and low extraction flour have lost most of their thiamin.

People whose diets are low in protein and high in carbohydrates are likely to show symptoms of thiamin deficiency. In the United States the condition is seen often among chronic alcoholics who get insufficient amounts of the right foods because of their displacement by alcohol.

The chief damages to tissues of the body seen in thiamin deficiency are found in the nerves and in the heart and blood vessels. Often these tissues become swollen with water. After about three months on a diet really deficient in thiamin the symptoms begin to appear. Gradually the person becomes tired and irritable and the muscles, particularly those of the calf of the leg become painful. Later serious inflammations of the nerves appear and these may go on to the point of loss of sensation and paralysis. When *neuritis* becomes so prominent the doctor must make sure that it does not result from some other cause since lead or arsenic poisoning or various infections may also cause neuritis.

As soon as a sufficient intake of thiamin is assured the patient begins to improve. Thiamin is now available in the form of tablets or capsules that can be taken internally and also in forms that can be injected into the body when prompt action is desired. If treatment is begun sufficiently early most patients recover rapidly and completely. If treatment is delayed until actual destruction of nerve tissue has occurred, results are doubtful. *See also* BERIBERI; SCURVY; PELLAGRA; RICKETS; XEROPHTHALMIA; KWASHIORKOR.

THOUGHT. *See* BRAIN; MEMORY; CEREBRUM.

THREE-DAY FEVER. *See* SANDFLY FEVER.

THROAT. The inside of the throat includes the *larynx* (voice box), the *pharynx,* the *fauces*—which is the space surrounded by the *soft palate,* a group of muscles used in swallowing—the *palatine arches* and the *base of the tongue.* On the outside, the front part of the *neck* is also described as the throat.

A sore throat is an inflammation of part of the throat. Inflammations are manifested by redness, swelling, and excessive discharges of mucus due to many different sources. Most common is exposure to cold, an extension of inflammation from the tonsils, adenoids, or the nose.

One form of sore throat, *pharyngitis,* may be an entirely separate disease or the symptom of another ailment, such as *scarlet fever, influenza, measles,* or *smallpox.*

Excessive use of tobacco, exposure to large amounts of dust, smoke, irritating fumes, and sudden changes in temperature or excessive dryness and similar atmospheric conditions may cause irritation of the throat. Persons who are sensitive to certain food substances frequently react with blisters on the tissues of the throat, which become infected and produce irritations and inflammation. Swelling and inflammation of the throat may produce pain in the ears, because of blocking of the tubes which pass from the nose to the ear. A sense of fullness or obstruction, with much spitting and hawking, can also develop.

In "strep" throat, which is *septic sore throat* caused by the *streptococcus* germ, a membrane, a thin layer of tissue, sometimes appears in the throat, the glands may swell, and the temperature may rise as high as 105° F. *Penicillin* generally cures this condition.

Application of an ice pack may relieve the pain of an inflamed throat. Most doctors feel that gargles are ineffective since they seldom reach into the throat, although they may help to remove mucus and to wash out infected material. Direct application of an antiseptic to the throat gives a specific effect. Either an atomizer or a cotton swab may be used. To be sure that the antiseptic reaches the back of the throat, it may be necessary to hold the tongue or use a tongue depressor.

The primary purpose of a mouthwash or throat wash is to clean and soothe. A good cleansing mouthwash is salt solution, made by adding a fourth of a teaspoon of salt to half a glass of warm water. If mucus is profuse, the addition of a quarter of a teaspoon of bicarbonate of soda, ordinary baking soda, may be beneficial. *See also* LARYNGITIS; QUINSY; SEPTIC SORE THROAT; SORE THROAT. *See* MEDIGRAPHS pages 515, 1269.

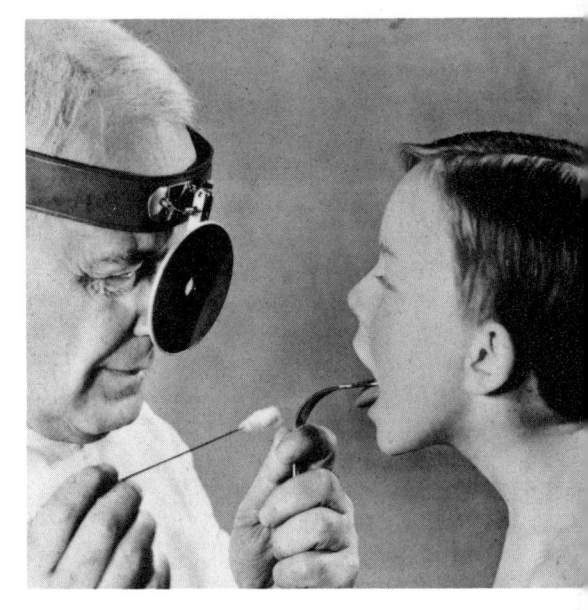

Throat—Inspection of the throat is an important part of physical examination. Changes in the throat or a sore throat may be symptoms of infection or a disease in another part of the body. To treat an infected area in the throat the doctor uses a tongue depressor and applicator.

THROMBO-ANGIITIS OBLITERANS. *See* BUERGER'S DISEASE.

THROMBOCYTOPENIA. People who bruise and bleed easily and who develop purple spots on the skin are often suffering with a condition called *idiopathic thrombocytopenic purpura*. This means that there is a deficiency of *blood platelets* in the blood and that the cause is not known. The condition may develop as a result of an infection or after the taking of various drugs. These drugs however affect only a few people in this way. The condition they cause usually disappears a few months after the drug is discontinued.

Chronic cases of this condition persist with ups and downs over the years. One theory holds that a chronic case is a result of a change in the person's blood in which the blood develops a substance which attacks its own platelets. This view has been confirmed by experiments which involved injection of the blood from a person who had the disease into a normal person. Such an injection made the number of blood platelets in the normal person decrease. The injection of normal platelets into people with *thrombocytopenic purpura* resulted in destruction of the normal blood platelets. *ACTH* and *cortisone* have been used in some of these cases with remarkably successful results. In fact the proper diagnosis of the condition and control treatment of this condition with ACTH and cortisone has been so successful that the operation which involved removal of the *spleen* as a life-saving measure in such cases has come into greatly diminished use. The emergency operation for removal of the spleen is now done in only the most severe cases which do not react favorably to the use of either ACTH or cortisone or both. *See also* SPLEEN; RADIATION SICKNESS; LEUKEMIA; RED BLOOD CELLS, DISEASES OF; WHITE BLOOD CELLS, DISEASES OF.

THROMBOPHLEBITIS. *See* PHLEBITIS.

THROMBOSIS, a clot formation inside a blood vessel; the clot is called a *thrombus*. Thrombosis is caused by failure of the mechanism in the blood which keeps it fluid. Such a disorder usually occurs in veins in which the flow of blood is slowed, as in a varicose vein of the leg, or in a leg vein of a person who must lie in bed for a long time. In some cases, thrombosis is associated with bacterial infection in the area affected, or in an actual inflammation of the vein, as in *thrombophlebitis*. Thrombosis may also occur in narrow arteries through which the blood passes with difficulty, but *arterial thrombosis* is much rarer than *venous thrombosis*.

Thrombosis does harm by obstructing the flow of blood to and from the part supplied by the vessel and as a source of traveling fragments of clots, or *emboli*. An *embolus* is especially dangerous when it affects the lung, and there is always danger of sudden death.

Thrombosis is often the source of *stroke,* although a stroke caused by thrombosis is less dramatic and severe than one from an embolism or with hemorrhage. Strokes from thrombosis have a better chance for recovery, but some permanent disability usually persists.

A clot in the main vein of a limb produces swelling. For example, a clot in a main vein of the leg, deep in the upper calf, will cause a swelling of the foot and ankle and probably most of the leg below the obstruction. The amount of harm done depends on what area the artery supplies and whether or not there are alternative routes for the blood. If there is no alternative route, all the living cells which compose the part supplied will die. The effect is exactly the same as that of an embolism or of complete blocking and obliteration of the artery by progressive hardening and narrowing.

Thrombosis is treated by certain *anticoagulants,* including *heparin, dicumarol,* and others, and in some cases surgery is employed to remove clots and help restore the flow of blood to the affected parts. Anticoagulants together with proper massage and exercise have been particularly effective for patients with swollen legs due to thrombophlebitis when infection is not a complicating factor. In some cases of varicose veins, a thrombus may change into fibrous or scarlike tissue and the inside of the tube is obliterated. In this way a natural cure is sometimes effected. *See also* APOPLEXY; COAGULATION; CORONARY THROMBOSIS; EMBOLISM. *See* MEDIGRAPHS pages 449, 1035.

THRUSH, a fungus infection of the mouth in infants and occasionally older persons. White spots form, then become shallow ulcers. Frequently fever and gastrointestinal disturbance are present. The fungus may spread to the buttocks, groin, and other areas of the body. *See* MEDIGRAPH page 665.

THUMB SUCKING. In a healthy happy baby, thumb sucking, if practiced in moderation, is normal and may be ignored. The child will discover new amusement with the passage of time. Persistent thumb sucking, authorities claim, may lead to malocclusion of the teeth. If the child ceases sucking his thumb before the age of five, however, this malocclusion has a tendency to cure itself.

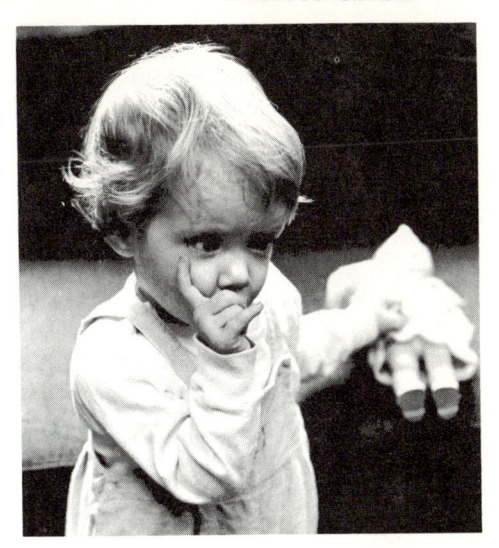

Thumb-Sucking—Before the coming of permanent teeth, thumb sucking will not harm tooth and jaw development. The habit is normal in the first two or three years of life, but in a five-year-old indicates unhappiness or anxiety that should be examined.

To cure a persistent thumb sucker is not easy. Painting the thumb with a bad-tasting medicine or forcing the child to wear a mitten have not been successful methods and are not recommended. The source of the habit lies in some kind of emotional disturbance or sense of insecurity. To cure thumb sucking, therefore, the source of the habit should be found. *See also* CHILD CARE.

THYMUS GLAND, a gland located in the chest near the heart. Its functions are not as yet established. This gland has an unusual part in the development of the body. Instead of growing like the rest of the physical structure, the thymus is largest during the first eight or nine months of life and after the second year normally shrinks almost to the point of disappearance and is replaced by other types of tissue.

If the gland does not shrink and its size and activity continue, the results can be serious. Occasionally, especially in infants, the gland enlarges so much that it interferes with circulation and breathing, because of its proximity to the heart and windpipe. X-ray treatment is often beneficial to reduce such an enlargement. Persons may develop thymic enlargement so suddenly, apparently in response to some stress or shock, that death results. This type of growth occurs in the condition called *status lymphaticus*.

The person whose thymus gland has failed to shrink has a soft complexion and, if male, will probably not have to shave, or infrequently. Such persons seem younger than their actual age. They lack body hair and may be subject to low blood pressure and fatigue.

In premature cessation of functioning of the thymus, aging seems to occur before the usual time, and blood pressure is apt to be high and body hair excessive.

In laboratory experiments in which animals have been administered thymus extract, their growth and development, both sexual and mental, have been precocious even into the second and third generations. However, giantism does not occur.

Investigation of the thymus is still in an early stage. The thymus is apparently implicated with development of the skeleton, the sex glands, and with metabolism of calcium. *See also* GLANDS.

THYROID GLAND. One of the most significant of the *endocrine glands* which produce secretions that regulate many basic processes of the body, the thyroid gland lies in the front part of the throat along the windpipe.

The thyroid secretion, *thyroxin*, is involved in the process of *oxidation* which occurs within the cells and by which the tissues generate the energy they require. Its importance is indicated by the serious consequences of excessive or deficient amounts of it in the body. A child born with insufficient thyroid activity becomes a *cretin*, physically undergrown and mentally an *idiot*. Thyroid deficiency in later life causes physical and mental coarsening and dulling. Excessive thyroid produces general restlessness, speeds up the heart, and may have other untoward effects. Both *hyperthyroidism*, too much thyroid, and *hypothyroidism*, too little, can be successfully treated.

The thyroid is susceptible to a variety of diseases, the most common being *simple goiter*, usually due to a lack of iodine. In *Graves' disease (exophthalmic goiter)*, overactivity of the thyroid causes a pop-eyed appearance and other serious symptoms. *Tumors* of lesser or greater malignancy may affect the thyroid. Surgical removal is indicated for most types of thyroid cancer. X-ray and radium treatment and radioactive iodine have also been

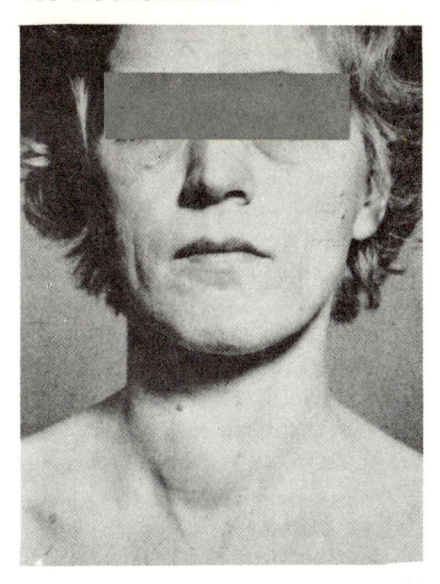

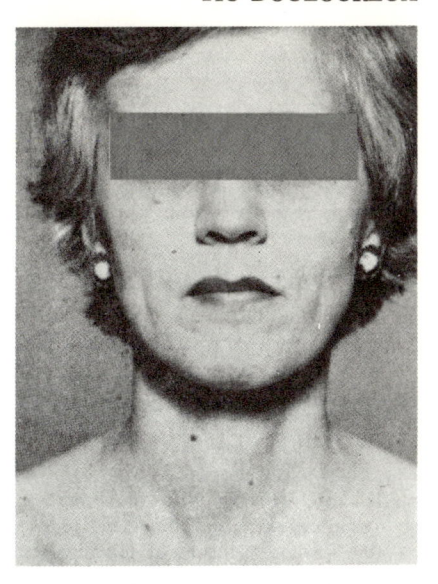

Thyroid—Moderate enlargement of the thyroid gland caused by a noninfectious disease (*left*). This type of inflammation affects men much less frequently than women. The gland enlarges gradually and one area may be more prominent than another. Photograph taken two months later, showing regression of the enlargement (*right*). Patient was treated with desiccated thyroid, a substance made from the thyroid of sheep. Desiccated thyroid is used to cure certain fairly common conditions affecting human beings.

beneficial in certain cases. A number of infectious and noninfectious diseases of the thyroid also respond well to treatment. *See also* BASAL METABOLISM; CRETINISM; GLANDS; GOITER; HYPOTHYROIDISM. *See* MEDIGRAPHS pages 465, 769, 1265.

TIC DOULOUREUX, or *trigeminal neuralgia,* one of the more common neuralgias or paroxysmal pains, usually beginning in the middle life and occurring more frequently in women. It is characterized by an intense stabbing pain which strikes one or a combination of three facial branches supplied by the *trigeminal (fifth cranial) nerve.*

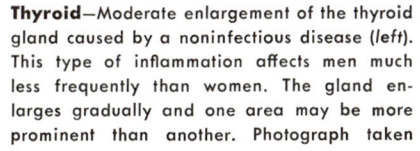

The attacks occur without warning, in violent, knifelike darts of pain. The face is twisted in spasms and there is a free flow of tears and saliva. The seizure lasts only a few seconds and may clear up spontaneously, with varying periods of relief. The pain may involve the first or ophthalmic division which includes the forehead and eye, the second division around the nose, or the third or side of the mouth. The second and third branches seem to be more frequently affected. The pain does not spread to the back of the head or across to the other side of the face. The attacks tend to increase in acuteness and extent and as the condition becomes worse the periods of freedom from pain become shorter. The seizures often are influenced by seasonal changes and occur more frequently during spring and fall. Pain may be prompted by touching

the disease and its causes This disease, which is the result of an overactive thyroid, is a less common form of chronic heart disease. The thyroid secretes an excess amount of hormone and causes other organs and tissues of the body to speed up beyond their normal pace. The heart attempts to keep up with the demands placed on it and pumps faster. The result is a change in the normal rhythm of the heart beat, and ultimately congestive heart failure. The age group affected is 35 to 50. Women are more susceptible than men.

symptoms Sometimes the overactive thyroid is overlooked because symptoms of the heart condition are more prominent. There is weakness, nervousness, and loss of weight. The patient may sweat profusely and always feel warm. Sometimes there are heart palpitations. The pulse is usually very rapid, even at rest, or else it is irregular. Blood pressure may or may not be higher than normal, but the heart is enlarged because of the heavier demands made on it. Usually there is some shortness of breath and swelling of the feet.

In addition, there are the symptoms of congestive heart failure, such as blue lips and fingernails, swollen neck veins, cough and breathing difficulty, fluid in the lungs and abdomen. As the condition worsens, it takes less and less exertion to produce these symptoms.

complications The usual complication of hyperthyroid heart disease is heart failure plus the abnormal rhythm previously mentioned.

prevention (or lessening of impact) Since the underlying cause of this disease is an overactive thyroid, measures must be taken to correct this. Surgical and medical treatment are both quite satisfactory, as well as radioactive iodine given orally. Every case must be considered individually and the most advisable approach used. Thyroid heart disease is a form of heart disease which may be cured permanently if it is recognized promptly and treated before excessive damage is done.

Thyroid Heart Disease

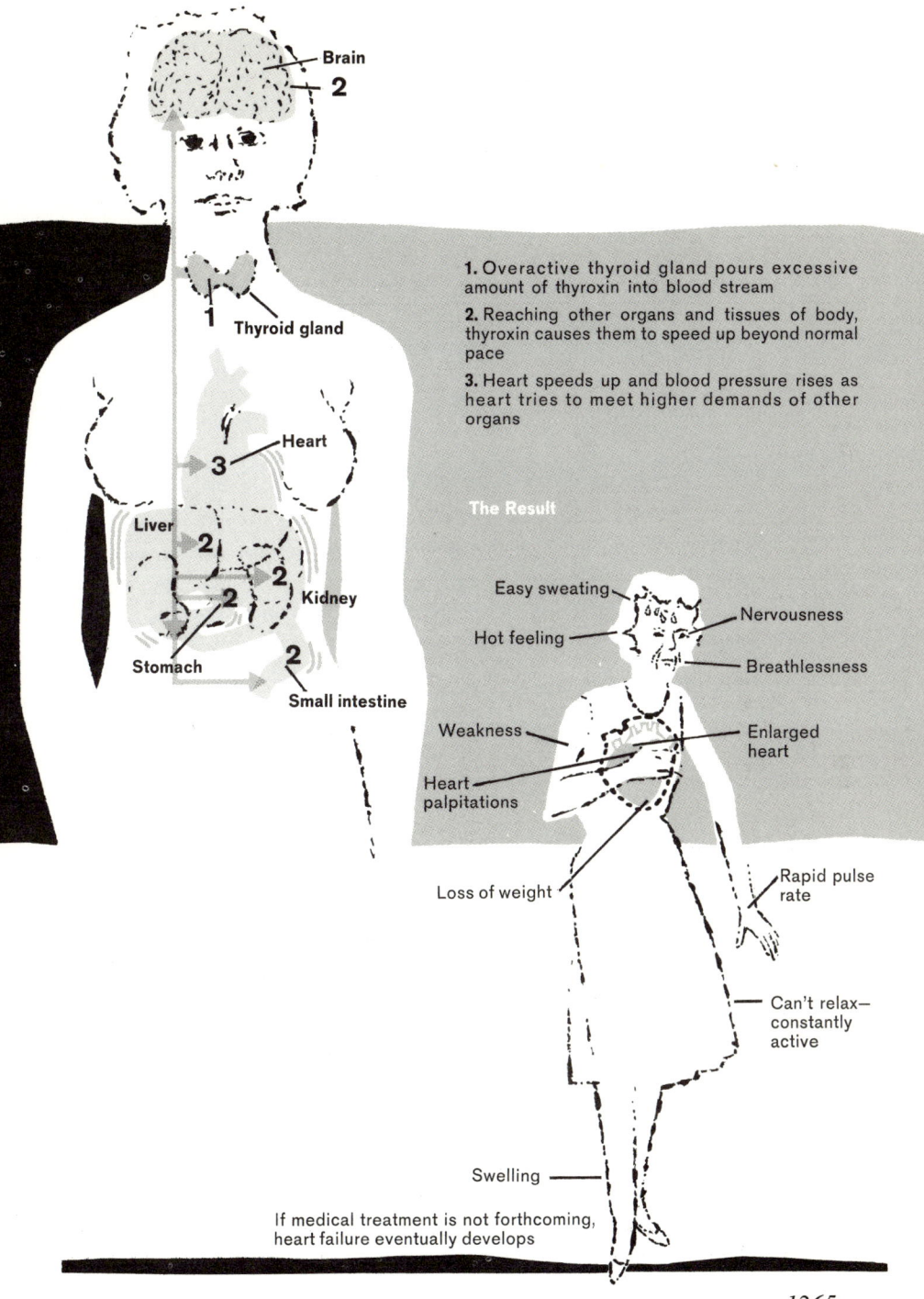

Brain — 2

Thyroid gland — 1

Heart — 3

Liver — 2
Stomach — 2
Kidney — 2
Small intestine — 2

1. Overactive thyroid gland pours excessive amount of thyroxin into blood stream
2. Reaching other organs and tissues of body, thyroxin causes them to speed up beyond normal pace
3. Heart speeds up and blood pressure rises as heart tries to meet higher demands of other organs

The Result

- Easy sweating
- Hot feeling
- Nervousness
- Breathlessness
- Weakness
- Enlarged heart
- Heart palpitations
- Loss of weight
- Rapid pulse rate
- Can't relax—constantly active
- Swelling

If medical treatment is not forthcoming, heart failure eventually develops

1265

the affected side of the face, by exposure to cold, washing, eating, drinking, or talking, and emotional tension or fatigue intensify the attack.

Treatment consists largely of measures to relieve individual attacks. *Nicotinic acid* and *trichlorethylene inhalations* give temporary relief. Alcohol injections, once widely used, have been discontinued because relief from pain is too often incomplete and the periods of relief between injections tend to become increasingly shorter. Alcohol injections are now given in some clinics before the *operation for trigeminal neuralgia* in order to accustom the patient to the facial numbness which generally follows the operation. The operation itself is now common and consists in cutting the branch or branches of the trigeminal nerve which carry the pain to the affected area of the face. In those cases in which the eye is involved and the first branch is cut, the patient is given special instruction in care of the eye, since sensation in this area is affected when the nerve is cut and the patient is unable to detect the presence of foreign bodies in the eye.

TINNITUS. *See* NOISE.

TOBACCO, a plant from which the leaf is especially dried, cured, and prepared for chewing or smoking in the form of cigars or cigarettes. Tobacco, especially in the form of cigarettes, is so popular that it takes a place on almost every family budget along with food, clothing, and shelter.

Many disorders of the human body such as respiratory infections, neuralgia, gastrointestinal difficulties, headache, inability to sleep, constipation, diarrhea, heart murmur, and cancer have been attributed to smoking. The cause-and-effect relationship cannot always be proved definitively.

Smoking does have a deleterious effect on the blood vessels and the circulation of the blood. A definite relationship has been determined between smoking and *Buerger's disease,* which is characterized by inflammation of the lining of the blood vessels.

Excessive smoking of cigarettes, according to recent evidence, is connected with cancer of the lung and is one of the most dangerous habits in which one can indulge. No evidence has been uncovered proving that filter tips *significantly* reduce the risk involved in excessive cigarette smoking. There is apparently less risk of lung cancer in the smoking of cigars and pipes, especially if inhalation does not occur. Cigars and pipe tobacco burn at a lower temperature than cigarettes, and this is probably an important factor. Evidence indicates that the higher temperature at which cigarette tobacco burns may catalyze certain carcinogenic chemicals which are not catalyzed at lower temperatures. *See also* CANCER. *See* MEDIGRAPHS pages 283, 865.

TOENAILS. *See* NAILS.

TONGUE, the movable muscular organ attached to the floor of the back of the mouth. Its chief functions are to help with chewing and swallowing food, with taste, and to form sounds in speech.

The *taste buds* are on the side of the *projections* (*papillae*) which lie across the tongue at the juncture of the mouth and the pharynx. A fold of membrane—the *frenum*—joins the undersurface of the tip of the tongue to the floor of the mouth. Sometimes the frenum is abnormally short and results in "tongue-tied" speech, which can usually be remedied by a simple operation.

Normally the tongue is pinkish white in color, moist and clean; a tongue that is dry, dark, and furry indicates disease. Among the most common of peculiar sensations that disturb persons is a burning painful tongue. The tongue, like all other tissue of the human body, is connected with the nervous system, and a burning sensation in the tongue is reflected through its nerves. In some cases, a relationship exists between this burning and vitamin deficiency, anemia, lack of iron, or even an allergy, but when no apparent physical cause exists, purely mental reasons are thought to be responsible—for example, a woman in menopause who is worried about developing cancer might experience a burning tongue.

Sometimes the tongue is inflamed through contact with edges of rough teeth, or ill-fitting false teeth. Frequently burning tongue is associated with difficulties of the digestive system. In such cases, the doctor will want to make a complete examination, which includes blood tests as well as checking the digestive system.

In a few instances, burning, and even ulcers, of the tongue have been found to be caused by the fact that different electric potentials have been used to fill teeth on opposite sides of the mouth. In a condition called *glossitis,* the tongue itself is infected and may have superficial or deep abscesses. The tongue may be subject to cancer or other specific diseases.

Sometimes the surface of the tongue, instead of being smooth, becomes marked by deep furrows and elevations. This condition, called *geographic tongue,* is not infectious and may be helped by mouthwashes, mild antiseptics, and a diet rich in vitamins and antianemic substances such as iron and liver. Black patches or hairlike projections can also form on the papillae. *See also* GLOSSITIS.

TONSILLECTOMY. *See* TONSILS.

TONSILS, masses of spongy lymphoid tissue located at the sides of the throat in the entrance to the digestive and respiratory tracts. They frequently become infected, with such symptoms as swelling, inflammation, pain, soreness, difficulty in swallowing, enlargement of the glands of the throat, fever, a rapid pulse, and general illness.

The person affected with *tonsillitis* should be put to bed and the doctor called. Ice packs or hot compresses may be applied about the throat and neck to relieve pain. The doctor will take steps to combat fever. Early administration of drugs, particularly antibiotics, greatly reduces the possibility of serious complications or aftereffects, which can include *deaf-*

the disease and its causes Many bacteria and viruses infect the tonsils, but it is the streptococcus which is the most common cause of tonsillitis—and from which it gets the alternate name of strep throat. The disease occurs most often in children, but affects every age group. Strep throat localizes on tonsils, stubs of tonsils, or in the pharynx. The incubation period can run from 1 to 10 days, but most generally lasts 2 to 4 days. The illness itself runs from 3 to 9 days without medication, and is shortened by treatment.

symptoms Acute tonsillitis begins suddenly with chills, aches and pains, headache, and sore throat. The temperature rises quickly to 102°-104°, and it may go as high as 106°. Nausea and vomiting are frequent with children, diarrhea less so. The disease reaches its peak quickly, usually within 24 to 48 hours. The sore throat is severe and persists until the infection is brought under control. Pain is likely to spread to the ear and the neck. Here glands behind the angle of the jaw, below the ears, are most commonly affected. One out of 2 cases shows cold symptoms, with nasal discharge, cough, and loss of voice. As shown in the Medi-Graph, the mucous membrane of the pharynx, soft palate, and tonsils may be red and swollen and covered partially or entirely with a yellow, white or grayish membrane. The tongue is usually gray and coated.

complications A frequent complication and disease to which tonsillitis is related is scarlet fever. It may appear 1 to 5 days after the onset of the infection and is identified by the rash. Other complications include sinusitis, ear infections, pneumonia, and a serious peritonsillar abscess called quinsy throat which occurs when the infection spreads about the tonsillar area. There is difficulty in swallowing, pain on opening the mouth, and very sore throat. Chronic tonsillitis can develop, with signs of the infection recurring in the same pattern every 2 or 3 weeks. Arthritis and meningitis are rare complications.

prevention (or lessening of impact) There is no specific vaccine against the streptococcus bacteria. Since the greater number of people with this illness carry the organism in their respiratory discharge for as long as 3 months, preventing its spread is a problem. Good hygiene must be observed. Those who come in close contact with a patient should be treated promptly with antibiotics. Susceptible people can be given protection over long periods of time with drugs prescribed by the doctor. Good medical care during the illness helps to prevent the patient from becoming a carrier.

Acute Tonsillitis (Strep Throat)

A. Red, swollen tonsils, pharynx, soft palate. Patches of yellow, gray or white membrane covers inflamed area. Tongue has heavy gray coating.

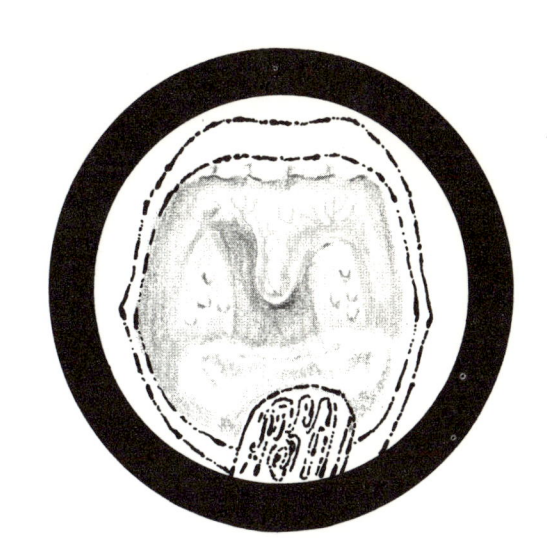

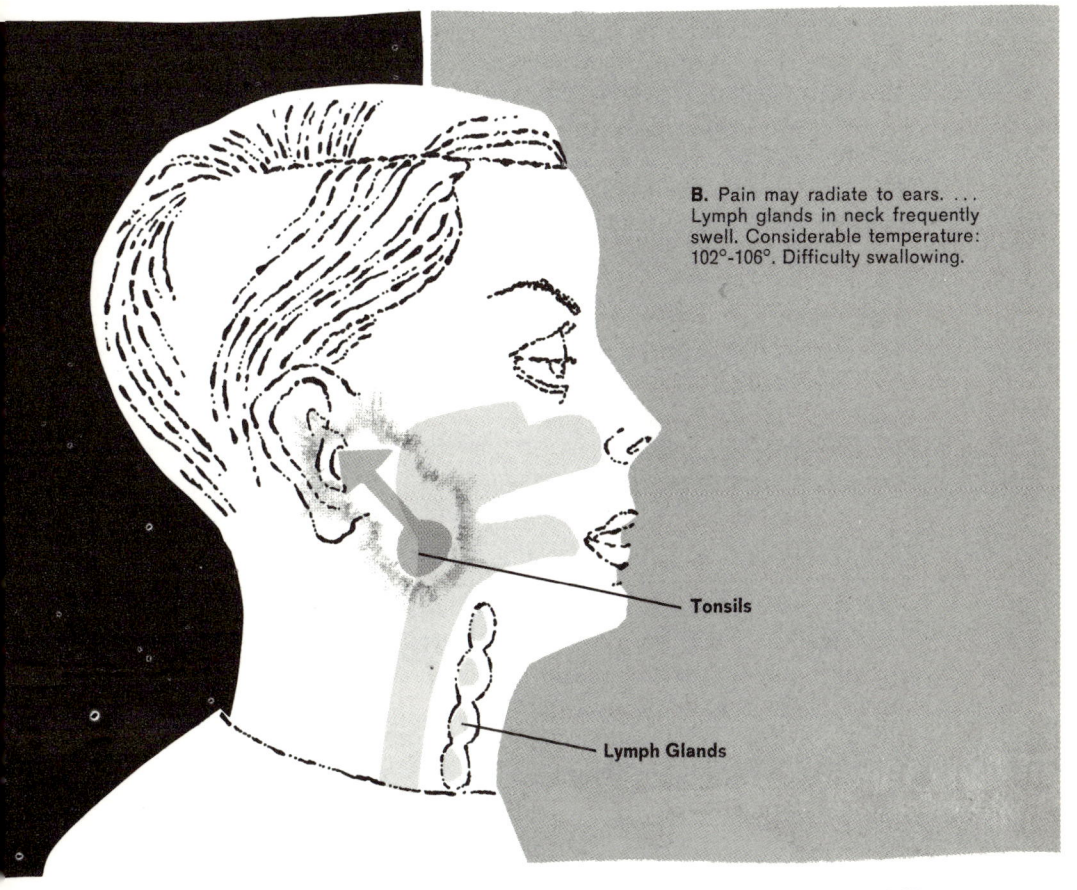

B. Pain may radiate to ears. ... Lymph glands in neck frequently swell. Considerable temperature: 102°-106°. Difficulty swallowing.

Tonsils

Lymph Glands

1269

ness, kidney disease, rheumatic fever and other *heart ailments.*

Extraction of diseased and enlarged tonsils and adenoids, which interfere with breathing, is usually beneficial not only in removing a source of infection but also in improving the child's general health, appearance, and disposition. Surgery to remove tonsils is advised in recurrent attacks of tonsillitis accompanied by swelling of the neck glands. The operation—*tonsillectomy*—is so common and has been so well perfected that complications are exceedingly rare.

In older persons or in the presence of heart disease and other cases in which anesthetic is not possible, tonsils are sometimes treated with *radiation* by x-ray. X-ray and radium are also occasionally used to treat fragments of tissue that may be left after tonsillectomy and when there is regrowth of secondary adenoidal tissue. *See also* ADENOIDS. *See* MEDIGRAPHS pages 1143, 1269.

TORTICOLLIS, commonly called *wry neck,* a spasmodic movement of the neck muscles which causes the head to be pulled toward one side. In some instances, shortening of neck muscles is present at birth or may occur from an injury, but in the majority of cases the origin of this disorder is unknown.

Wry neck begins suddenly without warning. The neck muscles unexpectedly contract and the head is pulled to one side in irregular jerks. It may follow a nervous reaction due to tension, worry, or anxiety. At this stage the movements can be suppressed by the person, but as the condition grows worse the movements recur involuntarily and cannot be controlled.

Psychotherapy has been successfully tried in treatment of some cases. In more stubborn cases, this treatment is combined with a *nerve block,* a procedure in which the *cervical nerves* are blocked with *procaine* or *novocaine.* Light exercises also help to relax the muscles. Frequent periods of spontaneous relief occur, but the condition generally returns, even after long intervals of relief. Use of collars or casts is not recommended. Medication includes drugs of the *belladonna* group and sedatives. Surgery has brought only temporary relief at best, and is not widely employed.

TOXEMIA, a condition in which the blood contains poisonous products, either those created by the body cells or those due to the action of microorganisms. It is a general infection in which the blood contains toxins but not bacteria.

TRACHEA, or *windpipe,* a tube about 4½ inches long which leads from the mouth and larynx to the lungs. It is susceptible to infections similar to those that attack any other part of the respiratory system. Inflammation of the trachea produces a hacking metallic cough, especially severe at night. This cough often produces considerable pain, particularly in the lower part of the neck and behind the breastbone. If the inflammation continues unchecked, mucus and sputum are eructed in coughing; and if the germ is *streptococcus,* pus may also be expectorated.

Treatment for ordinary inflammation of the trachea is rest in bed, warmth and quiet. A vaporizer, usually an electrical device which moistens and vaporizes the air the patient breathes, often brings relief. Medicated oil added to the water which is boiled in the vaporizer also has been found beneficial.

Ordinarily the inflammation will yield to proper treatment. In severe cases, which might often have become chronic in the past, the *sulfa drugs* or *penicillin* will usually eradicate the specific infection.

The tube may be obstructed by a physiological process, as in strangling, by a foreign object, or by disease. Surgical operation—*tracheotomy*—is performed in some instances to correct the condition. See MEDIGRAPH page 279.

TRACHOMA, a grave, highly contagious chronic disease of the eyelids, caused by a filterable virus. Trachoma was once an almost universal affliction and the most common cause of blindness. It is still widespread in countries where the standards of health and sanitation are low.

Trachoma is most contagious in the early stages and is spread by contact with infected persons, insects, or contaminated objects. The eyes become inflamed and congested, tears pour out excessively, and light is painful. Blisters and crusts appear on the upper lids and form scar tissue. Small gritty particles develop on the cornea, and in severe cases vision is so diminished that only light and dark can be distinguished.

Treatment of trachoma requires the care of a specialist. Each stage of the disease, from the first inflammation of the eyes to the development of granulations and finally scar tissue, demands expert handling. Rigorous hygienic measures must be observed to keep the eyes clean at all times. *Sulfonamide drugs* and *antibiotics* have made possible control of the spread of trachoma.

TRANQUILIZING DRUGS. See BARBITURATES.

TRANSMISSIBLE DISEASES. See AMEBIASIS; CHANCROID; DYSENTERY; ENCEPHALITIS; ERYSIPELAS; GLANDERS; GONORRHEA; LYMPHOGRANULOMA VENEREUM; MALARIA; PSITTACOSIS; RABIES; RAT-BITE FEVER; ROCKY MOUNTAIN SPOTTED FEVER; SYPHILIS; TETANUS; TULAREMIA; TYPHOID FEVER; UNDULANT FEVER; VINCENT'S ANGINA. *See also* INFECTIOUS DISEASES.

TRENCH FEVER, a mild acute rickettsial infection. During World War I, it was a major medical problem. It occurred during World War II also, but on a much smaller scale.

Trench fever is transmitted from person to person by the *body louse,* and causes headache and fever, vertigo, pain in the back, legs, and eyes. A distinctive rash appears on the chest, back, and abdomen which usually disappears in about twenty-four hours. Convalescence is prolonged. The pain and discomfort can be controlled by drugs prescribed by

1271

the disease and its causes Trichinosis is a roundworm infection which man contracts when he eats infected pork. The life cycle of the roundworm is such that the larval stage (the stage of the young worm just after it comes out of its egg) exists in the infected pig. When man eats raw or partially cooked infected pork, these larvae are freed in the course of digestion and pass into the small intestine. There they attach themselves, develop into adult worms, and reproduce. Their eggs pass through the walls of the bowel and are carried via the bloodstream to the muscles, where they form cysts. In occasional cases, the roundworms may find their way to the heart muscle and eventually the brain. Trichinosis is a quite common ailment, especially among people who eat ham or pork in a raw or partially cooked state.

symptoms The number of roundworms eaten determines the symptoms. In many cases, there are no symptoms at all. But when a patient has eaten a good many of the worms, there is usually abdominal pain, nausea, vomiting, and occasionally diarrhea. This is followed by chills and fever up to 102°-104°. The muscles become very tender and are painful on motion. There may be respiratory signs such as shortness of breath and hoarseness. Swelling around the eyes is not unusual. There may be a red rash over the body. In severe cases, this stage can last as long as eight weeks.

As convalescence sets in, the larvae become locked into the muscles and the symptoms subside.

complications Complications can be severe. They include pneumonia, involvement of the heart, and phlebitis—which is a vein inflammation in which blood clots form.

prevention (or lessening of impact) Trichinosis can be prevented simply by cooking all pork and pork products thoroughly. This destroys any larvae in the meat to be eaten.

Trichinosis

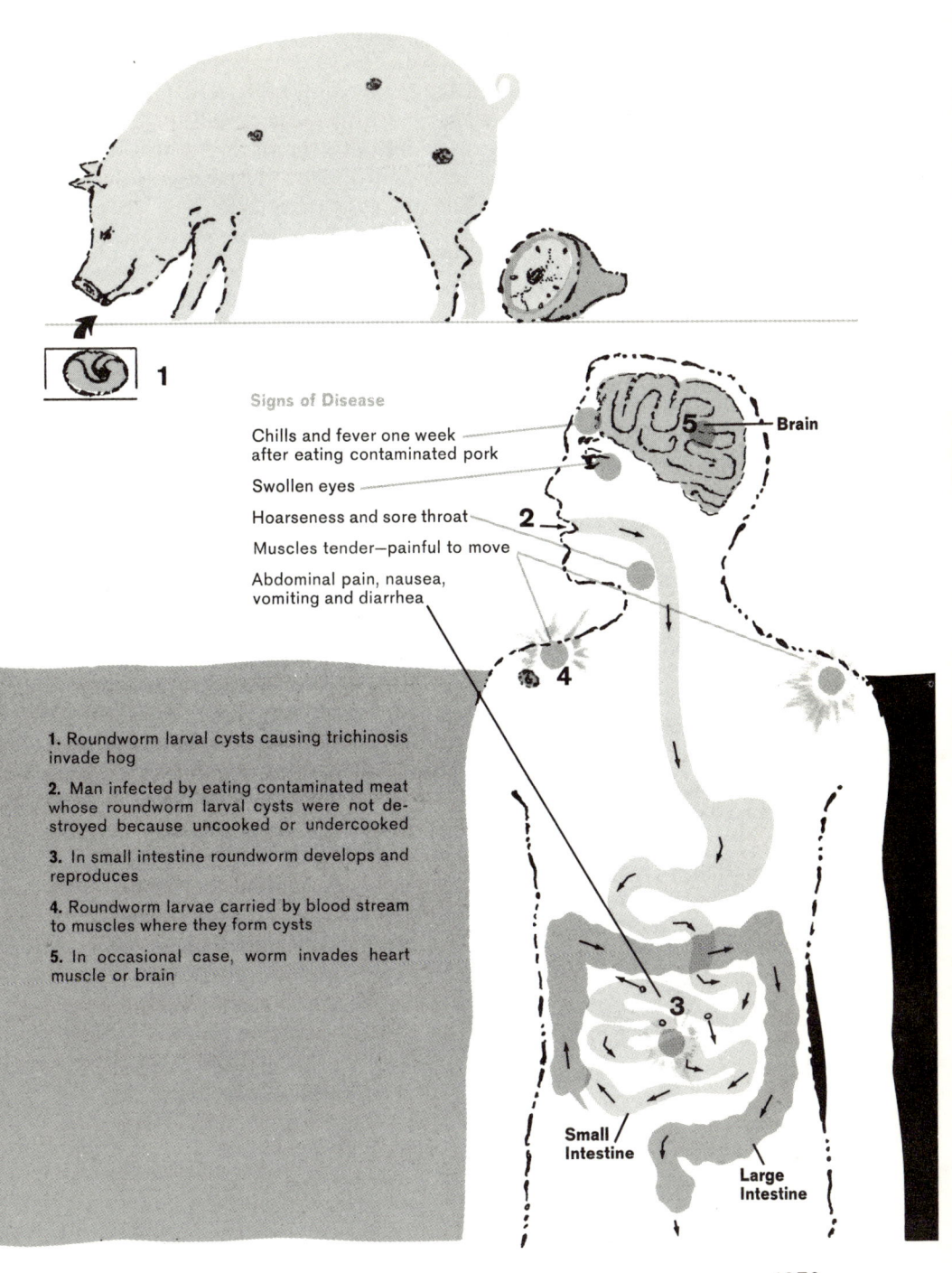

Signs of Disease

Chills and fever one week after eating contaminated pork

Swollen eyes

Hoarseness and sore throat

Muscles tender—painful to move

Abdominal pain, nausea, vomiting and diarrhea

1. Roundworm larval cysts causing trichinosis invade hog

2. Man infected by eating contaminated meat whose roundworm larval cysts were not destroyed because uncooked or undercooked

3. In small intestine roundworm develops and reproduces

4. Roundworm larvae carried by blood stream to muscles where they form cysts

5. In occasional case, worm invades heart muscle or brain

a physician, and bed rest and dietary measures help forestall a relapse.

Prevention of trench fever consists chiefly of delousing methods and sterilization of contaminated articles. The urine and sputum should be disinfected by chemicals or heat to prevent spreading the disease. *See also* RICKETTSIAL DISEASES; LICE.

TRENCH MOUTH. *See* VINCENT'S ANGINA.

TRICHINOSIS, a disease caused by eating pork or bear meat infected by *Trichinella spiralis,* a slender roundworm that is barely visible to the naked eye. If the worms have not been destroyed by proper cooking, they may develop in the intestines and later invade the muscle tissue, where they produce stiffness and painful swelling.

Tiny *cysts,* encasing immature worms, are present in contaminated pork. The human digestive process liberates them in the intestines, and they mature within a few days. The developed males fertilize the females, which then burrow into the intestinal wall and subsequently release larvae.

These larvae, carried through the blood circulation, lodge in the muscles, encysting themselves within a shell-like substance that they secrete. There they cause the pain and muscular irritation which are characteristic of the disease. Other symptoms are headache, fever, sore throat, general illness, and painfully swollen eyes. Specific treatment for the disease is not yet known. In time, the tissues of the body surround the organisms and wall them off.

Protection against trichinosis is possible in at least two ways. Since the *trichinae* cannot survive freezing or more than a certain degree of heat, they can be killed by freezing the meat at 0° F. for twenty-four hours or at 5° F. for twenty days, or by cooking at 140° F. or more for half an hour per pound of meat.

Another method of protecting against trichinosis is to prevent the infection in hogs. A principal source of trichinosis is uncooked garbage fed to hogs. Field-fed and grain-fed hogs have an infection rate of about .5 per cent, whereas animals fed on garbage which has not been heat-treated to kill trichinae have an infection rate of 5 per cent. Just as infected pork may be rendered safe for human consumption by proper cooking, so may garbage be made safe for pigs.

Epidemics of trichinosis are usually small and localized, and are associated with consumption of contaminated meat which can often be traced to one source. More than a quarter of pork consumed in the United States is processed without the close government supervision which is given in big packing plants and thus much pork offered for sale may harbor live trichinae. Most Americans probably consume contaminated pork at least once a year, but have no ill effects because the meat has been thoroughly cooked. The disease is, of course, more likely to occur when pork and pork products are eaten in a raw or semi-raw condition. *See* MEDIGRAPH page 1273.

TRIGEMINAL NEURALGIA. See TIC DOULOUREUX.

TRYPANOSOMIASIS. See CHAGAS' DISEASE.

TSUTSUGAMUSHI FEVER. See SCRUB TYPHUS.

TUBERCULOSIS, an infectious disease characterized by the production of *tubercles,* small rounded nodules which may appear on almost any part of the body. It is caused by the germ commonly called the *tubercle bacillus,* of which there are many varieties.

Recent decades have seen tremendous advances in the control and treatment of tuberculosis. The death rate in the United States has dropped from 250 out of every 100,000 persons to rates as low as 5 in many states. Nevertheless, it remains a serious threat which is far from having been eradicated.

Tuberculosis remains a chronic disease and if healing is not complete, relapse may occur. Although in the acute phases of the disease, the new drugs act quickly to promote healing, treatment of the tuberculous patient may require a long time. The discovery and application of new drugs, like *streptomycin, para-aminosalicylic acid,* and *isoniazid,* have virtually revolutionized the management of tuberculosis, and patients can now be treated by a combination of hospital and home care rather than being placed in sanatoriums. The closing of Trudeau at Saranac Lake, New York, was a dramatic indication of the change in approach to the treatment of tuberculosis. However, sanatoriums are still advisable in some cases where hospital and home care is not adequate.

In the past, tuberculosis was seldom suspected until severe coughs with expectoration, followed by loss of weight and night sweats, set in. With modern methods, the disease can be detected long before such serious symptoms have developed. X-ray pictures reveal changes which have occurred in the lung, and mobile units for lung x-rays are now common in many communities. Another method of detecting tuberculosis is the *tuberculin test.* A small amount of tuberculin, a material containing proteins of the *tubercle bacillus,* is applied to the skin or in some cases injected between the layers of the skin. A *positive skin reaction* indicates that the tissues have been sensitized to the tubercular germ, and that the germs are present and an infection exists somewhere in the body. Occasionally the reactions to the tuberculin test may be doubtful and additional tests, including *sputum* and *smear tests,* are necessary. Generally if the test is positive, other tests, such as the *bacteriological diagnosis,* are given to establish beyond doubt that tuberculosis is present. Tuberculin-positive cases showing chronic lung infection and confirmed by x-ray are usually considered as tuberculous, unless the bacteriological diagnosis indicates otherwise. Certain fungus diseases of the lung precisely imitate tuberculosis.

The germ causing tuberculosis was first described in 1882 by the bac-

the disease and its causes Tuberculosis is caused by the tubercle bacillus—found in humans, cows, and birds. These bacteria are spread by particles of dust or droplets which are expelled by a tubercular patient when he talks, coughs, laughs, or sneezes; or they are introduced into the intestinal tract by way of contaminated foods—such as milk from tubercular cows or objects placed in the mouth. Men and women between the ages of 20 and 40 are most susceptible. The exact incubation period is unknown and varies from days to many years.

symptoms Tuberculosis is a generalized illness affecting all organ systems. Pulmonary tuberculosis, discussed here, and the most common form, affects the lungs. The onset is usually abrupt, and there may be no history of exposure to the disease. A main symptom is a cough which can be either dry or productive. There is some spitting which varies in quality. Blood spitting may occur, and there may be pain in the chest. Frequently the voice box is involved and hoarseness results. Shortness of breath may be noted, often an indication of long-standing or advanced disease. There is almost always fever in active pulmonary tuberculosis, generally accompanied by night sweats, loss of strength, and loss of weight. When the gastro-intestinal system is involved there may be marked loss of appetite and symptoms of indigestion. Occasionally there is diarrhea.

complications The main complications are pleurisy, an involvement of the lining of the lung; pleural effusion, in which the chest fills with fluid; tuberculous laryngitis, the cause of the hoarseness; and pneumothorax, which is rupture of the lungs. A form of tuberculosis called miliary occurs when the infection is spread through the bloodstream to involve any part of the body, including the brain.

prevention (or lessening of impact) As yet, there is no really effective vaccine for the prevention of tuberculosis, although one has been undergoing extensive clinical testing for many years. A tuberculin test is available which shows whether or not an individual has been exposed to tuberculosis, or has had a healed case.

High hygienic standards and good health are necessary to maintain resistance to the disease. All contact with infected people or foods from contaminated sources should be avoided. Anyone exposed should have routine chest X rays so that the infection can be detected early and treated promptly. Specific medical and surgical treatment is available once the diagnosis is established.

Pulmonary Tuberculosis

1. Symptoms that sometimes appear are coughing, spitting up of blood, pain in chest, hoarseness, fever, night sweats, loss of weight and strength.

2. Bacterial infection causes inflammation, abscess and scarring of lung. May heal and then reinfect. X-rays reveal stage of infection, guide doctor in treatment.

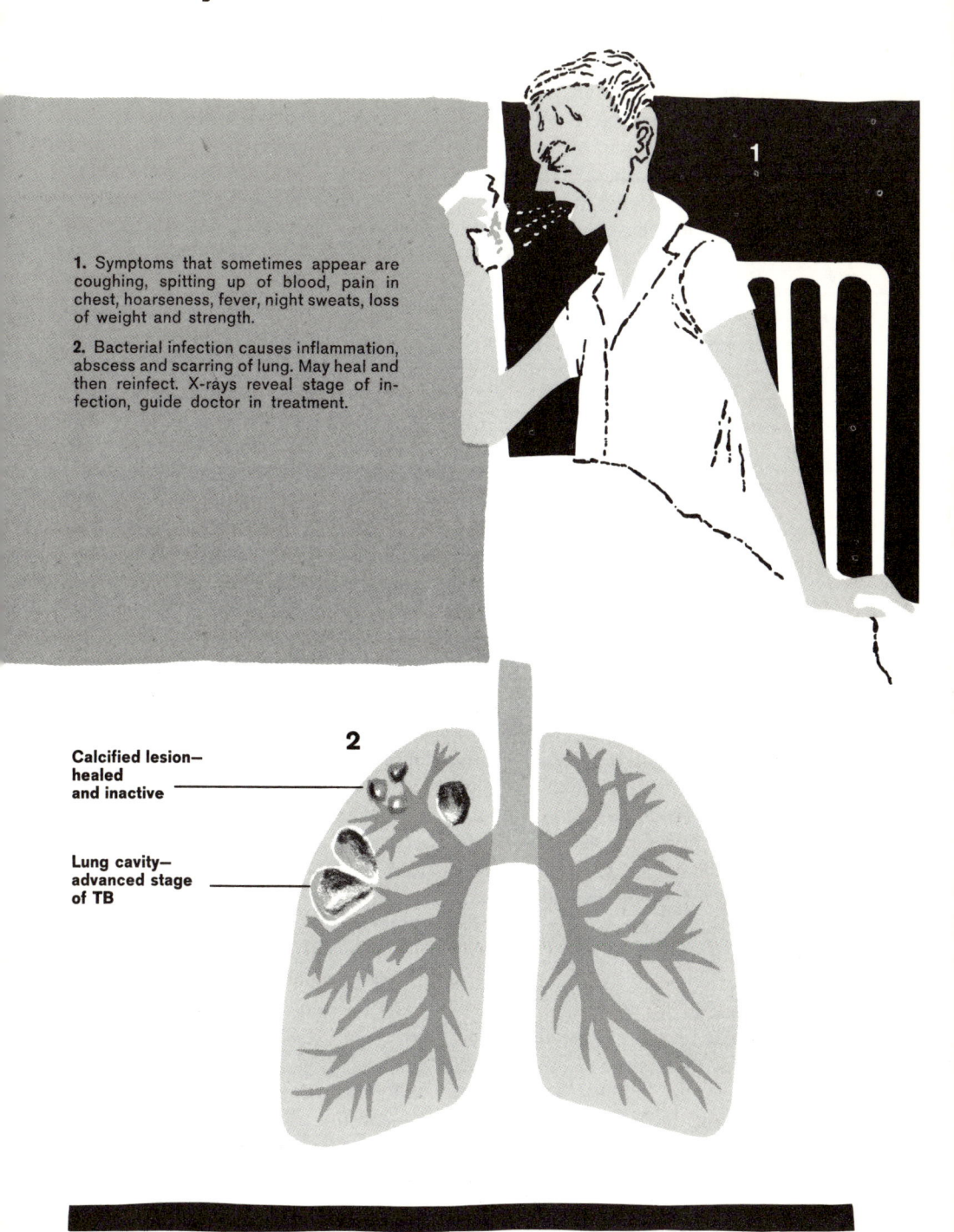

Calcified lesion—
healed
and inactive

Lung cavity—
advanced stage
of TB

teriologist Robert Koch. A variety of these germs exist, some affecting primarily human beings and others cattle, birds, or cold-blooded animals. The cattle type of germ may infect human beings, usually through the milk of infected cattle, and is largely responsible for *tuberculosis of the bones, joints,* and *lymph glands,* especially in children. However, the incidence of tuberculosis in cattle has been reduced to almost the vanishing point since the institution of tuberculin tests for cattle. In other countries, where the control of tuberculous cattle has not been so efficient, the disease continues at a high rate.

Although *pulmonary tuberculosis* is the most common form, the glands, covering of the brain (*meningeal tuberculosis*), the spinal fluid, the eye, the skin, and many other tissues may be affected. In acute *miliary tuberculosis* of the generalized type, the tubercle bacilli may be disseminated throughout the organs of the body. Acute active pulmonary tuberculosis—*galloping consumption*—may be difficult to diagnose at the onset. It may attack suddenly, with coughing of blood-stained sputum, and in such cases a doctor should be promptly consulted. This form, which was once rapidly fatal, has now yielded to modern drugs. *Tuberculosis of the abdominal region,* affecting the intestines and other organs, is rare in the United States. One of the most distressing forms, known as *Pott's disease,* after the British physician who first described it, causes crippling and curvature of the spine. A person may have tuberculosis of the lung and some other form of the disease at the same time.

The *cough* is the best-known symptom of tuberculosis, and is an indication of infection of the lungs by the tubercle bacillus or by some other germ. Any cough that persists for three or four weeks should always be brought to the attention of a physician. The cough is frequently accompanied by *expectoration,* and in some cases enough destruction of lung tissue has occurred for blood to be expectorated. Furthermore, fluid may pour out into the walls of the chest, an example of the way the body attempts to control infection. Another way the body tries to check the infection is to cover or wall off the infection with scar tissue, a process known as *fibrosis.*

The tuberculous person is generally sick, loses weight, and feels weak. A slight rise of temperature in the afternoon, or fever and an increase in the pulse rate, may also appear, and night sweats are common.

X-ray examination will reveal the extent of involvement of the lung, and a physical examination of the chest determines any changes that have taken place in its shape or contour and movement. By placing his hands on the chest, the doctor can determine the presence of spasms of the muscles or vibrations associated with the passing of air into or out of the lung. The doctor will also thump the chest and note whether the sound is dull, has increased resonance or a tympanic response. Sounds made by the air passing into the lung, as heard through a stetho-

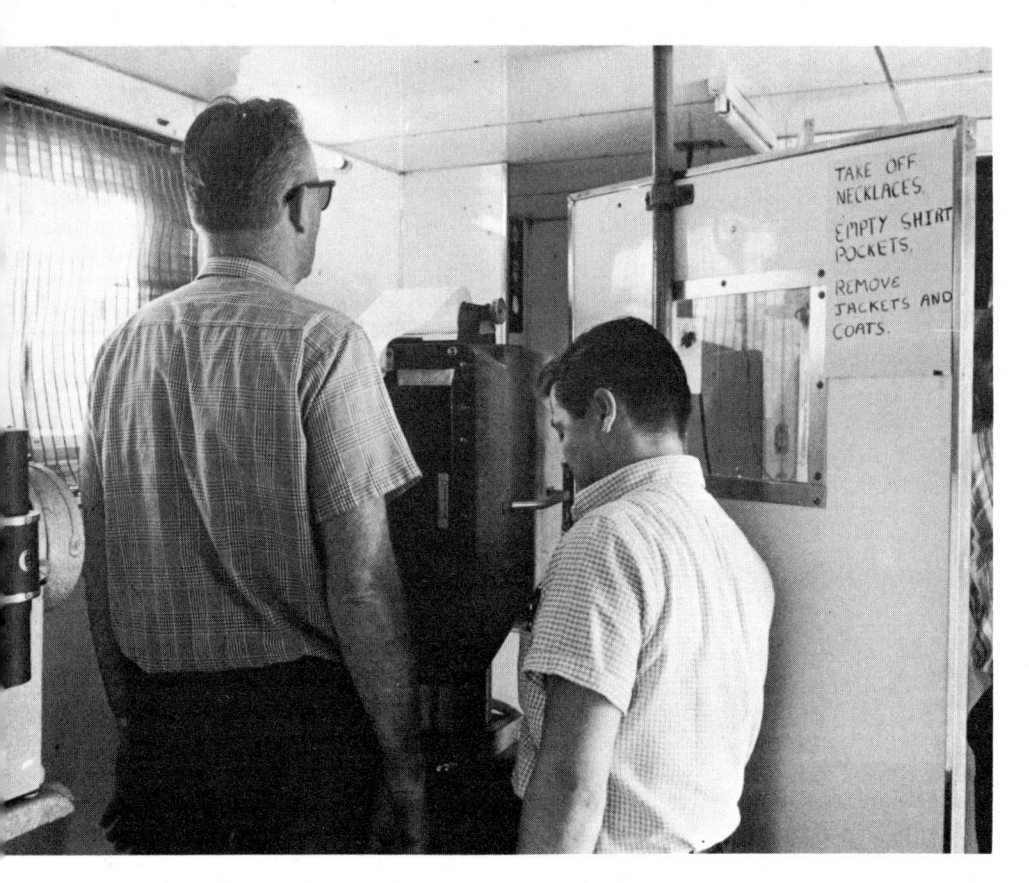

Tuberculosis, once one of the most dreaded killers, is now curable with the use of modern drugs and antibiotics such as streptomycin, isoniazid, and ethambutol. Nevertheless, thousands of people in the United States alone still die of tuberculosis each year, and an estimated 50,000 new cases still appear annually. These distressing statistics can be attributed largely to the neglect and carelessness of far too many individuals. Regular chest x-rays, provided free of charge in most communities, should be on everyone's agenda. A chest x-ray will reveal the presence of the disease, if it exists, in its incipient stages when it is most easily cured. Failure to detect tuberculoss in its early stages greatly magnifies the difficulties of its eradication. Above: a man submits to an x-ray. At right, a tuberculin skin test is administered. Such tests are another method of detecting the presence of tuberculosis.

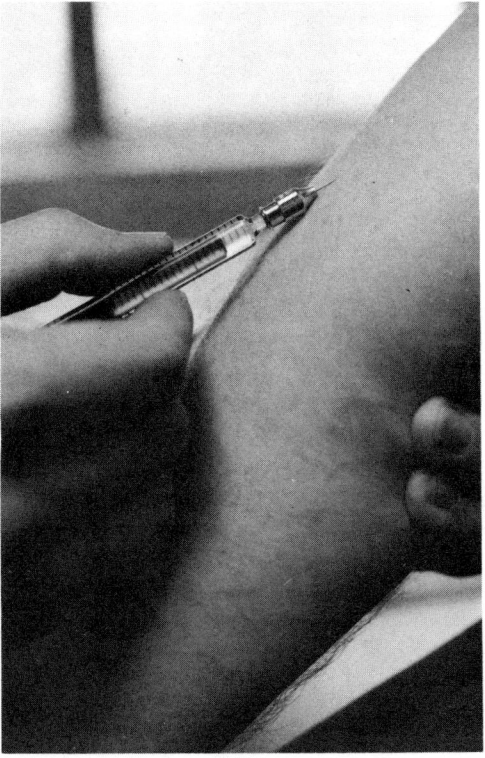

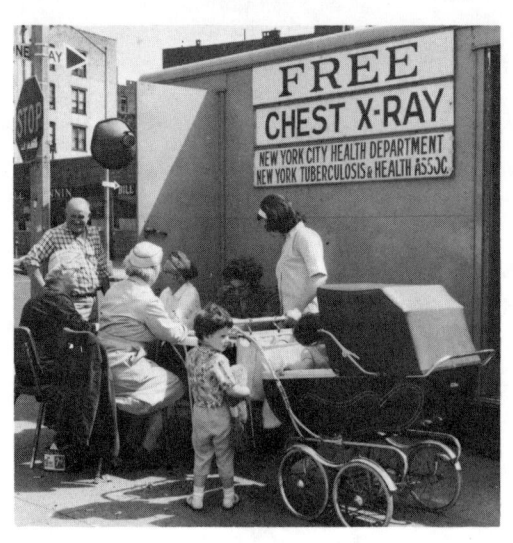

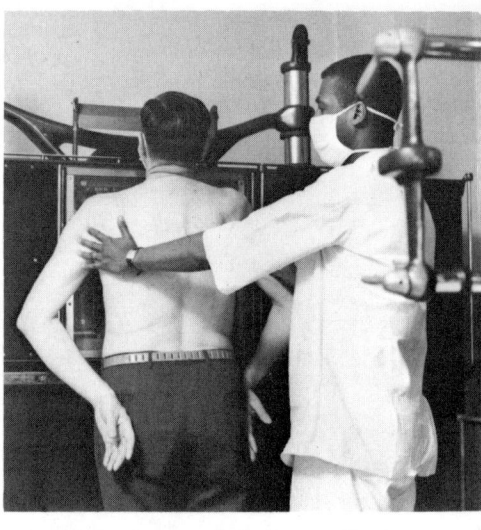

Above, left: a mobile chest x-ray clinic. X-rays are periodically administered free of charge to all volunteers by most municipal health departments. Extensive x-ray tests constitute one of the most effective weapons in wiping out this dreaded disease. Above, right, and below: a man suspected of having tuberculosis is examined.

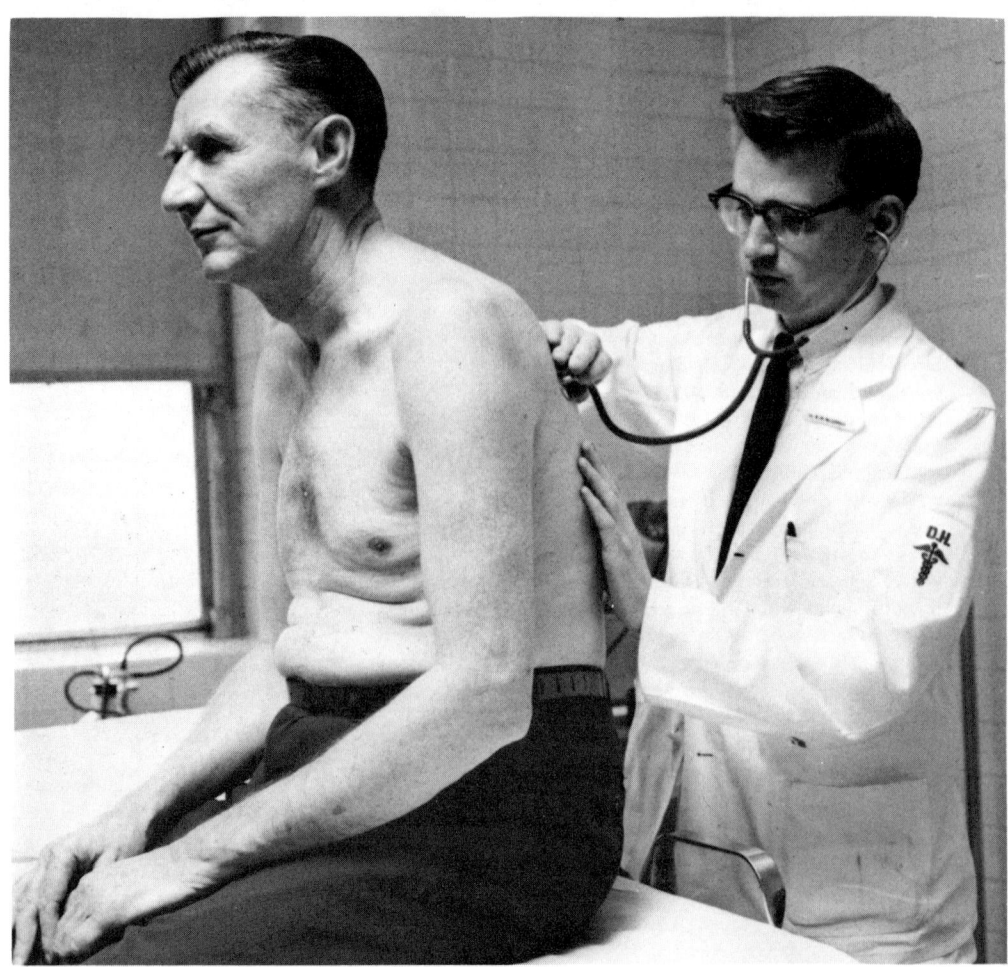

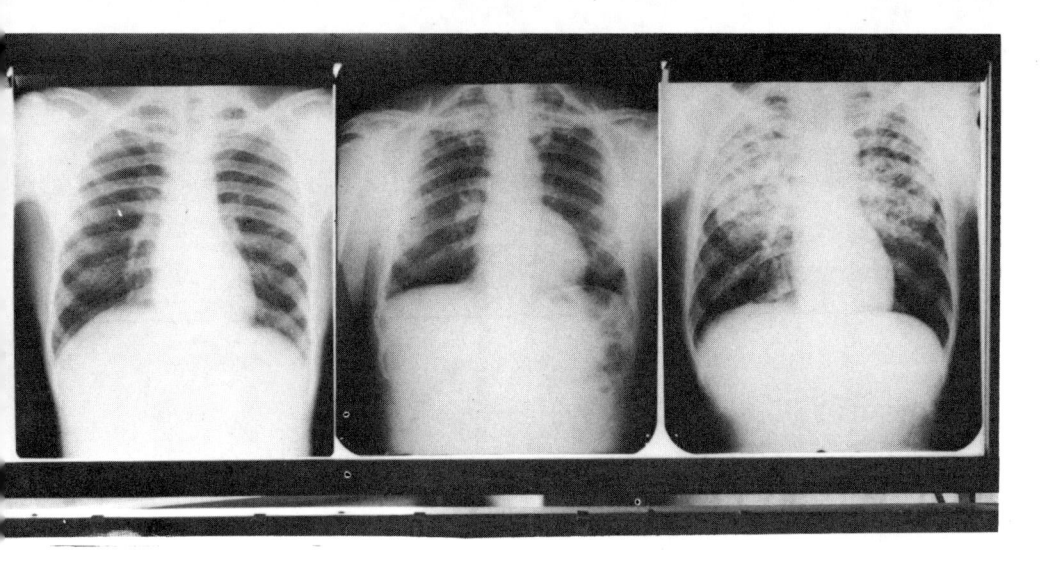

Chest x-rays reveal the physical condition of the lungs. Above, three x-rays reveal the following conditions: left, uninfected; center, cured of tuberculosis; right, infected with TB.

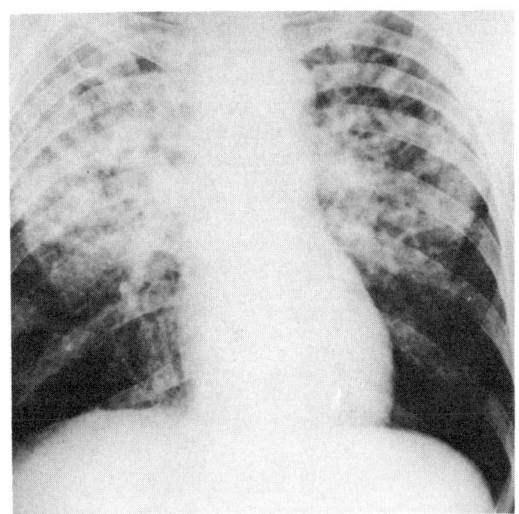

Right: a close-up of a lung infected with tuberculosis.

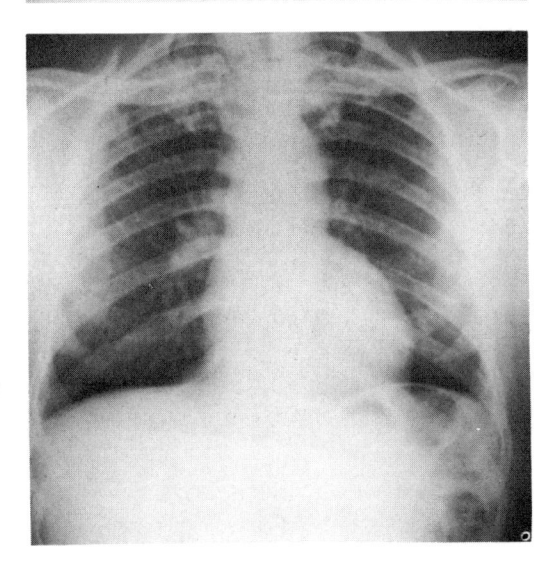

Right: this is an x-ray photograph of a lung undergoing treatment for cure of tuberculosis.

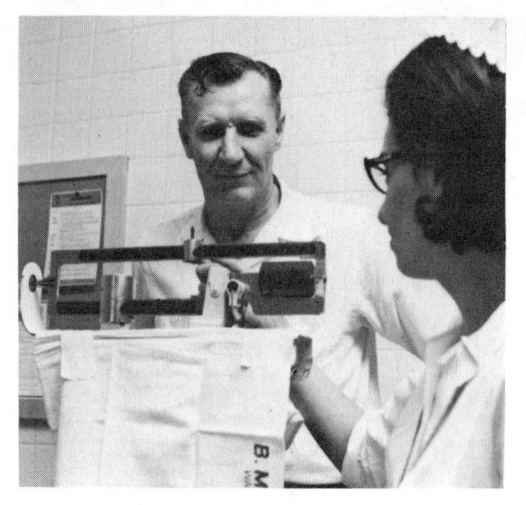

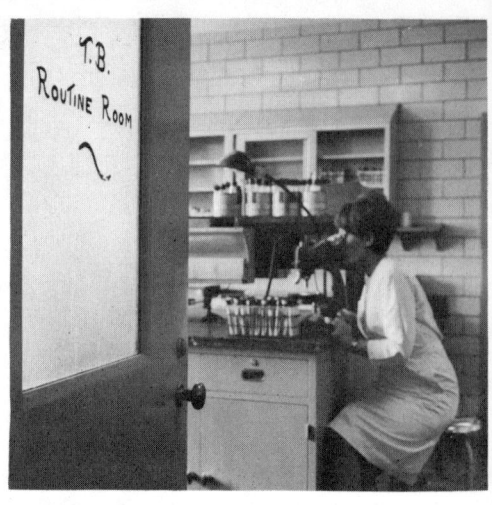

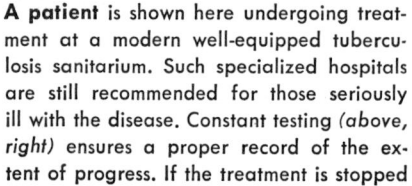

A patient is shown here undergoing treatment at a modern well-equipped tuberculosis sanitarium. Such specialized hospitals are still recommended for those seriously ill with the disease. Constant testing *(above, right)* ensures a proper record of the extent of progress. If the treatment is stopped too soon, the germs that have managed to resist any or all drugs will begin to multiply rapidly and may later prove insurmountable even if treatment is resumed. The drugs hamper the reproduction of the germs until the body's own antibodies can muster sufficient force to kill them.

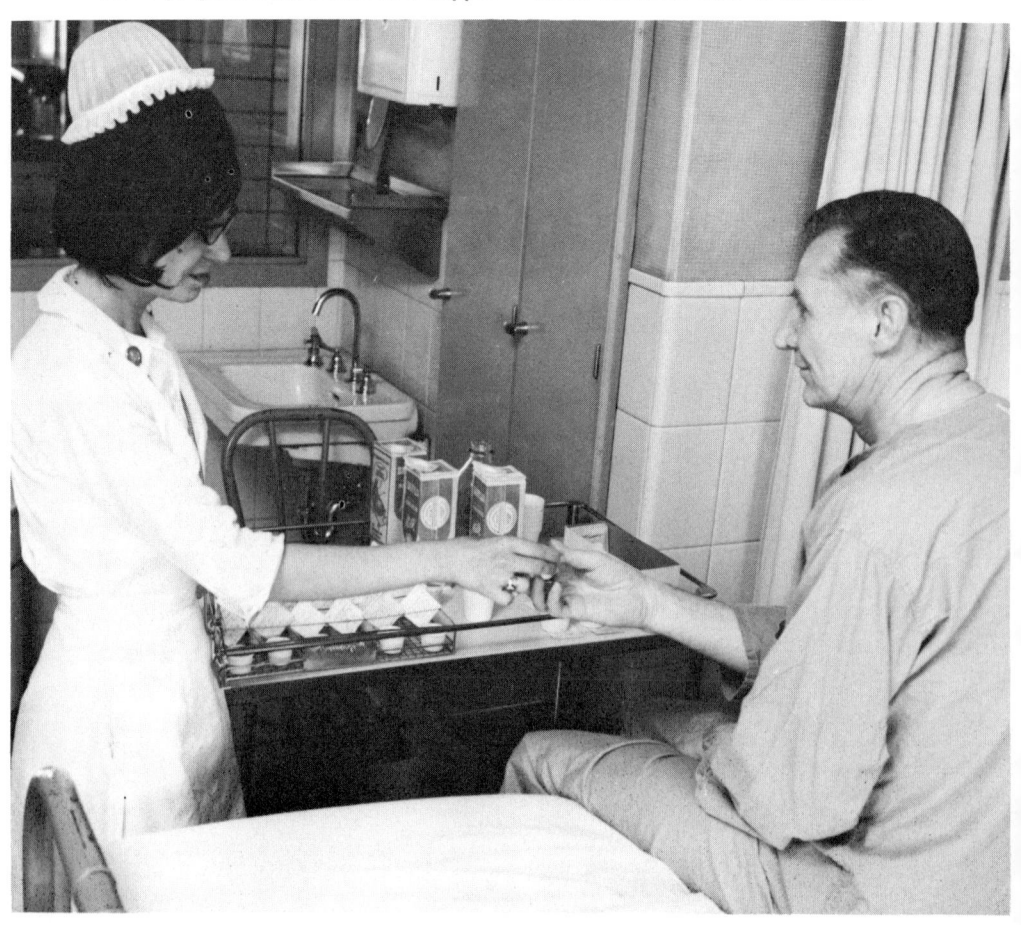

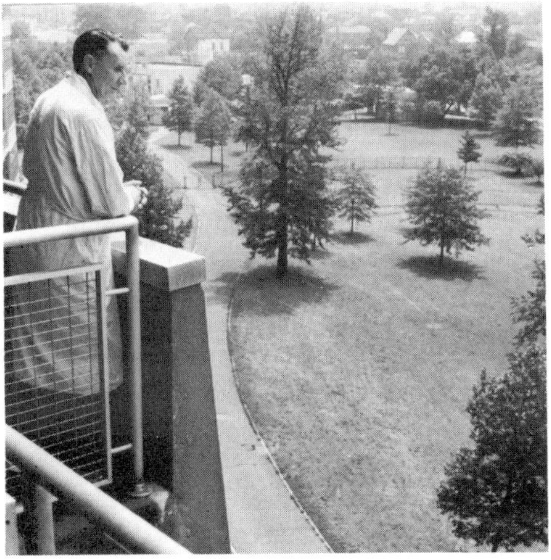
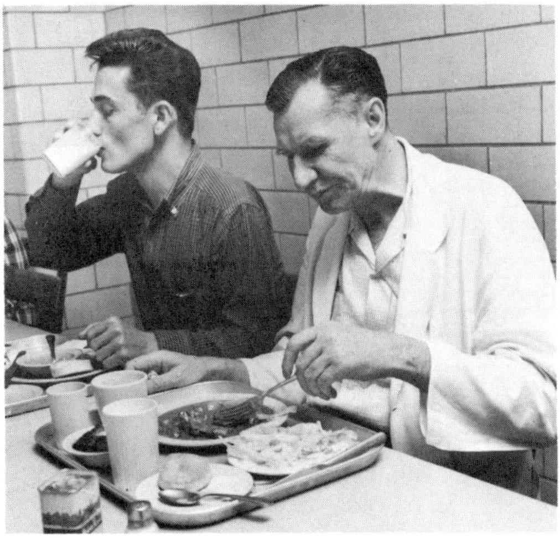
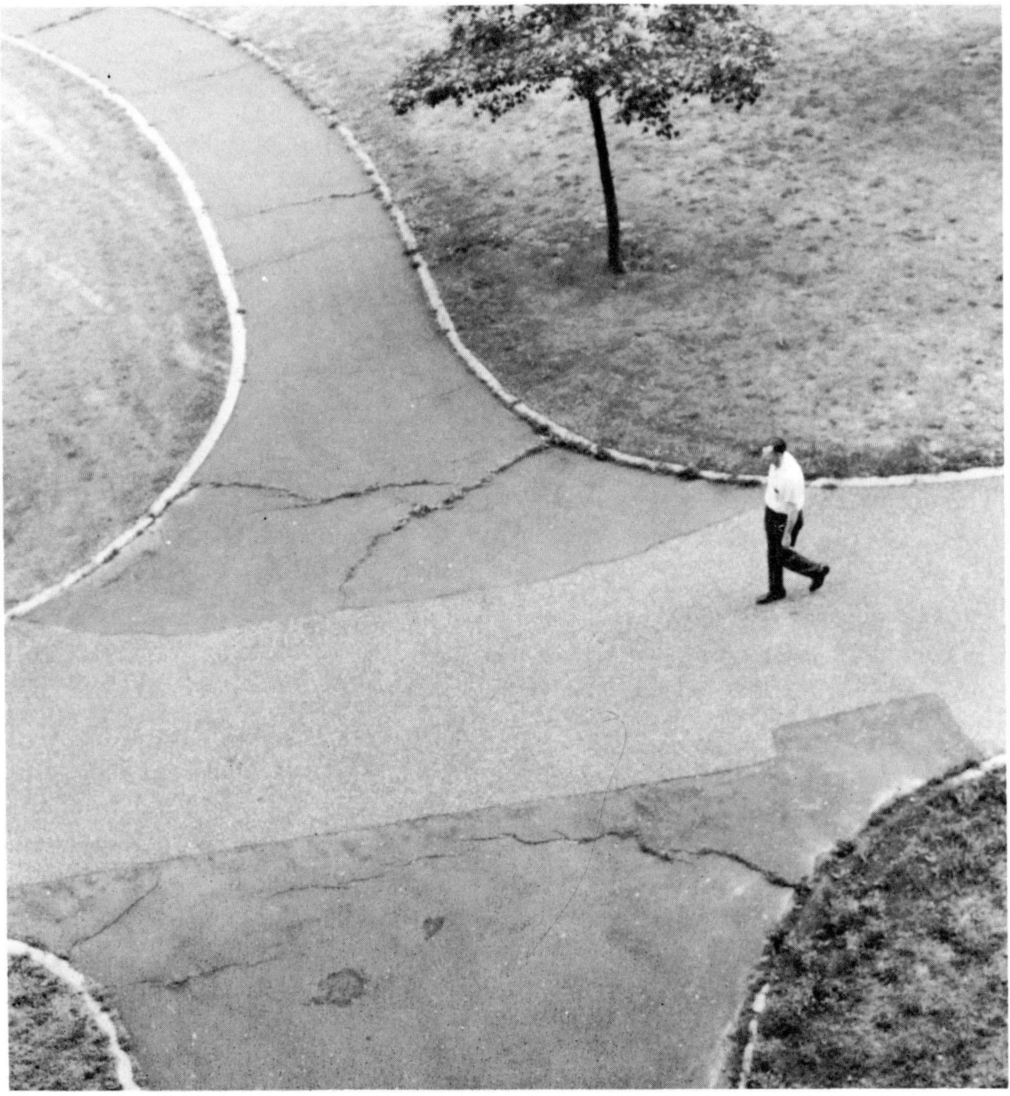

scope, indicate any interference with the passage of air, the presence of fluid or solid tissue, or other changes.

The sputum is examined to determine the presence of the tubercle germs, which conclusively point to tuberculosis. The absence of bacteriological evidence does not, however, exclude the disease, because in the earlier stages of the infection the germs may be absent in as many as 35 per cent of cases.

The success of the treatment depends largely on recognition of the disease at the earliest possible moment.

Once the doctor has determined the extent of the tuberculosis, the age of the infection, the portions of tissue involved, and other significant factors, he decides the course of management to be taken, not only medically but also personally with the patient. An understanding and healthy attitude on the part of the patient toward the disease may be a large contributing factor in the effectiveness of the treatment.

Social and economic problems arise in many families when some member develops tuberculosis, and social service departments in hospitals are often of great help in handling them. From a medical point of view, the principle of rest treatment requires as far as possible freedom from anxiety and worry, and by helping to alleviate these, the social service departments can help the physical state of the patient.

Once the diagnosis is established, almost without exception every case of pulmonary tuberculosis is treated with appropriate drugs for at least twelve months, and usually from eighteen to twenty-four months. Combinations of *streptomycin, isoniazid,* and *para-aminosalicylic acid* are prescribed in most cases. Bed rest of the sanatorium type is recommended at the onset of treatment in almost every case of active pulmonary tuberculosis, followed by a semiambulatory stage, and then an ambulatory period of limited activity.

In addition to isoniazid, streptomycin, and para-aminosalicylic acid, the drug *ethambutol* (MYAMBUTOL, LEDERLE) has given encouraging results. Combinations of ethambutol and isoniazid have been very successful in eliminating the tubercular organisms.

Although it was once believed that a high cool dry climate was most conducive for curing tuberculosis, it has now been established that the disease can be treated in any climate. The attention of a competent physician, the services of a good hospital or sanatorium, sufficient rest, good food, and administration of antituberculous drugs and other factors are primarily significant.

Because of the effectiveness of prolonged drug therapy, a combination of home and hospital treatment is recommended whenever possible. The American Trudeau Society has issued the following summary: "The management of tuberculosis today is a complex matter requiring the continuous supervision of a well-trained physician or physicians; the use of complicated laboratory facilities for proper evaluation; and long term, uninterrupted use of appropriate anti-tuberculous drugs; the availability of competent thoracic surgery in many cases; the opportunity for good nursing care and effective long-term physical rest and emotional relaxation; the availability of patient education and the proper proportion of recreation, occupational therapy and medical social service; and the proper facilities for isolation. It is concluded that in the majority of cases this service and treatment can best be offered in a hospital, during at least the acute phases of tuberculosis, and for the latter phases as well unless adequately supervised home care is available."

Reports indicate that good results are being obtained in those communities where the program of hospital and supervised home care is coordinated. Treatment is begun in the hospital and continued through the acute period, usually until cavities are closed, the sputum is negative, and the course of the disease is predictable. Then an appropriate supervised program of home care with continued drug treatment is established.

The employment of *artificial pneumothorax* for collapse of the lung has been almost completely abandoned, because of the high incidence of serious complications. However, when it is necessary to collapse the lung to rest it, *thoracoplasty,* an operation on the chest wall in which portions of the ribs are removed, remains an effective procedure.

The use of isoniazid to treat acute *miliary tuberculosis* and *tuberculous meningitis* has brought about a spectacular reduction in fatalities, and in some groups the survival is as high as 80 to 100 per cent. In general, tuberculosis affecting parts of the body other than the lung is treated with the same drugs as pulmonary tuberculosis.

The extensive knowledge of tuberculosis now available makes its complete prevention an ultimate possibility. Removal of those conditions which lower resistance and make the body more susceptible to tuberculous infection, such as slum areas where health and hygienic standards are low, can greatly decrease the incidence of tuberculosis. A more immediate measure is the detection of tuberculosis through periodic x-ray examination of the chest. Every person should have an x-ray examination of his chest and a general physical examination once a year. Active cases must be isolated, and persons who have been exposed should be particularly watchful. Anyone who has symptoms of tuberculosis—loss of weight and appetite, nausea, persistent fever, persistent cough and expectoration, a prolonged cold or spitting of blood—should immediately consult a doctor. *See also* LUNGS; MENINGITIS; BRONCHITIS; EMPHYSEMA; PNEUMONIA; ASTHMA. *See* MEDIGRAPHS pages 863, 995, 1047, 1277.

TULAREMIA, an infectious disease transmitted to man by infected rabbits or rodents, through their bite or through handling them.

An Arizona physician, Dr. Ancil Martin, first observed the infection in 1907 and traced it to the skinning and dressing of wild rabbits. In

1910, wild game in Tulare County in California were dying by the thousands; two investigators from the U. S. Public Health Service isolated the germ causing the disease, which came to be called *tularemia,* deriving its name from Tulare County. The medical director of the U.S. Public Health Service, Dr. Edward Francis, made further studies and discovered that human beings contracted the disease from contact with diseased rabbits and, in some rare instances, from bites of ticks and flies.

By far the most common source of infection is contact of the hands with the diseased rabbit. Rabbit meat, thoroughly cooked, is harmless when eaten, since a temperature of 130° F. will kill the germ of tularemia.

When tularemia appears on the body, an ulcerlike sore is usually found at the point where the germs have entered through the skin. This sore ordinarily appears several days after exposure. Following rapidly are headache, aching muscles and joints, weakness, chills, and fever.

The wild rabbit is the animal chiefly infected by tularemia, but the infection has been found in almost every type of small wild animal, including the muskrat, opposum, water rat, and squirrel. Cats and sheep have also been known to be infected.

Persons who handle rabbits for any purpose should wear protective rubber gloves. If they do not, they should wash their hands in a mild antiseptic before and after handling the rabbit. Contact of the rabbit flesh with a scratch, cut, hangnail, or sore should be carefully avoided, and the wrapping paper which has contained the animal burned. If any evidence of swelling or secondary infection around a cut or sore appears, a doctor should be seen promptly.

For those who hunt rabbits, it is well to remember that a rabbit which runs slowly is probably a sick rabbit and best ignored. Any rabbit which a child or dog brings home is likely to have been too sick to run.

In treatment of tularemia, *streptomycin* is rapidly curative, and other antibiotics including *aureomycin, chloromycetin,* and *terramycin* have been used effectively. Complications, including *pneumonia,* may arise and require hospitalization, intravenous feeding, and, for serious cases, blood transfusions and oxygen.

TUMOR, literally a lump or swelling, although the term is not used to describe the swelling of normal tissues such as occurs in inflammation or edema, or the enlargement of organs such as the spleen, liver, or kidneys. Specifically *a tumor is a mass of cells, resembling ordinary tissue, which develops independently as new growth and serves no useful function.* When such newly formed tissue occurs in blood vessels, it is called an *angioma;* in fatty tissue, a *lipoma* or fatty tumor; in cartilage, a *chondroma.* Tumors composed of tissue unlike the host organ may sometimes occur, such as cartilaginous or fatty tumors which develop in a gland—for example, the *carotid gland.* A *malignant tumor—sarcoma* —is composed of fleshy mass derived from connective tissue.

A large class of tumors do not have harmful effects, except as they produce pressure by their growth, and are designated as *simple, benign,* or *innocent*. However, a *malignant tumor* not only exerts pressure on adjoining tissue but actually invades and destroys it, or may disintegrate and produce new tumors in other parts of the body, a condition known as *metastasis*.

Any lump or swelling should be brought to the attention of a doctor who will diagnose it and determine the necessary treatment. Some tumors may be left undisturbed, whereas others should be removed. See also CANCER; CHONDROMA; LIPOMA; METASTASIS; POLYP; SARCOMA; XANTHOMA. *See* MEDIGRAPHS pages 259, 469, 995, 1007, 1081, 1311, 1315, 1349.

TYPHOID FEVER, an acute infection caused by the *typhoid bacillus*. As late as 1900, typhoid fever was among the most serious of diseases and responsible for numerous deaths each year. Today, although occasional cases still occur, the disease has been practically eliminated and deaths average around 200 a year throughout the United States.

The germ is found in the blood of a person seriously ill with typhoid fever, and in 80 per cent of the cases is also found in the material excreted by the bowels. The germ of typhoid fever is spread through excretions of the body, by contaminated food, clothing, water, and milk. In spite of improved sanitation, methods of treatment, and immunization by vaccination, a primary menace remains: the *typhoid carrier*—a person who has had the disease and recovered but who continues to propagate the germs and to spread them. Administration of *penicillin* and removal of the gallbladder of the carrier have helped curb the problem, but many typhoid carriers still exist.

Typhoid fever follows a long and serious course. From three to twenty-one days after the infection, which is known as the *incubation period,* the germs develop in the body and liberate their poisons. Typhoid fever begins with the usual symptoms of infection, such as headache, pains throughout the body, a feeling of exhaustion, and chills and fever. Frequently nosebleed occurs and almost invariably there is simultaneously a serious disturbance of the bowels, due to the fact that the typhoid germs produce ulcers in the bowels. As the disease progresses, the infected person becomes more and more ill. Clots may form in the blood vessels and rose spots appear on the skin at the end of the first week or beginning of the second. Because of the damage to the bowels, gas forms, causing bloating, and sometimes perforation of the intestines which may produce severe hemorrhage. Occasionally the infection also attacks the nervous system, resulting in not only pain but even delirium.

The doctor in examining the patient with typhoid fever makes his diagnosis on the basis of the history of the case, the nature of the symptoms, and by careful study of the blood. The *Widal test* of the blood determines, with reasonable certainty, the presence of typhoid fever.

the disease and its causes Typhoid fever is an acute, generalized infection caused by a specific type of bacteria. It is spread by infected water, milk, and other dairy products, other foods, or by direct contact with a typhoid carrier. It can occur at any season but appears most often in the fall. The incubation period is about 2 weeks. All age groups are involved, but the most frequent victims are young adults.

symptoms The disease usually begins as a mild, grippe-like infection, with headache and muscle aches. There may be nosebleeds, nausea, vomiting, constipation, or diarrhea. As the illness advances, the temperature goes higher, reaching levels of 104°-105°. The second week is marked by persistent high fever and an accompanying slow pulse. A rose-colored rash appears on the abdomen, back, and chest. The abdomen is distended and uncomfortable. By the 3rd or 4th week there is gradual decrease in the temperature and rash, and disappearance of symptoms.

complications There may be hemorrhage or perforation of the intestinal tract. The liver may become infected, resulting in jaundice. The gallbladder may become infected and remain as a source of infection. As a result of this condition, a person may become a carrier. Pneumonia and meningitis are also possible complications.

prevention (or lessening of impact) There is a typhoid vaccine which is highly effective but not an assured preventive. It is given in three weekly doses and followed by a booster at regular intervals. Hygienic measures and proper sewage disposal are important factors in preventing illness. In areas known to have typhoid fever, all water should be sterilized properly and particular precautions should be taken with foods fertilized with human excrement.

Food handlers should have stool examinations to rule out the possibility that they are typhoid carriers.

A patient with typhoid fever requires good nursing care. He should be isolated and his bed linen and dishes sterilized. Toilet facilities in contact with the patient's stools and urine should be carefully disinfected. The patient should be kept clean throughout and bathed daily if possible. His convalescent diet should include small amounts of low roughage-high calorie food at frequent intervals to maintain his strength and shorten his convalescence. Specific antibiotics are available for treatment. Booster shots of vaccine may be given in cases of epidemics or if a person has been exposed.

Typhoid Fever

1. First Week
Flushed face, glassy eyes, white or brownish coated tongue with reddened tip and edges. Chills, headache, other grippe-type symptoms. Fever mounting to 104-105°.

2. Second Week
Rash breaks out—usually on abdomen, sometimes on chest or back. 1-20 rose colored pimples appear in successive waves. Fade momentarily on pressure. Abdomen swells and is tender.

3. Third-Fourth Week
Rash disappears — leaving brownish stain. Fever declines and other symptoms gradually disappear.

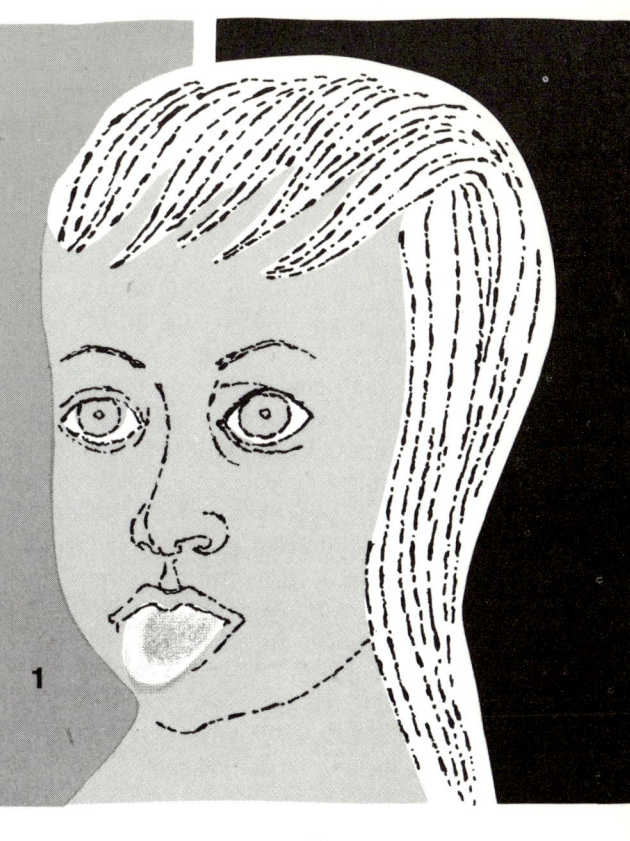

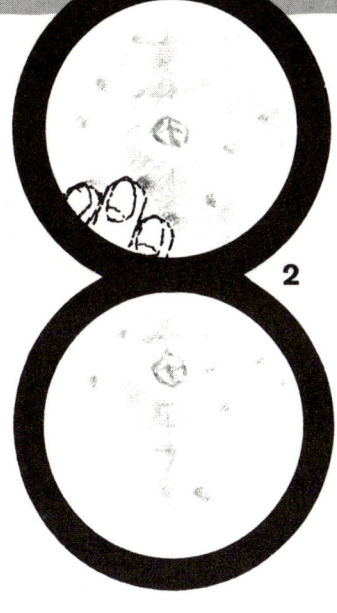

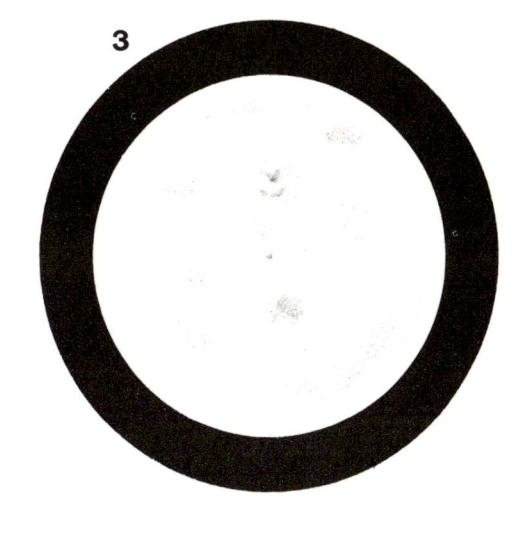

Isolation of typhoid fever patients and good nursing care by an experienced nurse are required. If the illness occurs during the summer when flies are common the sickroom should be screened. The most effective antimicrobial treatment is *chloramphenicol* or *chloromycetin,* which has induced earlier remission of symptoms and shortened the duration of the illness. Stools and urine of the patient should be disinfected with *cresol, formaldehyde,* or similar disinfectants. The patient's bed linen and dishes should be sterilized. He must be bathed at least once a day, be kept clean, and the mouth rinsed after eating to prevent secondary infection. Only a few restrictions in diet are necessary. Nourishing bland foods are given during the early part of the illness, but during convalescence a high-protein, high-calorie diet, containing from 3,000 to 3,500 calories, is recommended.

Typhoid vaccine is highly effective, but not absolutely preventive against typhoid fever. It is administered subcutaneously in three weekly doses by a physician or trained nurse. A booster injection at suitable intervals will maintain a high level of immunity and should be given to persons who because of occupation or travel may be exposed to typhoid-contaminated food or water.

Although areas still exist throughout the world where typhoid fever is a threat, persistent attention to water supplies, pasteurization of milk, disposal of sewage, control of typhoid fever carriers, and general education of the public in hygiene can eliminate the disease entirely. *See also* CARRIERS OF DISEASE. *See* MEDIGRAPH page 1289.

TYPHUS FEVER, an infectious disease caused by a rickettsial organism. Other names for it are *jail fever, ship fever, camp fever,* and *louse typhus.* It is carried by the *body louse* or *rat flea* and an epidemic may arise wherever overcrowding, famine, and poverty prevail. It occurs principally in cold weather and may follow in the wake of war and famine, and spread in slums, concentration camps, asylums, and prisons.

Typhus fever includes three diseases: the *epidemic louse-borne typhus, Brill's disease,* and *murine flea-borne typhus.* The three types differ from one another only in the intensity of the symptoms and the severity of the illness and fatality rate.

Epidemic louse-borne typhus is transmitted by the body louse. Dried louse feces on clothing or bedding can keep active rickettsial organisms for many months and be a source of contamination. Epidemic typhus is most frequent during winter and spring, when heavier clothing and less frequent bathing create ideal conditions for rapid multiplication of lice.

Symptoms appear about ten days after a person has been bitten by an infected louse. Severe headache, high fever, and aches and pains of the entire body develop. On the third to seventh day, a rash appears, first on the armpits and flanks, then on the trunk and later on the arms and legs. Mental faculties are dulled and prostration is severe. Odor from the mouth is foul and *bronchitis* and *pneumonia* often develop. In mild cases recovery is usually rapid, and one attack establishes long immunity.

In the past, the death rate from typhus epidemics was high. In the epidemic of eastern Europe and Russia between 1918 and 1922, thirty million cases occurred, with three million deaths. In Serbia, the mortality rate was between 30 and 80 per cent, and of some 400 doctors who contracted the disease, 126 died. An Egyptian epidemic in 1943 resulted in 40,000 cases and 8,000 deaths.

Brill's disease is a form of typhus found principally among emigrants from countries which have had epidemics of the louse-borne typhus. Though the same rickettsial organism is responsible for both forms of typhus, Brill's disease generally occurs in persons who have had epidemic typhus before emigrating. It is a milder form of typhus and generally is not fatal. Since the specific agent responsible for Brill's disease has not yet been isolated, the means for prevention and control have yet to be developed. Precautions are the same as for typhus.

Murine typhus is a flea-borne disease for which the *rat* is the breeding animal. Human beings become infected by the bite of an infected flea, or by eating food contaminated by flea feces or rat urine. The disease is not spread by man. It has occurred throughout the United States, but is most common in the Atlantic and Gulf states.

The incubation period is about twelve days, and the symptoms are similar to those of epidemic typhus, but are milder and of shorter duration. The rash is less extensive and fades sooner, and complications are fewer.

Treatment of the typhus fever group consists of good nursing care. *Antibiotics* have been effective in decreasing the severity of the disease and in controlling its spread.

Prevention of typhus depends largely upon elimination of the animal which breeds the disease and the insect which transmits it. Adult lice are destroyed with DDT, and the eggs are killed by steam sterilization. During World War II, prevention and control of epidemic typhus was one of the great medical accomplishments. Immunization was achieved by means of vaccines given to entire companies of men. Since rats are the primary source of murine typhus, prevention and control involves rat-proofing buildings, especially granaries and storehouses, and eliminating garbage dumps and other conditions conducive to breeding rats. *See also* IMMUNIZATION; RAT CONTROL; RICKETTSIAL DISEASES. *See* MEDIGRAPH page 851.

U

ULCER, any open sore, other than a wound, with an inflamed base. Such a lesion usually occurs in the skin or mucous membrane of some internal organ. Ulcers may result from infection, injury to the blood supply, damage to nerves, or from a wide variety of other causes. Ulcers require the attention of a physician who will not only endeavor to learn the specific cause but will plan the treatment accordingly. See PEPTIC ULCER. See MEDIGRAPH page 1297.

UMBILICUS, or *navel,* the depressed scar in the median (middle) line of the abdomen, which results from the separation of the *umbilical cord (placenta)* in childbirth.

UNDERWEIGHT, HAZARDS OF. The first problem encountered in a consideration of the hazards of underweight is that of *definition.* What is underweight? The answer is not easy because of lack of certain knowledge of what constitutes *normal weight.* It is clear that normal weight will depend on *age* and *sex.* It is also clear that it depends on *height* or *size.* The short person might be expected to weigh less than the tall person of the same age and sex. But this is not always true, and this brings in the factor of *constitution,* or *body build,* or *conformation.* All of us know the chunky, chubby, or tubby "type," the tall, lean, thin "bean pole," and the less extreme examples of these types. In technical terms, the chunky chubby type is referred to as *endomorphic,* the "bean pole" type as *ectomorphic* or *asthenic,* and individuals of more intermediate or "normal" weight and build as *mesomorphic.*

In the absence of any actual knowledge of what constitutes the proper weight of any individual in relation to height, age, sex, or other characteristics, dependence has of necessity been put on the *average weights of groups* of supposedly

1292

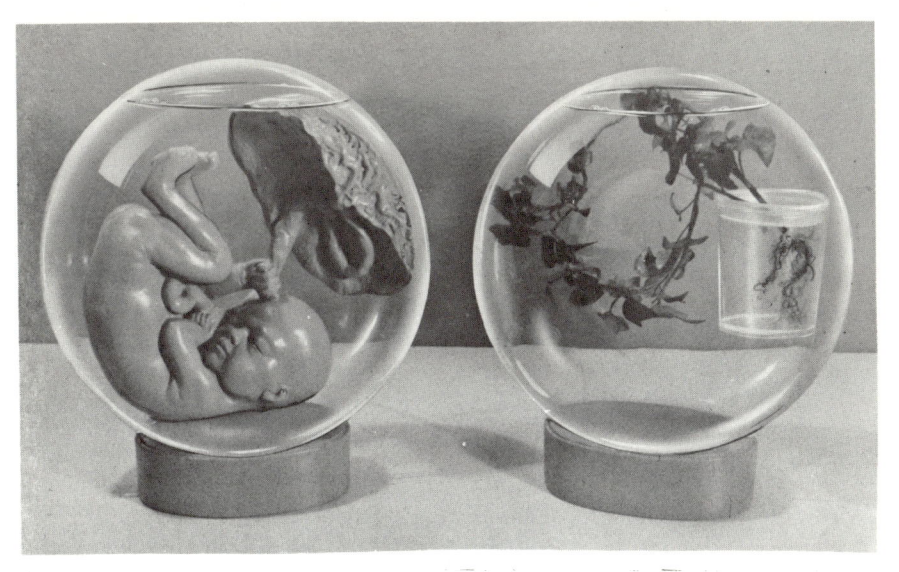

Umbilical Cord—The *umbilical cord* is the baby's lifeline before birth. Through it courses the baby's blood which picks up oxygen and food in the *placenta* (commonly called the afterbirth). The baby depends on the mother's blood supply in the placenta for its nourishment and removal of its waste products. The placenta and cord can be compared to the roots and stem of a plant. But it must be remembered that the placenta acts as a membrane through which substances are exchanged. The baby's and mother's blood never mix.

healthy persons *of like age, sex, and height.* These averages form standards with which the weight of a given individual can be compared. In some tables allowance is made for constitutional type, or body build, in use, and allowance is of necessity made for a permissable variation above or below the standard (average).

None of the standards available and in common use are altogether satisfactory. Variation between standards may exceed apparent limits of normality, and the range in some standards is so great as to make them of little value. Nevertheless, some weight tables are reasonably satisfactory.

What, then, is our criterion? When are we underweight? Disregarding as we must for the present the deficiencies in our standards, *we can define underweight as weight more than 10 per cent below the standard for the individual.* There are, however, certain modifying conditions which must be added if we are to avoid mistaking an individual characteristic for an abnormal condition. First, *such underweight is more likely to be significant in children,* and even more so if it persists and the child fails to increase in weight. It must be remembered, however, that growth, including increase in weight in children, is irregular and, to an extent, seasonal.

Second, *underweight of this degree is much more likely to be abnormal and represent a state of ill health if it is the result of loss of weight in an individual previously of*

1293

the disease and its causes Ulcerative colitis is a disease generally located in the rectal and the sigmoid portion of the large intestine. However, all of the colon may be involved, and occasionally this disease even extends into the end of the small intestine. There is ulceration, inflammation, and thickening of the bowel wall, and also a generalized inflammation involving joints and skin.

This disease is relatively common and is found equally in men and women. It can occur in childhood, but the usual age group is from 20 to 40. The cause is not known, but there are many theories. Various bacteria are thought to be responsible. Allergies, viral infections, and nutritional deficiencies have all been mentioned as possible causes. Emotional problems and anxieties have also been held responsible, particularly since they are definitely associated with flare-ups of this disease.

symptoms The illness may begin slowly or suddenly, and it may proceed haltingly or explosively. Few patients are permanently cured, and it tends to be chronic, flaring up frequently and then quieting down. Most patients are affected on and off throughout their lives.

Symptoms depend upon the extent and severity of the inflammation and its location. If it begins in the rectum, the only symptom may be the passage of bright red blood and mucus in the stool, along with some constipation or diarrhea. There may be a normal number of stools a day or up to 15 or 20. With a bowel movement there may be pus, accompanied by pain and cramps. There can be fever, loss of appetite, and marked loss of weight. There may or may not be discomfort in the abdomen.

As the disease progresses and becomes chronic, the patient becomes wasted and weak. His stools may now occur 3 to 5 times a day in a semi-solid form, with bright red blood. In severe cases, there is high fever, weakness, and other evidence of serious illness.

complications Serious complications are perforation (puncture) of the bowel wall, with peritonitis (infection), and massive bleeding. The patient is chronically ill and disabled.

Another complication in as much as 10% of the cases is the development of cancer in the area involved. Rectal fissures or abscesses can appear. And there are complications having to do with acute arthritis, skin changes, anemia, and phlebitis.

prevention (or lessening of impact) There is no known way of preventing this illness. Periodic examinations are essential to avoid some of the serious complications. Many symptoms can be controlled with the help of medicine and a suitable diet. Since repeated attacks are clearly linked to anxiety and frustration, psychotherapy is often mentioned and frequently used to help patients deal with their problems and thereby avoid recurrence of the disease.

Ulcerative Colitis

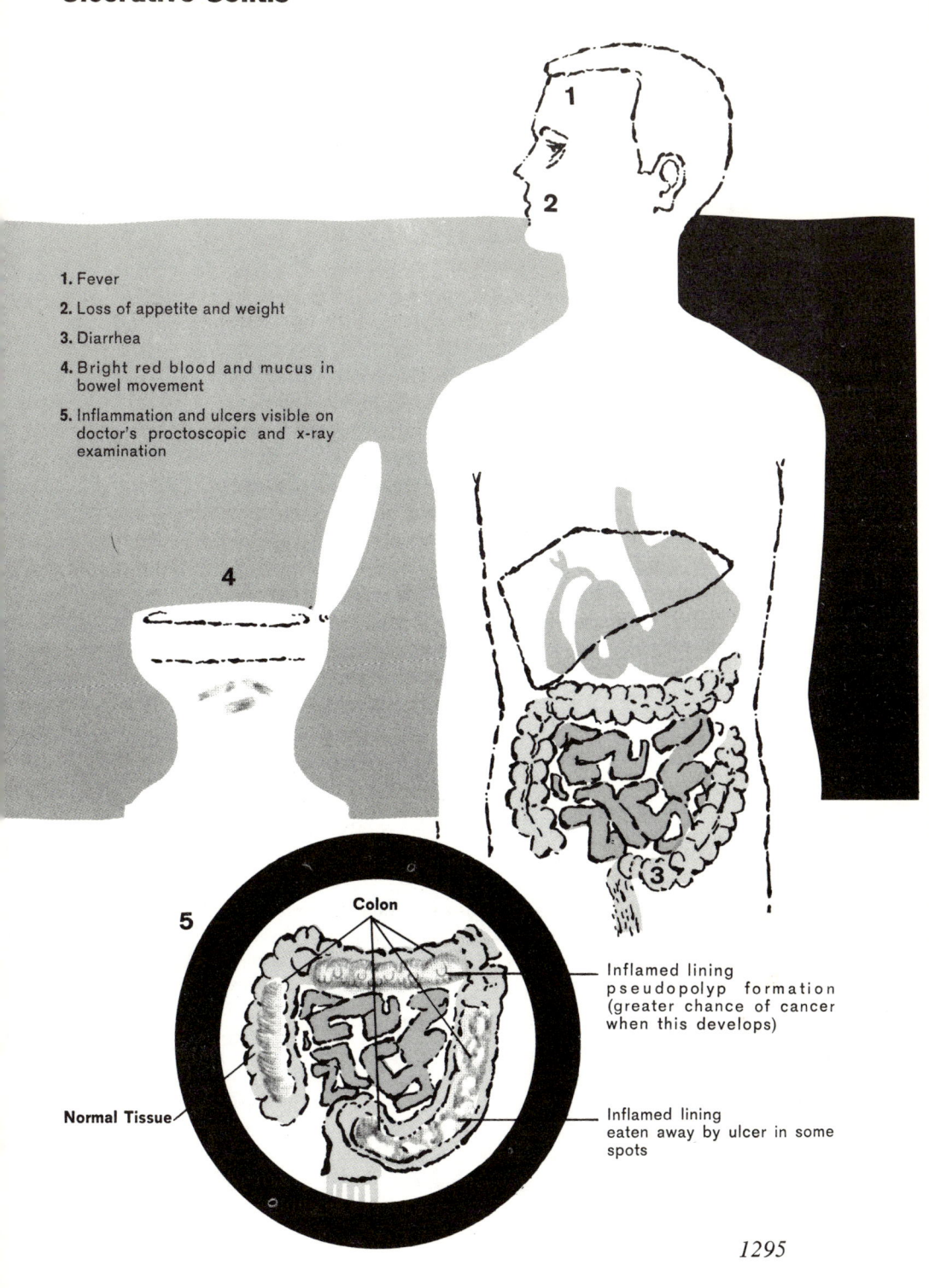

1. Fever
2. Loss of appetite and weight
3. Diarrhea
4. Bright red blood and mucus in bowel movement
5. Inflammation and ulcers visible on doctor's proctoscopic and x-ray examination

Colon

Inflamed lining pseudopolyp formation (greater chance of cancer when this develops)

Normal Tissue

Inflamed lining eaten away by ulcer in some spots

the disease and its causes Called stomach ulcers, gastric, peptic or duodenal ulcers, these are crater-like sores in the lining of the stomach and upper part of the small intestine (duodenum). Ulcers are believed to be caused by the stomach's producing an excess of digestive juices—pepsin and hydrochloric acid. In normal digestion, these juices break up food into forms that can be readily absorbed through the intestine. However, when the stomach produces too much hydrochloric acid, this may eat into the lining of the stomach or small intestine—causing ulcers. A majority of ulcers occur in the duodenum.

Tense, nervous people seem particularly prone to develop ulcers, as a result of a harmful cycle: emotional stress . . . leading to overproduction of stomach acid . . . leading to pain . . . leading to increased emotional stress . . . leading to ulcers.

symptoms During the digestive process food enters the stomach within several minutes after eating—but it takes a couple of hours to move on to the duodenum. Ulcer patients frequently have pain in the stomach area within minutes after eating (if they have stomach ulcers) or 2 to 3 hours after eating (if they have duodenal ulcers). This pain seems to be due to the effect on the ulcer of the digestive juices the stomach produces in response to the recently eaten food. The type of pain may vary from a mild upset stomach to a sharply gnawing or burning sensation. These ulcer pains are usually relieved if the patient takes an antacid, milk or other soft foods to neutralize the stomach acid. The pain is located high in the abdomen, as illustrated, and may radiate to the back.

However, some ulcer patients may experience no apparent pain or other symptoms for a long time after their ulcers have developed.

complications In the case of patients who are not warned by painful symptoms or who do not seek medical attention when these symptoms develop, an ulcer may eat all the way through (perforate) the wall of the stomach or duodenum. An ulcer may also break through the wall of a blood vessel, causing internal bleeding. Both these complications require immediate hospitalization and treatment.

If an ulcer patient finds his pain suddenly becoming much more intense than usual, and his usual medication doesn't relieve the pain, he can suspect perforation. Signs of possible internal bleeding would be vomiting of blood, or the passage of blood or black stool through the rectum. Stomach ulcers can become malignant.

prevention (or lessening of impact) Talking over emotional upsets and problems with a sympathetic or professional listener helps to get rid of the tensions which promote the formation of ulcers. Avoiding tobacco and other stimulants, developing relaxing hobbies, getting a good night's sleep regularly and following a doctor's advice regarding diet and medication help to prevent the formation of ulcers—or lessen the severity of attacks from ulcers, when they have developed.

Ulcers Of The Digestive Tract

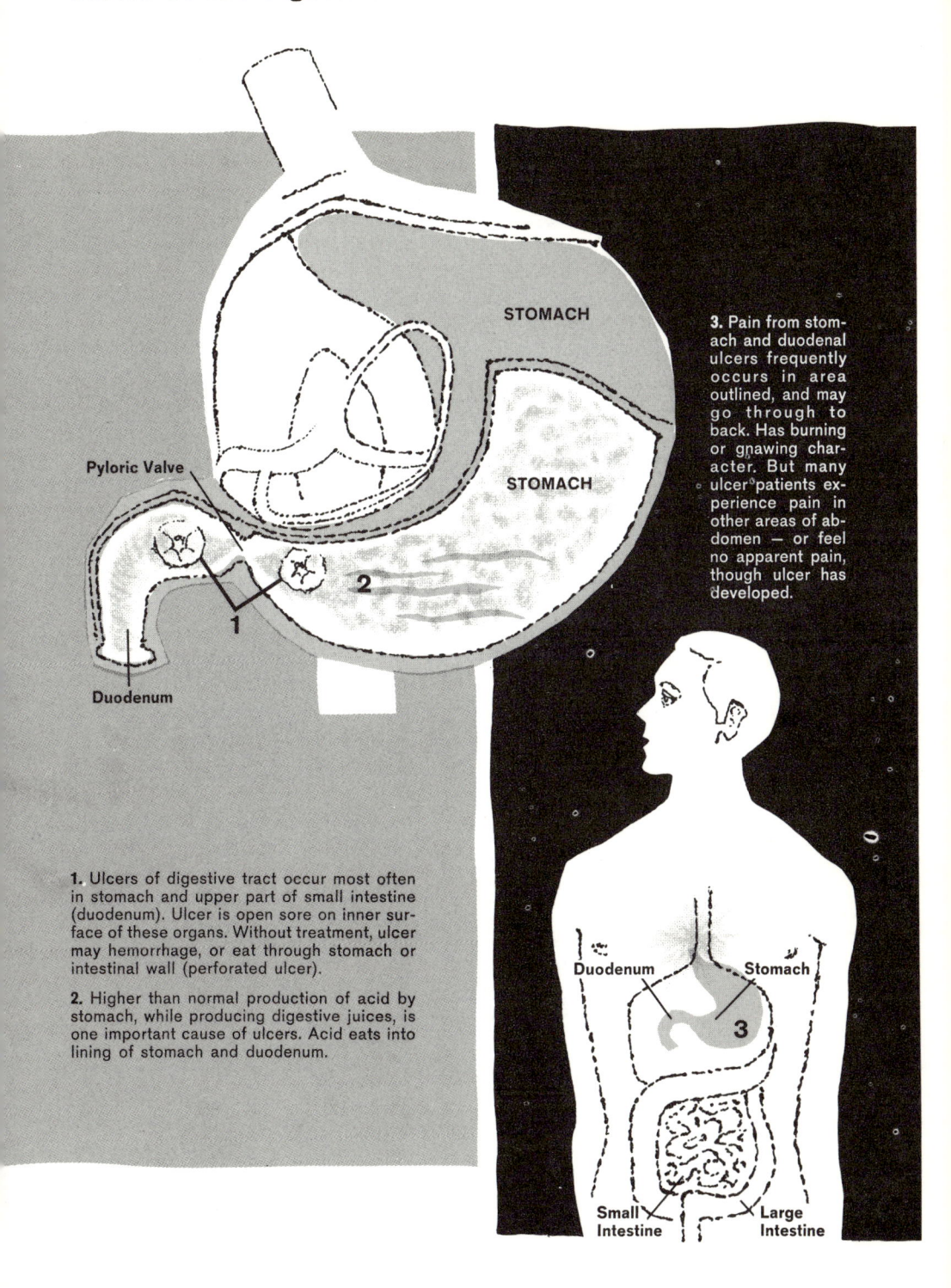

1. Ulcers of digestive tract occur most often in stomach and upper part of small intestine (duodenum). Ulcer is open sore on inner surface of these organs. Without treatment, ulcer may hemorrhage, or eat through stomach or intestinal wall (perforated ulcer).

2. Higher than normal production of acid by stomach, while producing digestive juices, is one important cause of ulcers. Acid eats into lining of stomach and duodenum.

3. Pain from stomach and duodenal ulcers frequently occurs in area outlined, and may go through to back. Has burning or gnawing character. But many ulcer patients experience pain in other areas of abdomen — or feel no apparent pain, though ulcer has developed.

standard weight. Underweight in an individual who has always or habitually weighed below his standard and who is in good health is most apt to represent an individual variation from the usual and to be without sinister significance. In fact, it probably reflects a fortunate state conducive to longevity.

Third, as may be deduced from the above, *underweight is much more likely to be significant to health if the individual concerned does not enjoy good health and complains of any one of many symptoms.* Finally, underweight becomes more worthy of attention if *it is the result of, or accompanied by, restriction of food intake,* particularly voluntary restriction as may occur with reducing or other forms of dieting.

A better understanding of the hazards of underweight will be had if physiological and biochemical conditions accompanying underweight are discussed. When food intake is reduced below that needed to maintain the existing weight the body draws on its own tissues. With the exception of very small reserves of sugar and animal starch (glycogen) the *body fat* is the first to furnish this food or fuel. For those who are overweight this is not objectionable; in fact, it is desirable and, of course, the basis for reducing. For those who are at their *physiological weight* (healthful weight) or below it means the encroachment on, and eventual loss of, the protection of their vital body substance, *protein.* The time it takes to lose the fat and expose the protein to loss depends, of course, on how deficient the diet is. If it is only slightly deficient it will take a long time to deplete the fat. Inevitably, however, the fat is lost if the deficient diet is continued, and under many conditions of dieting or reduced food intake the fat does not last long.

Some idea of the speed at which weight is lost can be gotten from a study which showed the loss of weight in a group of experimental subjects eating somewhat over half of the food they required. The group lost on the average approximately thirty-four pounds, or nearly a quarter of their original weight, within sixteen weeks. It can be assumed that none were significantly obese at the start. Under these conditions the greater part of the body fat must have been lost early, to be followed by serious inroads on their protein tissues leading to protein deficiency.

The body's reserves of protein are small. Any unusual loss must come from our tissues and organs, and, because of the nature of protein, it even comes from the vital tissues of the body. Much of the protein-containing tissue is muscle, and the muscle tissues and organs contribute their protein to be burned. The skeletal muscles such as our biceps and similar muscles are only a part of our tissues. Many organs such as the stomach contain muscles on the integrity of which much of their function depends. Furthermore, such a large and important organ as the heart is a muscular organ, composed almost entirely of muscle tissue. Protein makes up a large part of the substance of such organs as the liver and tissues not commonly thought of as such—the blood, for instance. Finally, protein is a principal constituent of many important hormones, secretions, and protective substances, some of which are manufactured by the body in relatively small but vitally important amounts, such as thyroid secretion, insulin, and the various antitoxins. Others such as milk are produced in relatively large quantities.

The sequence of events then is this: *Amounts of food insufficient to maintain weight are eaten. The body then draws on its own tissues. Fat being expendable without ill effect is used first, but, except in the obese, is relatively soon exhausted.*

Protein is then consumed. Protein being an indispensable tissue, a state of protein deficiency ensues, with the ill effects to be described below.

Perhaps the most evident and easily recognized effect of underweight is *weakness*. This is a direct result of the loss of muscle substance. The muscles shrink and become smaller, a change which can readily be observed. Actually a visible wasting of the exterior muscles of the body is one of the first signs of such nutritional deficiency. The weakness is most marked in terms of muscular endurance. Although strength for single muscular acts is somewhat lessened, it still is maintained surprisingly well in even rather extreme states of under-nutrition. But sustained muscular effort such as holding, squeezing, and pulling are much less well performed. Perhaps the best common example is found in climbing stairs, an act which becomes increasingly difficult.

With the weakness there is a disinclination to exertion, in part related directly to the increased effort needed, but, as we shall see, partly caused by other changes.

It is not only the skeletal muscles, however, which suffer. As previously pointed out, muscular tissue of all kinds all over the body is affected and, as it becomes smaller, displays evidence of its weakness. For instance, the heart becomes smaller and its contractions less forceful.

The weakening of the muscles of the front wall of the abdomen permits *hernias* or ruptures to develop more readily, and those which previously existed to a slight and insignificant degree may become enlarged to an extent which is disabling and requires treatment. From the esthetic point of view, there is a sagging and bulging of the abdomen with resulting sad effects on the figure. The muscles of the walls of the intestines weaken and allow the bowel to distend, diminish contraction and favor delayed passage of food through them.

One of the important structures to suffer with undernutrition is the *blood*. More than one of the elements of the blood is affected. Protein is involved in the formation of both the blood cells, red and white, and of the *plasma* (serum) in which the cells are suspended.

Anemia is a rather constant occurrence in underweight and undernutrition. This anemia, which is usually mild but may reach moderately serious proportions in severe and continued undernutrition, is *the result of both a reduction in the num-*

ber of red blood cells and the amount of hemoglobin. It is not the result of inadequate supplies of vitamins or minerals and appears despite an adequate supply of these substances. Its exact cause is unknown, but there is reason to believe that it, too, is related to the *loss of protein.* Protein is needed for both the manufacture of the red blood cells and the hemoglobin which they contain. Inadequate protein diets are known to impair blood formation in animals under experimental conditions. It is worth noting that recovery from the anemia of undernutrition is slow, even with a full and good diet. Restoration of the blood to normal may lay behind the recovery of body weight.

The white cells may be affected slightly. In the absence of intercurrent infections there is usually a slight-to-moderate decrease in their number. Changes in their character or in the proportion of the various cell types are not to be expected.

Another important constituent of the blood which may be affected is the serum, or plasma protein. There are two principal kinds of proteins in the blood plasma: *albumin* and *globulin.* Both serve the important function of holding water within the blood vessels, but in this the albumin is more important. Globulin is importantly concerned with immunity and resistance to disease as will be described below. Finally there is a small amount of a protein known as *fibrinogen,* which is required for the proper clotting of blood.

The quality of these proteins may be decreased as the result of undernutrition accompanying states of underweight, with resulting disturbance of the functions for which they are responsible. The reduction in the serum proteins may result in the condition known as *edema (dropsy),* which under these conditions is spoken of as *nutritional edema* or dropsy. In the ordinary mild states of underweight such swelling is slight in degree, confined usually to the feet and lower legs and more pronounced toward evening, often disappearing by morning. It may be displaced during the night and appear as puffiness of the face and hands in the morning. Locally this dropsy may impair the vitality of the tissues and interfere with healing. It is only fair, on the other hand, to point out that a slight swelling or increase in fluid in the tissues may serve to hide the haggard appearance that follows a loss of subcutaneous and muscular tissue. Such swelling should be distinguished from the normal or physiological swelling of the feet and even ankles which comes at the end of the day as a result of long sitting or standing and the fullness of the hands which is sometimes noticed in the morning. Actually these normal and abnormal changes in the amount of water in the tissues are of essentially the same nature, differing only in degree. As a rough guide the abnormal swellings are detected by the persistence of "pits" in the tissue when pressed on by the finger, but the exact interpretation in cases of swelling should be left to the physician.

A number of undesirable, if not injurious, changes take place in the surface tissues, skin, and hair with underweight. The least of these is a looseness, a sagging, a wrinkling, an accentuation of lines particularly in the face as the skin loses its support of subcutaneous and muscular tissue. In effect the envelope becomes too big for the contents and becomes "baggy." In younger people this may be compensated for to some extent by the elasticity of the skin, which after a time readjusts itself to the change. In older people in whom the elasticity of the skin is naturally decreased this fails to occur. At the same time the skin itself becomes drier, thinner and tends to be somewhat rough and scaly as its *turgor* and the blood flow through it are decreased. With the latter there is apt to be some grayish pallor and decreased warmth. Finally it has been observed that undernutrition is apt to be accompanied by a blotchy pigmentation, especially on the face. The hair tends to be dry, rough, and of poor quality. It is possible that all of these changes are related to a diminished blood flow through the skin, though the whole process is a complex one involving a lowered metabolic rate, a decreased surface temperature, and diminished action of the sweat glands and possibly of the sebaceous glands. In certain case studies, the eyes had a dull, glazed appearance, apparently because of decreased blood flow in the *sclera* (whites of the eyeball).

In underweight of a degree consistent with chronic undernutrition, the *basal metabolic rate* is reduced. The reduction, though only slight to moderate, is significant. The basal metabolic rate is a measure of the amount of heat produced by the body in relation to the individual's age, sex, and size, and the reduction is assumed to be a compensatory mechanism to conserve body heat and the wasting of body tissues when the food intake is inadequate to maintain normal weight. Direct ill effects from this reduction are not serious, but there is apt to be some *disinclination to physical activity* and an *unusual sensitiveness to a cool environment*. As already indicated, this reduction probably contributes indirectly to other changes, such as those in the skin, by reducing blood flow.

Because the lowered basal metabolic rate is mediated through the *thyroid gland,* there is reason to believe that other glands of internal secretion are affected, all such glands being closely interrelated. That this occurs in severe malnutrition is well known, and evidence of disturbances in the structure and function of certain of the *sex glands* has been observed. However, in these instances the diets have been deficient in many nutrients, and it has been impossible to say that simple undernutrition, as represented by underweight, can cause such effects. Nevertheless, temporary stopping of *menstruation* or shortened duration and diminished flow are common in undernourished populations and have been observed to occur in association with dietaries which were apparently not deficient except in calories and perhaps protein. If this is, in fact, an effect of simple undernutrition, it may be reasoned that possibly there is also an effect on *conception*. On the other hand very considerable losses of weight can occur in such diseases as *tuberculosis* without the amenorrhoea. Such occurrences illustrate the complexity of the situation and the many factors involved.

No special effects on the digestive tract are noted with underweight, with the possible exception of those described in association with the loss of muscular tones of the intestines. Unlike complete starvation in which the appetite is lost after a few days, under ordinary circumstances of *involuntary* restriction of food the appetite remains ravenous and the thoughts of food dominate the waking hours and even the dreams of night. But the factor of appetite is affected by so many factors, particularly psychological, that under many circumstances accompanying loss of weight, especially when the restriction of food is *voluntary*, appetite may actually be unaffected or diminished.

The effect of true underweight on the *heart and circulation* is a decrease in its size, a smaller output, a slowing of the pulse rate, especially during rest, and a lowering of the blood pressure. These changes, aided by others, cause a poor circulation through the skin and may lead to slight *lividity*, especially of the extremities. Such individuals often complain of giddiness or faintness. In themselves these cannot be considered serious ill effects and, in fact, such underweight and undernutrition have been used in the treatment of heart disease and high blood pressure. The incidence of certain types of heart disease and hypertension become much less frequent and severe in populations which have been subjected to undernutrition.

On the other hand the secondary effects of undernutrition on the nutrition of the heart may be deleterious, and a certain number of patients with heart disease suffer from undernutrition. With loss of weight and loss of muscle substance there probably is first a reduction in the size of muscle fibers and, if it continues, presumably in the actual number of fibers themselves.

The only *infectious diseases* for which a definite relation between underweight and resistance to the disease seems to have been established are *tuberculosis, pneumonia (lobar), and influenza*. Underweight is associated with an increased mortality rate from *tuberculosis* at all ages, being more than twice that for those of normal weight. Furthermore, the increase in the mortality rate is even greater as the degree of underweight increases.

Formerly the death rate from *lobar pneumonia* was significantly higher in the underweights, but the introduction of new and effective drugs in the treatment of pneumonia has greatly influenced the situation. Deaths from *influenza* were more frequent among the underweight group in the *pandemia* of 1918-20. Although the evidence is not clear, it is probable that the effect of undernutrition on tuberculosis is on preexisting but inactive infections, a state which may be found in a large proportion of adults. Lowered resistance to the initial infection with tuberculosis seems much less likely.

Theoretically the existence of diminished resistance to a large number of infectious diseases in states of underweight involving any significant degree of protein deficiency is highly probable. As has been pointed out, the *antitoxins* and other immune substances which our bodies manufacture as a protection against acquiring or succumbing to a large number of infectious diseases are made from *protein,* principally the *globulin fraction.* When protein deficiency exists there may be a defective or deficient manufacture of those substances and hence diminished resistance to those diseases, as has clearly been shown experimentally in animals. Practically this has been difficult to demonstrate unequivocally in man, but general observation on the incidence and mortality of many diseases such as *typhus fever, diphtheria,* and *dysentery* in undernourished subjects, except as modified by newer and powerful drugs, supports strongly the theoretical possibility. It is, however, to be pointed out that an exception must be made in many if not all diseases due to viruses in which undernutrition, at least in the sense of underweight, apparently exerts no unfavorable influence.

It might be thought that such solid and apparently indestructible structures as the *bones and teeth* would show no effect of the type of undernutrition and underweight being considered here. That is probably true of the teeth. It is also apparently true of the bones if the state of underweight is of relatively short duration, say several months. It may not be true with even rather mild underweight, however, if the condition is maintained over long periods. So-called hunger or famine thinning of the bones has been recognized and detected for many years. Usually the degree of undernutrition and underweight has been rather severe, but not always. Furthermore, it is now known that the bones are not the unchanging, static, almost inanimate things they were once considered to be but are dynamic, constantly changing structures with a continuous exchange of mineral salts and other evidence of a rather active metabolism. Thinning and demineralization of the bones occur associated with protein deficiencies and might be a cause under conditions which suggest long-continued, though mild, undernutrition. Though there is a loss of lime salts under such circumstances, the condition is not the result of a deficiency of calcium but more likely a protein deficiency. Particularly among the elderly it seems possible that the thinning and atrophy of the skeleton, although the result of other factors in many cases, may sometimes be the result of the chronic undernutrition and underweight not infrequent in these subjects.

Despite the occurrence of some actual structural changes in the *nervous tissue* in rather severe states of inanition and loss of weight, it is unlikely that they are present in the milder degrees of underweight. Nor are they likely to be the cause of the mental changes which may develop.

Included in this statement are the special senses, essentially nervous in structure and function, none of which show any significant effect with even severe loss of weight. The same is true of intellectual capacity, which remains unimpaired, although it may be unexercised because of the disinclination to exertion, physical or mental. This is not so true, however, of the *personality* and the *emotions*. As always, there are so many factors concerned with emotional responses and personality reactions that it is difficult to show that a single factor such as loss of weight and the undernutrition causing it are the causes of such changes, except under carefully controlled conditions which are difficult to have in ordinary living. For instance, the preoccupation with food and the emotional behavior associated with restriction of food which can be found in experimental subjects may be entirely lacking in the individual whose distorted thinking with regard to food and eating has been the actual cause of the underweight. The compulsive factor differs in the experimental subject and the individual who voluntarily or even on medical advice restricts his food intake. Nevertheless, the latter individual may suffer some of the effects on his or her emotional make-up and personality that have been shown to occur experimentally, even though they voluntarily stay underweight because of social custom or style. Such changes need not be extreme or even particularly evident. They consist of *lack of interest, depression* (though mild), and a trend toward *introversion*. *Irritability* is perhaps the most common and noticeable. In more severe restrictions there may be a trend to *hypochondriasis* and *hysteria*.

It will be apparent from what has been written that the dangers and impairments resulting from a moderate degree of underweight are not, with the exception of increased susceptibility to tuberculosis, serious. In fact, as already stated, a certain amount of underweight may be beneficial. However, there is here a rather fine distinction between what may be considered *beneficial underweight* and *harmful undernutrition*. The former refers to a state in which the weight is maintained slightly below the accepted standards but without progression downward and without encroachment on the healthy size or function of the organs and tissues. The latter refers to a state in which these structures have become actually deficient. With even the milder grades of the latter the effect on health, efficiency, and that precious asset, a sense of well-being, may be considerable. *See also* OBESITY; DIET, REDUCING; DIET, SPECIAL; ANEMIA; HYPOGLYCEMIA; WEIGHT, FACTORS WHICH INFLUENCE; WEIGHT, NORMAL FOR HEALTH; WEIGHT-REGULATING MACHINERY OF THE BODY.

UNDESCENDED TESTES. The development of the *testes (testicles)* takes place in the abdominal cavity. Normally they descend through the *inguinal canals* into the *scrotum* soon after birth. If this descent fails to occur, the abnormality is designated as *undescended testes*.

Undescended testes usually atrophy—that is, waste away. If this occurs in both testes, the person becomes *sterile*. Undescended testes through functional failure also hinder proper development of the *male secondary sex characteristics,* such as the beard, the low voice, and the flat chest.

The parents or pediatrician should, therefore, examine the child at an early age to be sure that the testes have descended into the scrotum. Ordinarily the testes can be felt. Rarely it may be possible to press them down gently to the proper position. In cases of any difficulty the advice of a doctor is absolutely essential. If the child is old enough to realize the situation, care should be taken not to arouse his curiosity or create anxiety.

Sometimes surgery is necessary to transplant the testes to their proper position in the scrotum. This operation should, if possible, always be performed before puberty. See also REPRODUCTION SYSTEM; TESTICLES; SCROTUM. See MEDIGRAPH page 1307.

UNDULANT FEVER, known medically as *brucellosis,* and in different sections of the world as *Malta, Mediterranean, Rio Grande, Texas,* and *goat fever*: a remittent febrile disease, caused by infection with *Brucella bacteria,* named after Bruce, a British physician who first isolated it on Malta. The infection may last weeks or months and during this time the fever rises and falls over periods of several days, and may be severe enough to cause death. Unfamiliar in the United States before 1927, undulant fever has now been reported in every state.

Undulant fever is also found in cattle, sheep, and goats, and human beings may contract the disease from infected animals, although more frequently from infected milk or milk products. Twelve to thirty-six days after exposure, fever and other symptoms are noted. The temperature rises steadily over a period of days, receding temporarily each morning, until a fever of 102°F. or 103°F. is reached. It remains at this point for a few days, then steadily drops down, and this cycle may persist for months. Fever periods are accompanied by general malaise, pain, constipation, sweating, and weakness. Undulant fever has occasionally been mistaken for other illnesses with somewhat similar symptoms, such as *malaria, typhoid fever,* and even *tuberculosis.*

Until recently, little could be done for the infection, but *vaccines* now exist which can effectively prevent it, and *sulfonamides* and *antibiotics* are helpful in some cases, and other measures, such as *heat treatments,* have yielded a certain amount of success.

UNIVERSAL ANTIDOTE. See POISONING.

UREMIA, the poisoning which results when the filtering and excretion of wastes from the blood by the kidneys is blocked so that these substances accumulate in the blood. It occurs in acute and chronic forms. The most extreme type is when both

the disease and its causes To function normally, the testicles, which are egg-shaped glands, must operate in their natural environment—the scrotum (or sac). Normally, the testicles descend at birth from the abdominal cavity through the inguinal canal to the scrotum. When they do not descend, they are in an abnormal environment where there is interference with their production of sperm and the male sex hormone testosterone. Undescended testicles can be found anywhere between the abdomen and the scrotum—as shown in the Medi-Graph.

Undescended testicles are found in about 10% of boys at birth. There are a variety of causes that are thought to be responsible for this disease: failure of the hormone supply to provide its normal stimulation of the testes to descend at birth; a refusal of the testicles to respond to such hormone stimulation; mechanical blockage such as adhesions or anatomical obstacles that prevent the normal descent of the testicles from the abdominal cavity to the scrotum.

Fortunately, by the time a boy born with undescended testicles reaches puberty, the condition has frequently corrected itself without creating any other problems.

symptoms When a testicle has not descended by the onset of puberty (the age when a boy matures sexually—usually between 12 and 15), it degenerates progressively. However, if the other testicle has descended, the only symptom observed as a rule is occasional pain over the undescended one—and even this symptom may not appear.

If both testicles do not descend and they fail to produce testosterone, the patient shows eunuchoid symptoms. The penis may fail to grow normally, the voice may remain high-pitched, and beard, armpit hair, and pubic hair may be absent. There is a tendency for the long bones to overgrow, and abnormal fat deposits may appear on the hips, buttocks, and breasts. This extreme picture appears only when there is a complete lack of hormone function. Very often an undescended testicle is capable of some hormone secretion.

complications Testicles which do not descend not only result in hormonal defects but also can be painful and be the site of cancer. When the testicles remain in the abdomen, cancer occurs most often. The greater the distance they travel toward the scrotum, the less likely is cancer to develop.

Another complication, as noted above, is the possible development of eunuchoidism.

prevention (or lessening of impact) If a diagnosis of the condition is made before a boy's puberty and the location of the undescended testicle established, it can be treated successfully. Testicles found in the inguinal canal usually descend by themselves. If not, they generally respond to specific hormone injections. When passage is blocked mechanically, surgery is used to relocate the testicle.

Undescended Testicles

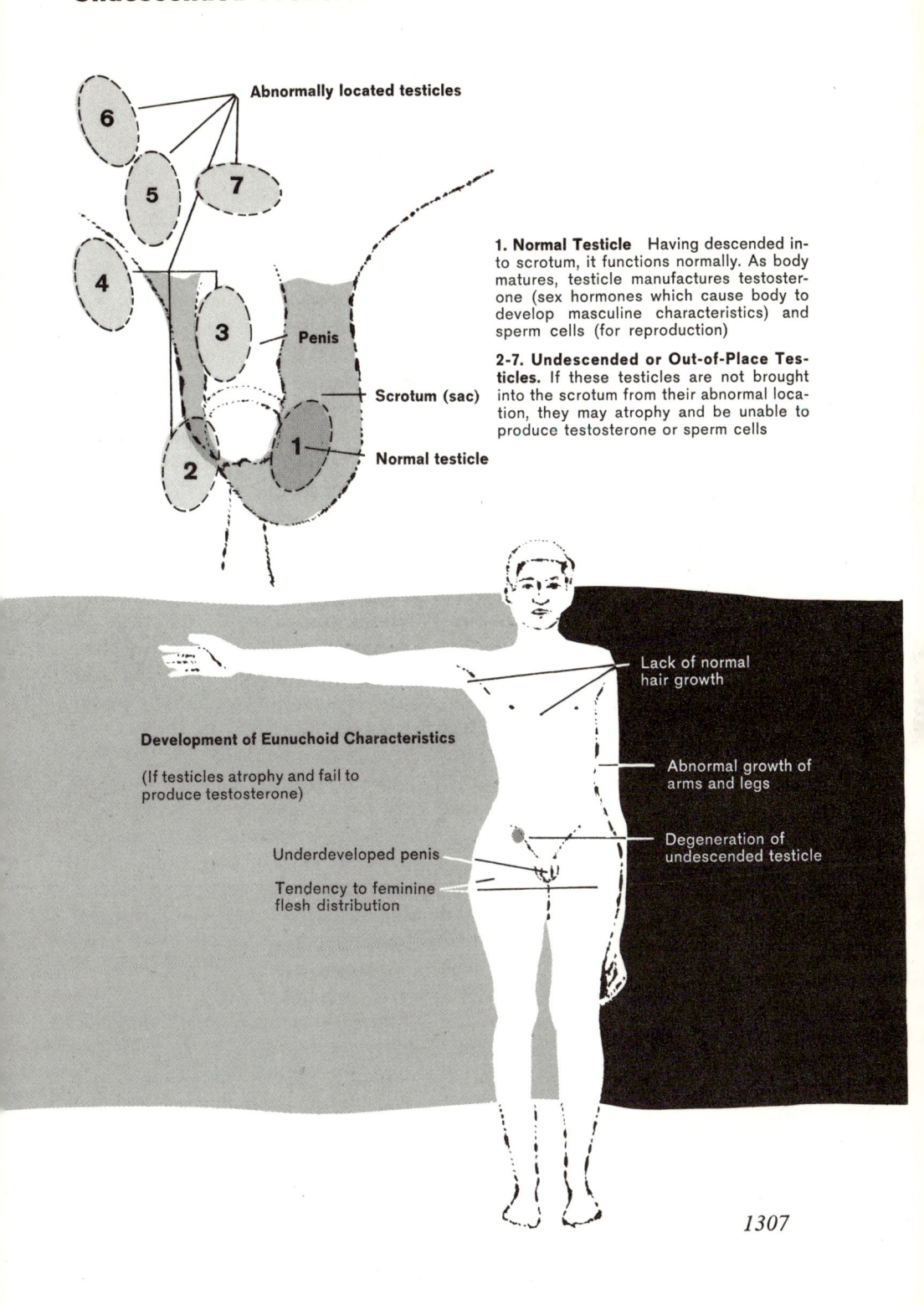

Abnormally located testicles

Penis

Scrotum (sac)

Normal testicle

1. Normal Testicle Having descended into scrotum, it functions normally. As body matures, testicle manufactures testosterone (sex hormones which cause body to develop masculine characteristics) and sperm cells (for reproduction)

2-7. Undescended or Out-of-Place Testicles. If these testicles are not brought into the scrotum from their abnormal location, they may atrophy and be unable to produce testosterone or sperm cells

Development of Eunuchoid Characteristics

(If testicles atrophy and fail to produce testosterone)

Underdeveloped penis

Tendency to feminine flesh distribution

Lack of normal hair growth

Abnormal growth of arms and legs

Degeneration of undescended testicle

kidneys are removed or their excretory channels are blocked. Death then follows in a few days.

An early symptom of uremia is headache, which may be present in annoying severity weeks before other indications of disturbance are perceptible. When the headache is accompanied by restlessness, difficulty in sleeping, nausea, and vomiting, the possibility of uremia definitely exists, and prompt medical attention is imperative.

In its *acute form,* uremia may attack without warning. A *convulsive epileptiform fit* followed by *coma* may be the first manifestation. Sometimes the coma occurs without a fit and in some instances *mania* seizes the patient. Inflammation of the kidney may occur in children during or after another acute infection, with similar sudden convulsions preceded perhaps by *rapid swelling of the tissues and face.* The attack may happen so quickly and violently that death ensues. Because of this, doctors watch carefully urine changes in children who have major infections such as *pneumonia, acute tonsillitis,* or *scarlet fever.*

In the more slowly developing uremia, the early symptoms are followed by *shortness of breath,* attendant on accumulation of toxic materials in the body. It is often difficult to distinguish between failing breath due to heart weakness and that accompanying the later stages of kidney disorder. The patient may grow apathetic, drift quietly into unconsciousness, and finally die. Occasionally fluid accumulates, presses upon the lungs, and affects breathing. Similarly fluid may intrude upon the brain and have to be withdrawn by spinal puncture.

In general, treatment of chronic uremia is the same as for chronic *nephritis.* Acute uremia is often relieved by inducing sweating and by frequent liquid bowel movements, both of which tend to help the body rid itself of excess fluid and liquid wastes. Many uremic patients, with obstructive lesions, are cured by proper treatment, which can include injections of *glucose* to correct dehydration.

Recent investigation indicates that uremia is probably not the result of accumulating urea in the blood as had been believed for more than a century. In one experiment, the ureters of animals were redirected to empty into the bowel. Some of the urine which would ordinarily be excreted by way of the urinary bladder entered the intestines and part of it was reabsorbed into the blood. Urea in the blood of the animals rose to a remarkable level of fifty times above normal without having any observable effect on them. A tentative conclusion from this experiment is that urea is not toxic enough to bring about the profound and sometimes drastic symptoms found in uremia. See also NEPHRITIS. See MEDIGRAPH page 1311.

URETER, a thick-walled muscular tube that conveys urine from the kidney to the bladder. There is one on either side of the pelvis. The ureter acts by a process of contraction (*peristalsis*) that forces urine down the tube in spurts. It is about twelve inches long and about one-fifth of an inch in diameter.

Sometimes a *stone* may block the ureter and require surgery for its removal. The tube may become twisted or infected, and occasionally it has been ruptured.

Disorders of the ureter or any part of the urinary tract are generally treated by a specialist known as a *urologist*. When the ureter is affected, x-rays are generally taken, after injection of a substance which causes the ureter to become visible. *See also* KIDNEYS; BLADDER DISEASES. *See* MEDIGRAPHS pages 825, 1311.

URETHRA, the passage from the bladder through which urine is voided. In the male, the urethra is approximately eight inches long, and in the female one and a half inches in length.

The *male urethra* begins with a *prostatic portion* which is surrounded by the *prostate gland*. The secretions of the prostate empty into the urethra—continuously in minute amounts but at a greatly accelerated rate during sexual activity. The two *ejaculatory ducts* also empty into the urethra at a proximate location, bearing (during sexual activity) the *spermatozoa* and the secretions of the *seminal vesicles* and the *epididymides*. (These secretions, the spermatozoa, and the prostatic fluid all combine to form the *semen*.)

The urethra then passes into the *penis*. There it receives the secretions of *Cowper's glands* (the *bulbo-urethral glands*). The walls of the urethra are here lined with mucus. The opening of the urethra at the tip of the penis is called the *meatus*.

Urethritis, inflammation of the urethra—most frequently the result of *gonorrhea*—causes a swelling which narrows and partly closes the urethra. The inflammation impedes the flow of urine and the emerging stream may fork or twist. Sometimes the urethra is clogged by a kidney stone or a foreign body which may have to be removed surgically.

Stricture of the urethra requires regular stretching with an instrument designed for the purpose, but sometimes surgical treatment may be needed to open the passage. A stricture of long duration can react on the kidneys and ureters and on the bladder too, causing it to dilate and enlarge abnormally.

The urethra may be ruptured by a severe blow or by an accident, causing urine to escape into nearby tissues.

Occasionally, congenital abnormalities of the urethra are present which render normal urination and normal sexual intercourse difficult or impossible. The most common of these is *hypospadias,* in which the meatus is on the underside of the penis instead of at the tip—sometimes as far back as at the point of junction between the penis and scrotum, or even on the *perineum* (area between the scrotum and anus). Less common is *epispadias,* in which the meatus is on the upper side of the penis. A surgical operation called a *meatotomy* is necessary to correct cases of hypospadias and epispadias.

In rare instances, complete epispadias is combined with *exstrophy*

the disease and its causes PYELITIS AND CYSTITIS Infections of the urinary tract are caused by a variety of bacteria. Common disorders which tend to recur, they may start in the urinary tract or as a secondary infection. Among the groups particularly subject to these infections are pregnant women, diabetics, patients subject to long periods of bed rest, and patients suffering from urinary tract problems such as kidney stones. Other sufferers are individuals with some neurological disorder that interferes with normal bladder function, and males in the older age groups who are subject to prostatic diseases which prevent free passage of urine.
TUMORS Malignant tumors of the kidney and bladder are fairly common. They are a source of concern because it is difficult to make early diagnosis. Except for one type which is seen in young children, kidney tumors occur most often after the age of 50, in both sexes, and in all races. The most common and most important sign that there may be a tumor present is the painless passage of blood in the urine. The amount may be microscopic or visible to the naked eye, and some time may pass before the blood appears again. On occasion there may be vague pains in the upper abdomen or flanks, and mild cramp.

symptoms PYELITIS AND CYSTITIS When the kidneys are infected, the disease is known as pyelitis. The onset is rapid, with the symptoms shown in the Medi-Graph. When the bladder is infected, the disease is called cystitis. In the latter disease the patient may have low-grade fever, chills, and aches and pains in addition to the symptoms noted in the accompanying Medi-Graph.
TUMORS Kidney tumor symptoms are somewhat similar—as shown in the Medi-Graph.

complications PYELITIS AND CYSTITIS Chronic urinary tract infection can lead to destructive changes in the kidneys. This in turn can lead to high blood pressure and, eventually, loss of ability of the kidneys to function, and uremia.
TUMORS Where there is a tumor, complications arise from infection and interference with urine flow. Severe pyelitis and the obstruction caused by a tumor can result in death. Spread of the tumor to other organ systems is a possible and serious complication.

prevention (or lessening of impact) PYELITIS AND CYSTITIS Pyelitis and cystitis require careful, prolonged treatment which should not be delayed. Fortunately, these urinary tract infections are usually highly responsive to proper care, if they are not neglected. The doctor will probably get urine cultures to identify the responsible bacteria, and will treat the patient with antibiotics or other specific drugs.
Infection in other parts of the body must be treated to prevent spread to the kidneys. Preventive measures are advisable for patients subject to long bed rest or catheterization.
TUMORS The only hope lies in early recognition and prompt surgery. Any neglect of any recognizable symptom can be calamitous.

Urinary Tract Tumors and Infections

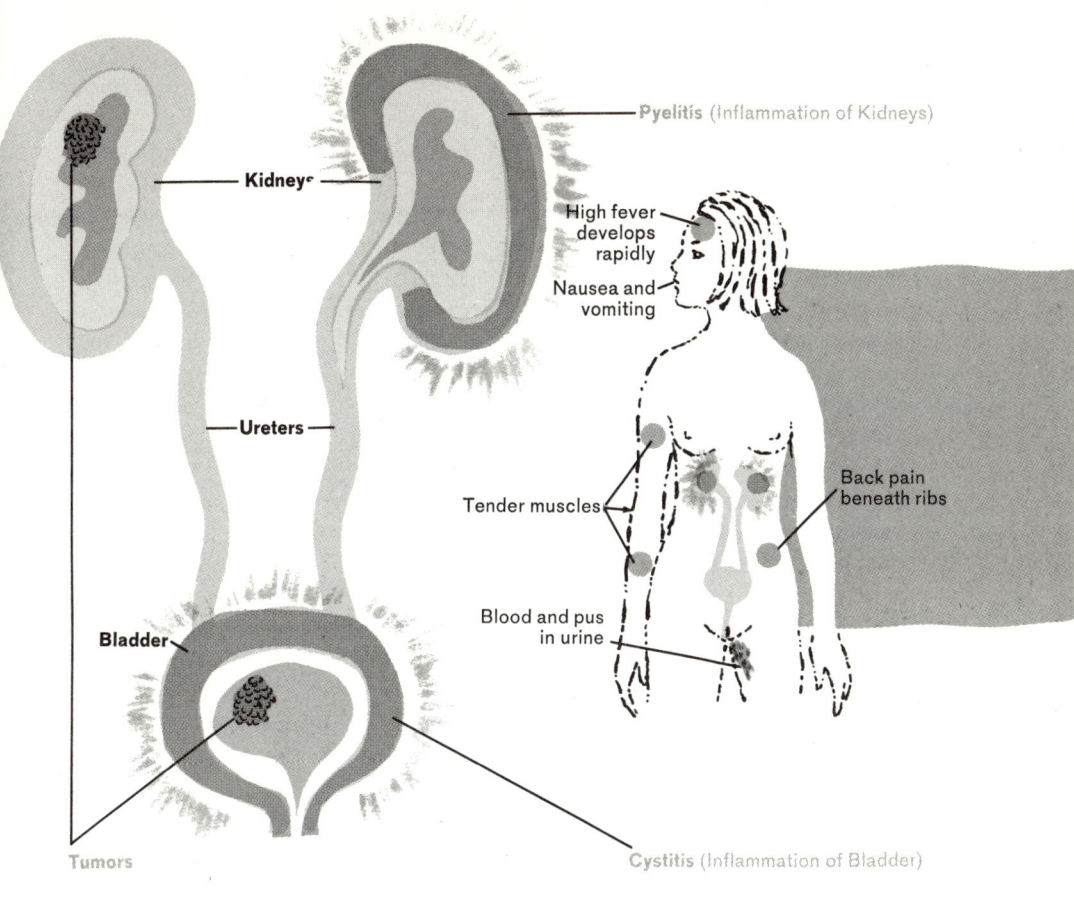

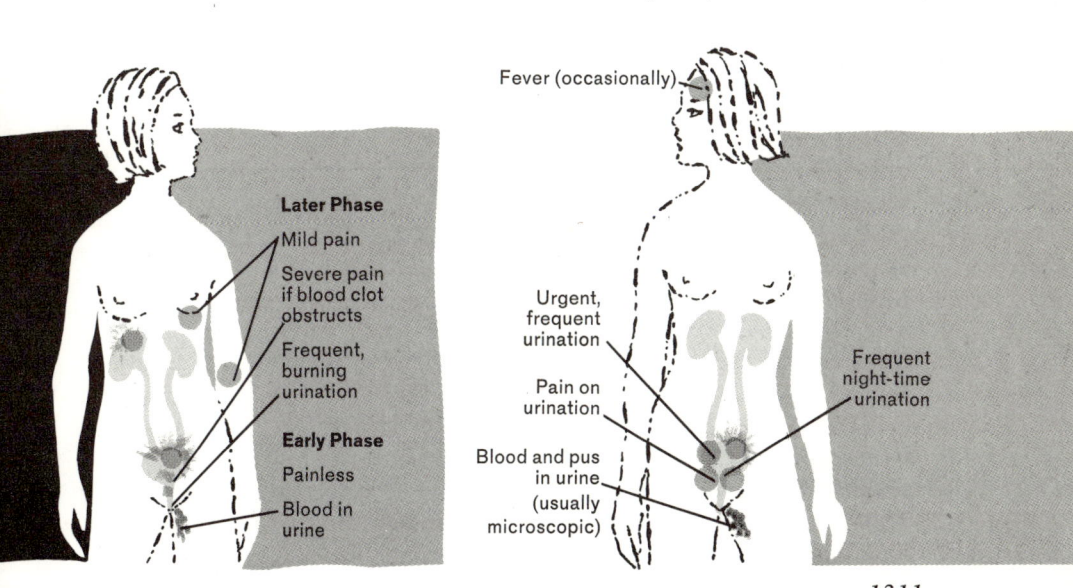

- Kidneys
- Ureters
- Bladder
- Tumors

Pyelitis (Inflammation of Kidneys)
- High fever develops rapidly
- Nausea and vomiting
- Tender muscles
- Back pain beneath ribs
- Blood and pus in urine

Cystitis (Inflammation of Bladder)
- Fever (occasionally)
- Urgent, frequent urination
- Pain on urination
- Blood and pus in urine (usually microscopic)
- Frequent night-time urination

Later Phase
- Mild pain
- Severe pain if blood clot obstructs
- Frequent, burning urination

Early Phase
- Painless
- Blood in urine

1311

of the bladder (protrusion of the bladder outside the abdominal wall), accompanied by total incontinence. In such cases, it is necessary to resort to radical surgery, sometimes transplanting the *ureters* so that they open into the rectum.

The *female urethra* is broader than that of the male and is subject to greater dilatation. *Urethral carbuncles* are small swellings peculiar to women, and if they do not give any discomfort are best left untouched. If they become tender and painful during urination, they can be removed surgically. *See also* PENIS; PROSTATE; SEMEN; SEMINAL VESICLES; REPRODUCTION SYSTEM; BLADDER DISEASES; KIDNEYS; NEPHRITIS; UREMIA; URINE; URINATION; VULVA; GONORRHEA; CHANCROID; GRANULOMA INGUINALE; SYPHILIS. *See* MEDIGRAPHS pages 825, 1311.

URINATION, technically termed *micturition,* the passing of urine from the body by the kidneys. A complicated muscular action is involved. The wall of the bladder and another related muscle are contracted. Then a circular muscle around the neck of the bladder—called the *sphincter* muscle—which keeps it shut and holds back the urine at all other times is released. The nervous regulation of urination is through a center in the spinal cord. Thus, even an unconscious person can urinate. Complete interruption of urination will bring death in a few days. The spinal center, however, is controlled by the brain, whether during sleeping or waking. Three or four times a day is a normal interval for micturition and ordinarily it is not necessary at night.

Many factors may increase the *frequency* of urination—for instance, *pregnancy* and *cold weather*. Since less moisture is lost from the skin during cold weather, a greater excretory load is thrown on the urinary system. Other factors may be *excitement; inflammation* or *irritation* of the kidney, bladder, or urinary passage; or a *growth* or *presence of a stone* within them. In addition, excessive urine may occur in *diabetes* and *nephritis,* and acid or other irritants be present in the urine itself.

Diminution of the flow of urine occurs when the prostate gland is enlarged, thus causing contraction of the *urethra,* the urinary passage leading to the exterior. Complete cessation may be due to feebleness of the bladder or to an obstruction or interruption of the kidneys' normal formation of urine.

Partially or wholly uncontrolled urination may also arise from several factors. The bladder may have reached its capacity and be unable to hold more, or nervous disorders may induce or permit involuntary urination. Apoplectic or epileptic fits as well as unconsciousness may affect micturition, and sometimes the brain loses its power to regulate the special spinal center.

Occasionally a sense of need to release urine develops when actually the bladder is empty. This condition, *dysuria,* may come from irritation of the urinary tract or from nervous sources in *locomotor ataxia,* a disease of the spinal cord. *See also* BED WETTING; BLADDER, URINARY.

URINE, the aqueous fluid extracted from the blood by the *kidneys,* stored in the *bladder,* and excreted through the *urethra.* In health, urine is amber-colored and contains *urea, inorganic salts, pigments,* and other end-products of the metabolism of both protein and minerals in the system. Urine has a somewhat disagreeable odor and when it stands for some time *ammonia* is produced, which is easily recognized by its stench.

The daily quantity of urine may vary in health. In cold weather it may be increased and conversely decreased in hot weather when perspiration removes a large amount of waste products. The quantity is also affected by certain diseases. In *diabetes,* pints of urine may be excreted each day. In fevers and acute *nephritis,* urinary output may be greatly lessened. If urine has an ammoniacal odor when excreted, it has undergone decomposition, as occurs in chronic inflammation of the bladder. In diabetes the odor may resemble that of new-mown hay. In certain diseases and disorders, it is essential to determine the quantity of both normal and abnormal constituents of urine, particularly urea. A diminution of urea occurs in nephritis and other disorders. *Albumin* in urine may be indicative of nephritis or another disorder, but sometimes, as in *albuminuria,* the cause is physiological. In diabetes the urine is tested to determine the amount of sugar, and another test indicates whether or not blood is present.

The acidity of urine is increased by an ample amount of meat in the diet; large amounts of vegetables make it alkaline. In *dyspepsia,* when copious amounts of soda are taken, it may also be quite alkaline.

Specific gravity is also tested in diabetes and in *diabetes mellitus* it is considerably raised. In *diabetes insipidus* or *cirrhosis of the kidney,* however, it is quite low. See also ALBUMINURIA; HEMATURIA. See MEDIGRAPH page 1311.

UTERUS, a hollow, pear-shaped organ in the female pelvis commonly known as the *womb.* Within the uterus, the unborn child develops and grows for nine months, nourished by the blood from the mother's body. In the nonpregnant woman, the uterus is about three inches long, but during pregnancy its elastic wall stretches. It returns to normal size after delivery. The uterus is suspended in the pelvis by ligaments and opens into the *vagina* by means of the *cervix,* a small hollow fibrous tubelike structure situated at the bottom of the uterus. The cervix is a protective passage which shields the rest of the uterus, especially during pregnancy. At delivery it distends to permit expulsion of the infant. The uterus is a muscular organ, but its lining is a soft glandular material known as *endometrium.* Bleeding at *menstruation* comes from this lining. The *ovaries* are near the uterus, on each side, but do not connect with it. Ova from the ovaries reach the uterus by passing from the top through two armlike projections known as the *Fallopian* or *uterine tubes* or as the *oviducts.*

the disease and its causes The most frequently found tumors in the female are fibroids, which are swellings that can appear in all parts of the uterine wall, extending to the outer surface as well as toward the uterine cavity. The cause is thought to be some kind of imbalance in the production of hormones by the ovaries. This theory is based on the fact that in all instances fibroid tumors shrink and rarely cause symptoms after menopause when the ovarian hormones cease to appear.

symptoms Many fibroids have no symptoms at all and are found only on routine examination. When symptoms do appear, they are usually related to the size and location of the tumor. When a fibroid tumor is near the region of the urinary bladder and exerts pressure on it, the patient needs to urinate frequently. When one exerts pressure on the rectum, constipation can result.

Bleeding is probably the most common symptom. It can either occur between normal menstrual cycles, or cause an unusually heavy menstrual flow, or extend the duration of the flow.

Fibroid tumors may degenerate, or calcify, or twist on a pedicle—which is a stalklike extension of the uterine wall. In the latter case, severe pain is the result.

Back pain is not unusual. When a tumor is unusually large, the patient herself can feel it easily through the lower abdominal wall. Or, it may even protrude in this area.

complications There are no serious complications to fibroid tumors and they almost never become malignant. However, bleeding during menstruation can become so profuse that treatment is necessary. Fibroids present a problem during pregnancy since, depending on their size and location, they can interfere with the development of the fetus and cause a miscarriage. They are also thought to be related to sterility in some women, but this probably applies to those cases where the tumors are multiple or very large.

prevention (or lessening of impact) There is no known method of preventing the development of fibroid tumors. Their presence is no cause for alarm unless there is severe bleeding, or the patient becomes pregnant.

When the fibroid tumors are detected they should be watched carefully to note how rapidly they are growing and their effects on the bladder or bowel. When nothing unusual is found, a woman close to menopause can wait safely for her fibroid tumors to shrink.

Surgery is indicated only in special cases and only on the advice of a trained gynecologist.

Fibroid Tumor

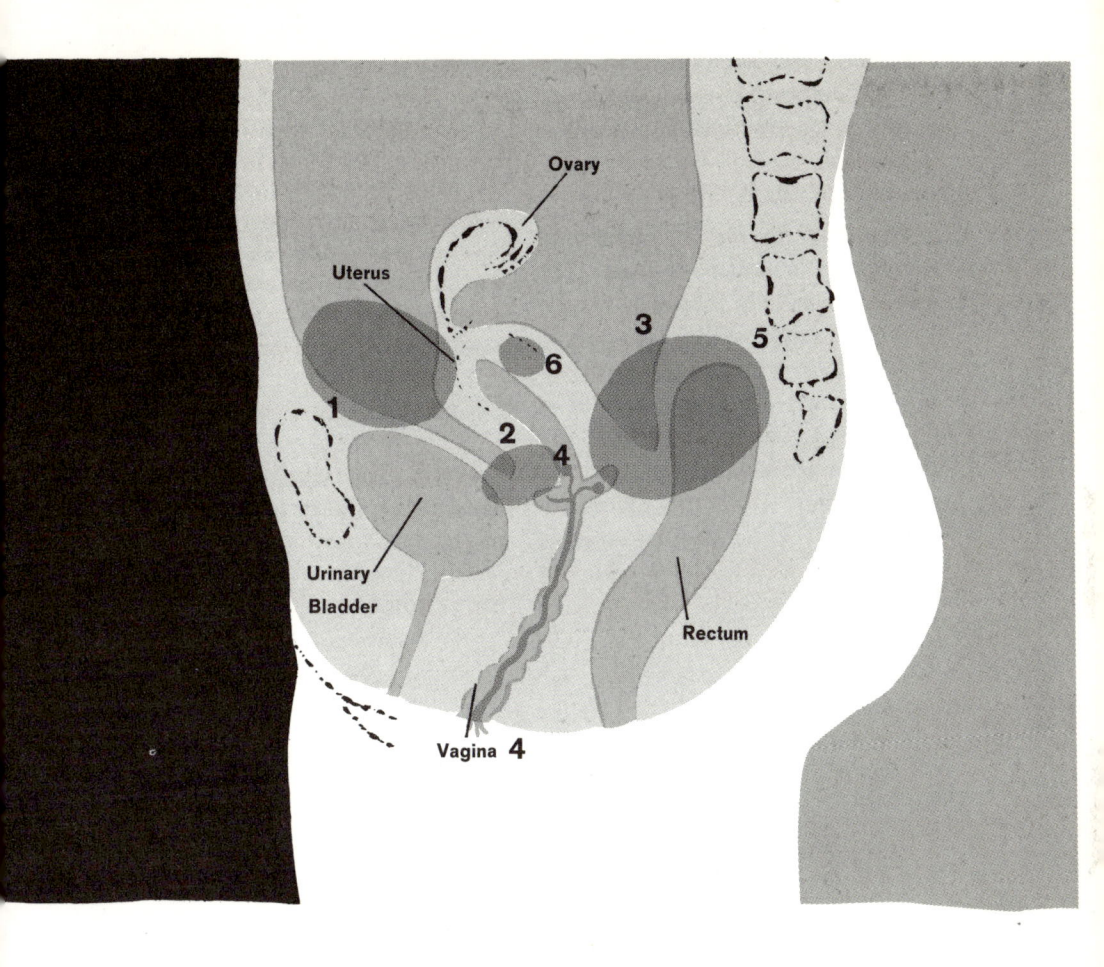

1. Large size tumors may be felt through abdominal wall
2. Tumor exerts pressure on bladder — increases frequency of urination
3. Tumor exerts pressure on rectum — constipation develops
4. Increased bleeding at menstrual period or between periods
5. Unusual pressure on nerves may result in back pain
6. But many fibroid tumors produce no symptoms

Fibroid tumors almost never become malignant. They shrink after menopause—and cease to cause symptoms

The uterus is prone to infection, especially after childbirth or abortion. Occasionally severe inflammation after abortion may result in permanent *sterility,* because of destruction of the uterine lining.

Cancer of the uterus occurs most frequently in older women. The symptoms include bleeding, usually between *periods* or after *menopause.* Bleeding may occur from less serious sources, such as *fibroid tumors* in the uterine wall. The doctor can usually make the diagnosis by removing tissue from the uterus for examination. This is done by scraping the lining of the uterus. In this procedure sometimes referred to as *curettage* the cervix is dilated and the uterus scraped or *curetted.* See also ABORTION; AFTERBIRTH; CANCER; CERVIX; CONCEPTION; CONTRACEPTION; HYSTERECTOMY; MENOPAUSE; MENSTRUATION; OVARIES; OVULATION; CHILDBIRTH AND PRENATAL CARE; PREGNANCY, SIGNS OF; REPRODUCTION SYSTEM; SEXUAL INTERCOURSE; VAGINA; VULVA. See MEDIGRAPHS pages 995, 1315.

URTICARIA. *See* HIVES.

UVULA, the small fleshy conical mass which hangs from the middle of the *soft palate* in the rear of the mouth. It seldom becomes infected or disturbed.

V

VACCINATION, inoculation with a preparation containing weakened or incapacitated disease germs or viruses for the purpose of engendering greater resistance or immunity to ailments caused by these organisms.

When the germs are grown from secretions or blood taken from a patient, so that it contains the strain of organisms responsible for the disease, the vaccine is called *autogenous*. Usually a vaccine contains killed germs, but sometimes living organisms are used, or a mixed vaccine of a variety of germs or viruses. A vaccine containing several strains of the influenza virus is used to prevent epidemic influenza. The *Salk vaccine*, which has been widely and effectively employed in immunization for poliomyelitis is an example of a killed virus. See also IMMUNIZATION; VIRUSES. See MEDIGRAPH page 1195.

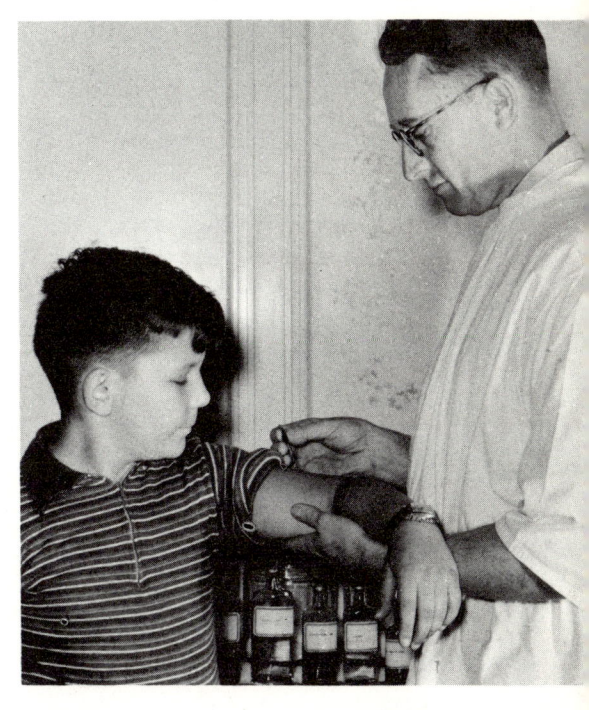

Vaccination—Immunity to certain diseases may be produced by vaccination. A weakened virus which will not produce the severe disease is injected. The child actually develops a slight case of the disease but he will recover and for a number of years be immune to the disease for which he was inoculated. Vaccinations are done on the upper arm or thigh because these areas are relatively free of friction by clothing. Some of the communicable diseases can be prevented by vaccination. The boy in the photograph is being vaccinated against smallpox.

VAGINA, the female genital passage or canal which extends from the outer sex organs (*vulva*) to the *uterus*. It consists of muscular tissue which is highly elastic. The vagina is lubricated by the secretions of *Bartholin's glands*.

Inflammation of the vagina occurs in certain venereal infections, such as *gonorrhea,* or it may be a complication of some other infectious disease, such as *scarlet fever* or *measles*. Vaginal discharge is commonly known as *leucorrhea* or *the whites*. *Vaginismus* is a painful spasmodic contraction of the muscles at the entrance to the vagina. See also DOUCHE; FISTULA; LEUCORRHEA; VULVA; UTERUS; REPRODUCTION SYSTEM; HYMEN; PENIS.

VALETUDINARIANISM, another word for *hypochondriasis*. See HYPOCHONDRIASIS.

VALLEY FEVER. See COCCIDIOIDOMYCOSIS.

VARICELLA. See CHICKENPOX.

VARICOSE VEINS, veins which become dilated so that they project in lumpy fashion above the surface of the skin. They are caused by a breakdown of the valves which ordinarily serve to maintain a continuous flow of blood to the heart. These valves cease to function properly, and the blood tends to accumulate at intervals, causing the appearance described.

Varicose veins appear most frequently in the legs, for in this area the blood is required to climb almost straight up on its way to the heart. For the same reason, varicose veins —*hemorrhoids*—often develop in the rectum.

People who suffer most frequently from varicose veins are those whose blood, for some reason, is failing to circulate in a normal manner. Fat people are susceptible and also pregnant women. After the birth of a child, the interference with normal circulation may terminate. By that time, however, the valves have been broken, and once broken do not repair themselves.

Varicose veins are dangerous because dilation leads to clotting of the blood and therefore to secondary infection.

Occasionally varicosity of the veins can be prevented by proper attention to clothing. The habitual wearing of tight belts or tight garters, for example, should be avoided.

The treatment varies with the patient. Small varicose veins are sometimes emptied of blood and then filled with a fluid which causes the walls of the vein to grow together. In treating the legs, the physician may block off a large vessel in the upper part of the thigh, and so prevent the downward flow of blood into veins which might otherwise become dilated. In some cases this condition can be controlled by the wearing of elastic bandages or stockings.

The current treatment of varicose veins is surgical removal, by stripping and segmental excision. This has largely replaced injection in severe cases; mild cases are generally left untreated. See also HEMORRHOIDS. See MEDIGRAPHS pages 743, 1321.

VARIOLA. See SMALLPOX.

VAS DEFERENS (plural *vasa deferentia*), the efferent duct of a *testicle,* leading from the *epididymis* through the *spermatic cord* and the *inguinal canal* to the *seminal vesicle,* with the duct of which it joins to form the *ejaculatory duct* emptying into the *urethra.* The *vasa deferentia* are to be distinguished from the *vasa efferentia,* which are the multiple tubes inside the testicles leading to the epididymides. The vasa deferentia convey the spermatozoa and the secretions of the epididymides to the seminal vesicles.

Sterilization is an operation in which the vasa deferentia are cut, so that the reproductive sperm cells cannot reach the outside, and the male cannot fertilize the female. See also SEMINAL DUCTS; SPERMATIC CORDS; EPIDIDYMIS; SEMINAL VESICLES; TESTICLES; SCROTUM; URETHRA; REPRODUCTION SYSTEM; STERILIZATION; CYSTIC FIBROSIS.

VEINS, vessels that return blood to the heart, as opposed to *arteries* which carry blood away from the heart. A vein has a structure like that of an artery, except that the three coats of a vein are thin and inelastic as compared with those of an artery. Many veins, especially those of the lower limbs, are provided with valves which open out when the blood tries to flow backward.

The blood in veins is a dark purplish color, except the blood of the *pulmonary veins* which is red (it is purified blood carried from the lungs to the heart). All the venous blood from the rest of the body is poured into the heart through two large veins, the *vena cava.*

Veins generally follow the same course as arteries and many are named after the arteries they accompany.

A wound of the vein is ordinarily less dangerous than a wound of an artery, because the bleeding can be controlled more easily. However, a wound of one of the large veins in the neck or in the armpit is dangerous not only because bleeding may be profuse but also because air may enter the vein and form an *embolus,* or obstruction. Breathlessness and discomfort may ensue, followed by death within a few seconds if the embolism reaches the lung.

Varicose veins are dilated, hardened, and twisted. Inflammation of a vein that is septic, affected by general reaction of certain bacteria, or simple is *phlebitis.* See also HEMORRHOIDS; PHLEBITIS; THROMBOSIS; VARICOSE VEINS; WOUNDS.

VENA CAVA. See VEINS.

VENEREAL DISEASE. See *separate entries for the five venereal diseases*: CHANCROID; GONORRHEA; GRANULOMA INGUINALE; LYMPHOGRANULOMA VENEREUM; SYPHILIS.

VENTILATION refers to the circulation or movement of fresh air through rooms and other areas such as halls and stairwells. It is also the process of supplying fresh air or of purifying air.

In *natural ventilation,* air from an

1319

the disease and its causes Varicose veins or varicosities are enlarged, twisted veins near the surface of the skin. They are caused by defective vein valves which can be present at birth; they can result from prolonged postural strain; or they can be the result of extra strain on the valves when the deep veins of the legs function ineffectively. Stagnation and back pressure on the vein result from these conditions, causing over-stretching, lengthening, and enlargement of the vein walls.

Varicosities are commonly seen in people whose work requires them to stand for long periods, and in women after pregnancy. Both men and women are subject to this disease, which usually appears in the legs and becomes more troublesome as age advances.

Sometimes only a short section of a single vein is involved; sometimes nearly all the veins in one or both legs are affected. Most cases involve the surface veins which lie just under the skin. If there are no other complications, these enlarged veins are not a serious threat to health. When varicose veins become severe, it may be the result of a disease or injury involving deep veins higher in the legs or in the body. In these cases, the underlying causes must be treated.

symptoms In the early stages there is no discomfort and the patient is generally more concerned with the unsightly appearance of the swollen veins. The first symptom is usually a feeling of heaviness in the legs. As the disease progresses, the feet swell. Still later there is pain, explained by the fact that the veins are close to the nerves of sensation.

Skin changes commonly result, and there is deep pigmentation in some areas. Skin ulcerations can appear, with craters that become quite large and heal slowly. Other symptoms are shown in the Medi-Graph.

Because all of these are also symptoms of other diseases or conditions, they cannot always be blamed on varicose veins. Only a doctor can decide in each case.

Another kind of vein which makes an appearance is called the "spider burst" type. These are tiny, purple veins seen under the skin in spidery clusters. They do not have the same significance as varicose veins, and in most instances doctors say that no treatment is necessary. Sometimes treatment to improve their appearance is tried, but this is rarely successful.

complications If varicose veins are not treated, eventually the enlarged veins, the ulcerated skin, and the swollen feet can disable the patient almost completely.

Phlebitis, which is an associated inflammation of the skin, and secondary infections related to the skin ulcers, are the complications of this disease. Rupture of the veins, with hemorrhage under the skin, is also seen frequently.

prevention (or lessening of impact) Elastic stockings and raising up the feet during periods of rest can limit the further development of varicose veins. Injection therapy has been useful in limiting the disease. Surgery offers the best hope for cure once the varicosities are well established.

Varicose Veins

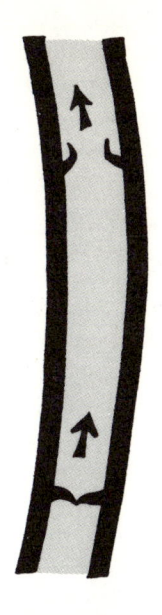

Operation of Normal Vein
Valves along your veins channel flow of blood. When valve above opens to guide flow toward heart, valve below closes to prevent backward escape of blood.

Varicose Vein
In varicose vein, walls swell out. Valves no longer close to prevent back flow of blood. Blood accumulates in vein.

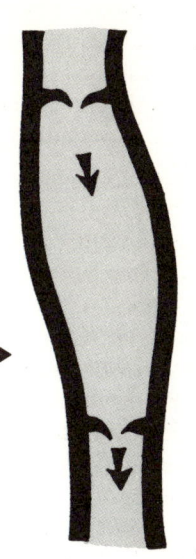

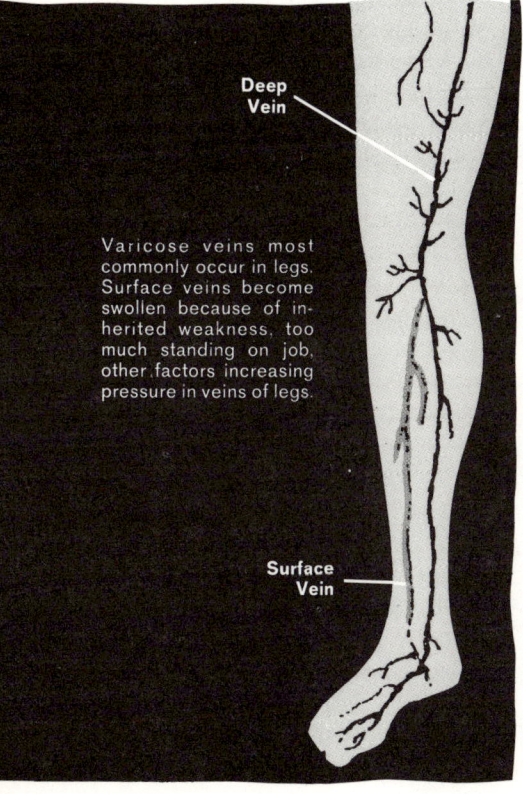

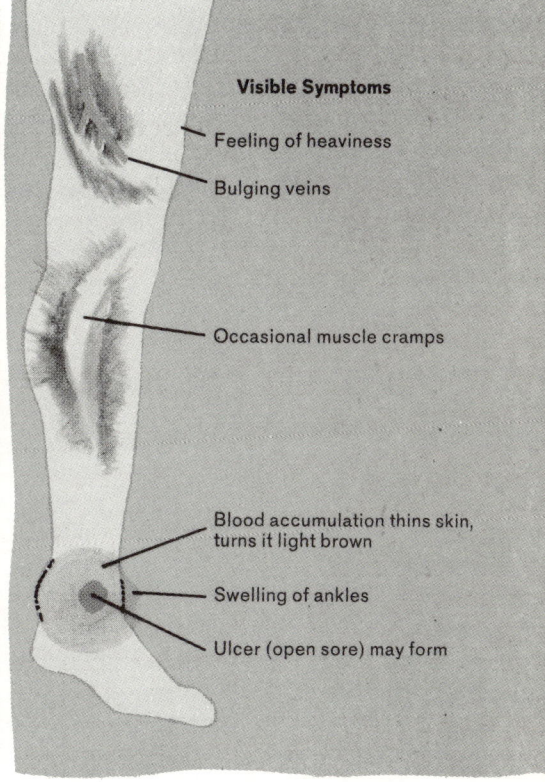

Varicose veins most commonly occur in legs. Surface veins become swollen because of inherited weakness, too much standing on job, other factors increasing pressure in veins of legs.

Deep Vein

Surface Vein

Visible Symptoms
- Feeling of heaviness
- Bulging veins
- Occasional muscle cramps
- Blood accumulation thins skin, turns it light brown
- Swelling of ankles
- Ulcer (open sore) may form

1321

open window, door, or other opening circulates throughout the rooms. If air is forced in or drawn out by a fan or similar apparatus, such as is used in air-conditioning and heating systems, it is described as *artificial ventilation*.

Good ventilation involves keeping the air free from dust, smoke, odors, and gases. Under normal circumstances, correct use of doors or windows provides a good supply of fresh air. Proper heating and provision of sufficient moisture in the air should be considered. A comfortable house temperature varies in summer from 70° to 85° F. and in winter from 68° to 70° F, with sufficient moisture in the air to produce a relative humidity of 30 to 60 per cent.

Investigations which studied the relationship between ventilation and occurrence of the *common cold* among school children revealed that colds were less frequent in naturally ventilated rooms than in those artificially ventilated. Of course, it is not possible to naturally ventilate many places, such as theaters and large office buildings; and for the person who suffers from *hay fever*, air conditioning has the advantage of keeping the air free of spores and dust.

VERMIFORM APPENDIX. *Vermiform* means *worm-shaped*, and *vermiform appendix* designates the worm-shaped tube or sac extending from the *cecum*. The vermiform appendix is commonly referred to simply as *appendix*. See also APPENDICITIS.

VERTEBRA, one of a number of small movable bones which make up the *spinal column (backbone)*. Each vertebra is an irregular bone, the parts of which are: the *body,* the neural arch through which runs the spinal cord; the *spinous process,* which is the tip that can be seen or felt by running a finger up and down the spine; and the *lateral projections* or *transverse processes,* which provide attachment points for the ligaments and muscles of the back.

The vertebrae have different functions and are described according to location. The seven *cervical vertebrae* constitute the neck; the twelve *thoracic vertebrae* form the chest region; and the five movable *lumbar vertebrae* are found in the middle of the lower back. The *sacrum* contains five vertebrae, fused together, and the *coccyx* consists of four vertebrae united as one bone at the end of the spine.

The vertebral joints have *cartilage* on their adjoining surfaces; and an *intervertebral disc,* composed also of plates of cartilage, lies between each of two movable vertebrae.

Various disorders involve the vertebrae and vertebral discs. Mechanical imperfections may affect the sacrum and the fifth lumbar vertebra. At the joining site, the nerves may become the seat of low back pain. *Spondylolisthesis,* also known as *swayback,* affects the stability of the lower spine, and a *slipped disc* or injury may affect the intervertebral disc, also causing low back pain. Fractures or protrusions may also occur in connection with intervertebral discs. *Tuberculosis of the spine* or *calcification* can implicate or even destroy the discs. *See also* DISC; SLIPPED DISC; SPINAL CORD; SPINE; SPONDYLOLISTHESIS. *See* MEDIGRAPHS pages 1211, 1221.

VERTIGO. When a person has the sensation that the outside world is revolving around him, or that he is moving in space, he has *vertigo*. There are various causes for vertigo. For example, a common type occurs when a person looks down from a height or up at a height. Other types are *epileptic vertigo* and *intestinal vertigo*. Vertigo is not the same as *dizziness* or *giddiness*, which designates a feeling of disturbed relation to the surroundings.

VINCENT'S ANGINA, variously known as *trench mouth, Borrelia,* and *ulcerative stomatitis,* an infection of the mouth and throat due to a peculiar spiral organism. It was first described in 1898 by Jean H. Vincent, a French physician, and since then the germ has been known as *Vincent's organism*. Apparently the infection is found only in man. Infants or adults who have lost their teeth are seldom affected.

In Vincent's angina, sores or ulcers occur on the lining of the cheeks and gums, sometimes also on the tonsils and in the back of the throat. The ulcers may become so large as to incapacitate the infected person. A typical unpleasant mouth odor accompanies the ailment. While the disease often begins with local symptoms, headache and a general feeling of illness may also be present. Pain in swallowing, membrane in the mouth and in the throat are characteristic. Because of this membrane, the disease was once often mistaken for *diphtheria*.

Vincent's angina is easily spread to other persons through kissing and through contaminated articles such as towels and eating utensils. Cases have been reported in which it has been spread by improperly sterilized dental instruments. An infected child should not go to school until he is cured, although isolation in the home is not necessary.

Prevention of Vincent's angina demands constant watchfulness of the condition of the mouth, teeth, and gums. Persistent bleeding of the gums, the appearance of an unpleasant odor, or occurrence of ulcers in the mouth demands consultation with a dentist or physician. Control of the infection is much easier in the early stages than later when the condition has become chronic.

Poor teeth and negligence of mouth hygiene are the prime causes of Vincent's angina. Conditions such as *scurvy, diabetes, lead* or *bismuth poisoning,* and *syphilis* may produce ulcers and damage to the mouth and gums, with Vincent's angina as a secondary condition.

The infection is treated according to the symptoms. *Crystalline penicillin* has proved beneficial, and solutions of *hydrogen peroxide* or *perborate of soda* are soothing as a mouthwash and of aid in destroying the Vincent's organism. In some instances, injections of *arsenical preparations* directly into the veins are beneficial. Care, however, is imperative, because of danger of chemical

the disease and its causes Trench mouth is an infection of the mucous membrane of the mouth and throat, caused by two types of germs working together in individuals whose resistance has been lowered. It is very common in young adults. At one time it was assumed that the disease was transferred by direct contact, such as kissing. However, since the germs are present in the mouth of most individuals much of the time, it is now believed that the disease takes hold when resistance is lowered because of poor vitamin intake, intestinal disorders, blood diseases, poor oral hygiene, associated dental problems, emotional stress, or fatigue.

symptoms The disease usually begins with soreness of the mouth, a metallic taste, pain around the teeth, and bleeding gums. There may be sore throat, headache, earache, and weakness. The breath usually has a foul odor. If the throat is involved as well as the regional lymph glands, there is usually temperature up to 102°-103°. The tongue will usually swell and become furry.

In weak and elderly patients, trench mouth may be more acute. There are high temperature and marked generalized effects. The mouth may have punched-out, grayish ulcerations around the edge, near the teeth. On pressure these will bleed readily. There may be similar ulcerations on the inside of the cheeks and on the pharynx. Because there is a grayish membrane in the mouth and throat, this disease was at one time confused with diphtheria. In cases with throat or tonsil involvement, the infection may last 10 to 14 days with persistent temperature and pain.

complications Complications are rare, since the infection tends to be mild and responds to therapy. However, neglect can result in infection at the roots of the teeth, with eventual loosening and perhaps loss of the teeth.

prevention (or lessening of impact) Trench mouth may be avoided with proper dental hygiene and the correction of any dental abnormalities that make for poor mouth conditions. Since there is a possibility of contagion, it is wise to use separate dishes and silverware for an infected patient. An infected child need not be isolated at home, but he should not go to school. And since observation suggests that lowered resistance plays a role in the onset of this disease, it is important to maintain good dental and general health.

Trench Mouth (Vincent's Angina)

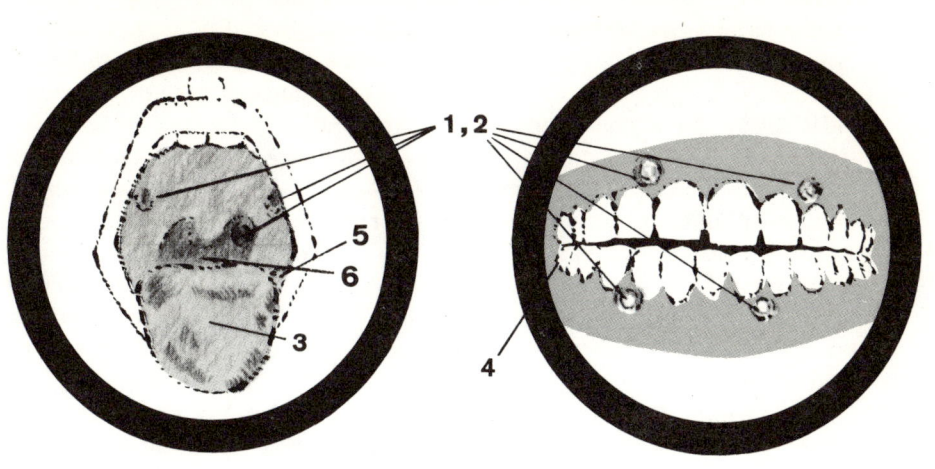

1. Sores (ulcers) appear on gums, throat, or lining of cheeks
2. Gray membrane covers sores
3. Swollen, furry tongue
4. Pain around teeth
5. Metallic taste
6. Foul breath

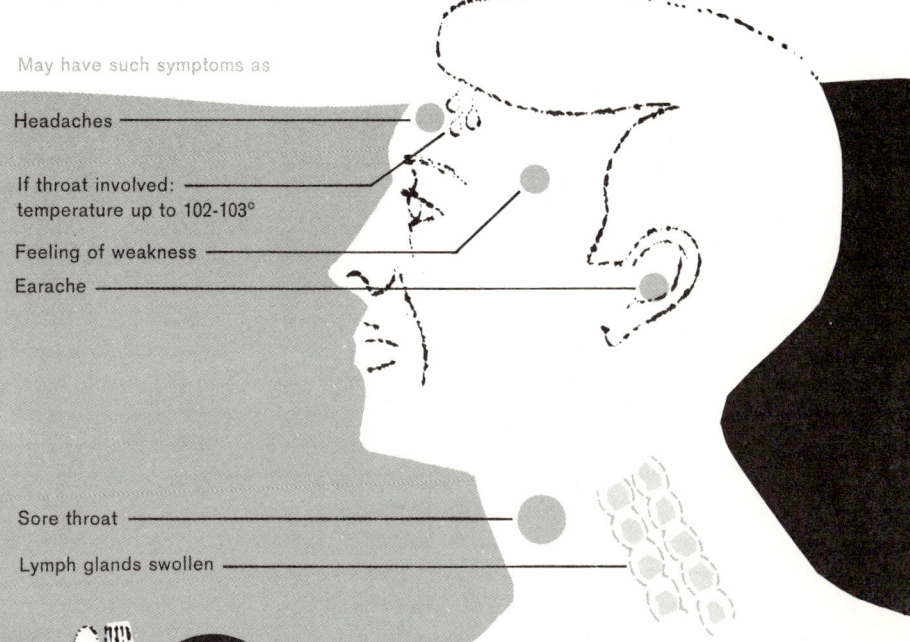

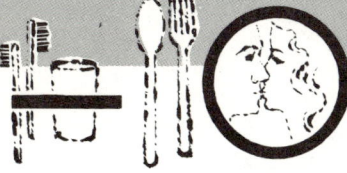

May have such symptoms as

Headaches

If throat involved: temperature up to 102-103°

Feeling of weakness

Earache

Sore throat

Lymph glands swollen

Spread by spirochete—bacillus via toilet articles, silverware, kissing, other contact with infected areas

1325

burns of the tender gums and lining of the cheeks. *See* MEDIGRAPH page 1325.

VIRUSES, the smallest and most elusive of the infectious agents, have been established as causative of more than fifty different infectious diseases of man. All forms of life may be affected by virus infection—animals, plants, birds, and insects, and even bacteria, are subject to injury and disintegration by viruses. The viruses which attack bacteria are known as *bacteriophages.*

Viruses are so infinitesimally small that they can pass through porcelain filters which hold back ordinary bacteria, though the larger viruses pass through with difficulty. Most of them can be seen only through a powerful *electron microscope.* Viruses are composed of tiny particles and differ from each other in total size, structure, and stability, from the smallest organism—responsible for *foot-and-mouth disease* and *poliomyelitis*—to the largest—which causes *parrot infection (psittacosis)* and which can be seen with an ordinary microscope to resemble the larger bacteria. The shapes vary from the spherical head and long tail of the bacteriophage to the sphere of the *influenza* virus and the cube of the *smallpox* virus.

Viruses thrive in the presence of living cells, becoming an intimate part of living body tissues which they damage, and are parasites, completely dependent for their existence upon this close intracellular association. They multiply only in young susceptible living cells and cannot be grown in artificial media unless living cells are present. This has made it difficult to study their growth habits, or to prepare vaccines for preventive treatment.

Each virus shows its specific type of action only upon certain tissues. For example, the virus of *rabies* does not become active in the body until it reaches the tissues of the nerves and brain. Different viruses which attack the human body are classified according to the part of the body for which they have an affinity. *Dermatropic viruses* affect the skin; *pneumotropic viruses* involve the lungs; *neurotropic viruses* attack nervous tissue; and *viscerotropic viruses* harm the internal organs (*viscera*). Among the more familiar diseases caused by viruses are the *common cold, measles, German measles, chickenpox, mumps, rabies, poliomyelitis, influenza, encephalitis, smallpox,* and *yellow fever.* A number of other ailments, among them the so-called *virus pneumonia, glandular fever,* and *epidemic nausea and vomiting,* have also been attributed to viral infections.

Virus diseases are conveyed in a variety of ways. The common cold, measles, smallpox, chickenpox, and influenza are probably transmitted by *direct contact,* as well as by airborne droplets of nasal and salivary secretions. Rabies is carried through the *bite* or *wound* produced by an infected animal. Mosquitoes, fleas, ticks, and other insects are *carriers,* as in yellow fever and in some of the encephalitic infections. Rarely have viral infections been spread by contaminated water or food, although transmission of *infectious hepatitis* has been traced to water, as well as milk, in some instances.

The fact that the virus becomes an intimate part of the cells of the body has made treatment of viral infections more difficult. Those substances which have thus far been found capable of destroying virus can, unfortunately, also damage body tissues and are too toxic for practical use. Some of the newer antibiotics, such as *aureomycin, terramycin,* and *chloromycetin,* have proved effective in treatment of *psittacosis* and *trachoma.* The antibiotics may have some value in treatment of *measles, chickenpox,* and *influenza,* if not directly upon the virus, at least in combatting any secondary invasion by bacteria, which often occurs in viral infections and aggravates the condition.

Until now, the most encouraging efforts to combat virus infections have been directed toward the *establishment of immunity* to viral diseases. *Immunity is the ability of living tissue to resist and overcome infection.* One way of acquiring immunity to a viral disease is to have had that infection previously. Measles, chickenpox, smallpox, and a few other viral diseases confer a lasting immunity. Immunity for flu, cold, and *herpes simplex (fever blisters)* has not yet been found.

Immunity may be produced artificially by two means. First is the introduction into the body of a *vaccine.* This substance is composed of *weakened viruses* which have been submitted to a chemical or other process and are called *attenuated viruses.* While the virus can still produce diseases in the body, this ability has been materially weakened. However, the vaccine stimulates development in the body of *antibodies,* a process known as *vaccination* or *active immunization,* and in general *it induces a high degree of immunity and tends to be lasting.*

The second means of producing an immunity is by injection of an *immune serum—gamma globulin,* or the *blood serum* of an immune animal or man. Production of immunity by this method is called *passive immunization* because the person involved does not take an active part in the development of resistance to the disease, but rather receives into his body a substance already containing the essential antibodies. *Passive immunity is temporary.*

In the search for drugs that can be used for the prevention and treatment of diseases caused by viruses, a substance called *interferon* (CIBA) has been discovered. Interferon is derived from viruses which have been inactivated with *hydroxylamine.* Such viruses not only reproduce themselves but also produce interferon in the process. Invasions of live viruses, microbial toxins, or polysaccharides induce the release of the interferon, which serves to combat their effects and effectively block viral action.

Other drugs which have been developed to combat viruses include *methisozone,* which is specific for *smallpox,* SYMMETREL® and AMANTADINE® which are used to combat the A_2 influenza virus, and the industrial dye *auriatricarboxylate,* which can block the entrance of RNA into body cells and thus prevent the proliferation of viruses. (RNA is the complex chemical substance of which viruses, like all other living cells, are constructed.)

The use of *gamma globulin* in measles, provided it is given early in the incubation period, has been successful in modifying the severity of that disease. It has also been helpful during the early stages of infectious hepatitis. In poliomyelitis, gamma globulin has been used in children in an attempt to prevent the disease or at least to avert the paralytic complications. The work of Dr. Jonas Salk and his associates has led to the historic development of a polio vaccine that furnishes active immunization—that is, the vaccine causes the body to set up its own defenses against the disease. This is the type of immunization that has overcome smallpox, diphtheria, and whooping cough. *See also* INFECTIONS; INFECTIOUS DISEASES; IMMUNITY; IMMUNIZATION; POLIOMYELITIS; VACCINATION.

VITAMINS, substances which are found in foods in minute quantities and which are indispensable to the normal functioning of the body. When they are deficient or lacking in the diet, or lost through cooking or processing, certain specific disorders, known as *deficiency diseases,* occur. About twenty vitamins are known, and deficiencies of about half of them are definitely causative of disease in human beings. The foremost vitamins are: *vitamins A, C (ascorbic acid), D, E, K, P,* and the members of the *B complex group,* including B_1 *(thiamine),* B_2 *(vitamin G or riboflavin), nicotinic acid (niacin),* B_6 *(pyridoxine), pantothenic acid, biotin, folic acid,* B_{12}*, choline, inositol* and *para-aminobenzoic acid.*

Vitamin A is manufactured in the body from *carotene,* which is found in fish liver oil, green vegetables, egg yolk, butter, and many orange- or yellow-colored foods. One of the first signs of a *vitamin A deficiency* is *night blindness*—reduced capacity of the eye to adapt to the dark. A characteristic disease of the eye, usually called *xerophthalmia,* results from this deficiency, and a thickening of the skin, *hyperkeratosis.* Splitting of the fingernails is another consequence of vitamin A deficiency.

Vitamin A deficiency usually occurs in persons who subsist largely on a starchy diet, but disturbances of the intestinal tract which prevent effective absorption of vitamin A can also be responsible as well as con-

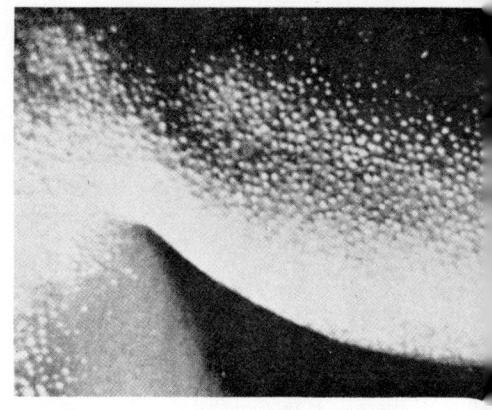

Vitamins—Deficiency of vitamin A in the body can cause the skin to become rough, dry and scaly, as shown in this closeup. Green leafy vegetables, carrots, squash, sweet potato, liver, crabmeat, and cod liver oil are excellent sources of vitamin A.

FOODS AS SOURCES OF
RIBOFLAVIN (Vitamin G)

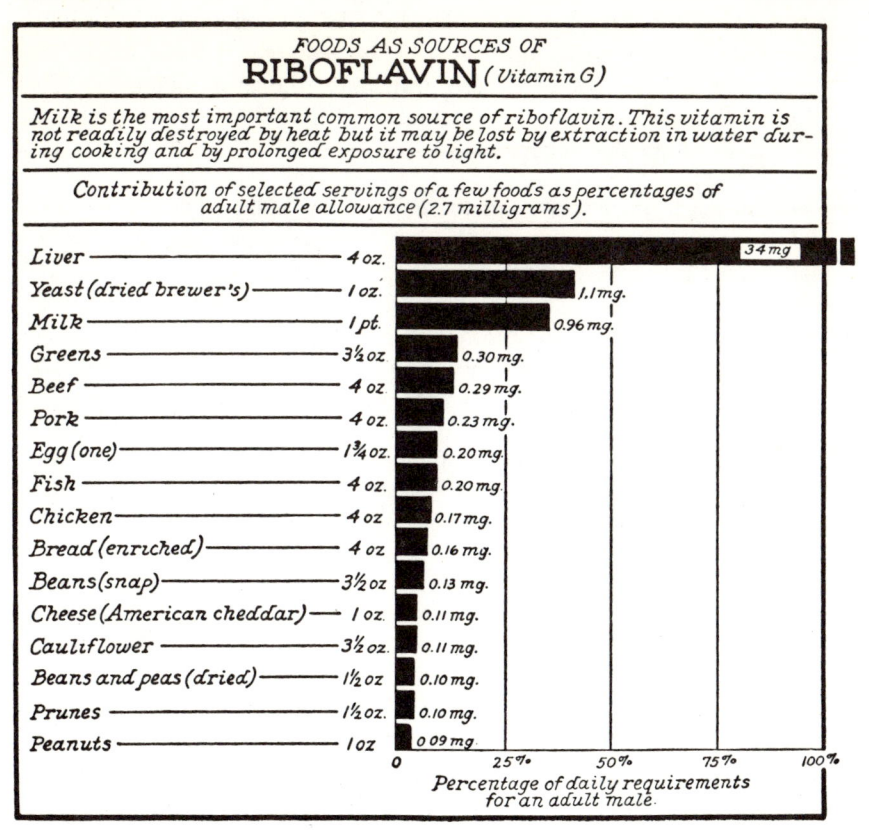

Milk is the most important common source of riboflavin. This vitamin is not readily destroyed by heat but it may be lost by extraction in water during cooking and by prolonged exposure to light.

Contribution of selected servings of a few foods as percentages of adult male allowance (2.7 milligrams).

Food	Serving	Amount
Liver	4 oz.	3.4 mg
Yeast (dried brewer's)	1 oz.	1.1 mg
Milk	1 pt.	0.96 mg
Greens	3½ oz.	0.30 mg
Beef	4 oz.	0.29 mg
Pork	4 oz.	0.23 mg
Egg (one)	1¾ oz.	0.20 mg
Fish	4 oz.	0.20 mg
Chicken	4 oz.	0.17 mg
Bread (enriched)	4 oz.	0.16 mg
Beans (snap)	3½ oz.	0.13 mg
Cheese (American cheddar)	1 oz.	0.11 mg
Cauliflower	3½ oz.	0.11 mg
Beans and peas (dried)	1½ oz.	0.10 mg
Prunes	1½ oz.	0.10 mg
Peanuts	1 oz.	0.09 mg

Percentage of daily requirements for an adult male.

ditions of pregnancy, infancy, and lactation, when the need for vitamin A increases. If a generous serving of a yellow or green leafy vegetable cannot be included in the daily diet, a teaspoon of fish liver oil instead insures an adequate supply of vitamin A.

B vitamins are found naturally in vegetables and grains, meat and milk. Each vitamin in this group has a particular function to perform in the complicated metabolism of the body. Part of these vitamins are destroyed by cooking or processing, but generous portions of vegetables and grains in the diet provide adequate amounts.

Thiamine (*vitamin B_1*) deficiencies—beriberi—result most frequently from *diets composed largely of refined or polished grain*—a diet reputed to have been formerly widespread among the laboring classes in China and other Asian countries. Acute beriberi is quite rare in the United States.

Thiamine is also useful to correct and prevent the *loss of appetite* that accompanies many forms of digestive disorder. Frequently conditions are noted in which thiamine, although taken into the body, is not properly absorbed. For example: in case of vomiting, when the person must be fed by tubes, when a paralysis of the muscles associated with swallowing

the disease and its causes Vitamin A is a fat-soluble vitamin found in large amounts in liver, eggs, cream, butter, fish liver oil, and green and yellow vegetables. When a diet does not include enough of these foods, the result is a disease which affects principally the eyes and skin. The severest changes occur in young infants, but milder forms can appear in individuals of any age or race.

symptoms The most serious effect is on the eyes of an infant. There is dryness and scaling of the cornea and the conjunctiva—which are the delicate membranes that line the eyelids and cover the eyeball. Vision is interfered with and there is extreme sensitivity to light. While adults with this disease show no positive signs when their eyes are examined, infants with severe cases develop some coloring or pigmentation of the eye membrane, and occasionally there are white spots around the cornea.

In the mild form there is night blindness or poor adaptation to the dark. The skin on the thighs, arms, and sometimes the face, thickens so that it resembles a permanent goose flesh. The hair tends to be dry and brittle. The tear ducts may waste away and dry out.

complications If the cornea is extensively involved and there is some secondary infection, blindness can result. In young infants, bronchial pneumonia is often a complication.

prevention (or lessening of impact) All that is necessary to prevent vitamin A deficiency is a diet that adequately includes the foods mentioned: liver, eggs, cream, butter, fish liver oil, and green and yellow vegetables. Supplementary doses of vitamin A can be bought commercially. For example, the simplest form is cod liver oil.

When the eyes of infants are involved, early recognition and treatment are important to prevent blindness.

Vitamin A Deficiency

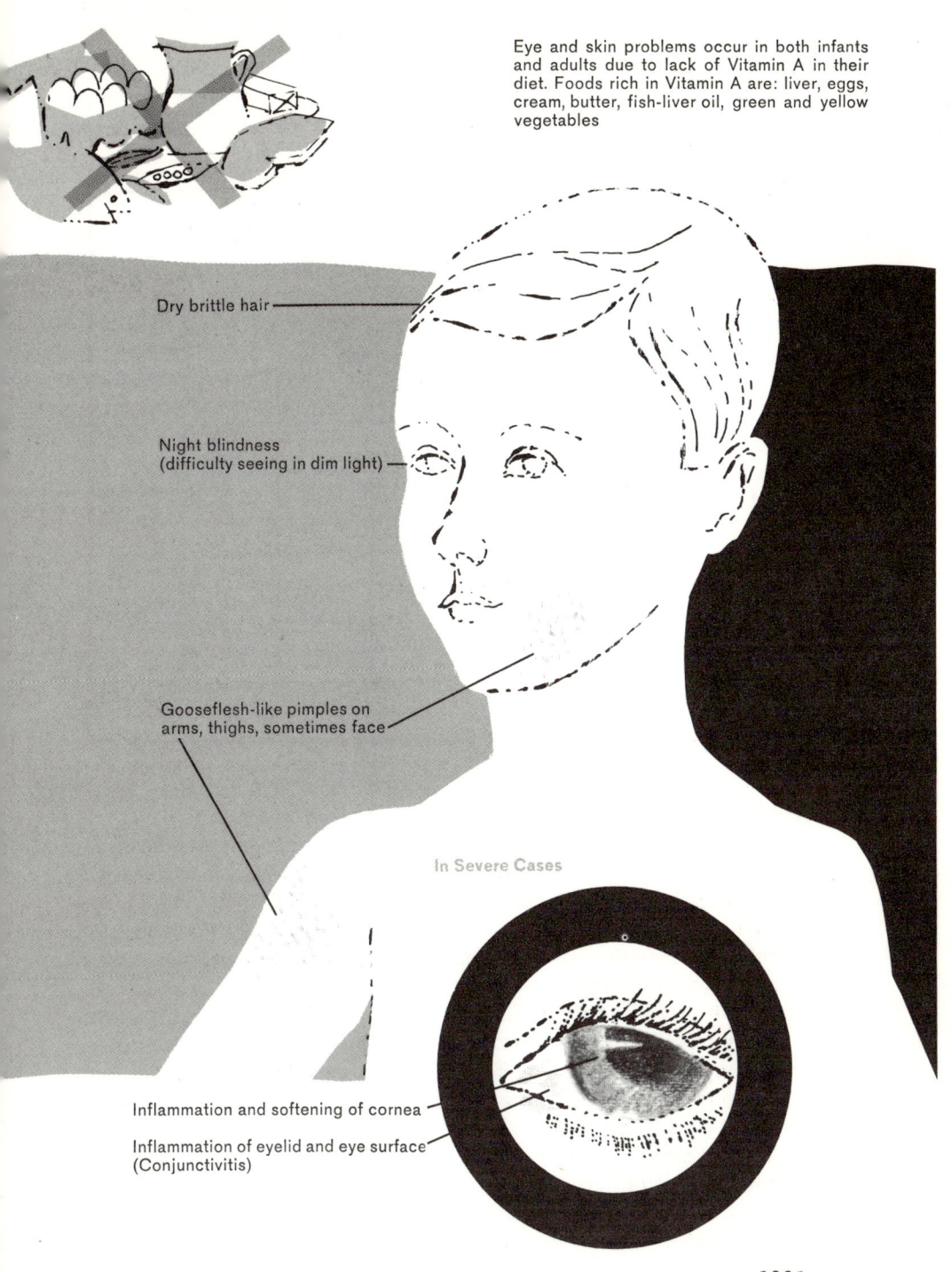

Eye and skin problems occur in both infants and adults due to lack of Vitamin A in their diet. Foods rich in Vitamin A are: liver, eggs, cream, butter, fish-liver oil, green and yellow vegetables

Dry brittle hair

Night blindness (difficulty seeing in dim light)

Gooseflesh-like pimples on arms, thighs, sometimes face

In Severe Cases

Inflammation and softening of cornea

Inflammation of eyelid and eye surface (Conjunctivitis)

FOODS AS SOURCES OF
NIACIN (Nicotinic acid)

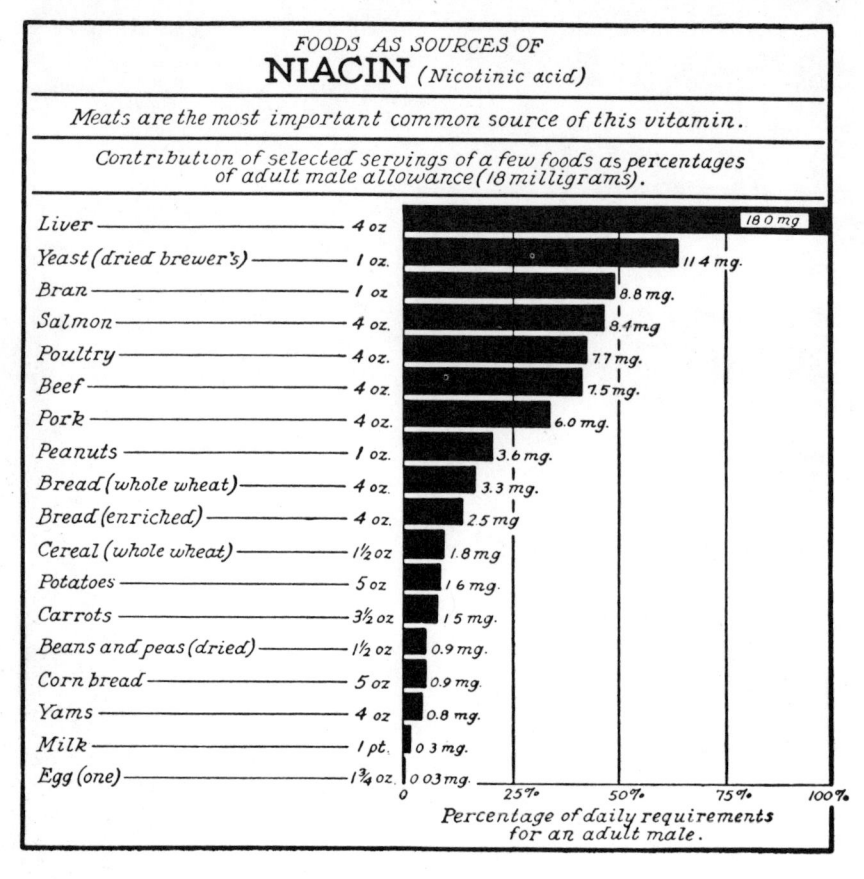

Meats are the most important common source of this vitamin.

Contribution of selected servings of a few foods as percentages of adult male allowance (18 milligrams).

Food	Serving	Amount
Liver	4 oz	18.0 mg
Yeast (dried brewer's)	1 oz	11.4 mg
Bran	1 oz	8.8 mg
Salmon	4 oz.	8.4 mg
Poultry	4 oz.	7.7 mg
Beef	4 oz.	7.5 mg
Pork	4 oz.	6.0 mg
Peanuts	1 oz.	3.6 mg
Bread (whole wheat)	4 oz.	3.3 mg
Bread (enriched)	4 oz.	2.5 mg
Cereal (whole wheat)	1½ oz	1.8 mg
Potatoes	5 oz	1.6 mg
Carrots	3½ oz	1.5 mg
Beans and peas (dried)	1½ oz	0.9 mg
Corn bread	5 oz	0.9 mg
Yams	4 oz	0.8 mg
Milk	1 pt.	0.3 mg
Egg (one)	1¾ oz.	0.03 mg

Percentage of daily requirements for an adult male.

is present, or in the case of excessive alcoholism, it may be imperative to inject extra amounts of thiamine directly into the body. Other conditions in which extra thiamine is required are excessive action of the thyroid gland, fever, or vigorous muscular activities, which use more thiamine than is ordinarily available.

Most symptoms of thiamine deficiency disappear when the vitamin in pure form in combination with other vitamins is administered. *Yeast, whole-grain cereals, liver* and *pork* are good sources of thiamine.

Vitamin B₂ (*riboflavin*) deficiencies are found most frequently among persons who live on *diets largely composed of starches.*

Symptoms of riboflavin deficiency may be *weakness* and *disturbances* of *the vision, skin, tongue, mouth, lips,* and *face.* To correct the deficiency, foods high in riboflavin, such as *liver, egg, milk* and *whole-grain cereals,* must be added to the diet. In treating acute cases, pure riboflavin alone is seldom effective, since, as in most deficiency conditions, more than a single vitamin is lacking.

An inadequate amount of *nicotinic acid (niacin)* in the diet can cause *pellagra,* which occurs in most areas of the world, and was once the major form of acute vitamin deficiency in the United States. Discovery that niacin is a specific in treatment of pellagra was a major step toward combatting this widespread deficiency. Administration of niacin helps to correct the condition and to cure the symptoms which involve the *skin, digestion,* and *nervous system.* Until the discovery that nicotinic acid could cure pellagra, two-thirds of all patients died from the condition. Today the death rate is low. In acute cases of pellagra, the vitamin is given in high-level doses. *Meat* — particularly *liver* — *whole grain cereals,* and *peanuts* are good sources of niacin.

Cobalt is a chief chemical ingredient of *vitamin B_{12},* which has a *blood-stimulating activity* similar to that of the *anti-anemic factor of liver.* It is therefore especially valuable in treating *pernicious anemia* and *sprue,* as well as anemia resulting from its deficiency. Although inadequate diets are occasionally responsible for deficiencies of *vitamin B_{12}* and *folic acid,* more often the deficiency is caused by some impairment in absorption or utilization of the vitamin in the body.

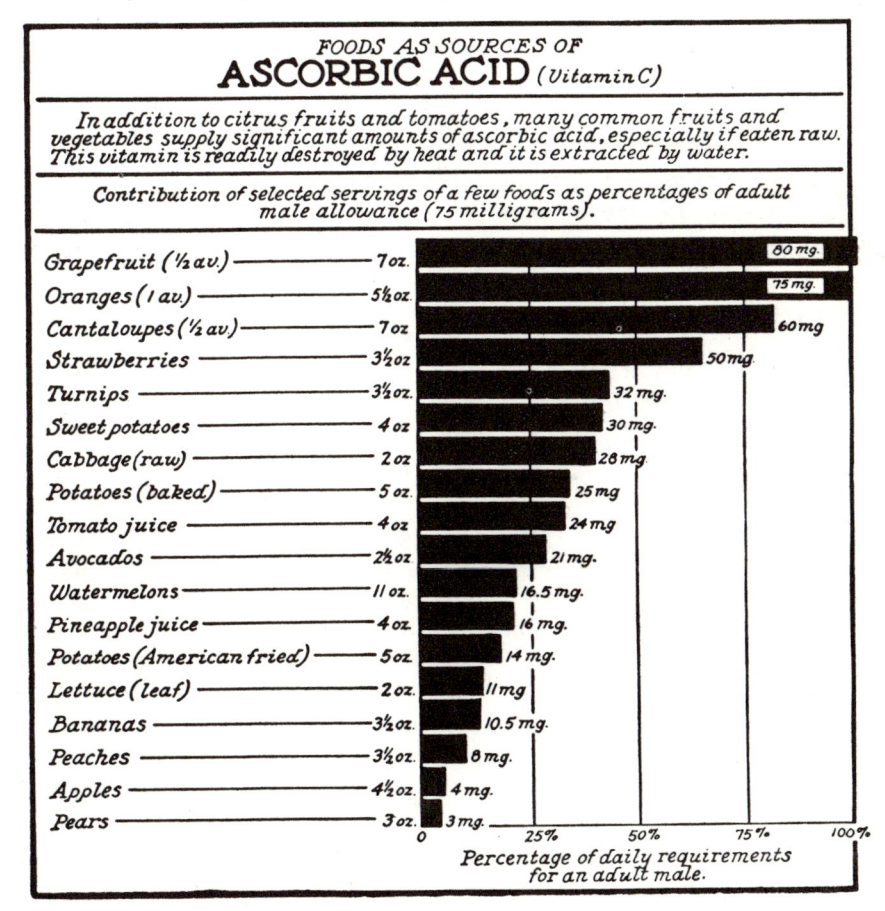

FOODS AS SOURCES OF
ASCORBIC ACID *(Vitamin C)*

In addition to citrus fruits and tomatoes, many common fruits and vegetables supply significant amounts of ascorbic acid, especially if eaten raw. This vitamin is readily destroyed by heat and it is extracted by water.

Contribution of selected servings of a few foods as percentages of adult male allowance (75 milligrams).

Food	Serving	Amount
Grapefruit (½ av.)	7 oz.	80 mg.
Oranges (1 av.)	5½ oz.	75 mg.
Cantaloupes (½ av.)	7 oz.	60 mg
Strawberries	3½ oz.	50 mg.
Turnips	3½ oz.	32 mg.
Sweet potatoes	4 oz.	30 mg.
Cabbage (raw)	2 oz.	28 mg.
Potatoes (baked)	5 oz.	25 mg
Tomato juice	4 oz.	24 mg
Avocados	2½ oz.	21 mg.
Watermelons	11 oz.	16.5 mg.
Pineapple juice	4 oz.	16 mg.
Potatoes (American fried)	5 oz.	14 mg.
Lettuce (leaf)	2 oz.	11 mg
Bananas	3½ oz.	10.5 mg.
Peaches	3½ oz.	8 mg.
Apples	4½ oz.	4 mg.
Pears	3 oz.	3 mg.

Percentage of daily requirements for an adult male.

FOODS AS SOURCES OF
CALCIUM

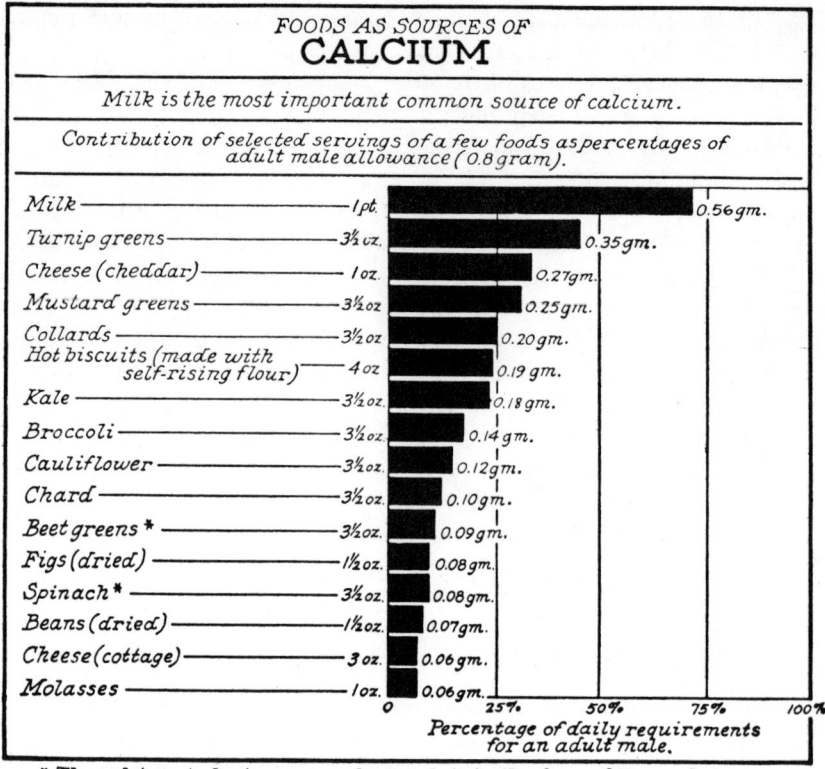

Milk is the most important common source of calcium.

Contribution of selected servings of a few foods as percentages of adult male allowance (0.8 gram).

Food	Serving	Amount
Milk	1 pt.	0.56 gm.
Turnip greens	3½ oz.	0.35 gm.
Cheese (cheddar)	1 oz.	0.27 gm.
Mustard greens	3½ oz.	0.25 gm.
Collards	3½ oz.	0.20 gm.
Hot biscuits (made with self-rising flour)	4 oz.	0.19 gm.
Kale	3½ oz.	0.18 gm.
Broccoli	3½ oz.	0.14 gm.
Cauliflower	3½ oz.	0.12 gm.
Chard	3½ oz.	0.10 gm.
Beet greens *	3½ oz.	0.09 gm.
Figs (dried)	1½ oz.	0.08 gm.
Spinach *	3½ oz.	0.08 gm.
Beans (dried)	1½ oz.	0.07 gm.
Cheese (cottage)	3 oz.	0.06 gm.
Molasses	1 oz.	0.06 gm.

Percentage of daily requirements for an adult male.

* The calcium in beet greens and spinach is in the form of the oxalate which is not assimilated by the body.

Other vitamins of the B complex group are *vitamin B₆, pantothenic acid, biotin, choline, inositol,* and *para-aminobenzoic acid.* A deficiency of vitamin B_6 can cause *neuritis, skin eruptions, excessive oiliness of the skin,* and *sore tongue, nervousness* and *depression.* It is widely employed in the treatment of nausea and vomiting in pregnant women.

Ascorbic acid (*vitamin C*), the *anti-scurvy vitamin,* is found abundantly in *citrus fruits* and *juices, tomatoes, potatoes,* and *leafy vegetables.* This vitamin is responsible for the manufacture by the body of the material which cements teeth into position. An infant with a *vitamin C deficiency* is likely to suffer from *fever, diarrhea, loss of weight, vomiting,* and have a generally *low resistance* and probably *intestinal bleeding.* In children, the bones may be malformed. Most of the symptoms of the deficiency disappear rapidly when the vitamin is administered. All fresh fruits and vegetables contain some vitamin C and to prevent recurrence of the deficiency the diet must include these foods.

Vitamin D (*ergosterol*) is manufactured in the body from a combination of chemically related substances,

VITAMINS

and is essential for the *formation and growth of bones and teeth* and for the *utilization of calcium and phosphorus* in the body. It is often called the sunshine vitamin because of the abundance supplied by the ultraviolet rays of the sun through their chemical action on the skin, and the person who gets enough sunshine each day receives sufficient amounts of vitamin D. *(See discussion at* PIGMENTATION.*)*

Vitamin D deficiency causes *rickets* in children, and in adults it results in *improper utilization of calcium* in the bones and produces a condition known as *osteomalacia.* These disorders can be corrected by adequate amounts of calcium and vitamin D. *Cod liver oil, vitamin D concentrates,* and *sunshine* or *ultraviolet irradiation* are effective in promoting a rapid improvement in rickets. Other good sources of vitamin D are *eggs, salmon, tuna fish, milk* and *butter.*

Vitamin E is found abundantly in *wheat germ oil,* and in adequate amounts in *liver, eggs, whole-grain cereals,* and *lettuce.* Experiments with animals have indicated that a deficiency of vitamin E may be associated with *sterility* and *miscarriages;*

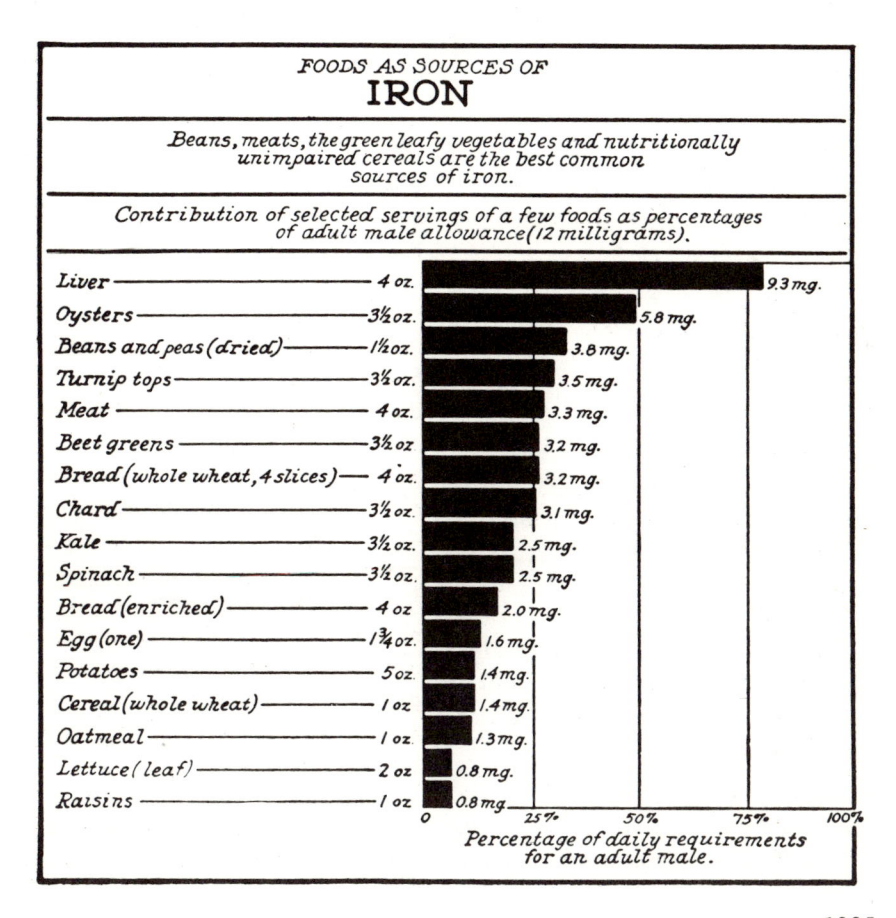

FOODS AS SOURCES OF
IRON

Beans, meats, the green leafy vegetables and nutritionally unimpaired cereals are the best common sources of iron.

Contribution of selected servings of a few foods as percentages of adult male allowance (12 milligrams).

Food	Serving	Amount
Liver	4 oz.	9.3 mg.
Oysters	3½ oz.	5.8 mg.
Beans and peas (dried)	1½ oz.	3.8 mg.
Turnip tops	3½ oz.	3.5 mg.
Meat	4 oz.	3.3 mg.
Beet greens	3½ oz.	3.2 mg.
Bread (whole wheat, 4 slices)	4 oz.	3.2 mg.
Chard	3½ oz.	3.1 mg.
Kale	3½ oz.	2.5 mg.
Spinach	3½ oz.	2.5 mg.
Bread (enriched)	4 oz	2.0 mg.
Egg (one)	1¾ oz.	1.6 mg.
Potatoes	5 oz.	1.4 mg.
Cereal (whole wheat)	1 oz	1.4 mg.
Oatmeal	1 oz.	1.3 mg.
Lettuce (leaf)	2 oz	0.8 mg.
Raisins	1 oz	0.8 mg.

Percentage of daily requirements for an adult male.

FOODS AS SOURCES OF
PROTEIN

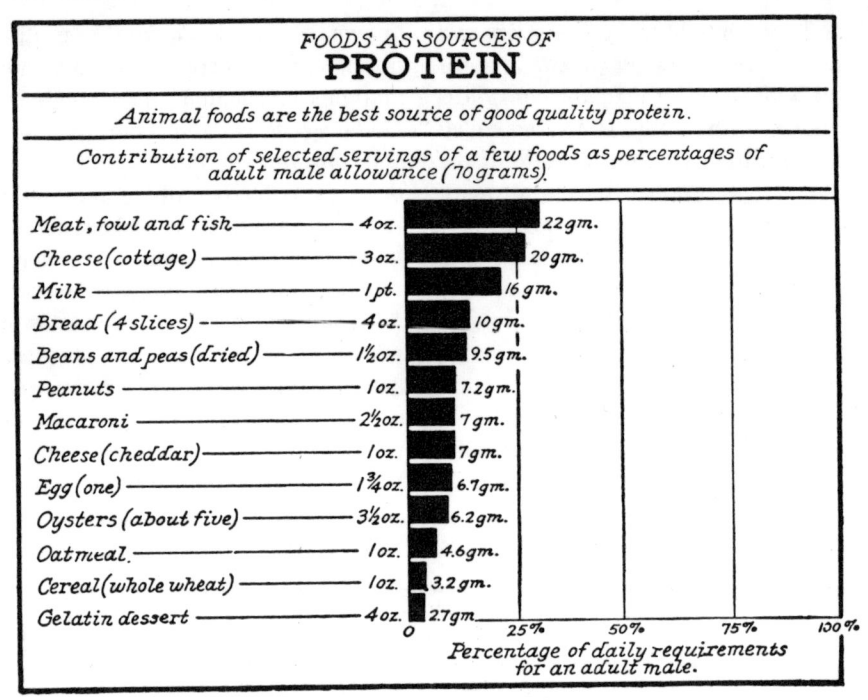

Animal foods are the best source of good quality protein.

Contribution of selected servings of a few foods as percentages of adult male allowance (70 grams).

Food	Serving	Amount
Meat, fowl and fish	4 oz.	22 gm.
Cheese (cottage)	3 oz.	20 gm.
Milk	1 pt.	16 gm.
Bread (4 slices)	4 oz.	10 gm.
Beans and peas (dried)	1½ oz.	9.5 gm.
Peanuts	1 oz.	7.2 gm.
Macaroni	2½ oz.	7 gm.
Cheese (cheddar)	1 oz.	7 gm.
Egg (one)	1¾ oz.	6.7 gm.
Oysters (about five)	3½ oz.	6.2 gm.
Oatmeal	1 oz.	4.6 gm.
Cereal (whole wheat)	1 oz.	3.2 gm.
Gelatin dessert	4 oz.	2.7 gm.

Percentage of daily requirements for an adult male.

however, it has not been determined whether or not vitamin E deficiencies occur in human beings.

Vitamin K has significant *antihemorrhagic properties*, and deficiencies of it usually involve the clotting of blood. It is useful in treating *obstructive jaundice, hemorrhage* which results in certain intestinal disorders, and in hemorrhagic conditions affecting newborn infants. In treating *coronary thrombosis*, vitamin K together with the drug *dicumarol* is also of value, since dicumarol affects the action of vitamin K and consequently the *clotting of blood*. *Green vegetables* are rich in this vitamin.

Also known as *hesperedin*, vitamin P is found in the *rind of citrus fruits*. Whether a deficiency of vitamin P can exist has not yet been determined. The vitamin has been used *in connection with vitamin C in cases of abnormal bleeding.*

The significance of vitamins cannot be overemphasized, and certain basic foods should appear in the diet each day, notably *milk or milk products such as butter, cheese or yogurt, meat, green leafy vegetables, citrus fruits,* and *whole-grain products.* If the diet furnishes adequate quantities of vitamins, vitamin supplements are not necessary for the average person. A doctor should be consulted if any deficiency exists. *See also* NUTRITION; PROTEIN; AMINO ACIDS. *See* MEDIGRAPHS pages 195, 1019, 1149, 1167, 1331.

VITILIGO, a pigmentary disorder in which the coloring matter disappears in spots from the skin. These spots then appear white, in contrast to the normal coloring of the rest of the skin. Sometimes this condition is an indirect result of another disease of the skin, but usually it occurs without apparent cause.

Vitiligo usually occurs in individuals of African origin. While not generally considered dangerous, it is often badly disfiguring. This disease sometimes disappears spontaneously.

In about 15 per cent of the cases of vitiligo, *repigmentation* can be induced by a drug derived from an Egyptian plant called *Ammi majus,* together with treatment by exposure to *sunlight* or *artificial ultraviolet rays.* This must be prescribed by a physician. Persons who have been so treated have relatively small areas of depigmentation when the spots have been present less than five years.

If 80 per cent of the skin surface is depigmented, it is often practical to extend the condition to the entire body by treating the skin with a special compound. The hair and eyes are not affected as in *albinism. See also* SKIN; PIGMENTATION; MELANOSIS.

VOCAL CORDS. *See* LARYNGITIS; LARYNX.

VOICE BOX. *See* LARYNX.

VOMITING, the forceful ejection of the contents of the stomach through the mouth. The possible causes are innumerable. Vomiting by a person who is seasick is probably caused by a disturbance in the organs of balance. Vomiting may be set off by a severe pain, such as a sharp blow to the abdomen. Psychological factors related to the senses may also produce vomiting, such as an unpleasant smell, a displeasing sight, or even an unkind remark.

When vomiting is imminent, certain nerves are stimulated and a valve—called the *pylorus* or *pyloric sphincter*—in the lower part of the stomach, customarily employed to pass food to the bowels, is then automatically closed. Following this, a chain of waves passes through the wall of the stomach, moving not downward as usual but upward. The person inhales deeply and the climax is a powerful contraction of both the *diaphragm* and stomach. Whatever happens to be in the stomach is then thrown through the *esophagus* and out of the *mouth.* Vomiting may happen so suddenly that some of the material emerges through the *nose.*

While vomiting is not a disease, it is often a symptom of illness. If vomiting persists, or the matter ejected has traces of blood, a doctor should be consulted to locate and treat the cause.

VULVA, the external sexual organs of the female. The vulva consists of the *mons pubis, labia majora, labia minora, clitoris, vaginal opening, urethral meatus, Skene's glands, Bartholin's glands,* and (in virgins) the *hymen.*

The *mons pubis* is the term given to the triangular mound of fatty tissue covering the pubic bone between the groins. It is also called the *mons veneris* (mount of Venus). It is covered with hair in adult women. In back, it merges with the *perineum*.

The *labia majora* (major lips) lie within the *mons pubis* and consist of folds of tissue surrounding the *vaginal* and *urethral orifices* and the *clitoris*. The *labia majora* normally conceal these inner vulval organs.

The *labia minora* (minor lips) consist of folds of tissue surrounding the *vestibule* on which the vaginal and urethral orifices are situated. The *clitoris,* which lies at the apex of the vestibule, is a small organ of erectile tissue homologous to the penis in the male. Under sexual excitement, it becomes engorged with blood and highly responsive to stimulation. (In *masturbation,* it is manipulated until the production of a sexual climax or *clitoral orgasm*. A total orgasm, however, can only be induced in the inner recesses of the *vagina,* normally by the intromission of the penis.)

Skene's glands, which open just below the clitoris, secrete alkaline substances which neutralize any vestiges of urine remaining in the vestibule during sexual intercourse and thus protect the spermatozoa, which are highly vulnerable to damage from the acid urine. These secretions also reduce the acidity of the vagina. *Bartholin's glands* are located near the vaginal orifice and secrete a mucous substance which lubricates the vagina during sexual intercourse, facilitating the intromission of the penis.

The *hymen* is a thin membrane of skin covering the vaginal orifice in young girls. It gradually becomes perforated during adolescence, particularly if masturbation occurs. It disappears altogether in adult women after repeated sexual intercourse.

Inflammation of the vulva (*vulvitis*) may result from infection, but often is associated with various skin disorders. In children and in obese women, acute vulvitis results from uncleanliness and from constant irritation. It is characterized by redness, swelling, burning, irritation, and sometimes by itching which may spread to the surrounding areas. The treatment depends on the cause.

In *leukoplakia,* white thickened areas of the skin are found, usually in the region of the clitoris, labia, or perineum. This condition may also be accompanied by itching. Proper medication is needed promptly to cure these conditions.

In the rare cases of *cancer of the vulva,* leukoplakia is often the forerunner. Early diagnosis is essential for a successful treatment by x-ray, radium, surgery, or combinations of these methods. *See also* REPRODUCTION SYSTEM; VAGINA; HYMEN; PERINEUM; URETHRA; CLITORIS; MASTURBATION; ORGASM; SEXUAL INTERCOURSE; PENIS.

W

WARTS, small, usually hard growths on the skin. Warts seldom produce any symptoms except when they are on the soles of the feet, in which case they may become painful. It has been found that when warts are picked, the blood or material from the wart may spread over the skin, causing the appearance of new warts by *autoinoculation*.

There are many different methods used to treat warts including injections of *bismuth* directly into the wart, destruction of the warts by strong *chemicals,* freezing with *carbon dioxide snow,* electric dessication of the wart, and *surgical removal* if the warts are large or multiple in any one spot. *Radium* and *x-ray treatment* are also used, especially when there are many warts around the fingernails. When warts appear on the scalp, it is customary to soften them first with various acids and then to remove them by electric needle or by freezing with carbon dioxide snow. These methods or materials should not be used except by those trained in the technique.

Warts on the soles of the feet tend to resist treatment strongly. Surgery is often the best method to remove them. After the horny material has been cut away, *caustics* are used on the base of the wart to prevent regrowth. In these cases x-ray is frequently used as additional treatment to destroy the wart-bearing area and to prevent the growth of new warts. Although warts have been known to disappear spontaneously in many cases, it is not recommended that a person postpone medical treatment in the hope that this will happen.

In addition to the common wart, there are similar growths associated with venereal infections. These are called *venereal warts*. They develop around places where the mucous membranes join the skin. They are usually aggregate collections of overgrowths like warts. Because of irritation, friction, heat, moisture, and a large supply of blood they grow luxuriantly and spread rapidly. Such warts demand special, prompt treatment to prevent their spreading over other areas.

the disease and its causes Warts are elevations of the skin that can occur on any part of the body but occur most often on the fingers, face, and soles of the feet. They are caused by a virus and are moderately contagious, spreading from one area to another in the same person, or to several members of one family. They are extremely common in children. It is hard to say how long warts will last. Their response to medication is uncertain and, in fact, it is reported that cases of warts have been cured by suggestion or hypnosis! Often they disappear without any treatment at all.

symptoms They appear at first as rather flat masses about the size of a pinhead. Rapidly they develop into raised, hard, rough-surfaced, horny bumps, usually grayish brown in color. It is not unusual to find a central large wart surrounded by a ring of small ones. There may be some local tenderness, but as a rule there is no real pain.

When warts occur on the feet (plantar warts) they are not usually raised because the constant pressure of walking flattens them and drives them under the skin. Because of this pressure, however, they can be quite painful and make walking difficult.

complications There are no serious complications, and there is no relationship between warts and cancer. When they occur on the feet and attempts are made to root them out surgically, the healing can be slow and the patient can be somewhat handicapped during the healing process.

prevention (or lessening of impact) There is no way to prevent warts from developing, nor is there a sure way to evaluate how effective treatment is. Plantar warts which are painful and disable the patient are treated by a variety of medical and surgical techniques. One method—where the doctor paints the affected area with acid as long as the wart is visible—is credited with some success without being painful to the patient.

Warts

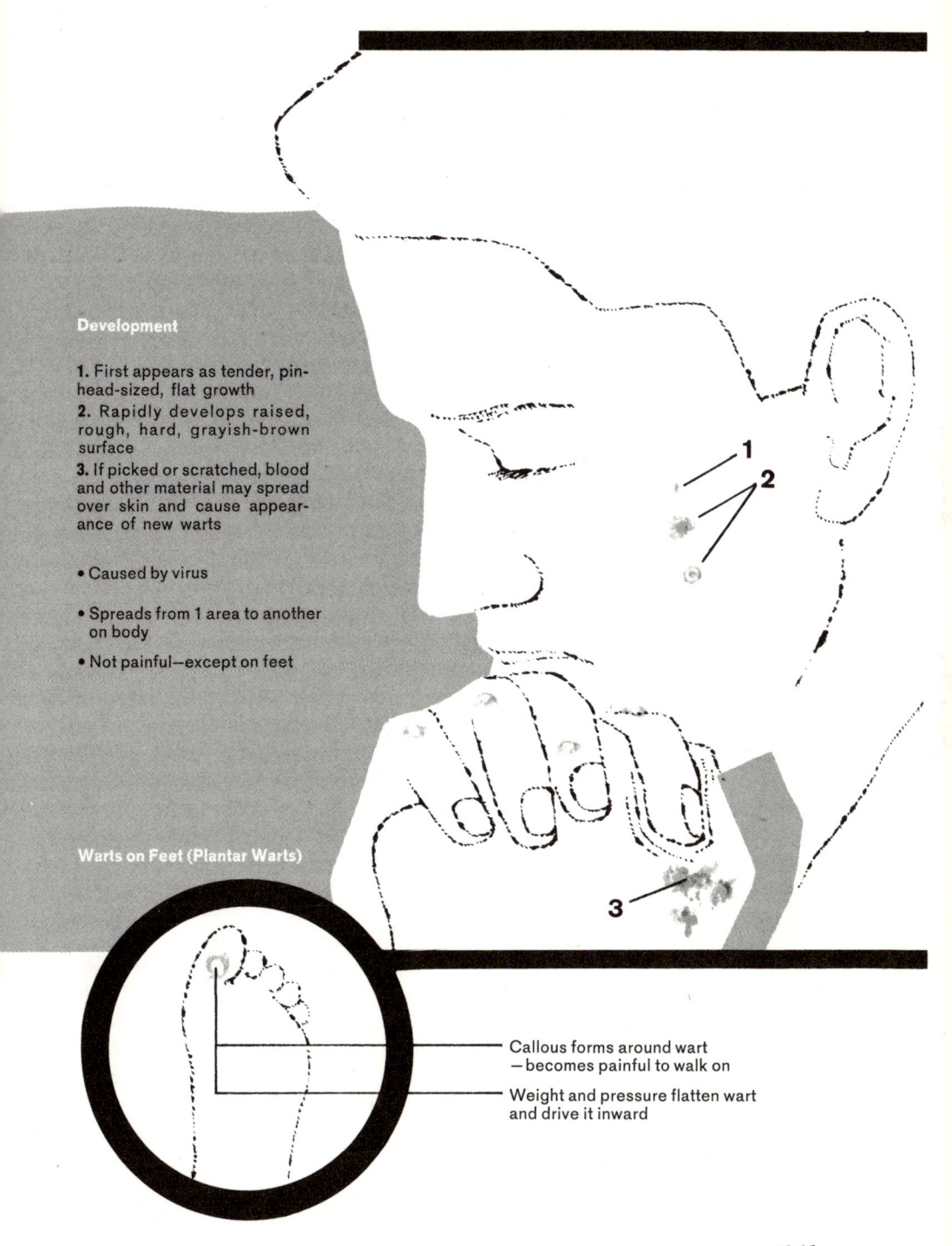

Development

1. First appears as tender, pinhead-sized, flat growth
2. Rapidly develops raised, rough, hard, grayish-brown surface
3. If picked or scratched, blood and other material may spread over skin and cause appearance of new warts

- Caused by virus

- Spreads from 1 area to another on body

- Not painful—except on feet

Warts on Feet (Plantar Warts)

— Callous forms around wart — becomes painful to walk on

— Weight and pressure flatten wart and drive it inward

1341

Old people have a special form of wart known as *senile wart*. These also demand prompt attention because continued irritation may cause them to develop a malignant growth that is characteristic of *cancer*. It is best in such instances to have each wart removed as it develops and to have a careful study made of the tissues under the microscope to make certain that cancerous changes have not occurred. Such warts develop most often on the body rather than on the hands or the exposed skin. As far as is known, this type of wart never disappears spontaneously. See also WEN; CYST; FURUNCLES; CARBUNCLES. See MEDIGRAPH page 1341.

WASSERMANN TEST, a test used to determine whether or not a person has *syphilis*. Only a modification of the original test is now used. The test was named after the German physician August von Wassermann. Various modifications, such as the *Kahn test,* the *Eagle test,* and the *Hinton test,* are also used.

In the test, the blood serum and sometimes the cerebrospinal fluid are examined. A positive reaction indicates the presence of syphilis. Tests are also made at frequent intervals during the course of the disease, to determine its progress and the effectiveness of treatment. *See also* KAHN TEST; TESTS.

WATER, the chemical combination of *hydrogen* and *oxygen,* H_2O. Two-thirds of the weight of the body is water and about 75 per cent of the *protoplasm*—the material surrounding the nuclei of the cells—is composed of water. Water is essential to life and is found in large proportion in most foods. In the body, water transports food elements to the cells. It is removed from the body as waste by the action of the kidneys and the urinary system, the sweat glands, the lungs, and the bowels.

Insufficient production of certain types of hormones in the glands results in a disturbance of the distribution of water and salt in the body. This disturbance is reflected by an excessive loss of water in the urine, a condition known as *diuresis,* which results in *dehydration* of the body.

Water may be a carrier of disease-producing bacteria, notably bacteria causing *typhoid, cholera,* and *dysentery*. When a dependable municipal water supply does not exist, the individual must insure the purity of his own water. Boiling the water to destroy disease-producing organisms is often the simplest method. Aeration and filtering with charcoal help to remove undesirable tastes and odors. Chlorine tablets can be dissolved in water to purify it, and home filter systems that utilize sand beds several feet thick through which the water passes are also effective.

Spring water should be used only after the spring has been cleaned and the water tested for bacteria. Shallow wells must be walled and a good pumping system installed. Deep well water is generally pure but its source and purity must be tested and expert advice on sanitation sought. Cisterns should be screened against mosquitoes and the water boiled or purified in some way before it is used. Proper sewage disposal is always necessary to safeguard the purity of any water supply system, whether public or private. See also FLUORIDATION.

WEIGHT, FACTORS WHICH INFLUENCE. Neither *body build* (physique, or body shape) nor *body size* (body surface area), taken by itself, is a good indication of the appropriateness of a person's weight. Individuals of many different shapes may be the same size, that is, have the same *body surface area*. The tall thin man and the short chubby woman may be peers in this respect; yet the weight of neither one may be desirable. Conversely, individuals of assorted sizes may resemble one another in *body build* or *shape*. A six-sided solid block is a cube, whether it be a dice or a cornerstone. During the growth period the healthy child shows a tendency to preserve the same physique, or shape, through the changes in size which occur at successive ages. However, among adults, it is seldom that we see miniature or greatly enlarged replicas of various body types. It is only when we relate body build to body size that we can get a useful conception of the suitability of a person's weight with respect to health and good looks.

Influence of framework on height and build. Body build is largely a matter of bony structure. We are as tall and as broad as our skeletons. The skeletal pattern is set by heredity and roughed in by the forces which bring the body to maturity. The dimensions of the long bones and the spinal column, which largely determine *height*, are little susceptible to fluctuations in dietary fortune (except in cases of marked *calcium* and *vitamin D deficiency*) but are greatly susceptible to fluctuations during the growth period in the amounts of certain *hormones* secreted, particularly those of the *anterior portion of the pituitary gland*. Upon reaching maturity the skeleton stops growing. Hence height and the contributions made to weight by the skeleton become stable features of the human body.

The trunk with its powerful bone structure and tightly packed visceral contents contributes more to weight than do the head and limbs. Hence a person with a long and roomy trunk, with broad shoulders, and wide pelvis would be classified as having a heavy frame irrespective of total height. And the individual with a medium or short trunk would be classified as medium or slight in build, depending upon the ruggedness or delicacy of his skeleton.

Unlike *height*, which is a stable feature of the mature body, *weight* is a variable feature. This is true because total weight, which is a measure of mass, is made up partly of the weight of soft tissues, and the substantial proportion of body weight contributed by these tissues can be added to or reduced according to our living habits and circumstances.

Influence of musculature on weight. The type of skeletal build with which a person is endowed appears to be related in some measure to the amount of muscular tissue allotted for the operation and support of his bones. A person with a large bony framework requires large muscles for its operation, while a lighter framework requires smaller muscles. Also a big frame is well equipped structurally speaking to carry a relatively large amount of muscular tissue, whereas the slight frame is built for smaller loads.

In general, *muscle tissue* makes up about 40 per cent of body weight. In the adult, degree of activity probably has the biggest influence on muscular development. Given the raw materials (food elements) required, each tissue tends to produce more like itself when it is actively engaged in doing its proper work. Hence the extent to which a person uses his muscles in work and play will have a great deal to do with the comparative heaviness or lightness and the comparative strength or weakness of his musculature.

How much the bulkiness or flabbiness of one's muscles ought to be taken into consideration as a factor influencing desirable weight for health is a debatable question. Nevertheless, insurance studies have shown that the solidly built large-boned overweights do have better longevity records than the flabby overweights.

Exercise, while it enlarges and toughens muscles and improves nerve-muscle tone and posture, cannot make up for a lack of the food materials required for muscle building, nor can the increased energy output occasioned by exercise adequately counterbalance the excessive storage of fat resulting from overeating. For example, a man weighing 300 pounds who walked a mile on level ground would use up only about the amount of extra energy contained in a piece of chocolate fudge.

The influence of body fat on weight. The least stable factor affecting body weight is *fat*. Hence it is by far the most controllable factor. So firmly entrenched in the popular mind is the idea that excess fat is chiefly to blame for overweight that the terms *fatness—obesity—*and *overweight* are practically synonymous. And obesity is closely associated, even etymologically, with overeating; the word *obese* comes from the Latin *obesus* (the past participle of the verb *obedere,* to devour), which literally means *having eaten itself fat.*

In the average well-nourished person fat makes up from 10 to 15 per cent of the body weight. It has a more or less passive but none the less important role. It is found in every cell, tissue, and organ of the body, but in certain regions great numbers of specific fat-containing cells are normally packed closely together to form the storehouses of fat, or fat depots, of the body. The largest internal fat depots are located in the abdominal cavity, around joints, and between muscles. Most of the fat under the skin (*subcutaneous fat*) is found in the abdominal wall, in the lower part of the back, and in the buttocks. However, fat is normally present with few exceptions in all other subcutaneous regions.

The relative fullness or emptiness of the fat depots is a matter of great concern in body economy. Fat is stored in them because the body sets aside a store of fuel food to be used in time of hunger so that it will not perish through hunger.

The contents of the *fat depots* may be compared to goods placed in dead storage. They consist of *fat droplets* produced from the fuel food (chiefly *fats* and *carbohydrates*) remaining over and above the amount required by the body for immediate use and for live storage in the liver and muscles.

The fat held in storage primarily to take care of possible shortages in the body's fuel supply serves many other useful purposes in the body. The internal fat depots form soft elastic shock absorbers between various organs, and the fat deposits beneath the skin help to regulate body temperature, cushion blows, and round out body contours. The chubbiness of some children and the streamlined curves of youth owe their existence, in part at least, to the paddings of fat below the surface of the elastic skin. And the thinning out of these paddings is usually responsible for the baggy wrinkled skin seen in many old persons and in persons who have lost a great deal of fat quickly as a result of illness or of too drastic a reducing diet. *See also* WEIGHT, NORMAL FOR HEALTH; UNDERWEIGHT, HAZARDS OF; OBESITY; DIET, REDUCING.

WEIGHT, NORMAL FOR HEALTH. This question can be answered only for the individual and even then only when the answers to several other questions are known. For example: How tall are you? Is your framework, small, medium, or large? How long is your trunk in relation to the length of your appendages? Has your weight pendulum tended to swing back and forth within rather narrow limits after attaining maturity? Or are you a great deal heavier—or lighter—than you were at twenty-five? For a person younger than twenty-five the question, "How old are you?" would also have to be answered, because physical growth obviously is accompanied by increase in size. Terminal stature is reached in the average girl at about age sixteen and in the average boy at about age seventeen, but there are many individual variations. To allow for these variations and also to give the structural pattern of the body time to settle, so to speak, twenty-five is the age generally accepted as marking the arrival of full-blown physical maturity.

Height-weight-age tables. In tables showing average weights for height of men and women cognizance is taken of the age factor. In constructing such tables the *average—mean —weight* for height at various ages of very large numbers of individuals is computed, and the average weight for a particular height and age is then set up as the standard of comparison for any individual of that height and age.

On the next page are shown *simplified tables of optimum weight averages*. A person is considered over- or underweight if he varies more than 15 per cent from these averages. There have been numerous medico-actuarial studies of hundreds of thousands of insured men and women which conclusively prove that

IDEAL WEIGHTS FOR MEN. AGES TWENTY-FIVE AND OVER

These tables are based on numerous medico-actuarial studies of hundreds of thousands of insured men and women. Weight in Pounds According to Frame (as ordinarily dressed)

Height (with shoes on)

Feet	Inches	Small Frame	Medium Frame	Large Frame
5	2	116-125	124-133	131-142
5	3	119-128	127-136	133-144
5	4	122-132	130-140	137-149
5	5	126-136	134-144	141-153
5	6	129-139	137-147	145-157
5	7	133-143	141-151	149-162
5	8	136-147	145-156	153-166
5	9	140-151	149-160	157-170
5	10	144-155	153-164	161-175
5	11	148-159	157-168	165-180
6	0	152-164	161-173	169-185
6	1	157-169	166-178	174-190
6	2	163-175	171-184	179-196
6	3	168-180	176-189	184-202

Weights for men in the age group eighteen to twenty-five can be estimated by subtracting one pound for each year under twenty-five from the limits at each height. Examples:

Age	Feet	Inches	Small Frame	Medium Frame	Large Frame
18	5	2	109-118	117-126	124-135
	5	10	137-148	146-157	154-168
19	5	2	110-119	118-127	125-136
	5	10	138-149	147-158	155-169

IDEAL WEIGHTS FOR WOMEN. AGES TWENTY-FIVE AND OVER

Height (with shoes on)

Feet	Inches	Small Frame	Medium Frame	Large Frame
4	11	104-111	110-118	117-127
5	0	105-113	112-120	119-129
5	1	107-115	114-122	121-131
5	2	110-118	117-125	124-135
5	3	113-121	120-128	127-138
5	4	116-125	124-132	131-142
5	5	119-128	127-135	133-145
5	6	123-132	130-140	138-150
5	7	126-136	134-144	142-154
5	8	129-139	137-147	145-158
5	9	133-143	141-151	149-162
5	10	136-147	145-155	152-166
5	11	139-150	148-158	155-169

Weights for women in the age group eighteen to twenty-five can be estimated by subtracting one pound for each year under twenty-five from the limits at each height. Examples

Age	Feet	Inches	Small Frame	Medium Frame	Large Frame
18	4	11	97-104	103-111	110-120
	5	6	116-125	123-133	131-143
19	4	11	98-105	104-112	111-121
	5	6	117-126	124-134	132-144

body weight plays a leading role in influencing one's health. All in all, those who stay within the average weight range have the best longevity record, the frank overweights the worst. Also, it is known that, irrespective of age, but allowing for differences in body build, the most favorable weights for health and longevity for adults are those which come closest to the averages observed at ages twenty-five to thirty.

These findings make it possible to answer *no* to the question *Is it all right—desirable—for men and women to make sizable gains in weight after attaining complete physical maturity at about twenty-five years of age?* They have also made it possible to construct tables showing the range of desirable weights for men and women of various heights and body build, irrespective of age, after reaching or passing their twenty-fifth birthday. *These tables are intended as a guide for judging correctness of weight rather than as a standard to which all individuals must conform.*

Although the classifications of *slight, medium,* and *heavy body build* are used in the tables, it must be remembered that there are many graduations in body build, or physique. The classification into which an individual falls will depend upon the characteristics that are predominant. See also WEIGHT, FACTORS WHICH INFLUENCE; UNDERWEIGHT, HAZARDS OF; WEIGHT-REGULATING MACHINERY OF THE BODY; OBESITY.

WEIGHT - REGULATING MACHINERY OF THE BODY. The body is equipped with a great many automatic checks and balances for preserving healthy conditions in its internal environment and for safeguarding its vital processes. Is there any self-regulating machinery for stopping the storage of fat when the depots are comfortably full? It would seem that regulation of the deposition of fat would be an important task, since both the reduction of fat reserves below the danger mark and the accumulation of fat to the extent of making the body "a bloated bondholder" are detrimental to health.

The regulation of body weight by automatic control over the amount of fat deposited in the fat depots would mean the application of a simple mathematical formula. *Food intake* (in terms of *calories*) must exactly equal *energy output* (in terms of calories) to maintain body weight at a constant level. To gain weight food intake must exceed energy output. To lose weight food intake must be less than energy output so that the body will use, or burn, its excess fat to make up the difference between food income and energy expenditure.

The assumption that the body does have an automatic weight-regulating mechanism is based on the fact that a great many people, especially those of slender and medium build, maintain practically the same weight throughout adult life. Although medico-actuarial tables show that the *average* man or woman has a tendency to gain weight year after year, it has been pointed out that these average increases were arrived at by measurements obtained from a mixed population including some in-

1347

the disease and its causes WENS Wens are cysts or sacs which form when the fatty material produced by the oil glands of the skin is unable to reach the surface of the skin.

MILIUM A milium is a nodule the size of a pinhead, which appears often on the face, especially in the region of the eyelids. The cause is unknown.

LIPOMA A lipoma is a tumor made up of an abnormal collection of fatty cells beneath the skin. It is quite common and may appear on any part of the body singly or in number. The growth is round, feels rubbery, and has a normal skin covering.

symptoms WENS They are found, as a rule, on the scalp, behind the ears, and on the back. Their size varies. Wens may appear singly or in combination with others.

MILIUM The nodules are yellowish white and usually hard.

LIPOMA Characteristically, they are soft masses that move freely. Usually they are painless, but they can be tender.

complications WENS Occasionally wens will become inflamed. Once open, they empty out a foul-smelling, cheesy material. However, they can be removed surgically and present no serious problems. They never become cancerous.

MILIUM The only complication is the unfavorable effect these have on one's appearance. However, milia are easily removed surgically and present no serious problems.

LIPOMA A lipoma never results in cancer and is easily removed surgically. Occasionally it becomes infected.

prevention (or lessening of impact) There is no way to prevent their development, but in cases where such growths have become infected, surgical removal is indicated to prevent further problems.

Wens, Milium and Lipoma (Non-malignant Skin Growths)

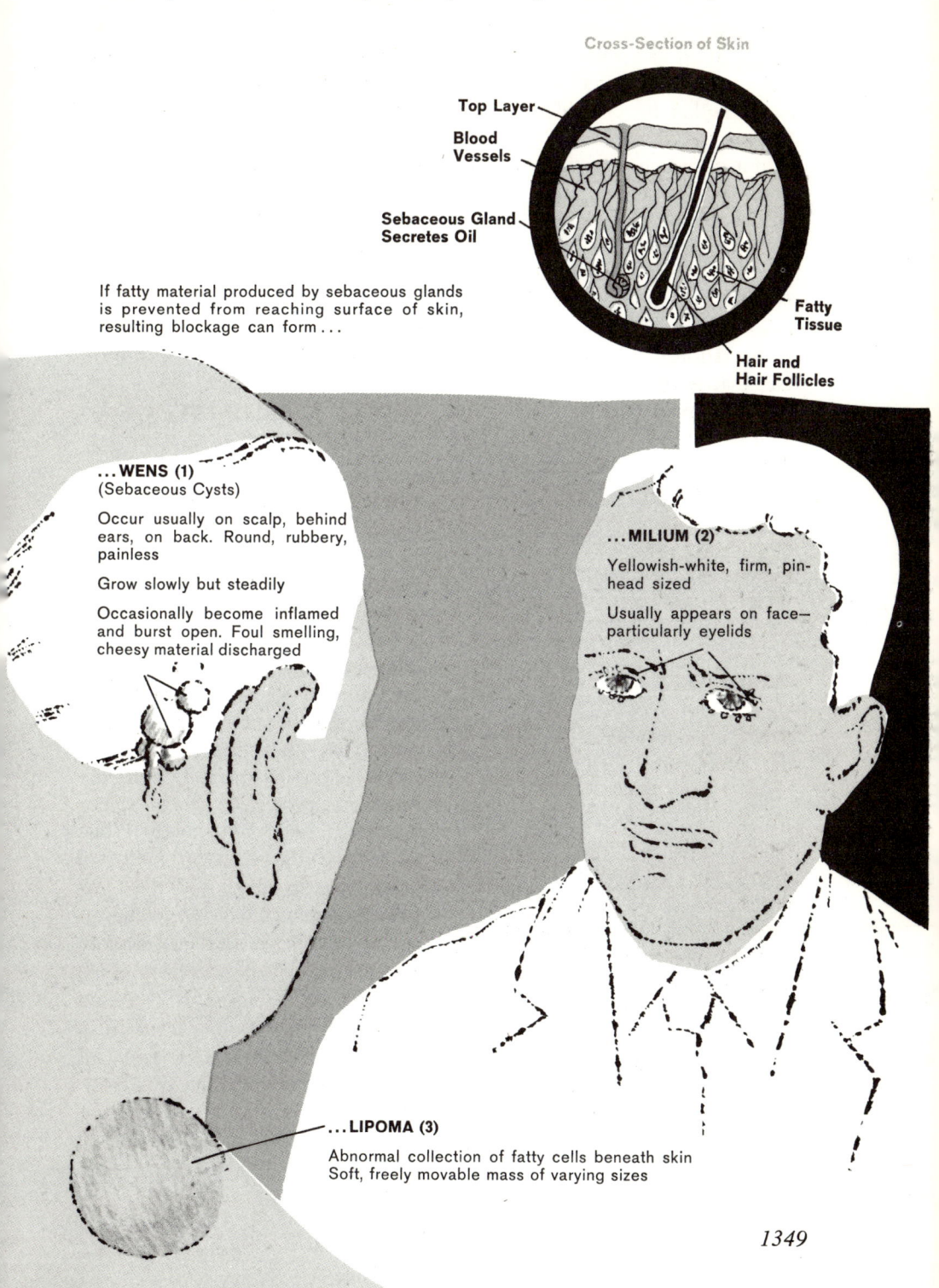

Cross-Section of Skin

- Top Layer
- Blood Vessels
- Sebaceous Gland Secretes Oil
- Fatty Tissue
- Hair and Hair Follicles

If fatty material produced by sebaceous glands is prevented from reaching surface of skin, resulting blockage can form...

...WENS (1)
(Sebaceous Cysts)

Occur usually on scalp, behind ears, on back. Round, rubbery, painless

Grow slowly but steadily

Occasionally become inflamed and burst open. Foul smelling, cheesy material discharged

...MILIUM (2)

Yellowish-white, firm, pinhead sized

Usually appears on face—particularly eyelids

...LIPOMA (3)

Abnormal collection of fatty cells beneath skin
Soft, freely movable mass of varying sizes

dividuals who do not change their weight at all and others who gain in weight at a faster rate than the average. Another bit of evidence is the fact that the frankly obese, who seem to put on weight easily, do reach a limit—that is, a point at which their weight remains static.

The nature of this weight-regulating mechanism is obscure. Both *heredity* and the *nervous* and *endocrine systems* undoubtedly influence its operation. It is a well-established fact that stoutness and leanness are hereditary variations of body build.

And endocrine or nervous-system disturbances, or both, whether inherited or acquired during life, have been found in many cases of generalized obesity and of grotesque distributions of body fat. *See also* WEIGHT, FACTORS WHICH INFLUENCE.

WEIL'S DISEASE. *See* JAUNDICE.

WEN, a sac formed in the skin when the *sebum,* the fatty material excreted by the skin's sebaceous or oil glands, is obstructed and cannot escape to the skin surface normally. Physicians call such a sac a *sebaceous cyst.* If not removed, the material within the sac or cyst interacts with the blood and changes from a rather solid mass to one that is semifluid, and may develop an offensive odor.

Since a wen may continue to grow as long as the blockage continues and infection does not occur, it may reach the size of a golf ball or even larger. With a minimum of surgery a doctor can drain the material from the cyst and eliminate the blockage.

If, however, infection has occurred, merely cutting an opening for drainage is insufficient. Sebaceous matter will continue to be secreted by the inner wall of the sac which will harden, collect, and repeat the initial process. Removal of the entire internal wall of the cyst by surgery may be essential to prevent recurrence of an infected wen. *See also* CYST; WART; FURUNCLES; CARBUNCLES. *See* MEDIGRAPH page 1349.

WHEAT SENSITIVITY. *See* ALLERGY; CELIAC DISEASE.

WHITE BLOOD CELLS. *See* BLOOD.

WHITE BLOOD CELLS, DISEASES OF. White blood cells number from 5,000 to 10,000 per cubic millimeter of blood. White blood cells are not all alike. *Granulocytes* are the most numerous of the white cells. They, as well as red cells, are produced in the marrow. *Lymphocytes* are produced in the spleen and lymph nodes of the body. White cells have the unusual ability of being able to leave and enter the blood stream at will. *Granulocytes* act as *scavengers* and are able to remove bacteria and debris or dying tissue from damaged or infected areas. *Lymphocytes* are involved in production of *antibodies.* A count of the number of white cells indicates whether this mechanism of bodily defense is at work; that is, in cases of infection, the white count will be elevated.

WHITE BLOOD CELLS, DISEASES OF

Leukemia is one of the most serious blood disorders. *Acute leukemia* is the most rapidly fatal blood disease. Young forms of white cells suddenly are produced which mature abnormally. These may appear as abnormal cells in large quantities in the blood and bone marrow. Over-production of the leukemic cells crowds the marrow and *platelets* and *red cells* may not be produced. Absence of platelets produces severe bleeding which in turn may produce *anemia*. Part of the anemia is due to insufficient production of red cells.

Acute leukemia is more common in children than in adults. Many drugs are available which help to control this malignant disease, at least for a while. Such drugs as the hormone *cortisone* help stop the bleeding tendency and may have a direct effect on production of leukemic cells. Other drugs have a specific effect on the marrow. These latter drugs are quite toxic and must be given only under close supervision of a patient by a hematologist.

The *chronic leukemias* tend to have a much longer and milder course than the *acute*. Chronic leukemia almost never occurs in children. Persons with this type of leukemia may live fifteen to twenty years from the onset of symptoms, if given proper care.

In either acute or chronic leukemia, the number of white cells does not indicate the severity of the disease. Leukemia may occur with a low or normal count. Severity of the disease is dependent on such factors as the degree of enlargement of the spleen, liver, or lymph nodes; extent of the anemia; or bleeding phenomena. Invasion of tissues by leukemic cells may be the only symptom of the disease. Marrow examination usually is necessary for proper diagnosis.

Infectious mononucleosis is a benign disturbance usually found in adolescents and young adults. It must not be confused with leukemia. The disease is caused by a virus. Epidemics in college dormitories and military barracks have occurred. It is most frequently transmitted by kissing; hence, it is sometimes called the *kissing disease*.

The disease usually starts with a sore throat and enlargement of lymph nodes in the neck. The person has some pain, fever, and tenderness in the left side of the abdomen. The latter symptom is due to enlargement of the spleen. An afflicted person frequently complains of being tired and, in fact, tires very easily. *Infectious hepatitis* may be a part of the picture. Specific treatment is not known. Measures to counteract any secondary bacterial infection may be taken, such as injections of antibiotics. Bed rest and drugs to make a patient feel more comfortable are helpful. The disease may last from one week to many months. In almost all cases complete recovery occurs. The blood shows an increase in the number of lymphocytes. These cells differ in appearance from normal lymphocytes and are termed *atypical lymphocytes*. They may persist for many months after a person apparently shows no further symptoms.

Lymph nodes have already been mentioned. These small structures are strategically placed throughout the body. Their function is twofold: they produce the lymphocytes, and they function as a filtering system for bacteria and tissue debris. The spleen frequently is called a lymph node of the blood. An example of the anti-infection activity of lymph nodes frequently occurs in persons with bacterial infections of the throat and tonsils. In these persons, nodes in the jaw swell, producing visible tumor masses under the jaw.

Malignant diseases of lymph nodes and the spleen are termed *lymphomas*. Not all lymphomas are fatal. Such diseases as *Hodgkin's disease, lymphosarcoma,* and *reticulum cell sarcoma* are included under the name of lymphoma.

Hodgkin's disease has three forms. *Hodgkin's paragranuloma* is the least malignant of the forms and persons afflicted with it have been known to live many years. Often the disease does not recur after surgical removal or x-ray treatment. *Hodgkin's granuloma* and *Hodgkin's sarcoma* are more serious forms of the disease. Much research has been done on the cause and treatment of lymphomas and leukemias and great strides have been made in control of these diseases. People afflicted with these cancer-like disorders live longer and more comfortably than was previously possible.

Sometimes it is necessary to remove the spleen. Actually, the spleen is an organ which in mankind does not seem to be indispensable for normal life. In a way, it is analogous to the appendix, except that certain *harmless* changes in the blood do occur following removal of the spleen. In *hereditary spherocytosis, idiopathic thrombocytopenic purpura,* unexplained *enlargement of the spleen,* and certain other conditions, removal of the spleen may be necessary. Families of patients should not be afraid of this operation because of what they may have been told by unauthoritative persons. *See also* BLOOD; LEUKEMIA; MONONUCLEOSIS, INFECTIOUS; HODGKIN'S DISEASE; SPLEEN; SPLENIC DISEASE; ANEMIA; ANEMIA, PERNICIOUS; RED BLOOD CELLS, DISEASES OF; THROMBOCYTOPENIA. *See* MEDIGRAPH page 845.

WHITFIELD'S OINTMENT, a preparation compounded of *salicylic* and *benzoic acids* and *petrolatum.* The mixture is useful as a *fungicide* following mechanical removal of the nail in *ringworm of the nail,* and also in other fungus infections of the skin such as *athlete's foot.* Whitfield's ointment is quite strong and should be used with care. It should not be applied to acutely inflamed oozing lesions of the skin, and is best reserved for use in older, scaly lesions.

WHOOPING COUGH, or *pertussis,* a disease characterized by a convulsive cough, and infecting the mucous membrane of the respiratory system. The cough leaves the patient out of breath and the resultant deep inhalation produces the whooping sound.

WHOOPING COUGH

The disease is not a trivial affliction of childhood. Coupled with a secondary infection, such as *bronchopneumonia,* whooping cough can be fatal, especially in young children or the aged. The most frequent victims are children under five.

During the first ten days of this disease, the incubation period, the victim exhibits the symptoms of an ordinary cold. The cough, however, does not improve. The second stage begins with the onset of the whooping sound. During a coughing spell the face may grow scarlet while the facial veins swell and tears appear in the eyes. The cough may be followed by vomiting.

Whooping cough is caused by the germ *Hemophilus pertussis.* To ascertain the presence of this germ, modern science requires the child to cough on a special culture plate on which the germs are then examined. The same test may be used as a proof that the child is finally free of the germ and no longer needs to be isolated. This is the primary purpose of the test. Diagnosis, as well as pronouncement of cure, may be determined by other means. A blood test may be made, since one of the characteristics of whooping cough is an increase in the number of single-nucleus white blood cells. However, the whooping sound in itself is a fairly reliable guide for a doctor.

The prevention of whooping cough primarily involves *immunization* which is now accomplished by a series of injections which combine immunity against *diphtheria* and *tetanus* as well. Only infants and children need to be injected.

If a child develops whooping cough, isolation of the child is necessary, chiefly to prevent secondary infection in the child and exposure of other children. In some cases of children under two or three years of age, antibiotics are used, but older children generally recover without the use of drugs. If convulsions occur, as sometimes happens, the doctor may place the child in an oxygen tent and sedative drugs such as *phenobarbital* may be given. Treatment requires complete rest as well as constant protection of the patient's lungs from atmospheric irritants such as tobacco smoke or cold drafts of air. The *inhalation of steam* is sometimes advised, as well as certain drugs which relieve the severity of the coughing attacks. If coughing places a great strain on the stomach muscles, a *rubber binder* may be worn around that area. It is better to praise the child for coughing less than to pity him for coughing more. Commiseration is not the best medicine.

Finally, special attention should be given to the patient's diet, particularly to that of children, who are susceptible to vomiting and therefore to undernourishment. Generally speaking, the child requires nutritious food which is also easy to digest. The best time for meals is approximately a quarter of an hour after a coughing spell. The child should eat in small amounts, perhaps several times a day. To feed him a large amount of food at any one time is likely to stimulate coughing, whereupon the food which has been eaten will be regurgitated.

the disease and its causes Whooping cough is a contagious disease involving the respiratory tract and is caused by a specific type of bacteria. It gets its name from the whooping sound produced by a patient taking a deep breath inward after a prolonged coughing seizure. It is a childhood disease primarily, and can be fatal to very young children if complications become severe. One attack gives lifelong immunity.

symptoms It may begin with low-grade fever and mild cold-like symptoms. This is followed by a dry, hacking cough which becomes worse at night. By the 3rd week the typical explosive cough, followed by the long whoop, has developed. A coughing spell usually continues until the characteristic stringy mucus can be expelled. During this stage the child's face may become bluish, the eyes bloodshot, and he is most uncomfortable. This stage may go on for as long as a month. The final stage resembles an ordinary bronchitis and may continue another 3 or 4 weeks.

complications Bronchopneumonia is a frequent complication because the thick mucus plugs block the bronchial tubes. Lung collapse and other destructive lung changes can also occur. Ear infections are another possibility. Sometimes intestinal problems are brought on by the repeated vomiting which follows severe coughing. The resulting loss of important chemicals in the blood can lead to serious problems. One is the development of a condition in which the muscles go into painful and prolonged spasms accompanied by tingling, numbness and sometimes twitching. This is called tetany. Meningitis and encephalitis are rare complications.

prevention (or lessening of impact) Fortunately, a vaccine that prevents whooping cough is available and should be given to every child before he or she reaches school age. It consists of a series of three injections. Exposure to known cases of whooping cough should be avoided, but if a child does become exposed he should be given booster shots.
Antibiotics are used to prevent complications and control the long course of the illness. Sedation is used to control the cough and the distress of the patient. Oxygen is sometimes provided during severe, choking coughing.

Whooping Cough

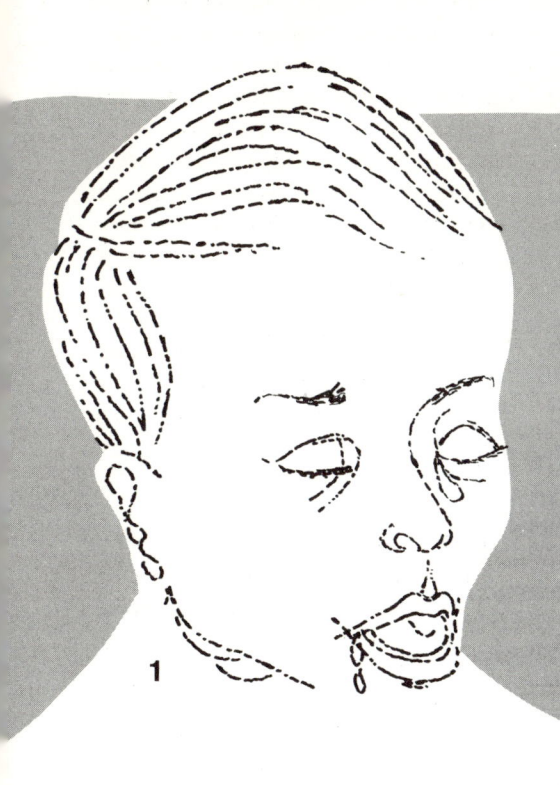

1. Puffy Face
3-4 days after heavy coughing stage starts, child's face becomes puffy and blueish in color. Eyes tear, tongue is pushed out and mucus is expelled during coughing spell.

2. Bloodshot Eyes
Around 5th day, heavy coughing causes bloodshot eyes because of breaking of some blood vessels in lining of eyes.

3. Sore Under Tongue
Rubbing of tongue against teeth during coughing spells usually produces sore under tongue by 6th day.

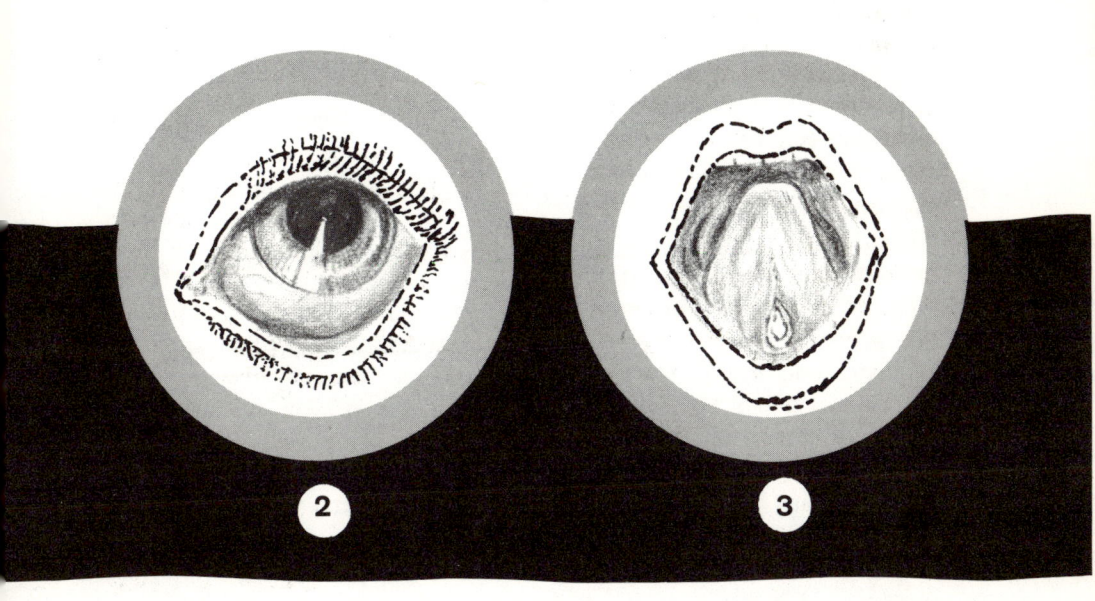

1355

Starchy foods—bread, pastries, and potatoes—should be avoided, as well as any dry and crumbly foods which might tickle the throat and produce a cough. Vegetable soup is recommended, and also meat in small amounts, provided that it is carefully chopped or strained. Fresh fruit juices and plenty of plain drinking water are also to be given. See also DIPHTHERIA; INFECTIOUS DISEASES. See MEDIGRAPH page 1355.

WILM'S TUMOR, a malignant growth that affects the kidneys of children, usually under six years of age. It may grow to great size and cause the child's abdomen to protrude. Sometimes the doctor can feel the tumor with his fingers before such symptoms as pain or blood in the urine appear. Other symptoms are weakness and vomiting.

Removal of the affected kidney followed by radiation is the best means of curing this condition. If the tumor is large, it may be necessary first to treat it with radiation, then follow with surgery and postoperative radiation.

WOMB. See UTERUS.

WOOD ALCOHOL OR METHANOL POISONING. Poisoning with this industrial solvent may lead to *blindness* and *death*. Since it has been used as an antifreeze many deaths of alcoholics have resulted from drinking antifreeze solution. The symptoms of wood alcohol poisoning are like those of ordinary drunkenness except for the symptoms that include blurring of vision or blindness. In treating wood alcohol poisoning, the stomach is washed out by having the person drink copious amounts of *salt solution* which is then vomited back. Afterward a *saline cathartic* is taken to wash out the bowel. *Thiamin* and *nicotinamide* and *vitamin K* are given to protect the nervous system. The pain, restlessness, or delirium should have prompt medical attention. The doctor may provide oxygen for breathing and necessary stimulation. See also POISONING.

WORMS. Several types of worms live parasitically in the human body, usually in some part of the digestive tract. Although the United States has relatively high sanitation and hygienic standards, various kinds of worm infestation still occur in some areas. A study of children in the District of Columbia, for example, revealed that 35 to 65 per cent of certain groups had *pinworm infestation,* and another study reported that 50 to 60 per cent of children in different parts of the United States had *intestinal worms.*

Some worms attain remarkable size, such as the *beef tapeworm* which may reach a length of fifteen feet; whereas others—such as the worm which causes *trichinosis*—are so thin and small that they are barely visible to the naked eye. Often worms are present in the bowels without causing any serious symptoms. However, sometimes they may produce general and far-reaching disturbances.

Pinworm. The pinworm is easily

the most widely distributed of worms which live as parasites in human hosts. Known also as the *seat worm* or *threadworm,* it exists only in the form of a human parasite. The adult worm, which is white, may be as long as half an inch down to a quarter of that size. Infestation occurs when worm eggs are taken into the body. They may enter through the mouth from fingers which have touched some contaminated surface or may be inhaled, for the eggs are so small and light that they can float in the air. From the mouth the eggs pass to the small intestine where they hatch and begin a life cycle that takes about two months. They mature in the intestine and eventually mating occurs. The males then leave the body of the host, but the females migrate to the large bowel where the eggs develop. Finally, when the eggs are ready to be deposited for hatching, the female passes out of the body through the anus, leaving behind several thousand eggs on the skin surface just outside the anal opening.

The itching in and around the affected areas is usually the most disturbing symptom of pinworm infestation. In females, the worms sometimes travel to the genital area. The eggs may be widely distributed in the bed, bedclothes, pajamas, and other clothing. When the person scratches the affected area, the worms get under the fingernails and the infection process begins again. Pinworms sometimes become so troublesome that they affect appetite and thus cause loss of weight.

Scrupulous cleanliness is absolutely necessary in the elimination of pinworm, and a daily bath is essential. Since the eggs, the source of infection and reinfection, are distributed so widely and so easily, the entire family should be placed under the doctor's care at the same time, so that reinfection does not pass constantly from infected to uninfected persons.

The drugs used against pinworm can be given only by a doctor's prescription and under his care. Enemas with a chemical called *hexylresorcinol* are given; a dyestuff—*gentian violet*—may be given internally; and *antiseptic ointments* for affected external areas may be prescribed by the doctor. The amount and manner of application of these remedies will vary with each case and must always be determined by the doctor.

Roundworm. After the pinworm, the parasite which most frequently infests the human body is the *giant intestinal roundworm,* scientifically known as *Ascaris lumbricoides.* The female reaches a length of ten to fifteen inches and the male is about half that size. Like the pinworm, it lives in the digestive tract.

Normally the symptoms of roundworm infestation are not serious, except that sometimes, particularly when another illness is present, sensitivities resembling those of an allergy may appear. If, however, the affected person becomes ill enough to develop a fever, or if he is treated with drugs, the worms may migrate within the body to places quite remote from their usual habitation. They may appear in the nose, mouth, and have even entered and

1357

the disease and its causes This is a small, round worm which infects the small and large intestines of humans. It is found most often in children, but frequently all the members of one family can be infected.

The eggs of the worm enter the body through contaminated food or water and pass into the small intestine where they develop into adult worms. Then the fertilized females wander to the anus and deposit a new crop of eggs there. Sometimes they even enter the vagina and Fallopian tubes.

symptoms There is intense itching and irritation of the anus and the surrounding area. Since the adult female pinworms migrate and lay their eggs in the anal area at night, the symptoms are much more marked at that time.

complications There are no serious complications. This is a mild but annoying illness. Occasionally there is secondary infection around the anus.

prevention (or lessening of impact) Personal hygiene is the most important factor in controlling this disease. After bowel movements the anus should be carefully cleaned and the hands thoroughly washed. Infected children should have their nails clipped short and scrubbed before eating, because when they scratch the anal area, they embed the microscopic-sized eggs under the fingernails. Then, in eating, the pinworm eggs can come off the fingernails onto the food, starting the infection cycle again. Children should also be warned to keep their hands out of their mouths.

Stool examinations or rectal smears should be taken, as directed by the physician, to make certain no living worms remain after treatment. Pinworm infestation responds well to drug therapy, but reinfections are frequent unless the entire family is treated.

Pinworm

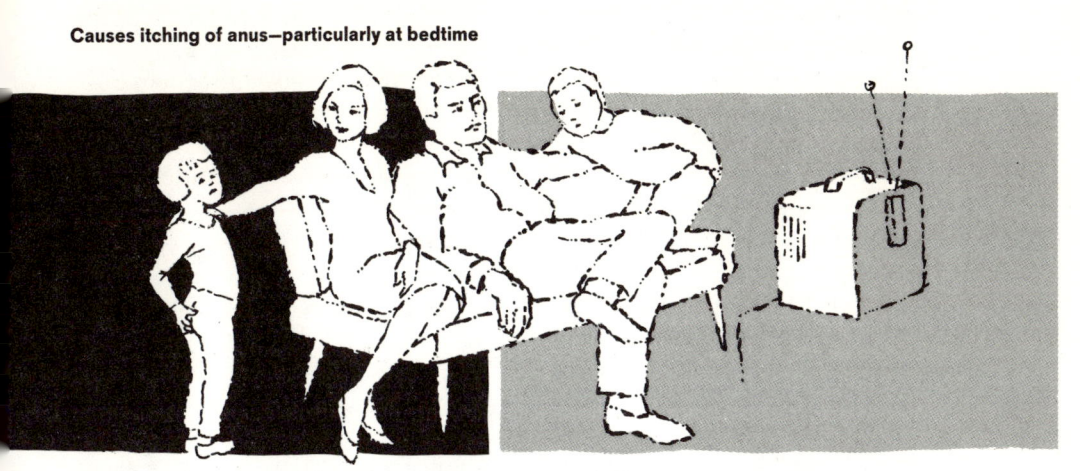

Causes itching of anus—particularly at bedtime

Pinworm generally spreads throughout family, starting with children

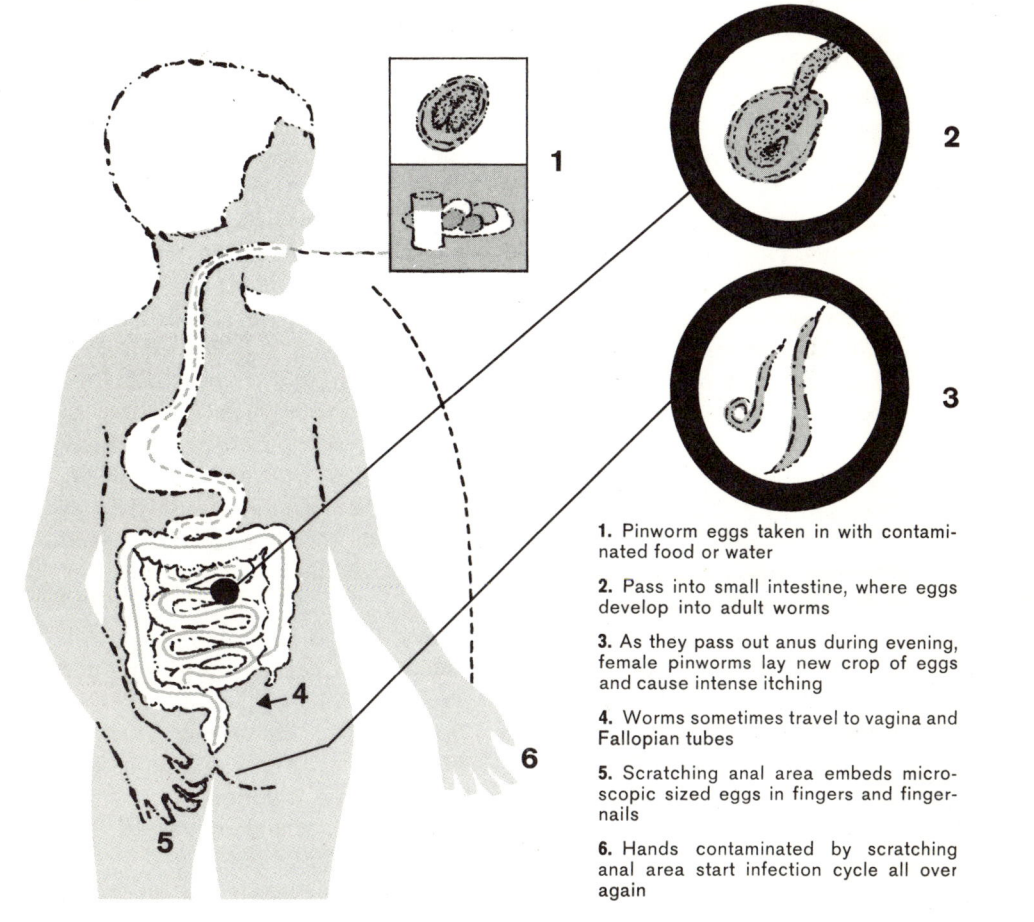

1. Pinworm eggs taken in with contaminated food or water

2. Pass into small intestine, where eggs develop into adult worms

3. As they pass out anus during evening, female pinworms lay new crop of eggs and cause intense itching

4. Worms sometimes travel to vagina and Fallopian tubes

5. Scratching anal area embeds microscopic sized eggs in fingers and fingernails

6. Hands contaminated by scratching anal area start infection cycle all over again

blocked the appendix, the bile duct, and the Eustachian tubes which connect the throat and the inner ear. If for no other reason, this makes it obviously desirable to rid the body of these parasites.

The worms live within the intestine, where in a single day the females produce as many as 200,000 eggs, a million and a half each week. Once outside the body of the host, these eggs are ready to hatch in from two to four weeks. On the surface of the ground and in moist shaded spots they can and do survive in this state for months. When the eggs are taken into the human body, almost always because of lack of simple sanitary precautions, they pass first to the small intestine where they hatch. The larvae burrow through the intestinal wall, reach the liver, and finally pass to the lungs. From the lungs they are coughed up into the mouth, swallowed again, and are returned to the intestines where they remain. The total period of development is from four to six weeks and the worm may live in the body for another six months.

Although the consequences of infestation are not particularly alarming, the possible secondary effects are such that the condition should be eliminated. Here again, treatment is strictly the responsibility of a doctor. *Hexylresorcinol* has been found to be especially effective against the giant roundworm. The stomach is first emptied of its contents by purgation and abstinence from food for at least twelve hours. After the drug is given, the person must not eat for another five hours or more, and only semifluid foods are recommended for the next five hours. At the end of twenty-four hours, a cathartic is taken to wash all residual material from the bowel. Ordinarily one such treatment satisfactorily disposes of worms.

Hookworm. Infestation by hookworm — *necator americanus* — presents a more serious situation than that of the pinworm or roundworm. The hookworm does specific and substantial damage within the body. In extreme cases it may permanently disable a person or even bring about death. There are still sizable areas of the United States where it is a real public health problem.

The organism itself is about the size of the pinworm, a little less than half an inch long, and the female is slightly larger than the male. The most serious damage that the hookworm does is to fasten itself by its teeth to the bowel wall and secrete a *poisonous fluid* which at the same time dilates the small blood vessels there and prevents coagulation of the blood. The worm feeds by drawing blood, of which it uses only a small amount for its own nourishment, letting the remainder pass through its system, relatively unaffected, and then out with the digestive waste of the host. When the number of parasitic worms is large, the person will suffer from *anemia, weakness,* and *lassitude.* Although his appetite may be increased, he usually loses interest in activity, his face is dull and his hair lusterless. If left untreated, the condition may in time cause invalidism or death.

This worm may have other ad-

1360

verse effects on the human body, as it makes its way from the surface inward by a route much more complex than that of the roundworm. The female hookworm lays from 6,000 to 15,000 eggs daily and these pass from an infected human being to the ground. Most infested persons have picked up the worms by exposure to infected soil. The larvae penetrate the skin and produce, first of all, a severe local condition on the skin called *ground itch*. At the point of entry, they penetrate a blood vessel and are carried in the blood stream to the lungs. Within the lungs they break out in the open space, climb the bronchial tubes to the throat and are swallowed, and eventually reach the small intestine where the adult worm finally develops. Here the females begin to lay eggs and when these appear in the person's excretions the developmental process of the worm is completed. The cycle takes about six weeks from the time the larvae penetrate the skin. During passage through the lungs, the larvae may induce a bronchial inflammation accompanied by fever.

Fortunately hookworm is easily diagnosed and treated. Examination of the patient's bowel waste by the doctor will readily reveal the eggs. A number of remedies which will eradicate the worms from the digestive tract, including *hexylresorcinol, tetrachlorethylene,* and *oil of chemopodium,* are effective. All of these drugs are toxic and must be administered only by a physician.

In areas where hookworm is most prevalent, it is possible to avoid infestation by taking simple precautions. Shoes should always be worn, and excrement should be disposed of in such a way that the larvae from the excreted eggs are not scattered about. This can easily be done by providing places for disposal that are sufficiently deep, since the larvae cannot climb vertically to any considerable height. In urban areas with adequate sewage disposal and running water facilities, this is no problem.

Tapeworm. Of several types and sizes, tapeworms are among the most common intestinal worms which invade human beings. They vary in size from the *beef tapeworm,* which can reach a length of fifteen feet, to the *dwarf tapeworm* which never measures more than a few centimeters. More than thirty species affect human beings, but only six are really common.

Tapeworms are not actually single worms, but are in fact colonies of worms. The first segment serves as the head and other members are separate and hitched to each other, end to end. Each of these individual segments, called *proglottids,* contains little more than the required equipment of sexual reproduction, since feeding by absorption of predigested nutriment from the host eliminates the need for digestive apparatus. Fertilization may be between a male and female element of a single proglottid or between one proglottid and another. Fertilized eggs remain within the worm and eventually the proglottid breaks off and is passed to the outside with the waste material.

The most common way in which

the disease and its causes The tapeworm is a parasite that infects hogs, steers, and cows. When a person eats contaminated meat that is raw or undercooked, the tapeworm larvae (young worms just out of the egg) that are present in the meat can pass into the person's small intestine. There, the tapeworms grow into mature worms from 6 to 20 feet long.

symptoms As a rule, tapeworm infection causes no unusual disturbances. A patient may not know he has it until segments of the worm are discharged into his feces and he observes them. In occasional cases there can be some abdominal discomfort, nausea, vomiting, or a change in bowel habits. An outstanding characteristic of the infection is the patient's ravenous appetite. (Thus, there are good grounds for the folk saying "He eats so much and stays so thin—you'd think he had a tapeworm!")

complications Generally there are no serious complications from beef tapeworm. The worm may live for years before it is detected, with no effect on the general health of the patient. Occasionally, a moderate anemia (loss of red blood cells) develops.

However, pork tapeworm larvae can cause serious complications by invading the muscles in general, the heart muscle, brain, eye, and nervous system.

prevention (and lessening of impact) To prevent this infection it is essential that pork and beef be cooked thoroughly in order to destroy the larvae of the tapeworm. Once a patient is infected, the entire worm, including the head, must be removed, and this can be done medically. Removing the head is important because when it remains attached to the intestinal wall, it regenerates itself and the infection cycle starts all over again.

Tapeworm

1. Tapeworm larvae invade hog, steer or cow

2. Man infected by eating contaminated meat whose tapeworm larvae were not destroyed because uncooked or undercooked

3. In small intestine, adult tapeworm develops. Some grow long as 15-20 feet

4. Mild stomach pain, nausea, constipation or diarrhea are sometimes felt

5. Segments of tapeworm can frequently be seen in feces

6. Pork tapeworm larvae can also invade muscles in general, heart muscle, brain, eye, nervous system—with potentially very serious results

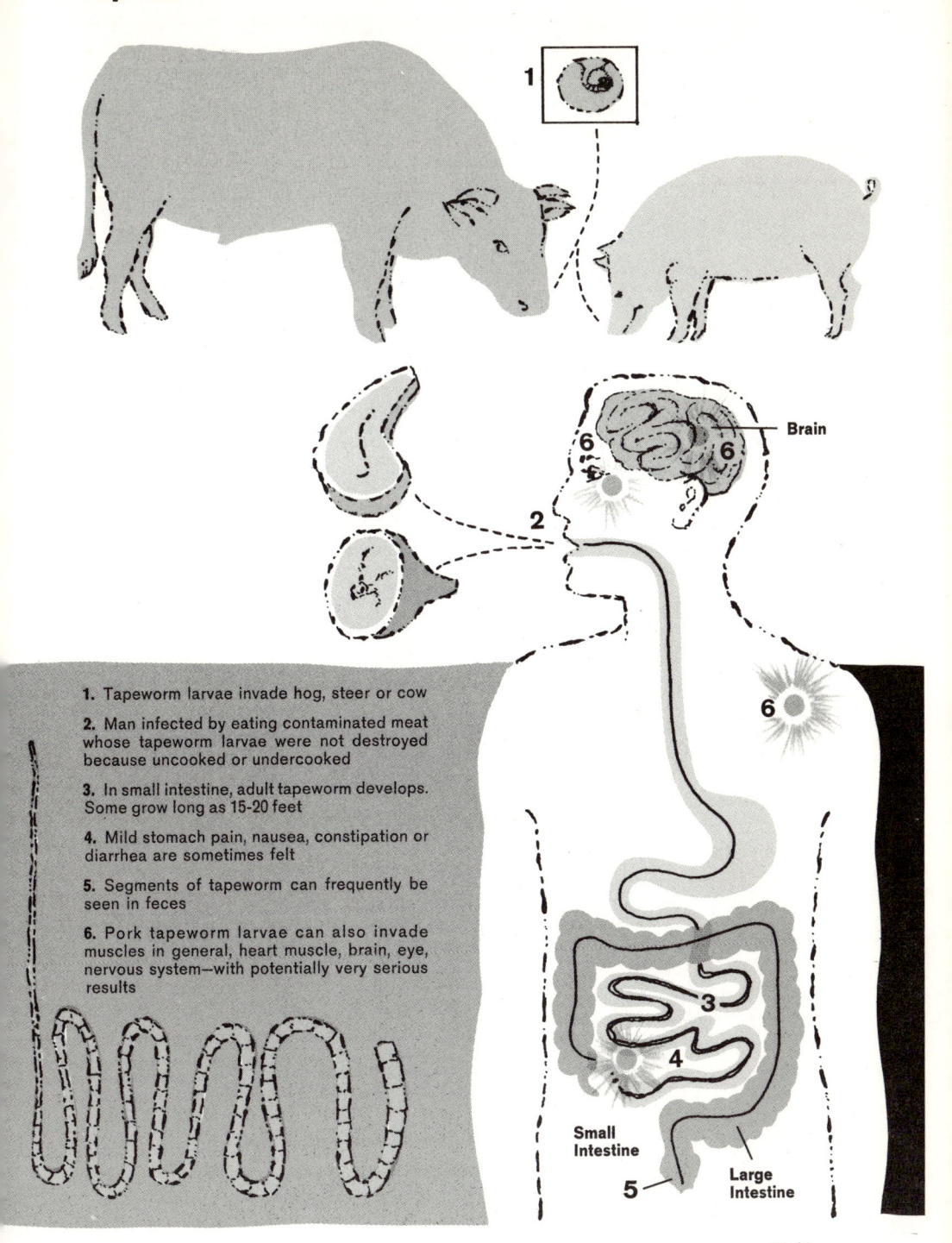

1363

human beings are infested by tapeworm is by eating the meat of animals that have eaten either the fertilized eggs or a discharged proglottid, then incubated the eggs in their intestine where later the tapeworm larvae develop and finally invade the muscle tissue. The same sequence of development may ensue with the beef tapeworm when cattle have been pastured where there is contaminated human excrement. If beef from such cattle is consumed either raw or partially cooked, the live worm may be taken into the person's body. The beef tapeworm reaches fifteen feet in length and the numbers of its separate parts may be as many as 2,000, of which approximately the lower half will at any one time be bearers of fertilized eggs.

The life history of the *pork tapeworm* is essentially the same, with some biological variations. Its maximum growth is usually ten feet and the number of parts about 1,000. Infestation is from eating improperly cooked meat from hogs which have consumed infected human sewage.

The *fish tapeworm,* with somewhat more substantial differences, experiences the same life cycle within a fish as the other types. This worm does not release whole pregnant proglottids but mature individual eggs which discharge embryos capable of swimming. They enter the water through infected human waste. The embryos are eaten by water fleas and the water fleas by fish. The fish become infected and, if eaten raw, will transmit the infection to man. Sometimes there is an intermediate stage, in which the infected fish is eaten by a larger fish which in turn becomes human food and transmits the infestation.

Dwarf tapeworms, which measure less than an inch, affect children more often than adults. *Dog* and *rat tapeworms,* are so rare as to be of little concern to laymen.

Several effective substances are available which can be used by the physician to rid the host of tapeworms. As in the other treatments, the person must abstain from food for a day or a few days while taking the drug. Recovery of the top end of the worm from the bowel waste usually is considered to constitute elimination of the worms. A person who has a tapeworm may have only a few mild symptoms or he may have more severe attacks. The condition often begins with *diarrhea,* which then alternates with *constipation. False hunger pains* are characteristic, although the appetite may sometimes diminish. The person *loses weight* and *secondary anemia* appears, and still later symptoms may disappear entirely. The victim of beef tapeworm is likely to experience discomfort when the proglottids pass through the rectum. In every case, the diagnosis can be made easily and with certainty by examination of the excrement. *See also* FILARIASIS; BILHARZIASIS. *See* MEDIGRAPHS pages 1359, 1363.

WOUNDS. Any injury that breaks the skin, mucous membrane, or inner surface of the tissues of the body is a wound. Although *fractures* and *bruises* are wounds, the term usually is applied to the following:

Cut or incision, a slash or slit in the skin caused by a sharp cutting object, such as a razor blade. This type of wound bleeds profusely, since all the blood vessels are cleanly severed. There is usually little tissue damage, and less danger from infection than in other wounds. A deep cut may possibly sever tendons and nerves.

Laceration or torn wound, an irregular tearing of the tissue by a rough or blunt or jagged-edged object. A laceration might result from a fall against an angular object or piece of machinery. Bleeding is usually not severe, as the blood vessels are irregularly torn, but *danger of infection* exists because bleeding is often slight and body tissues are damaged at the edge of the wound.

Puncture and stab wound, caused by a penetrating object, such as a nail, bullet, or splinter. Unless a large blood vessel is injured, puncture wounds do not bleed profusely. They are *especially liable to infection,* since they are difficult to clean.

Abrasion, rubbing off or scraping of skin or mucous membrane, commonly called *floor burn* or *mat burn* although not a true burn. They usually cover a wide surface and so are easily infected.

Severe bleeding or hemorrhage and infection are two dangers to be considered with wounds. If a wound is bleeding profusely, the first step is to attempt to control the bleeding. Bleeding may be from a vein, an artery, or both. When an artery is cut, the blood spurts out. Blood from a cut vein comes in a steady flow, since the blood is under much lower pressure than arterial blood.

Venous bleeding is easier to control than arterial bleeding. Pressure should be applied to the edges of the wound until a compress can be obtained. Usually venous bleeding can be stopped by placing a compress over the wound and bandaging it snugly. If necessary, hand pressure firmly applied directly on the compress will help a clot to form. The injured area should be elevated, unless a fracture accompanies the wound.

In *arterial bleeding,* if someone is present who has knowledge of the pressure points of the body, this method of controlling hemorrhage is first attempted. A pressure point is some point between the wound and heart where the main artery of the injured area lies close to a bone; hand or finger pressure against the bone may stop bleeding. A dressing or other material is pressed firmly against the wound. If the bleeding stops, the dressing should be bandaged into position and left undisturbed.

If the firmly pressed gauze dressing does not stop bleeding, a tourniquet may be necessary. *Since a tourniquet cuts off the total blood supply to the area, it is applied only when other methods fail.* In the absence of a ready-made tourniquet, a rolled handkerchief, belt, or other substitute may be used. Anything which would cut the skin, such as wire or cord, should not be used. If circulation is stopped for too long, there is danger of *gangrene,* and so the tourniquet should never be left in place for more than an hour.

In all cases of serious hemorrhage, the injured person should be kept lying down and quiet, since movement might disturb the blood clot. He should be treated for shock, which is nearly always present, and a doctor called.

Most cases of serious infection and blood poisoning develop from a seemingly insignificant wound which has not been correctly treated. Since danger of infection is present any time the skin is broken, even the smallest wound should receive proper attention. In cases of severe bleeding, the first step is, of course, to control the hemorrhage. Infection is characterized by heat, pain, swelling, redness, and often pus formation, and if these symptoms are present in a wound a doctor should be consulted. Minor wounds can be treated with various antiseptic preparations, such as *tincture of iodine, metaphen, merthiolate, boric acid,* and others, and then covered with a clean snug bandage or compress. If the wound is more serious, only the bandage should be applied and the cleansing and disinfection of the wound done by a doctor, since amateur efforts can cause serious damage. *See also* SNAKEBITE; INSECT BITES; BEE STINGS.

WRY NECK. *See* TORTICOLLIS.

XYZ

XANTHOMA, a flat yellow tumor which may develop on the surface of the skin. Xanthomas are caused by the deposit of a fatty substance which the body has failed to dispose of in the normal manner. Most frequently they are seen in the vicinity of the eyes, especially on the inner part of the lower lid. A surgeon can remove these *yellow spots* with relative ease, leaving only slightly visible scars. Xanthomas may tend to recur, but are seldom cancerous. See also TUMOR.

XERODERMA, a disorder in which the skin becomes rough and dry, and sometimes discolored, with fine scaly shedding.

XEROPHTHALMIA, a disease in which a severe dryness of the eye occurs, resulting from a *deficiency of vitamin A*. The cornea becomes clouded and inflamed; ulcers of the cornea may develop. Permanent blindness may result in the advanced stages of this disease if it is not promptly and properly treated. The administration of vitamin A is effective for this condition. *See also* NUTRITION; DEFICIENCY DISEASES; VITAMINS; SCURVY; BERIBERI; PELLAGRA; KWASHIORKOR. *See* MEDIGRAPH page 1331.

XEROSIS, a disease in which abnormal dryness of the skin caused by vitamin A deficiency is a symptom. This condition may be corrected by taking liver oil extracts and making sure that the diet includes enough leafy green and yellow vegetables, as well as egg yolks, butter, or vitamin A-enriched margarine.

XEROSTOMA, decreased salivary flow; it is a symptom which arises from a number of causes rather than a disease. In many instances it is temporary, as in fever or in a state of fear or anxiety. *Atropine,* a drug often administered to patients before a surgical operation, may produce a dry feeling in the mouth.

In chronic cases, lack of saliva may cause the mouth to become rough and dry, and painful cracks

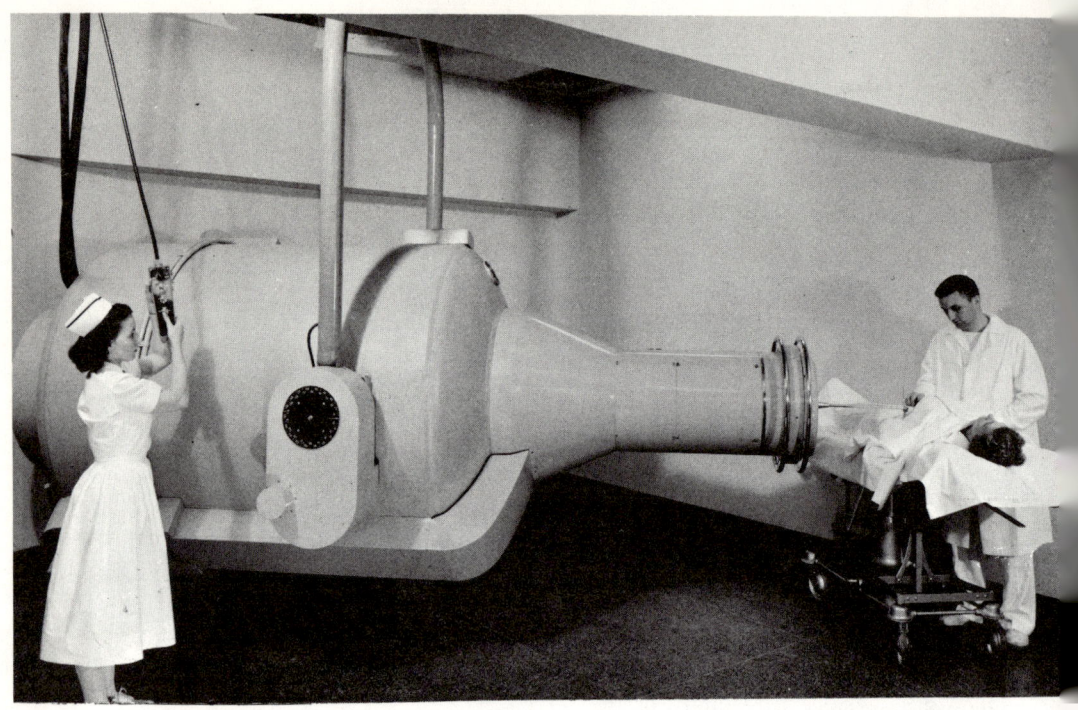

X-ray—This x-ray therapy unit visibly suggests its powerful two-million volt force, harnessed to treat the sick. Although this unit is large, it is balanced as delicately as a watch. It can be directed and positioned for best alignment for the individual patient.

and fissures which bleed easily may develop. A stone in the duct of the salivary glands may cause obstruction, swelling, and pain that will interfere with the intake of food and predispose the gland to infection. Surgery is the only means then of removing the stones. See also SALIVA.

X-RAYS, radiation produced by the vacuum tube, similar to light but of much shorter wave length and possessing special penetrating and tissue-ionizing power. First announced in December of 1895 by the German physicist Wilhelm Konrad Roentgen, the x-ray has since become one of the most important adjuncts in the practice of medicine and surgery.

One of the chief uses of the x-ray continues to be for the *diagnosis of broken bones*. Today pictures are made from different angles so that the exact relationship of the broken bones to the tissues may be determined.

An x-ray of the skull shows the presence of disease of the bone, sometimes the presence of a tumor or changes in the blood vessels in the brain.

It is also now possible by the use of accessory materials to visualize various organs and tissues. These substances include various dyes which may be taken into the body and which localize in certain organs and tissues. Then by the use of the x-ray these tissues and organs are made visible. One dye substance is used in taking x-rays of the gall-bladder; others are used for the kidney and urinary bladder; still others for the female genital system or the spinal column. A substance called *lipiodol* may be injected into the lungs or sinuses to make them visible. For the investigation of the alimentary tract an *opaque meal of barium* is given and the progress of the meal along the intestinal tract is studied to detect ulcers and obstructions. A *barium enema* is given to study the large intestine and other organs in the lower abdominal region.

By the use of the x-ray the exact size of the heart may be determined. The x-ray is also used in the treatment of disease, particularly in the treatment of tumors, conditions affecting the skin, inflammations of various kinds, and for a wide variety of purposes where radiation therapy is called for.

The x-ray is also widely employed in *dentistry,* and is invaluable in providing a precise indication of the nature and extent of tooth decay, particularly in cases where such decay may be hidden by pre-existing fillings. It is also used to reveal the location of impacted wisdom teeth, and to determine the presence of abscesses.

Since the introduction of x-ray equipment innumerable improvements have been made. Portable apparatus is now available that can be

X-rays—(Left) Diagram of an x-ray tube. A is the *cathode;* B, the *anode;* and C, the *vacuum regulator.* (Right) Chest x-ray of a nine-year-old child, showing pathology in the left lung.

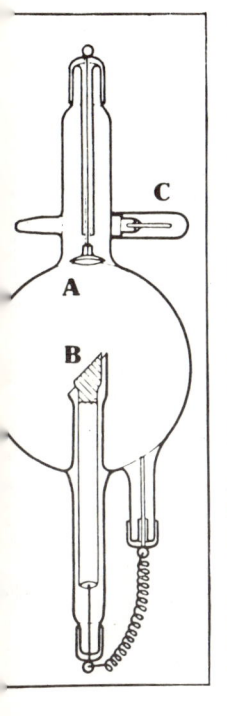

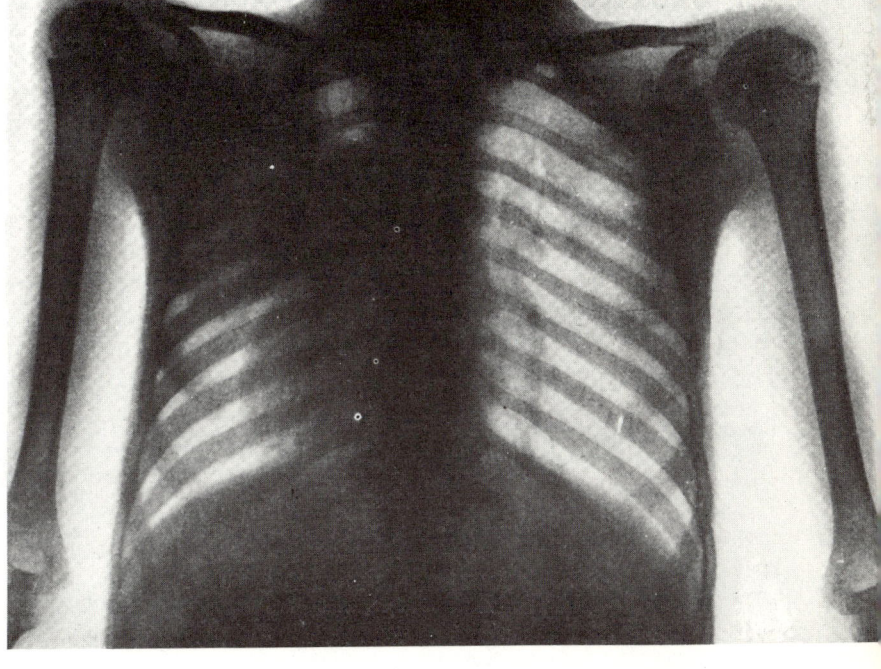

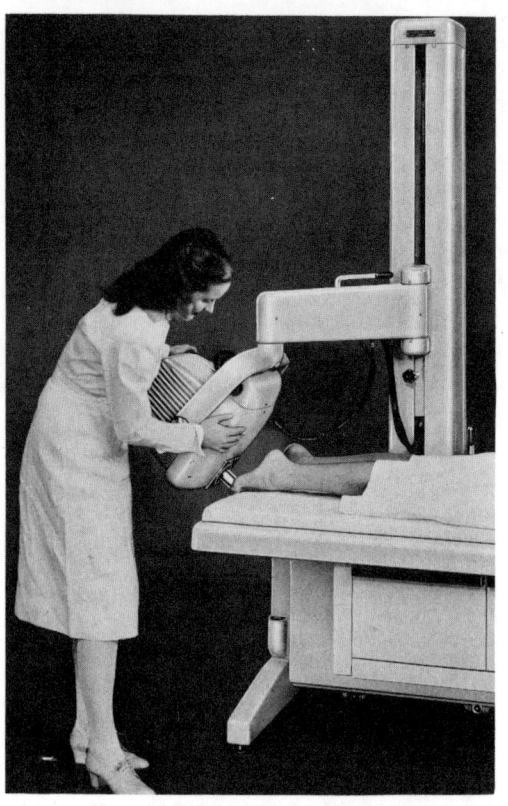

X-rays—Operator is adjusting a small x-ray therapy unit so the rays will be directed to a small growth on the patient's foot. Treatments such as this, aimed specifically at the surface skin, are known as superficial x-ray therapy.

taken directly to a patient's bedside. One of the most important developments in the use of the x-ray on a mass scale has been the introduction of mobile units as a means of taking chest films of school children and of the general public in order to determine the presence of tuberculosis and cancer of the lung. *See also* RADIATION; FLUOROSCOPY.

YAWS, also called *frambesia, pian,* and *bubas,* a disease which is caused by a spiral microorganism, the *treponema pertenue*—related to the *treponema pallidum,* the agent of *syphilis.* Yaws is rarely found in the United States but is a disease of tropical regions, especially where sanitation is poor. Raspberry-colored growths on various parts of the body, especially the face, feet, legs, hands, and around the external genitals are characteristic signs. The growths may join to form large masses and may become ulcerated. *See also* JUNGLE ROT; LEPROSY.

YEAST. In the compressed form with a starchy or absorbent base, yeast is used medically because of its richness in the water-soluble vitamins, including *thiamine, riboflavin, pyridoxine, nicotinic acid,* and *pantothenic acid.* Dried yeast or *brewer's yeast* is frequently fortified with vitamins of the B complex group.

YELLOW FEVER, an acute infectious disease caused by a filterable virus which is transmitted by the bite of an infected mosquito, *aëdes aegypti,* in whose system the virus lives and breeds. The illness strikes suddenly, usually three to six days after the mosquito bite. The face becomes flushed and swollen, the eyes suffused, the lips and tongue a bright red, and a high fever appears, with pain in the head and back, and a feeling of extreme exhaustion. In two or three days, the temperature drops below normal, the pulse slows down, and the skin grows cold and assumes the yellow jaundiced hue, which gives the disease its name. A characteristic *black vomit* occurs, indicating *intestinal bleeding.* As the patient recovers, the temperature returns to normal, generally by the seventh or eighth day, and convalescence begins, leading to rapid, complete recovery. Complications are rare, and one attack gives lifelong immunity.

Until the twentieth century, large areas of Central and South America were considered uninhabitable because of the disastrous effects of yellow fever. A considerable portion of the population along the southern Atlantic and Gulf seaboard was wiped out in one of the yellow fever epidemics. The first indication that the disease was transmitted by the bite of a mosquito came from Dr. Carlos Finlay, a Cuban, in 1881. Two decades later, Dr. Walter Reed, an American army surgeon, proved that yellow fever was transmitted solely by the bite of an infected mosquito. This led to such effective mosquito control that today yellow fever has been eradicated in much of its former domain.

Studies show that yellow fever is present in the jungles of South America and Africa. It is found in monkeys and possibly in other jungle animals. Human beings are also affected by the germ, which is easily transmitted where poor sanitary conditions prevail.

International health authorities have concerned themselves with preventing the spread of yellow fever into urban communities. In 1951, the Nobel Prize was awarded to Dr. Max Theiler of the Rockefeller Foundation for his development of a vaccine, *17-B*, for yellow fever. The vaccine was given to more than 8,000,000 members of the armed forces during World War II.

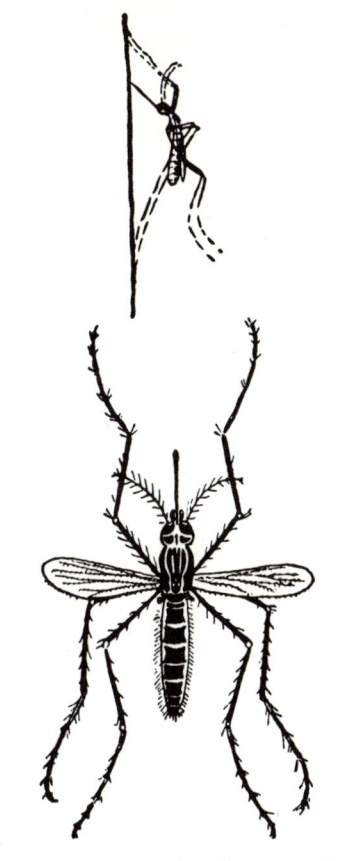

Yellow Fever—Female aëdes aegypti mosquito (enlarged). These mosquitoes transmit the yellow fever virus from infected persons to uninfected persons. Vaccinations against yellow fever have helped to control the disease.

The greatest precautions are taken to prevent introduction of infected mosquitoes onto airplanes and ships. Crews are vaccinated against the disease and ships are fumigated. Persons who are infected are isolated in a screen-protected room for at least the first four days after development of symptoms of yellow fever. The United States Public Health Service, the World Health Organization, and quarantine agencies all over the world are constantly alert to the threat of mosquito disease carriers. Breeding places are sprayed with DDT or oil to kill the larvae, and such measures in recent years have kept the spread of yellow fever at a minimum. *See also* MALARIA; DENGUE.

YELLOW JAUNDICE. *See* JAUNDICE.

ZINC, a metallic element which occurs naturally as *silicate* and *carbonate* and is known as *calamine* in these forms. The uses of zinc in medicine are chiefly as a component of *zinc chloride* and *zinc oxide* and similar preparations used in treating the skin. These are combined with ointments and dusting powders.

A poisonous compound of zinc and phosphorous is used as an ingredient of *rat poison*.

ZYGOMA, that part of the temple bone of the skull that lies beneath the cheek; it is also known as the *zygomatic arch*. Some of the muscles involved in mastication of food are attached to it. It is sometimes involved in fracture of the skull.

ZYGOTE, a *fertilized ovum*—in effect, a new living individual. A zygote is produced by union of a spermatozoon with the nucleus of the ovum. *See also* REPRODUCTION SYSTEM; OVULATION; PREGNANCY, SIGNS OF.

ZYME, a word derived from the Greek, meaning *ferment*. Many different forms of ferment are used in medicine—for example, to dissolve secretions. The *zymogenic cells* of the stomach are those which secrete *pepsin*, which is useful in digesting the protein foods.

Index

A

abasia, 17
abdomen, 17, 19
abdomen, distention, 1049
abdomen, enlargement of, 940
abdomen, increased size in pregnancy, 1076
abdominal examination, 19
abdominal hernias, 752-53
abdominal pain, 17-19
abdominal region, tuberculosis of, 1278
abdominal supports, 20
abductor, 20
abductor auris, 20
abductor position, 1180
ablation, 20
ABO system, 1116
abortion, 20-21
abortive poliomyelitis, 1057
abortus fever, 21
abrasion, 21, 1365
abruptio, 21
abruptio placentae, 21
abscess, 21-22, 853, 1049
abscess, lung, 862-63, 866
abscess, liver, 855
abscess, teeth, 1249
absorption, 22
absorption system, 745
abulia, 22
Acarus scabiei, 1158
accessory sex organs, 22
accessory spleens, 1215
accidents, 22-24

accommodation, 24, 592
accumulators, 883
acetanilid, 24, 107, 884, 966-67
acetanilid poisoning, 1054
acetazoleamide, 503
acetest, 25
acetic acid, 24, 25
acetone, 25, 967, 1155
acetophenetidin, 81
acetylene gas, 967
acetylene welding workers, 803
acetylsalicylic acid, 25, 81, 884
ache, 25
Achilles' tendon, 25, 928
achlorhydria, 25, 26
acholia, 25-26
achondroplasia, 26, 739
Achromycin, 26
achylia, 26
acid, 26
acid intoxication, 403
acid poisoning, 26, 1053
acidosis, 25, 26-27, 67, 480, 489, 823, 978, 986, 1198
acids, inflammation from, 962
acids, swallowing, 26
acne, 27-33, 612, 1090, 1190
acne rosacea, 33, 612, 777
acne vulgaris, 28
aconite, 34, 852
acoustic nerve, 34
acoustical heartbeat analyzer, 883
acquired cretinism, 931
acquired hemolytic anemia, 34, 1115
acriflavine, 34

acrodynia, 34
acromegaly, 34-37, 739, 817, 1040, 1191
acrophobia, 35
ACTH, 35, 53, 70, 78, 137, 147, 157, 287, 691, 761, 764, 766, 843, 867, 942, 1021, 1041, 1097, 1115, 1139, 1164, 1184, 1215, 1260
actinomyces, 35
actinomycosis, 35, 38, 663, 964
active immunization, 1327
acupuncture, 38, 39
acute bacterial endocarditis, 170
acute benzene poisoning, 193
acute bronchitis, 278-79
acute catarrhal jaundice, 856
acute diseases, 910
acute ear infection, 528
acute gastritis, 674
acute glomerulonephritis, 232, 937, 940
acute hepatitis, 855
acute illness, 39
acute infectious jaundice, 856
acute intussusception, 812
acute laryngitis, 837
acute lead poisoning, 840
acute leukemia, 843, 1351
acute nephritis, 938-39, 940
acute obstructive laryngitis, 466
acute otitis, 991
acute pain, 39
acute pancreatitis, 1006-7

acute perforation, 1028
acute peritonitis, 812
acute pharyngitis, 1032
acute tonsillitis, 39-40, 817, 1032, 1268-69, 1308
acute uremia, 1308
acute viral hepatitis, 856
Adam's apple, 40
addiction, 40
addiction, narcotic, 522, 896, 914-15, 935
Addisonian syndrome, 1240
Addison's disease, 40-41, 42-43, 53, 887, 1041
adductor, 41
adenitis, 41
adenocarcinoma, 45
adenoidal virus, 112
adenoidectomy, 41, 427
adenoid face, 44-45
adenoids, 41-45, 399-400, 530, 951, 991, 1198, 1227
adenoma, 45, 262, 293, 684
adenosis, 46
adhesiectomy, 46
adhesions, 46
adhesive tape, 885
adiposis, 46
adiposis dolorosa, 46
adjustment problems of the school-age child, 46-48
Adler, 1085
adnexa, 48
adnexa oculi, 48
adnexa uteri, 48
adolescence, 48-50, 636-38, 897
adolescence, feminine hygiene, 636-37

adoption, 50-52
adrenal cortex, 53, 226, 684, 765, 1040
adrenal cortical extract, 456
adrenal cortical insufficiency, 1008
adrenal cortices, diminished function of, 1008
adreno-cortico-trophic hormone, 1041
adrenal glands, 40, 137, 226, 684, 1157
adrenal medulla, 684
adrenalin, 52, 70, 142, 226, 232, 270, 571, 774, 805
adrenals, 52-54
adrenocortico-trophic hormone, 35
adventitia, 409
aëdes aegypti mosquito, 54, 482, 871, 872, 915, 1108, 1370, 1371
aero otitis media, 54, 428
aerobic, 54, 169
aerophagia, 54
affect, 54
affection, 897
afferent nerves, 54, 943
African sleeping sickness, 563, 792
after baby arrives, 640
afterbirth, 55
afternoon fever, 951
afterpains, 55
agalactia, 55
agar, 55, 323
agar-agar, 55
age and weight, 1292

1373

INDEX

age-weight-height tables, 1345-47
agglutination, 55
agglutinin, 239
agglutinogen, 239
aging, 55-58
agnosia, 58
agoraphobia, 58
Agote, Luis, 238
agranulocytosis, 58-59, 150, 867
agricultural sprays, 899
ague, 59
ainhum, 59
air bacteriology, 961
air cells, dilation of, 866
air conditioning, 59-61
air conduction, 476
air pollution, 61
air sickness, 61, 916-17
air suction, 1237
air swallowing, 61
akinetic, 61
albinism, 804, 1337
albino, 61-62
albumin, 62, 219, 908, 937, 1083, 1300, 1313
albuminuria, 62, 402, 827, 937-40, 1313
alcohol, 62-64, 89, 349, 518
alcohol intake, excessive, 505, 857
alcoholic psychosis, 896
alcoholism, 64-66, 481, 896
alcoholism, chronic, 948
aldosterone, 41, 52
alexia, 66
alimentary canal, 66
alimentary tract, 1224
alimentation, 66
alkalemia, 66, 67
alkali, 66-67
alkali inflammations, 962
alkali poisoning, 1053
alkalinity, 67
alkaloid, 67
alkalosis, 67
allergenic substances, 1184
allergens, 68, 436
allergens, removal of, 1097
allergic asthma, 141-47
allergic diseases of skin, 440-41
allergic salute, 68
allergy, 67-71
allergy and emotions, 560-61
allergy in children, 71-72
allergy to protein, 1097
alloys, 484
aloes, 72
alopecia, 72, 171, 697
alopecia areata, 72, 171, 174
alopecia cachetica, 72

alpha emanations, 974
altitude sickness, 72-73, 1199
alum, 73
aluminum, 73
aluminum acetate, 73
aluminum dust, 803
aluminum hydroxide, 74, 1024
aluminum hydroxide gel, 73
aluminum phosphate gel, 74
aluminum powders, colored, 969
alveolar, 817
alveolar abscess, 695
alveolar bone, 1246
alveoli, 74, 861
amanita muscaria, 929
amanita phalloides, 929
amaurosis, 74
ambivalence, 74
ameba, 788
amebiasis, 74-75, 76-77, 505, 855
amebic dysentery, 74, 75, 76-77, 164, 789, 792
amebic hepatitis, 74
amenorrhea, 75
amentia, 75
American Heart Association, 75
American trypanosomiasis, 334-35
amidopyrine, 58
aminion, 79
amino acids, 78, 954, 1083
amino acid deficiency, 1083
aminophylline, 78
aminopterin, 78-79, 305
aminopyrine, 708
Ammi majus, 858, 1337
ammonia, 67, 79, 852, 1169, 1313
ammonia, dilute, for insect bites, 805
ammonia gas, 967
ammoniated mercury, 782, 1085
ammoniated mercury ointment, 911
ammonium chloride, 889
ammonium hydroxide, 79
amnesia, 79, 950
amnesia, auditory, 79
amnesia, post-traumatic, 79
amobarbital, 178
amog, 79-80
amphetamine, 80, 177, 192, 914, 935
amplifiers, 883
amputation, 80
amylase, 80
amylnitrate, 96
amylnitrate inhalation, 1055
amyloid diseases, 1214
amyotrophic diseases, 80

amyotrophic lateral paralysis, 948
amyotrophic lateral sclerosis, 80, 643
amyl alcohol, 967
Amytal, 178, 885, 1054
anacidity, 26
anaerobic, 54, 169
Anahist, 108
anal canal, 811
anal fistula, 648
anal sphincter, 741
analgesia, 80-81
analgesics, 80, 178, 884, 948
anaphia, 81
anaphylaxis, 81
anastomoses, 456
anatomy, 1237
anatomy of teeth, 1245-46
ancylostoma duodenale, 81
androgen, 81, 893
androgyny, 81
anemia, 81-85, 612, 718, 790, 843, 894, 1024, 1111, 1299, 1351, 1360
anemia, hemolytic, 82, 573, 740, 1111
anemia, hemolytic, acquired, 34, 1115
anemia, hemolytic, of newborn, 241
anemia, cerebral, 257
anemia, chronic infection, 1114
anemia, Mediterranean, 886, 1114
anemia, pernicious, 18, 84, 85-87, 222, 858, 1029, 1114, 1214, 1333
anemia, pregnancy, 83
anemia, secondary, 50, 1364
anemia, severe, 953
anemia, sickle cell, 83, 1114, 1181
anemias, nutritional, 83
anemic, 1116
anesthesia, 87-90, 1232, 1237
anesthesia, spinal, 87
anesthesia, closed system administration, 89-90
anesthetics, 178
aneurysm, 90, 92-93
angina pectoris, 91-96, 233, 450, 718, 996, 1106, 1239
angina, Vincent's, 96
angioma, 1286
angiotonin, 226
angular cheilosis, 479
angular stomatitis, 480
aniline, 24, 96-97, 975
aniline dye, 974
aniline oil, 966, 967
animal bites and wounds, 97
aniseikonia, 97-98
ankle, 98
ankylosis, 98, 536, 819, 820
anodontia, 1247
anodyne, 99, 852

anopheles mosquito, 54, 482, 871, 872, 915, 1108, 1370, 1371
anorexia, 99, 1008
anterior chamber, iris, 591
anorexia nervosa, 99, 121
anosmia, 99, 1196
anoxemia, 99
Ansolysen, 108
Antabuse, 64, 65, 99, 812
antacid, 99, 1024
antenatal, 99
antepartum, 99
anterior choroidal artery, 949
anterior pituitary, 1040, 1343
anterograde amnesia, 79
anthrax, 99-100, 787, 960-61, 964, 1214
anti-anemic factor of liver, 1333
antibacterial ointment, 815
antibiotics, 663, 691, 790, 797, 843, 853, 876, 885, 892, 985, 991, 993, 1029, 1052, 1082, 1153, 1184, 1192, 1219, 1225, 1231, 1271, 1291, 1305
antibody(ies), 67, 107, 216, 780, 781, 855, 1064, 1083, 1327, 1350
anticoagulant, 107, 418, 1110, 1261
antidotes, poisoning, 107, 1052-56
antifebrin, 107
antifever drugs, 402
anti-friction agents, 971
antigenic, 1116
anti-hemorrhagic vitamin, 1336
antihistamines, 70, 147, 761, 949
antihistaminic drugs, 107-108, 427, 522, 1184
antihistaminic lotions, 815
anti-hypertensives, 108
antimalarial drugs, 108-109
antimicrobe action of blood, 780
antimicrobial therapy, 427
antimony, 109, 197, 842
antimony compounds, 822
antimony poisoning, 899
antiperspirants, 637
antipyretic, 402, 884
antirabies serum, 1103
antirabies vaccine, 1103
anti-Rh factor, 241
antirickettsial vaccines, 1150
antisepsis, 1232
antiseptics, 109-110, 885
antiseptic ointments, 1357

anti-scurvy vitamin, 1334
antispasmodics, 949
antithrombin, 855
antitoxin, 110, 169, 781, 804, 1303
antivenom serum, 1197
antrum, 110, 1184
ANTU, 1110
Anturan, 131, 691
anuria, 110
anus, 111, 1110
anxiety, 111, 558, 621
anxiety attack, 111
aorta, 91, 111, 112, 175, 223, 224, 407
aorta, coarctation, 232
aortic valve, 714
apathy, 559
APC viruses, 112
aphasia, 66, 112-113, 1206
aphonia, 113, 1206
aphrodisiac, 113
aplastic anemia, 113, 150, 1115
apocrine, 243
apocrine glands, 113, 1187
apoplexy, 113-114, 233, 1009, 1198, 1226, 1228-29
appendectomy, 910
appendicitis, 114-121, 217, 232, 420, 463, 519, 804, 1029
appendicular bones, 1184
appendix, 18, 1322
appetite, 121-122
appetite loss, 921, 940, 1024, 1329
Apresoline, 108, 236
aqueous humor, 122, 591
arachnodactyly, 122
arachnoid, 889
arches, fallen, 122
Arctic health, 122-124, 706
arginine, 78
Argyrol, 122, 124
argyrosis, 124, 978
Aristocort, 457
arm(s), 124, 248, 1184
aromatic cascara, 884
arrector muscle, 1187
arrhythmia, 718
arsenic, 505, 887, 977, 1054, 1115
arsenic poisoning, 816, 899, 948, 962, 967-68, 969, 973, 979, 1054
arsenical compounds, 74
arsenical preparations, 1323
artane, 949
arterial bleeding, 1365
arterial blood, 408
arterial thrombosis, 1260
arteriolar nephrosclerosis, 937
arterioles, 223, 407
arteriosclerosis, 94, 108, 124-30, 234, 404, 418, 450, 620,

INDEX

699, 804, 950, 953, 954, 1173
arteriosclerosis, cerebral, 233, 328, 896, 1173
arteriosclerosis obliterans, 129
arteriosclerosis, peripheral, 129
arteriovenous aneurysms, 227
artery(ies), 130, 223, 407, 408, 611, 714, 1091, 1319
arteries, contraction, 1239
arthritis, 130-138, 819, 1049, 1173, 1185
arthritis, degenerative, 136
arthritis, degenerative, sacroiliac joint, 860
arthritis, painful migratory, 1138
arthritis, rheumatoid, 131, 134-35, 834, 860, 1145
articulation, 1206
artificial kidney, 828-34
artificial limbs, 138
artificial pneumothorax, 477, 1285
artificial respiration, 139, 140-41, 1053, 1133
artificial ventilation, 1322
artificially radioactivated iodine, 1106
asbestos, 963, 968
asbestos corns, 139
asbestos fiber, 803
asbestosis, 139, 524, 803, 968
ascarid, 139
Ascaris lumbricoides, 1357
ascending colon, 253, 811
Aschheim-Zondek test, 139, 342, 1041, 1252-53
ascites, 651
ascorbic acid (vitamin C), 139, 908, 1328, 1334, 1336
ascorbic acid, food sources of, 1333, 1334
asepsis, 139
ash, 908
asparaginase, 308
asphalt, 968
asphyxia, 139-141
asphyxiant, 967, 970, 972, 973
asphyxiation, 979
aspiration, 141
aspirin, 25, 81, 108, 138, 141, 708
assassin, 875
astasia, 141
astasia-abasia, 141
asthenia, 141
asthenic, 1292
asthenopia, 141
asthma, 67, 68, 141-47, 157, 612, 1088
astigmatism, 97, 147-48, 447, 592, 593, 597, 610
astragalus, 98, 628

atabrine, 109, 148, 872, 1100
ataxia, 148
atelectasis, 148-149
athlete's foot, 149-150, 789, 792, 1238, 1352
atomic bomb, 150-151, 1104
atomic energy in medicine, 151-155
atomic fallout protection, 613-17
atomizer, 886
atopic dermatitis, 156-157
atrophic pharyngitis, 1033
atrophic rhinitis, 1002
atrophy, 157, 855, 928, 1191
atropine, 157, 473, 603, 805, 929, 1367
attenuated viruses, 1327
atypical lymphocytes, 1351
auditory amnesia, 79
augmentation of heartbeat, 1239
auditory canal, 526
auditory nerve, 157
auditory tube, 576
aural vertigo, 889
aureomycin, 40, 75, 101, 120, 157, 564, 754, 826, 842, 870, 885, 911, 1022, 1052, 1118, 1174, 1286, 1327
auriatricarboxylate, 1327
auricle, 157, 406, 710
auricle, left, 408
auricle, right, 407
auricular diastole, 714
auricular dilation, 714
auricular fibrillation, 643, 1092
auricular systole, 714
auriculo-ventricular node, 718
auscultation, 156, 157
autogenous, 1317
autoinoculation, 1339
autonomic nervous system, 157, 943, 1239-40
autopsy, 157
average weight, 1345
average weight of groups, 1292
axial bones, 1184
axilla, 636
axons, 943

B

babies, premature, 158-64, 1077
baby, care of in hot weather, 394-95
bacillary dysentery, 74, 164-65, 505
bacilli, 165
bacillus, 789
bacillus anthracis, 961
bacillus, common colon, 1225
bacillus subtilis, 106

bacitracin, 101, 783, 842
backache, 165-67, 799
backache, abdominal supports for, 20
backbone, 167, 1192, 1208, 1322
bacteremia, 167-69, 790, 1174
bacteria, 169-70, 788, 792, 1005, 1225
bacterial endocarditis, 170-71
bacteria culture, 168
bacterial endocarditis, acute, 170
bacterial endocarditis, subacute, 172-73
bacterial infection, 855, 1244
bacterial infections of skin, 314-15
bacterial pneumonia, 1052
bactericide, 171
bacteriological diagnosis, 1275
bacteriophages, 171, 1326
bacteriostatic, 171
bad breath, 699
bagasse dust, 803
bagassosis, 803
bakelite, 968
baking soda (bicarbonate of soda; sodium bicarbonate), 27, 67, 404, 507, 547, 885, 1198-99
baking soda and water paste, 805
BAL, 899, 900
balance, 526
balance sense impaired, 1008
balanitis, 171
Balantidial colitis, 171
balantidiasis, 171
balantidium, 171
baldness, 171-75, 697, 804
baldness gene, 804
baldness, hereditary, 697
baldness, temporary, 697
ball-and-socket joints, 250, 818
ballistocardiography, 175-76
bananas, ripe, 1212
Bancroft's filariasis, 176, 645
bandage, 176
bandages, ready-made sterilized, 885
bandages, sterile gauze, 885
bandaging, 545
Banting, Frederick G., 807
Banti's disease, 176, 1214
Banti's syndrome, 1215
barber's itch, 176-77
barbiturate poisoning, 177, 1054-55

barbiturate(s), 177-79, 708, 1054
barbiturate sedatives, 948
barbituric acid, 177, 885
bare nerve endings, 1187
barium, 298, 1024
barium enema, 1368
barium, opaque meal of, 1368
barium sulphate, 179
barium sulphide, 179
barium sulphite, 179
barium test, 518
Barlow's disease, 179
Barnard, Christian N., 985
Bartholin's glands, 180, 1318, 1337, 1338
basal ganglia, 180
basal metabolic rate, 1301
basal metabolism, 180, 341
basal metabolism test, 689, 770, 1106, 1252-53
base, skull, 1191
base, tongue, 1258
Basedow's disease, 180, 1017
basidiomycetous fungi, 929
bathing, 181
bathing, baby, 367-68
bathing, during menstruation, 638
bauxite, 803
BCG vaccine, 181
BCG vaccination, 477
beard, ringworm of, 1153
bed and bedding, 181-83
bed rest, 802, 941
bed sores, 184-85
bed wetting, 185-86, 364-65
bedbug, 183-85, 805, 1118
bedpan, 886
bee stings, 97, 186, 549
beef, 882
beef tapeworm, 1356, 1361
beers and malt liquors, 63
behavior, 186-89, 1088
behavior, criminal, 896
behaviorists, 186
belching, 189
Bell, Charles, 189
belladonna, 189, 473, 852, 949, 1042, 1270
Bell's palsy, 189-92
Benadryl, 108, 131, 186, 192
"bends," 192, 288-89, 429, 787
beneficial underweight, 1304
Benemid, 131, 691
benign fibromas, 644
benign growths or tumors, 293, 1286
benign tertian malaria, 109

benoquin, 858
benzathine penicillin G, 106
Benzedrine, 121, 177, 192-93, 914, 935
benzene, 967, 968, 979, 1054, 1115
benzene hexachloride, 1158
benzene poisoning, 193, 1054-55
benzine, 968, 973
benzoic acid, 1352
benzol, 968, 979
benzyl benzoate, 1165
benzyl benzoate emulsion, 847
beriberi, 193-96, 478, 948, 954, 1257, 1329
beryllium, 968-69
beryllium copper, 969
beryllium disease, 803
beryllium glass, 969
beryllium poisoning, 899
Best, Charles, 807
bestiality, 196, 1199
beta emanations, 974
bicarbonate of soda (baking soda; sodium bicarbonate), 27, 67, 404, 507, 547, 885, 1198-99
biceps, 196, 928
bichloride of mercury, 196, 901, 1056
bichromates, 969
biconcave lens, 842
biconvex lens, 842
bicuspid, 196
bifocal, 196-97
bifocal lenses, 196
bile, 197, 208, 435, 854
bile acids, 435
bile ducts, 817, 854
bile excess, 816
bile passages, obstruction of, 816
bile pigments, 854
bile salts, 197, 854
bilharziasis, 197-98, 792
biliary colic, 197, 668
biliary disease, 1005
biliousness, 198
bilirubin, 198, 1111, 1116
Binet, Alfred, 199
Binet-Simon test, 198-99
Binet-Stanford intelligence test, 809
binocular, 594
biomicroscope, 600
biopsy, 199, 262, 298, 1157
biotelemetry, 1205
biotin, 1328, 1334
birth, caul at, 327
birth certificate, 199
birth control, 199-202, 1146
birth injuries, 202-4, 807
birth, multiple, 205-6
birthmark, 204-5
bismuth, 206, 1152, 1339

1375

INDEX

bismuth poisoning, 1323
bismuth subcarbonate, 207
bissynosis, 803
bisulphide of carbon, 969
bite, (animal), 1326
bite wounds, 549
biting flies, 805
black damp, 979
Black Death, 1044
black eye, 607
black fever, 207, 822
black vomit, 1370
black widow spider bite, 97, 207, 549, 805
blackheads (acne), 27-33
blackwater fever, 207, 792
bladder, 208, 1313
bladder diseases, 208-10
bladder, exstrophy of, 1309-12
bladder, urinary, 207-8
Blaiberg, Philip, 985
blasting workers, 976
blastomycosis, 210-11, 663, 961
bleeder's disease, 740
bleeding, 211, 257, 1092
bleeding, abnormal, 1336
bleeding, arterial, 1365
bleeding peptic ulcer, 814
bleeding, prolonged, 843
bleeding tooth socket, 545
bleeding, vaginal, 21
blepharitis, 211-12
blindness, 1241
blisters, 211-12, 484, 662
bloating, 212
blocking polyps, 1184
blood, 212-20, 1299
blood, abnormal states of, and itching, 815
blood, antimicrobe action of, 780
blood bank, 220-21
blood cholesterol, decline in, 1008
blood, circulation, 903, 943, 1213
blood clot(ting), 217, 417, 854, 1252-53, 1336
blood clot(ting), spontaneous, 1115
blood coagulation, 221-22
blood conditions, 222-23
blood cross matching, 466
blood cultures, 564
blood groups, 1116
blood groups, incompatible, 910
blood loss, 814, 1177
blood, oxygen-carrying power of, 970
blood plasma, 219-20
blood platelets, 217-18, 221, 741, 1092, 1259
blood poisoning, 223
blood pressure, 223-25, 586
blood pressure, control of, 225-26
blood pressure, elevation in, 940
blood pressure, high, 226-36, 605, 755, 1173
blood pressure, low, 236-37, 860, 1008
blood pressure, normal, 237
blood pressure test, 1252-53
blood serum, 1327
blood shunting, surgery for, 237-38
blood sugar, 685, 814
blood supply, 924
blood transfusion, 83, 137, 213-15, 219-20, 238-39, 843, 1219, 1232
blood types, 239-41
blood vessel(s), 223, 224, 1191, 1246
blood vessel destruction, 1028
blood vessels, dilation, 1177
blood vessel grafts, 225
blood vessel, nerves, 943
blows, 953
blue baby, 241-42
blue discoloration, skin, 966-67
blushing, 242
body, 242-43
body (spinal cord), 1322
body build, 1292, 1343
body fat and weight, 1298, 1299, 1344
body (louse) lice, 243, 847, 1271, 1290
body muscle, 924
body odor, 243-44
body odors, feminine hygiene and, 637, 639
body, ringworm of, 1152
body surface area, 1343
Boeck's sarcoid, 244
boil(s), 22, 244, 314-15, 529, 534, 666, 1022, 1238
bolus, 253
Bonamine, 349, 889, 916
bone bank, 244
bone cancer, 153
bone conduction, 476
bone marrow, 248, 1092
bone marrow deficiency disease, 84
bone(s), 244-51, 1246, 1303
bones, broken, 545, 1368
bones, diagnosis of broken, 1368
bones, formation and growth, 1335
bones, pain in, 843

bones, tuberculosis of, 1278
booster dose, 251
borax, 251, 1169
boric acid, 251, 1366
boric acid poisoning, 1055
boric acid, saturated, 109, 150
Borneholm disease, 251, 486
boring pain, 1003
Borrelia, 1323
botulism, 110, 251-52, 654
boutonneuse fever, 1153
bowel, 252
bowel control, 365-66
bowels, infections, 1239
Bowen, John T., 253
Bowen's disease, 253
box elder blossom, 704
brachial, 254
brachial artery, 225
brachial nerve, 945
brachycardia, 1092
brachydactyly, 254
Braille, Louis, 254
Braille system, 254
brain, 254-56, 408, 900, 943, 1191, 1207
brain blood vessels, distention of, 905
brain center, vision, 591
brain concussion, 256-57
brain hemorrhage, 257, 1009
brain injury at birth, 807
brain lesions, 949
brain tumor 257-62, 308-9
brain, water on, 766
brain waves, 262
brass, 969
brass chills, 979
brass dust, 969
brass founders' ague, 59
brass workers' ague, 979
Brassica, 930
breast, 262-68, 682, 921
breast cancer, 262, 266-67, 295, 1003
breast feeding, 368-69, 624-25
breast, self-examination, 264-65
breasts, pendulous, 263-64
breastbone, 1184
breath, bad, 699
breath, shortness of, 1308
breathing, 268-69, 587
breathing, rapid, 799
brewer's yeast, 1370
Bright, Richard, *937, 942*
Bright's disease, 270, 313, 505, 666, 783, 827, 937, 940
Brill's disease, 270, 1290, 1291
British anti-lewisite (BAL), 899, 900

broken bones, 545, 1368
bromide(s), 236, 270, 570, 944
bromidrosis, 243-44, 270, 1032
bromism, 270
bromouridine, 309
bronchi, 337, 910
bronchial asthma, 270-71, 272-73
bronchial tubes, 268
bronchiectasis, 271-76, 861, 976
bronchioles, 337, 861
bronchitis, 276, 277, 278-79, 425, 612, 799, 866, 930, 976, 978, 1291
bronchitis, chronic, 278-79
bronchopneumonia, 276-77, 426, 880, 1049, 1196, 1353
bronchoscopy, 217, 298
bronchus, 861
bronze powders, 969
bronze workers, 969
brow ague, 59
Brucella bacteria, 1305
brucellosis, 277, 961
bruises, 277-80, 401, 546, 953, 1364
bubas, 280, 1370
bubo, 280, 335, 870
buboes, 870, 1044
bubonic plague, 280, 797, 1044, 1109
Buerger's disease, 280-81, 282-83, 852, 1266
bulb, 281
bulb, hair follicle, 1187
bulbar, 281
bulbar poliomyelitis, 281
bulbo-urethral glands, 281, 462, 1126, 1309
bulimia, 935
bulk laxatives, 884
bullae, 1190
bumps, 418
bumps, the, 281
bundle of His, 718
bunion, 281-86, 628, 633
burning pain, 1003
burns, 286, 547, 934
burns, acid, 26
Burow's solution, 150, 815
burrs, 1244
bursa, 286, 633, 820, 1178
bursae, knee, 834
bursitis, 284-85, 286-87, 820, 834, 1145
butacaine sulphate, 287
Butazolidin, 131, 691
butter, 1335, 1336
buttocks, 287
butyl alcohol, 969-70
butyn, 287

C

cachexia, 764
cadmium, 956, 970
cadmium oxide fumes, 899
cadmium poisoning, 656, 899

cadmium workers disease, 804
Caesarian operation, 288, 289
Caesarian section, 289, 334, 349
caffein(e), 177, 419, 884
Caisson disease, 288-89, 787
caking, 368
calamine, 289, 1372
calamine lotion, 150
calcification, 1323
calcium, 155, 289-90, 348, 771, 908, 934, 956, 1147, 1245, 1249
calcium carbonate, 245
calcium deficiency, 1343
calcium fluoride, 652
calcium, food sources of, 1334
calcium gluconate, 900
calcium lactate tablets, 1219
calcium magnesium silicate, 968
calcium oxide, 852, 973
calcium phosphate, 245
calcium propionate talcum powder, 150
calcium-phosphorus ratio, 290
calcium salts, 1147
calcium triphosphate, 1036
calcium utilization, 1013, 1335
calculi, 403, 1016
calculus, 290-92
callipygian, 287
callus, 249, 291, 292, 628
calomel, 292, 901
calorie(s), 292, 293, 348, 1347
calorie deficiency, 873, 954
cancer, 293-305, 505, 804, 846, 964, 979, 993, 1044, 1082, 1114, 1173, 1185, 1342
cancer, bone, 153
cancer, breast, 262, 266-67, 295, 1003
cancer, cervix, 333-34
cancer, diagnosis, 199, 294
cancer, larynx, 189, 295, 838, 839
cancer, lung, cigar smoking and, 1197
cancer, lung, cigarettes and, 1197
cancer, colon and rectum, 300-1
cancer, lip, 853
cancer, lung, 864-65
cancer, mouth, 295
cancer, pancreas, 302-3, 1005
cancer, prostate, 1080-81
cancer, rectum, 300-1
cancer, skin, 1188-89
cancer-stimulating substances, 304

1376

INDEX

cancer, stomach, 296-97, 298, 1224
cancer, thyroid, 153
cancer, vulva, 1338
cancer, treatment of, 305-9
Candida albicans, 910
canine teeth, 196, 1247
canker sore, 309, 484
canned whole milk, 908
cantharides, 309-10
cantharidin, 309-10
Cantharis vasicatoria, 309
capillaries, 223, 310, 407, 408, 861, 1185
capillaries, increased permeability, 1104
capillary fragility, 954
capsule, 250
capsule, knee, 834
carbohydrates, 310, 954, 1345
carbolic acid, 109, 970
carbomycin, 101
carbon, 956, 1083
carbon bisulphide, 977
carbon dioxide, 212, 268, 310-11, 578, 970, 974, 977, 979
carbon dioxide snow, 1339
camp fever, 1290
camoquin, 872
camphor, 108, 292-93, 852, 1196
carbon disulfide, 311-12
carbon monoxide, 312-13, 548, 970, 974, 977, 979
carbon monoxide poisoning, 996
carbon, radioactive, 1108
carbon tetrachloride, 313, 886, 967, 970, 972, 977, 979
carbonated waters, 310
carbonylchloride, 976
carbuncles, 313-16, 853
carcinogens, 316
carcinoma, 316
cardiac, 317
cardiac and coronary, 317-18
cardiac catheterization, 715
cardiac cycle, 715
cardiac muscle, 924
cardiac neurosis, 734-35
cardiac treatment, 316
cardiovascular disease, 318
carditis, 318
care of baby in hot weather, 394-95
caries, dental, 318, 483, 1249
carminative, 318, 650
caronamide, 318, 564
carotene, 318, 956, 1328
carotid arteries, 408
carotid gland, 1286
carpal bones, 318

carriers of disease, 318-20, 1326
carrying injured, 546, 547
car sickness, 318, 916-17
cartilage, 250, 321, 834, 1192, 1322
cartilaginous discs, 1212
cascara, 321, 326
cascara sagrada, 321
casein, 321, 908
caseinogen, 321
cast, plaster, 928, 1180
castor oil, 321, 326, 884
castrati, 321-22
castration, 321-22, 1126, 1223
catalyst, 1088
cataplexy, 935
cataract, 322-23, 324-25, 594, 605, 1172
cataract glasses, 605
cataract, senile, 605
catarrh, 323
catarrhal jaundice, 816
catarrhal jaundice, acute, 856
catgut, 852
cathartic drugs, 505
cathartics, 323-26, 884
catheter, 208, 326, 1082
cathode-ray oscilloscope, 326-27
caudal anesthesia, 89
caul at birth, 327
causalgia, 327
caustics, 1339
cavernous hemangioma, 739
cavities, 327
cecum, 327, 422, 811
celiac disease, 327-28
cell, 328
cellulitis, 328
cement, tooth root, 1246
Centigrade, 1257
centipede, 549
central incisors, 1247
central nervous system, 943, 1207
ceramics, 484
cereals, whole-grain, 1332, 1335, 1336
cerebellum, 254, 260, 328, 333
cerebral, 328
cerebral anemia, 257
cerebral arteriosclerosis, 233, 328, 896, 1173
cerebral cortex, 328, 537
cerebral dysrhythmia, 328
cerebral hemispheres, 328
cerebral hemorrhage, 112, 113, 328, 418, 1173
cerebral palsy, 148, 204, 328-29, 330-31, 948, 949
cerebrospinal fluid, 329-32
cerebrospinal fever, 332
cerebrospinal meningitis, 332

cerebrum, 257, 260, 328, 332-33
cerumen, 530
cervical nerves, 1270
cervical rib, 1147
cervical vertebrae, 1322
cervix, 333-34, 638, 894, 1079, 1313
cesium-137, 154
cessation of menstruation, 1077
chafing, 334
Chagas' disease, 334-335, 792
chancre, 335, 1240
chancre, hard, 335
chancroid, 335, 792
change of climate, 1164
change of life, 892-93
changes in breasts, 1076
changes in skin, 1075-76
changes in uterus, 1076
changes in vagina, 1076
chapped skin, 335-36
chapping, lips, 853
characteristic of living matter, 1083
cheatinine, 826
cheek, 1191
cheese, 1190
cheilosis, 336-37, 479, 480
chemical poisoning, 816
chemicals, anti-microorganism, 797
chemicals, wart destroying, 1339
chemistry of skin, 336-37
chemopodium, oil of, 1361
chemotherapy, 308, 337
chemotherapy, cancer, 306
chest, 337
chickenpox, 337-40, 792, 793, 837, 1150, 1326, 1327
chiggers, 340, 805
chilblains, 340-41
child care, 353-401
child, adoption of, 50-52
childbirth afterpains, 55
childbirth and prenatal care, 341-52
childbirth, painless, 89
childhood, 634
childhood, second, 1117
children, adjustment problems of school-age, 46-48
children, allergy in, 71-72
children, lead poisoning, 900
children, mouth-to-mouth resuscitation, 1136
children, psychometric tests, 359-62
chill(s), 401-2, 799, 921, 1099
chiropractic, 402
chloasama, 402, 611, 858

chloral, 236
chlorambucil, 309
chloramphenicol, 101, 911, 1290
chloraquine, 109
chlordane, 1155
chloride of lime, 109, 517, 971
chlorinated hydrocarbons, 970, 972, 979
chlorine, 507, 971, 1157
chlorine, liberated, 971
chloroform, 89, 970, 1155
chloroform liniments, 852
chloromycetin, 101, 564, 1118, 1286, 1288, 1327
chlorophyll, 485
chloroprene, 174
chlorosis, 50, 402
chlorothiazide, 236
chlorpromazine, 65
chlorprophenpyridamine maleate, 108
chlortetracycline, 101, 157
Chlortrimeton, 108
chocolate, 1190
choice grade meats, 882
"chokes," the" 429
cholecystitis, 402, 669
cholecystography, 402-3
cholelithiasis, 403
cholera, 164, 403-04, 505, 782, 792, 796, 1342
cholesterin, 197
cholesterol, 404, 620, 1107
cholesterol, blood, decline in, 1008
choline, 1328, 1334
chondroma, 404, 1286
choraquine, 872
chordee, 405
chorea, 48, 405, 1205
chorion, 405
choroid layer, 591
chromates, 969
chromic acid, 969
chromidrosis, 1032
chromium, 969
chromium-51, 309
chromium, radioactive, 309
chromoblastomycosis, 406
chromosomes, 1130-31
chromosomes, sex, 1104, 1130-32
chronic, 406
chronic alcoholism, 948
chronic benzene poisoning, 193
chronic bronchitis, 278-79
chronic diseases, 910
chronic ear infection, 528
chronic gastritis, 64, 675
chronic glomerulonephritis, 937, 941
chronic hepatitis, 857

chronic illness, 39
chronic infection, anemia, 1114
chronic inflammation of nose and sinuses, 1238
chronic interstitial nephritis, 409
chronic intussusception, 812
chronic laryngitis, 838
chronic lead poisoning, 840
chronic leukemia, 843, 1351
chronic mastitis, 876
chronic osteoarthritis, 817
chronic otitis, 991
chronic otitis medea, 991
chronic pancreatitis, 1005
chronic pharyngitis, 1033
chronic prostatitis, 1079
chronic pyelonephritis, 232, 937
chronic rheumatoid arthritis, 820
chronic valvular disease, 1138
chrysanthemum buds, 971, 973
chrysarobin, 406, 1084
chymotrypsin, 605
CIBA, 1327
cigar smoking and lung cancer, 1197
cigarettes and lung cancer, 1197
cilia, 406
ciliary body, 591
ciliary muscle, 591
cimex lectularis, 183
cinchona, 1100
cineplasty, 138
circulation, blood, 903, 943, 1213
circulation stimulants, 852
circulation, systemic, 406, 407
circulatory disorders, 934
circulatory system, 218, 406-9
circumcision, 409, 1022
cirrhosis, 409-12, 855
cirrhosis, kidney, 1313
cirrhosis, liver, 409, 410-11, 954
citric acid, 26, 412
citrus fruits and juices, 1334, 1336
citrus rinds, 1336
claudication, intermittent, 852
claustrophobia, 58, 412
clavicle, 337, 412, 1185
cleaning fluids, 886
cleanliness, 391-92, 766-67
cleft palate, 412, 413, 1206
climate, 412-14
climate and skin color, 1038
clinitest, 414
clitoral orgasm, 1338

1377

INDEX

clitoris, 414, 1130, 1337, 1338
clonic convulsion, 446
clonic spasm, 504, 1205
closed fractures, 1191
Clostridium, 252
Clostridium botulinus, 252
clothes louse, 847
clothing, 414-16
clothing, baby, 394
clot(ting), blood, 217, 417, 854, 1252-53, 1336
clot(ting), blood, spontaneous, 1115
clotting time test, 1252-53
clubfoot, 416-18, 1243
coagulation, 1092
coagulation, electric, 853
coagulum, 417
coal oil poisoning, 1055
coal-tar distillation, 968
coarctation of aorta, 232
cobalt, 153, 956, 1333
cobalt-60, 153, 1107
cobalt-60 needle, 152
cobalt, radioactive, 152
cobra bite, 549, 1197
cocaine, 89, 192, 418
coccidioides immitis, 418
coccidioidomycosis, 418-19, 666, 755, 789, 792
coccus, 789
coccyx, 249, 419, 1322
cod liver oil, 349, 392, 419, 1339
codeine, 81, 419
coenzyme A, 1008
coffee, 419-20, 518
coitus, 420, 1177
colchicine, 131, 153, 420, 691
cold (disease), 399, 420, 530, 1032
cold, hazards of, 705-6
cold cream, 420
cold, neuritis and, 948
cold, sensation, 470, 1003, 1186
cold, sensitivity to, 932, 1301
cold sore, 420, 754, 756-57
cold vaccine, 426
cold weather, urination and, 1312
colic, 420-21
colic, biliary, 420
colic, intestinal, 420
colic, mucous, 421
colic, renal, 420, 421
colic, stomach, 421
colitis, 422, 1088
colitis, ulcerative, 1294-95
collagen diseases, 422-23, 457
collarbone, 412, 423, 867
collodion, 423

colloid, 688
colon, 422
colon, cancer, 300-1 431-36, 893, 1008, 1024, 1077, 1364
colon bacillus, common, 1225
color blindness, 423, 595-97, 804
color, eyes, 599
colored rings, seeing, 599
coloring, abnormal, 842
colostomy, 423
colostrum, 263, 350, 385, 625, 1076
Columbian spirits, 974
coma, 423-24, 986, 1308
comedos, 424
comma bacillus, 403
commercial grade meats, 882
common cold, 399, 424-27, 1145, 1198, 1199, 1322, 1326
common colon bacillus, 1225
common throat infection, 1022
common wood tick, 1153
communicable disease(s), 318, 427-28
compazine, 349
compensation, 903
compensatory hypertrophy, 773
complement fixation test, 1252-53
complemental air, 269
complete fistula, 648
complete proteins, 1083
compound fracture, 428, 1191
compress, 428
compresses, hot wet, 138
compression, 428-29
compression air disease, 288-89
compulsion, 429
computers, 429
concave lens, 842
conception, 343, 429, 1130, 1302
concussion, 429-30, 709, 1198, 1208
condensed milk, 908
conditioning, 430-31
condom, 201, 431, 443
conformation, 1292
congenital heart disease, 716-17
congenital polycystic kidneys, 232
congenital syphilis, 447, 1241
congestive heart failure, 1106
conjunctiva, 431, 560, 591, 984, 1040
conjunctival virus, 112
conjunctivitis, 251, 431, 432-33, 600-61, 880, 967, 977, 1196
conjunctivitis, allergic, 431
connective tissue, 1246

constant-flow bath, 1037
constipation, 323, 431-36, 893, 1008, 1024, 1077, 1364
constitution, 1292
constrictor fibers, 591
contact dermatitis, 149, 436-42, 934
contact lenses, 442
contagious, 318, 427
continuous bed rest, 1144
contraception, 442-43
contraction, arteries, 1239
contraction, heart, 1091
contrast bath, 633
control of disease, 1213
control of fluid, 1232
contused wound, 443
contusion, 443, 709
convalescence, 444-46
conversion hysteria, 111
conversion reactions, 776, 950
convex lens, 842
convulsion(s), 446, 648, 900, 1205
convulsions, babies, 401
convulsions, infantile, 649
convulsions in pregnancy (eclampsia), 532-33
convulsive epileptiform fit, 1308
cooking utensils, aluminum, 73
Cooley's anemia, 1114
copper, 855, 956
copper refining, 899
copper sulphate, 447
copperhead bite, 1197
copulation, 429, 755
coral snake bite, 549, 1197
corium, 1186
cornea, 147, 447, 591
corneal transplantation, 447, 606-7
corneal ulcer, perforated, 1079
cornified layer, 1186
Corning, J. L., 89
corns, 447, 628, 633
coronary, 317
coronary arteries, 219, 408, 418
coronary artery disease, 448-49
coronary circulation, 408
coronary disease, 317
coronary infarction, 317
coronary occlusion, acute, 447
coronary sclerosis, 317
coronary thrombosis, 233, 317, 404, 418, 447-56, 1336

corpora cavernosa, 1022
corpus cavernosum urethrae, 1022
corpus luteum, 909
corpus spongiosum, 1022
corpuscles, red, 417
corpuscles, white, 417
corrosive poison, 1052
cortex, 52, 235, 1157, 1206
Corticotropin, 457
cortin, 41
cortisone, 35, 41, 52, 70, 78, 137, 147, 157, 192, 257, 287, 456-57, 608, 691, 754, 761, 764, 843, 867, 942, 985, 990, 1008, 1021, 1041, 1097, 1115, 1157, 1164, 1184, 1215, 1219, 1260, 1351
coryza, 457
coryza, allergic, 457
cosmetic poisoning, 459-60
cosmetics, 457-60
cosmetics, allergy to, 71, 458, 459
costume jewelry sensitivity, 460-61
cotton fiber inhalation, 803
cotton, sterile, 885
cottonmouth bite, 1197
cottonwood, 704
cough, 461, 951, 1278
cough, persistent, 799
Cowper's glands, 462, 1126, 1309
cow's milk, 387-88, 1114
Coxsackie virus, 486
crab (louse) lice, 462, 847
cradle cap, 368
cramps, 462-63
cramps, night, 950-51
cranial nerve, fifth, 945, 1263
cranium, 818
cramps, 462-63, 1219
cranial nerve(s), 943, 1191
cranial nerve, fifth, 945
cranium, 1191, 1239
cream, 908
creams and lotions, cosmetic, 458-59
creams, contraceptive, 443
cremasteric muscles, 1207
cresol, 463, 517, 1290
cresylic acid, 870
cretin, 26, 774, 1262
cretinism, 247, 463, 464-65
cretinism, acquired, 931
criminal behavior, 896
criminal behavior, chromosomes and, 1131-32

Crohn's disease, 463, 780
cross-eyes, 466, 597
cross matching, blood, 466
croup, 466-67
crown, 1246
crust, 418, 1191
crying, 363, 467
cryptorchism, 1256
crystalline lens, 591
crystalline penicillin, 1323
culex mosquito, 915
cultural environment, 1088
cultural standards, 897
cunnilinction, 467, 764
curd, 417
curettage, 21, 298, 467, 871, 1316
curette, 467
curetted, 1316
Curie, Marie, 1108
Curie, Pierre, 1108
curvature of spine, 1185
Cushing's disease, 467, 1044
Cushing's syndrome, 467, 468-69, 1240
cusps, 196, 1246, 1247
cutaneous nerve(s), 470, 1186
cutaneous senses, 470
cuticle, 934, 1185
cuts, 401, 470, 1365
cutting occupations, 965
cutting pain, 1003
cyanide(s), 971-72, 979, 1055
cyanide poisoning, 470, 1055
cyanosis, 141, 470, 975, 1049
cyclizine hydrochloride, 108
cyclopropane, 90, 470
cycloserine, 477, 523
cylindrical lens, 842
cyst(s), 470-71, 775, 870, 894, 1274
cysts, pancreatic, 1005
cystic fibrosis, 471
cystitis, 208, 471-72
cystoscope, 209, 472

D

dactinomycin, 309
damp working conditions, 963
dandruff, 175, 473, 1168
daraprim, 109
dark skin, 1038
Darkfield method, 1241
Davy, Sir Humphry, 89
DDT, 473, 1155
DDT emulsion, 847
DDT powder, 847
DDT solution, 847
deadly nightshade poisoning, 473
deaf mutism, 473-74
deafness, 474, 921, 1241, 1267-70

1378

INDEX

death rates, fall in, 476
DeBakey, Michael, 733
debility, 1185
Decadron, 457
decay, dental, 477
decibel, 965
deciduous teeth, 1247
decreased elasticity of arteries, 227
defecation, 477
deficiency diseases, 477-80, 1190, 1328
deficiency disorders, 18
deformities, 1241
degenerative arthritis, 136
degenerative arthritis, sacroiliac joint, 860
degenerative diseases, 290, 480
degenerative joint disease, 987, 1145
dehydration, 480, 823, 1342
delinquency, 896
delirium, 480-81
delirium tremens, 64, 65, 481, 812
delivery, 481
delousing agents, 481
delusions, 481
dementia, 481, 1173
dementia paralytica, 1016
dementia praecox, 482
demulcent, 482
demyelinating diseases, 949
dendrons, 943
dengue (fever), 482-83, 915, 1157
dental antrum, 110
dental caries, 318, 483, 1249
dental health, 1249
dental research, current, 483-84
dentifrice, 484-85
dentin(e), 485, 1246
dentistry, 1368
dentition, 1246-47
denture, 485
deodorants, 109, 637
depilatory, 485-86, 637
depression, 486, 559, 1304, 1334
depressive reaction, 950
Dercum's disease, 46, 486
dermatitis, 486, 533, 815, 846, 967, 968, 971, 1190
dermatitis, contact, 149, 436-42, 934
dermatitis, seborrheic, 175, 1168, 1169, 1170-71
dermatomyositis, 423, 486
dermatophytid, 150
dermatophytosis, 149
dermatropic viruses, 1326
dermis, 1185, 1186
dermis, projections on, 1186
dermoid cyst, 486

descending colon, 253, 811
desensitization, 70, 701, 761
desert fever, 418, 486
desoxycorticosterone acetate, 41, 53
dessication, electric, 1339
detachment, retina, 605, 1137
determination of prothrombin time, 218
detumescence, 986
devil's grip, 486
Dexedrine, 121, 935
dextrose, 486, 685
dhobie itch, 487, 1151
diabetes, 27, 313, 342, 480, 487-503, 603, 605, 666, 783, 804, 948, 951, 1033, 1107, 1173, 1198, 1312, 1313, 1323
diabetes insipidus, 487, 503, 699, 1313
diabetes mellitus, 227, 487, 503, 806, 814, 986, 1005, 1313
diabetic coma, 489
diabetic shock, 1180
Dial, 1054
dialysis of kidneys, 828-34
diamox, 503, 518
diaper rash, 251, 503-4, 809
diaphenadione, 404
diaphragm, 116, 337, 504-5, 1337
diaphragm (contraceptive), 443
diaphragm with jelly or cream (contraceptive), 201
diaphragmatic hernia, 750-51
diarrhea, 74, 165, 505, 940, 1219, 1334, 1364
diarrhea, acute, 505
diarrhea, chronic, 505
diarrhea, infantile, infectious, 796
diarrhea, transitory, 505
diathermy machine, 1037
diastolic hypertension, 227
diastolic pressure, 223-24
diathermy, 138, 819, 1118
dichloro-difluoromethane, 972
dichlor-diphenyl-trichloro-ethane, 473
Dick test, 1252-53
dicumarol, 219, 221, 456, 1036, 1261, 1336
diet, 506
diet, Arctic, 123-24, 707
diet deficiency, 814
diet, digestive disorders, 506-7
diet, faulty, 1223

diet, high-caloric, 511
diet, high-carbohydrate, 511
diet, high-fat, 511
diet, high-protein, 511
diet, low-carbohydrate, 511
diet, low-protein, 511
diet, low-salt, 235, 507-8, 942
diet, nursing mothers, 369-85
diet, reducing, 508-9
diet, roughage in, 509-10
diet, salt-free, 511
diet, smooth, free from roughage, 510-11
diet, special, 511
dietary deficiencies, 791, 855
digestion, 511-12, 943, 1333
digestive disorders, diet in, 506-7
digestive disturbances, 512, 858
digestive glands, 682
digestive process, 854
digestive system, 512-13
digestive tract, 408
digestive tract ulcers, 1296-97
digitalis, 153, 513, 518, 643, 1108
dihydrocortisone, 52
dihydrochysterol, 771
dilantin, 270, 513
dilation, 333
dilation, auricular, 714
dilation, blood vessels, 1177
dilation, pupil, 1239
dilator, 591
dimenhydrinate, 520
dimethyl ketone, 967
dimethyl phthoilate, 916
dinitrobenzene, 972
Dipaxin, 404
diphenhydramine hydrochloride, 108
diphenylhydantoin sodium, 513
diphtheria, 466, 467, 513-16, 530, 782, 792, 793, 948, 991, 1303, 1323, 1353
diphtheria antitoxin, 110
diphtheria, toxin of, 513
diphtheria toxoid, 110, 516
diplegia, 1009
diplopia, 594
direct contact, 1326
disc, 516-17
discharges, respiratory tract, 799
discoloration, 841
discoloration, skin, 799
discoloration, skin, blue, 966-67
discoloration, teeth, 1248

disease, carriers of, 318-20, 1326
disease, control of, 1213
diseases, chronic, 910
disinfectants, 109
disinfection, 517
dislocation, 517-18, 536, 658-59, 818-19, 948, 1178, 1185
disordered functioning, 791
disorders and diseases of teeth, 1247-49
dissection, electrical, 1082
dissociative reaction, 950
distended stomach, 1219
distention of abdomen, 1049
distribution system, 745
diuresis, 518, 942, 1342
diuretics, 518
Diuril, 236
diver's palsy, 288-89
diverticula, 518
diverticulitis, 518-19
diverticulosis, 518
diverticulum, 519
divorce, 896
dizziness, 519, 548, 737, 893, 916, 917, 1323
dog bites, 519-20
dog rabies, 1102
dog tapeworm, 1364
dog tick, 1153
dominant eye, 594-95
DONV, 308
double focus, 196
double vision, 520
douches, 443, 520, 639
Down's syndrome, 520-21
Dramamine, 349, 520, 889, 916
dreams, 888
dressings, 521
dried milk, 908
dried skim milk, 908
drinking tube, glass, 886
dropsy, 507, 513, 521, 823, 841, 937, 1157, 1300
drowning, 521-22, 548
drowsiness, 548
drug addiction, 522
drug allergy, 522
drug inflammation, 962
drug injection, 804
drug management, 304
drugs, 948
drugs in tuberculosis, 523
dry gangrene, 673
dry heat, 138
"dry" pleurisy, 1045
dry skin, 458
DT, 523
Dumdum fever, 523, 822
duodenal ulcer, 523
duodenum, 253, 337, 523, 810, 817,

1004, 1024, 1097, 1224
dura, 256, 709
dura mater, 889
dust, 71, 523-24, 866, 963
dwarf tapeworm, 1361, 1364
dwarfism, 27, 247, 524, 661, 684, 739
dye inflammation, 962
dynamite head, 976
dyschesia, 435, 524
dysentery, 524, 1239, 1303, 1342
dysentery, amebic, 74, 75, 76-77, 164, 789, 792
dysentery, bacillary, 74, 164-65, 505
dysentery group, organisms of, 1230
dysmenorrhea, 524-25
dyspepsia, 525, 1313
dyspnea (dyspnoea), 91, 525, 975
dysuria, 1312

E

Eagle test, 1342
ear, 526-31
ear, drainage, 991
ear, external, 526
ear infection, 528, 1138, 1238
ear, internal, 526
ear, middle, 526
ear, pain under, 921
ear speculum, 529
ear polyp, 1064
ear stuffiness, 531-32
earache, 526
eardrum, 526
eardrum, surgical incision of, 991
ears, care of, 400
ears, lop, plastic surgery for, 859-60
early adolescence, 897
eating habits, 766
ecchymosis, 532
eccrine, 243
eccrine glands, 1187
echeosis, 951
eclampsia, 532-33, 817
ectomorphic, 1292
ectopic pregnancy, 533, 613
eczema, 68, 69, 270, 533-35, 612, 777, 841
edema, 219, 513, 535, 651, 841, 942, 971, 1083, 1157, 1300
edema, eyelids, 977
edible portions, meats, 882
education, sex, 1175-77
efferent nerve, 943
eggs (as food), 535, 1128, 1332, 1335
egg cells, 992
egg white, 901
eight- to ten-year-old, pictorial guide to needs of, 378-79
Eijkman, Dr., 193
ejaculation, 986, 1128

1379

INDEX

ejaculatory ducts, 1169, 1172, 1309, 1319
elastic fibers, 1185
elbow, 535-36, 820
electric arc workers, 803
electric coagulation, 853
electric current, 1070
electric current, high-frequency, 1037
electric dessication, 1339
electric needle, 1164
electric pad, 886
electric shock, 548
electric shock treatment, 537
electric stimulation, 192
electrical dissection, 1082
electrical injuries, 536-37
Electro Stethograph, 156
electrocardiogram, 537, 719
electrocardiograph, 450, 537, 538, 719
electrocardiograph tests, 1139
electroencephalograph, 538
electroencephalography, 537
electrolysis, 33, 637, 772
electron microscope, 1326
electronic medical aid, 538-43
elephantiasis, 543, 645, 789, 870
eleven- to thirteen-year-old, pictorial guide to needs of, 380
elimination, 943
emaciation, 543
emboli, 1260
embolism, 543-44, 1009, 1033
embolus, 543, 1260, 1319
embryo, 544
embryonic development, 343
emergencies, home, 544-50
emergencies, medical 550, 551-57
emergency responses, 1040
emery wheels, 1244
emetic, 550, 840, 930, 1157
emetine, 74, 197
emissions, 1089
emotion, 558
emotional changes, 1008
emotional disorders, 1085
emotional disturbances, 558-59, 783, 896, 1223
emotional grasp, 1085
emotional health, 559-60
emotional stimulus, 1088
emotions, 1304

emotions and allergy, 560-61
emphysema, 561-62, 866, 976
empyema, 21, 562-63, 1045, 1049
enamel, 1246
encephalitis, 563-64, 881, 978, 1012, 1326
encephalitis, postinfection, 563
encephalitis, St. Louis, 563
endamoeba histolytica, 74, 75
endarteritis, 564
endocarditis, 318, 544, 564, 710, 1049
endocarditis, acute bacterial, 170
endocarditis, bacterial, 170-71
endocarditis, malignant, 564
endocarditis, subacute, 544
endocarditis, subacute bacterial, 172-73
endocardium, 318, 564, 710
endocrine glands, 52, 564, 682-84, 765, 945, 1005, 1089, 1223, 1262
endocrine system, 745, 772, 1040, 1350
endocrinologist, 247
endocrinology, 564
endometritis, 564-65
endometrium, 893, 1313
endomorphic, 1292
endothelium, 408, 710
enema syringe, 886
enemas, 326, 565
energy, 348, 928
energy output, 1347
energy, transformation of, 956
enlargement, 1082
enlargement, abdomen, 940
enlargement, liver, 950
enlargement, muscle of pyloric valve, 1224
enlargement, prostate, 1080-81, 1173
enlargement, spleen, 950, 1214, 1352
enteric fever, 565, 1214
enteritis, 565, 1225
enuresis, 185, 364-65, 566
enzyme(s), 566, 641, 1004
enzymes, pancreatic, 954
ephedrine, 70, 147, 177, 427, 532, 566
ephedrine sulfate, 931
epidemic bacillary dysentery, 164
epidemic louse-borne typhus, 1290
epidemic nausea and vomiting, 1326
epidemic septic sore throat, 1174

epidemic sore throat, 110
epidemic typhus fever, 1150
epidermis, 572, 1185
epididymis (epididymides), 22, 566, 1126, 1164, 1169, 1207, 1251, 1309, 1319
epididymitis, 1256
epigastric, 19
epiglottis, 566, 685, 838
epilepsy, 178, 328, 559, 566-71
epileptic vertigo, 1323
epinephrine, 52, 142, 226, 270, 571, 1184
epinephrine hydrochloride, 761
epispadias, 1024, 1309, 1125
epistaxis, 571
epithelial cells, 1185
epithelioma, 572
epithelium, 572
Epsom salt, 326, 572, 884
epyphisis, 536
equilibrium, 572
equine encephalomyelitis, 563
erection, 1022, 1126
ergosterol (vitamin D), 908, 956, 1147, 1328, 1334-35
ergot, 572
ergotamine, 708
ergotamine tartrate, 905
ergotism, 572
erosions, 333
erysipelas, 73, 110, 572-73, 777, 792, 1225, 1244
erythema, 68, 573, 867
erythema solars, 1231
erythematosus, lupus, 423, 511, 573, 867, 868-69
erythroblastosis (fetalis) foetalis, 573, 1116
erythrocytes, 216, 466, 573
erythromelalgia, 573
erythromycin, 101
eschar, 1165
esophagus, 337, 573-76, 1224, 1337
essential hypertension, 108
essential hypotension, 236
estradiol, 894, 992, 1129
estrogen(s), 33, 175, 304, 576, 893, 1129
ethambutol, 1284
ether, 89, 576, 1155
ethmoid sinus, 1184
ethyl alcohol, 62
ethyl benzene, 972
ethyl chloride, 29, 755
ethyl nitrate, 972
ethylene, 90
ethylene dichloride, 970, 971, 972, 973
eucalyptus oil, 576
eunuch, 576, 1256

European relapsing fever, 183
Eustachian tube, 526, 576, 991
evaporated milk, 908
Evipal, 90, 1054
evipan sodium, 178
exanthem, 577
exanthematous disease, acute, 577
excretion, 577
exercise, during menstruation, 638
exercise(s), 138, 366-67, 430, 577-88, 632, 959, 1065-69, 1071-73
exercises, child, 364-65
exercises, faulty posture, 1074
exercises, therapeutic, 981-83, 1037, 1058-59, 1125
exhalation, 310, 337
exhaustion, 588, 619, 799
exhibitionism, 588-89
exogenous hormones, 956
exophthalmic goiter, 589, 688-89, 695, 768-69, 770, 1262
exophthalmos, 589
expectoration, 589, 1278
exstrophy of bladder, 1309-12
external ear, 526
external ear, otitis of, 991
external forces, infection due to, 791
external secretion glands, 682, 765
extosis, 526
eye, 589-610
eye banks, 606, 610
eye, foreign bodies in, 546-47, 609
eyeglasses, 610
eye injuries, safety rules, 609
eyelids, edema of, 977
eyes, accommodation, 24
eyes, color, 599
eyesight, guarding 608
eyestrain, 599-600
eye worm, 645

F

5-diazo-4-oxo-L-norvaline, 308
fabrics, man-made, 977
face, 611-12, 1191
face, disturbances of, 1332
face powders, 457
facial ague, 59
facial massage, 192
facial nerve, 611
facial neuralgia, 612
facial paralysis, 921
facial vein, 611
Fahrenheit, 1257
failure to descend, 1257
fainting, 548, 612-13
falciparum malaria, 872

fallen arches, 122, 613, 628
falling fit, 776
falling hair, 1104
Fallopian tubes, 613, 1313
fallout protection, 613-17
falls, 544
false aneurysm, 90
false hunger pains, 1364
false ribs, 1147
familial hemolytic jaundice, 1114
Faraday, Michael, 89
farcy buds, 682
farsightedness, 592, 595, 596, 610, 617, 1077-78
fast breathing, 548
fasting, 617
fat, 197, 617-19, 1344-45
fat depots, 1345
fat droplets, 1345
fat globules, suspended, 908
fat necrosis, 853
fat, subcutaneous, 1344
fatigability, 1008
fatigue, 602, 619-20, 940, 1077
fatness, 1344
fats, 348, 620, 908, 954-55
fats, unsaturated, 620-21
fatty material, 1186
fatty tumors, 293
fauces, 1258
faulty diet, 1223
favoritism, 898
favus, 1152
fear, 621-23
febrile, 623
febrile disease, 1138
febrile disorders, 951
febrile pemphigus, 1022
feces, 253, 623, 811
fecundation, 429
Federal Food and Drug Administration inspections, 1093-96
feeble-mindedness, 623-24, 684
feeding, breast, 368-69, 624-25
feeding, frequency of, baby, 386-87
feeding, older child, 392
feeding, spoon, cup, 389
feet, 625-33
feet, frozen or frostbitten, 123, 124, 706
feet, numbness and tingling of, 1008
fellation, 634, 764, 814, 1199
felon, 634
female organs, cancer of, 298
female sexual anatomy, 1128
female urethra, 1312
feminine hygiene, 634-40
feminine hygiene products, 202
femur, 818

1380

INDEX

fenestration, 475, 992
ferment, 641
fermentation, 641
ferrosilicon, 977
ferrous iron, 814
fertility, 641
fertilization, 429, 1177
fertilized ovum, 343, 1372
fetal heartbeat, 1077
fetal movements, 1077
fetal outline, 1077
fetid perspiration, 243-44
fetus, 342, 641
fever, 398-99, 641-43, 666, 799, 843, 921, 986, 1099, 1109, 1334
fever blisters, 643, 745, 756-57, 1327
fever, high, 799
fever, infection and, 788
fever pemphigus, 1022
fibers, 818, 1239
fibers, nerve cell, 943
fibrillation, 643
fibrin, 219, 221, 417
fibrin foam, 219
fibrinogen, 219, 221, 417, 855, 1083, 1300
fibrinogen deficiency, 644
fibroid tumor, 894, 1314-15, 1316
fibroma(s), 262, 293, 644
fibroma(s), benign, 644
fibroneurosarcoma, 1157
fibrosis, 1278
fibrosis, lungs, 978
fibrositis, 644, 929, 1145
fibrous capsule, 591
fibula, 98, 841
field mice, 1165
fifth cranial nerve, 945, 1263
filaria, 543, 644
filariasis, 543, 644-45, 792, 915
filterable virus, 1102
filterable viruses, 1150
finger, 645-46
finger muscles, weakness of, 1008
fingernails, 646
fingers, extra, 804
fingers, loss of, 842
Finlay, Carlos, 1371
first aid, 646-47, 885
first aid, poisoning, 1052-56
first molar, 196
first six years, 357-63
fish, 647
fish skin disease, 777
fish tapeworm, 1364
fish tapeworm, infestation with, 85
fissure(s), 647-48, 742-43
fistula, 648
fistula, complete, 648
fit, 446, 648-49, 1205
fits, hysterical, 649
five- to seven-year-olds, pictorial

guide to needs of, 376-77
flaccid paralysis, 1009
flat bones, 247
flatfoot, 649
flatulence, 649-50
Fleming, Sir Alexander, 101, 1022
flies, 650-51
floating ribs, 337, 1147
floating spleen, 1215
floor burn, 1365
flu, 651, 798, 800-1
fluid, control of, 1232
fluid retained in the body, 651-52
fluids, absorption of, 22
fluorescent lamp manufacture, 803, 899
fluoridation, 652
fluorides, 652
fluorine, 485, 1246, 1248
fluoroscope, 1024
fluoroscopy, 450, 652
folic acid, 305, 1111, 1219, 1328, 1333
folic acid antagonists, 78
follicular fluid, 1129
follicles, 1128
folliculitis, 314-15
fontanelles, 355, 1191
food, 212
food, absorption of, 22
food, acid-forming, 27
food, alkaline-forming, 27
food allergy, 652
Food and Life, 290
food, basic requirements, 652-53
food deficiencies, 505
food fats, 653-54
food intake, 1347
food poisoning, 19, 549, 654-56, 1109
food restriction, voluntary, 617, 1302
food restriction, involuntary, 1302
food sources, ascorbic acid, 1333
food sources, calcium, 1334
food sources, iron, 1335
food sources, niacin (nicotinic acid), 1332
food sources, protein, 1335
food sources, riboflavin, 1329
foods, solid, 389-90
foot-and-mouth disease, 656, 1326
foramina, 249
forced nutrition, 1106
forceps, 1155
foreign bodies, 656-57
foreign bodies, first aid, 546-47, 609
foreign bodies, nose, 952

foreign substances, infection due to, 791
foreskin, 409, 1022
formaldehyde, 968, 972, 1290
formalin, 972, 973
formula, preparing, 388-89
forty, 1100
foundry work, 803
four-year-old, pictorial guide to needs of, 374-75
fourteen- to sixteen-year-old, pictorial guide to needs of, 382-83
fracture(s), 657-60, 1180, 1185, 1364
fractures, closed, 1191
fracture, compound, 428, 1191
fractures, skull, 1191
frambesia, 1370
framework and body build and height, 1343
Francis, Edward, 1286
fraternal twins, 206
freckles, 660
freckle and blemish removers, 459, 660
free silica, 978
free-floating anxiety, 111
Frei test, 870
frenum, 1267
Freon, 1244
Freon bomb, 663
frequency of urination, 1077, 1312
fresh air, 766
Freud, Sigmund, 89, 1085
Friedlander's bacillus, 277
Friedreich's ataxia, 660-61
Froehlich's syndrome, 661, 1044
frontal bone, 1191
frontal lobes, 256
frontal sinus, 1184
frostbite, 124, 661-62, 934, 948
frozen shoulder, 1180
functional headache, 707, 708
functional murmur of childhood, 719
functioning, disordered, 791
functions, paralysis of, 257
fumigation, 662-63
fungi, 788, 792, 866, 929
fungicide, 1151, 1352
fungus, 663-66
fungus diseases, 1150
fungus infection, 815
fungus infections of skin, 820
furacin derivatives, 826
Furadantin, 209, 471
furor, 559
furuncles, 314-15, 666
future generations, 1104

G

gait, 667
galerina venenata, 929
gall duct, 688
gallbladder, 197, 208, 668-72, 854
gallbladder, infected, 18
galloping consumption, 1278
gallstones, 197, 670-71, 672, 854
galvanizing workers, 967
gamma emanations, 974
gamma globulin, 219, 672-73, 679, 881, 1327, 1328
game (meats), 881, 883
ganglia, 1239
ganglions, 673
gangrene, 114, 662, 673-74, 842, 853, 986, 1365
Gantrisin, 1230
gargle, 674, 1157
gas gangrene, 673
gasoline, 968
gastrectomy, 674
gastric, 674
gastric distress, 1008
gastric juice, stoppage of flow of, 1239
gastric juices, 954
gastric juices, stimulation of flow of, 1239
gastric polyp, 1064
gastric ulcer, 674
gastritis, 674-75
gastritis, chronic, 64, 675
gastrocnemius, 25
gastroenteritis, 674, 675
gastro-intestinal system, 675
gastroscope, 674, 1024
gastroscopy, 298
gastroptosis, 675, 1224
gatophobia, 675
gauze bandages, sterile, 885
gauze pads, sterile, 885
Geiger counter, 1104
gelatin, 245, 675
general anesthesia, 87
general headache, 707
general infection, 788
general paralysis, 1016
general paralysis of insane, 1016
general paresis, 896, 1016, 1241
genetics, 678, 748, 1130
genes, 745, 748
genitals, 678
gentian violet, 911, 1357
genito-urinary system, 678, 1128, 1129
genito-urinary tract, 1126

genius, 678
geographic tongue, 1267
geriatrics, 55-58, 676-77, 678
German measles, 678-79, 680-81, 793, 881, 1326
germination, 992
germicide, 109, 679
germ plasm, defective, 909
germs, 679
giant intestinal roundworm, 1357
giant molecules, 1083
giantism, 34-37, 247, 679, 684, 739
Gibraltar fever, 961
giddiness, 1323
Gila monster bite, 1197
Gilchrist's disease, 210-11, 679
gin fever, 804
gingivitis, 679, 695
glacial acetic acid, 25
gland, swelling in front of ear, 921
glanders, 682
glands, 682-84, 1250
glandular deficiency, 909
glandular fever, 857, 867, 911, 1326
glandular substances, 1082
glans, 1022
glass tubes, 1108
glasses, cataract, 605
glaucoma, 447, 601-2, 684-85, 686-87
gleet, 685
gliding joints, 250
glioma, 685
globin, 740
globin insulin, 807
globulin, 219, 1300
globulin fraction, 1303
globulins, 1083
glomeruli, 826
glomerulonephritis, acute, 232, 937, 940
glomerulonephritis, chronic, 937, 941
glossitis, 685, 1267
glossopathy, 685
glossopharyngeal neuralgia, 685
glottis, 461, 566, 685, 1198
glucose, 685-88, 814, 1308
glucose injection, 817, 1055
glucose tolerance test, 685
gluteal, 287
glycogen, 487, 578, 854, 1169
glycerin suppositories, 326
gnawing pain, 1003
goat fever, 688, 1305
goiter, 478, 688-90, 767, 804, 813
gold needles, 1108
gold poisoning, 899, 900
gold, radioactive, 153, 309, 1106
gold refining, 901
gold salts, 867, 890

1381

INDEX

gonads, 690, 1089, 1118, 1128
gonococcus (gonococci), 101, 604, 690
gonorrhea, 169, 566, 984, 993, 1022
gonorrheal epididymitis, 566
good grade meats, 882
gout, 691, 692-93, 694, 819, 1145
gouty arthritis, 136
grades of meats, 882
grain itch, 972
grain, refined or polished, 1329
grand mal, 566, 570
granite, 972
granulocytes, 216, 1350
granulocytopenia, 58, 691
granulocytosis, 846
granuloma, 899
granuloma inguinale, 691-95
Graves' disease, 589, 695, 768-69, 1017, 1262
gray matter, 943
greenstick fracture, 660
green vegetables, 1336
grippe, 695, 798, 800-1
groin, ringworm of, 1151
ground itch, 1361
growth, 1040
growth charts, 384, 390-91, 393
growth factor, 84
growth hormone, 765, 1040
guanidine, 971
gullet, 573, 1224
gum diseases, 484
gums, 695, 1098, 1246
gums, thickened, 843
gumboil, 695
gumma, 1240, 1241
Guthrie, Samuel, 89
gym, 406
gym itch, 1151
gynecology, 695
gynecomastia, 262, 695

H

habit spasm, 696, 1205
hair, 696-99
hair dyes, 459-60
hair follicles, 1185, 1187
hair loss, 931
hair remover, 699
hair, superfluous, 637-38, 698
halitosis, 434, 699
hallucination, 699
Halsted, William S., 89
hammertoe, 633
hamstring tendons, 928
hand, 248
handicapped, aids for, 1119-25
hands, numbness and tingling of, 1008

Hand-Schuller-Christian disease, 699
hangnails, 934
Hansenosis, 842
Hansen's disease, 699, 842
hard chancre, 335
hard palate, 917, 1004
hardening, arteries (arteriosclerosis), 94, 108, 124-30, 234, 404, 418, 450, 620, 699, 804, 950, 953, 954, 1173
hardening, nervous tissue, 1164
hardening, skin, 1191
harelip, 412, 699, 853, 1206
harmful undernutrition, 1304
Harvey, William, 222
hashish, 875
Haverhill fever, 1109
Haversian canals, 249
hay fever, 67, 68, 157, 270, 524, 701-5, 1198, 1322
head, 408
head banging, head rolling, 708-9
head injuries, 709-10
head louse, 847
headache, 706-8, 737, 799, 893, 916, 917, 921, 940, 1099
heads, babies, 203
hearing, 526
hearing aid(s), 475, 476
hearing and retardation, 809
hearing, difficulty in, 917
hearing, hardness of, 710, 917
hearing, inherited difficulties, 804
heart, 217, 223, 337, 406, 710-19
heart ailments, 1270
heart and circulation, underweight and, 1302
heart block, 719
heart contraction, 1091
heart damage, predilection to, 1138
heart disease, congenital, 716-17
heart disease, hypertensive, 230-31
heart disease, pulmonary, 730-31
heart disease, rheumatic, 1142-43
heart disease, thyroid, 1264-65
heart diseases, 1173
heart dysfunction, 976
heart failure, 712-13, 714, 1049
heart failure, congestive, 1106
heart murmur, 719-20
heart palpitation, 718, 893
heart, slowing of, 1239

heart surgery, 721-29, 1232-36
heart surgery, artificial, 720-36
heart troubles, symptoms of, 736-37
heart valves, plastic, 710
heartbeat, 714
heartbeat, acoustical analyzer, 883
heartbeat, augmentation of, 1239
heartbeat, fetal, 1077
heartburn, 719
heart-lung machine, 720-32
heart transplants, 736, 985
heat, 470, 517
heat absorption, 1037
heat, and occupational diseases, 972
heat cabinet, 137
heat cramps, 737, 738
heat, dry, 138
heat exhaustion, 737, 738
heat loss, 1249
heat production, 1249
heat rash, 1078
heat, sensation of, 1003
heat sickness, 737-38
heat stroke, 548
heat treatment, 132, 1305
heatstroke, 737, 738
Heberden's nodes, 987
height, 738-39, 1292, 1343
height charts, 384, 390-91, 393
height-weight-age tables, 1345-47
heliotherapy, 739
Helmholtz, Hermann von, 984
hemangioma, 739
hemathrosis, 818
hematin, 740
hematoma, 277
hematuria, 739
hemianosmia, 99
hemiplegia, 776, 1009
hemiplegia paralysis, 934
hemispheres, 256
hemodialysis, 739
hemoglobin, 81, 216, 740, 813, 970, 1107, 1111, 1116
hemoglobin determination test, 1252-53
hemoglobinuria, 740
hemolytic anemia, 82, 573, 740, 1111
hemolytic anemia of newborn, 241
hemolytic disease of newborn, 1116
hemolytic jaundice, 83
hemophilia, 222, 418, 740-41, 748, 804, 953
hemophilus pertussis, 1353
hemorrhage, 545, 741, 968, 1214, 1336

hemorrhage, cerebral, 112, 328, 418, 1173
hemorrhage, brain, 257, 1009
hemorrhage, lung, 546
hemorrhagic jaundice, 1109
hemorrhagic pancreatitis, advanced, 1007
hemorrhoids, 323, 741-44, 1318
heparin, 221, 418, 1261
hepatic vein, 408
hepatitis, 744-45, 746-47, 816
hepatitis, acute, 855
hepatitis, acute viral, 856
hepatitis, amebic, 74
hepatitis, chronic, 857
hepatitis, infectious, 792, 856, 1327, 1351
hepatitis, secondary, 857
hepatitis, serum, 856
hepatitis, toxic, 857
hereditary factors in overweight, 745-48
hereditary spherocytosis, 748, 1114, 1352
heredity, 748, 1350
hermaphroditism, 748
hernia, 20, 399, 504, 748-54, 984, 1207, 1299
heroin, 754
herpes, 854
herpes simplex, 754, 756-57, 1327
herpes zoster, 754, 758-59
hesperedin, 1336
heterosexuality, 754-55
HETP, 977
hetrazan, 543, 645
"hex," 968, 973
hexaethyl-tetraphosphate, 977
Hexamethonium, 236
hexamethonium tartrate, 108
hexamethylene-tetramine, 968, 973
hexylresorcinol, 1357, 1360, 1361
hexylresorcinol solution, 109
hiatus hernia, 750-51
hiccoughs, 755
hiccups, 504, 549, 755
hickory stick fracture, 660
high altitudes, oxygen at, 428
high blood pressure, 226-36, 605, 755, 1173
high-caloric diet, 511
high-carbohydrate diet, 511
high-fat diet, 511
high-frequency electrical current, 1037

high-pressure oxygen therapy, 996-1002
high-protein diet, 511
hinge joints, 250
Hinton test, 1342
hip lift, 1134
hip lift-back pressure, 1136
hip roll-back pressure, 1136
hirsutism, 772-73, 755
His, Wilhelm, 718
histamine, 68, 107, 186, 192, 755, 905
histidine, 78
histoplasma capsulatum, 755
histoplasmosis, 666, 755-60, 792
hives, 68, 524, 760-61, 762-63
hoarseness, 761
hoarseness, pronounced, 932
Hodgkin, Thomas, 761
Hodgkin's disease, 761-64, 1214, 1352
Hodgkin's granuloma, 1352
Hodgkin's paragranuloma, 1352
Hodgkin's sarcoma, 1352
Holger method, 1133
homogenized milk, 908
homosexuality, 764-65
hookworm, 765, 788, 789, 792, 964, 1360-61
hormonal therapy, 308
hormone treatments, 304
hormones, 212, 304, 692, 765-66, 893, 992, 1223, 1343
hospital, child in, 397
hot flush, 893
hot-water bottle, 886
house mice, 1150
housemaid's knee, 766, 834-35
humerus, 535
humidity, home, 336
hunger pains, false, 1364
hyaline, 941
hyaluronidase, 98, 823, 842
hydatid diseases, 1214
Hydergine, 236
hydralazine, 108
hydrathrosis, intermittent, 818
hydrocephalus, 766, 1191
hydrocephaly, 1207
hydrochloric acid, 25, 26, 507, 814, 954, 1157, 1224
hydrochloric acid, absence of, 86
hydrocortisone, 28, 157, 456, 766, 990, 1097, 1139, 1181
hydrocortisone acetate, 673
hydrocyanic acid, 972, 973

1382

INDEX

hydrogen, 973, 974, 1083
hydrogen, phosphureted, 976-77
hydrogen peroxide, 109, 484, 1055, 1323
hydrogen sulphide, 973, 977, 979
hydronephrosis, 826
hydrophobia, 766, 1102
hydroquinone, 973
hydrotherapy, 1037, 1059
hydrothorax, 651
hydroxylamine, 1327
hygiene, 766-67
hygiene, nursing, 385-86
hygiene, sick child, 397-98
hymen, 638, 767, 1130, 1137, 1138
hyoscine, 949
hyperacidity, 767
hyperactive reflexes, 1008
hyperbaric (high-pressure) oxygen therapy, 996-1002
hyperglycemia, 767, 814
hyperhydrosis, 767
hypermetropia, 592
hyperparathyroidism, 1014-15
hyperkeratosis, 1328
hyperkeratotic athlete's foot, 149
hyperosmia, 99
hypersensitivity, 67
hypertension, 108, 226-36, 767
hypertension, essential, 108
hypertensive heart disease, 230-31
hyperthyroidism, 227, 689, 767-72, 774, 1262
hypertrichosis, 772-73, 698
hypertrophic pharyngitis, 1033
hypertrophy, 263, 773
hypertrophy, compensatory, 773
hypnosis, 773, 887
hypnotics, 806
hypochondriac, left and right, 19
hypochondriasis, 773-74, 1304, 1318
hypodermic injection, 805
hypogastric, 19
hypoglycemia, 52, 774, 814, 1005
hypogonadism and Simmond's disease, 1178-79
hypomania, 873
hyposmia, 99
hypospadias, 1024, 1309
hypotension, 236-37, 774
hypotension, essential, 236
hypotension, postural, 236
hypotension, secondary, 236
hypothalamus, 255

hypothyroidism, 774, 1262
hysterectomy, 775
hysteria, 475, 775-76, 1206, 1304
hysterical dysphagia, 576
hysterical fits, 649
hysterical paralysis, 776

I

ice bag, 886
ice cap, 777
ichthyol, 777
ichthyosis, 777
icterus, 777, 816-17
identical twins, 205, 206
idiopathic thrombocytopenic purpura, 1259, 1352
idiot, 623, 777, 1262
ileitis, 777-80
ileocecal valve, 812
ileum, 777, 810, 817
iliac, left and right, 19
ilium, 1156
illness, acute, 39
imbeciles, 623, 780
immune globulin, 881
immune serum, 1327
immunity, 81, 780-81, 1327
immunization, 781-82, 961, 1353
immunization and infectious disease, chart of, 793-95
immunization, passive, 1327
immunology, 222
impacted teeth, 1249
impetigo, 534, 612, 782-83, 784-85, 847
implanted pacemakers, 883
impotence, 783
impregnation, 429
incision, 783, 1365
infantile diarrhea, infectious, 796
infertility, male, 783
infestation with fish tapeworm, 85
inflammation, 798, 1223, 1224
inflammation, eye, 1238
incisors, 1247
incomplete proteins, 1083
incomplete fistula, 648
incontinence in women, 783
incubation period, 1287
indigestion, 783-87, 951
indium 113m, 883
individual responses to given stimuli, 1088
induced abortion, 20
industrial health, 787
infancy, 634
infantile convulsions, 649
infantile paralysis, 787, 1057-64

infantile spinal paralysis, 934
infantilism, 787-88
infarct, 317
infection(s), 505, 788-91, 986, 1223, 1256
infection, prevention of, 397
infection, secondary, 790
infection, severe, 1178
infection, susceptibility to, 1008
infection, throat, 1022
infections, blood, 1225
infections, bowels, 1239
infections, ear, 528, 1138, 1238
infections, urinary tract, 1310-11
infectious, 318, 427
infectious cirrhosis, 412
infectious diseases, 791-96, 816, 915, 1302
infectious diseases and immunization, chart of, 793-95
infectious diseases, control of, 796-97
infectious hepatitis, 792, 856, 1327, 1351
infectious infantile diarrhea, 796
infectious jaundice, acute, 856
infectious mononucleosis, 18, 797, 857, 867, 911, 912-13, 1351
inferior vena cava, 407
infertility, 797-98
inflammation, joint, 819
inflammation, nerve, 945
inflammation, retina, 604-5
influenza, 277, 505, 530, 789, 798-802, 910, 948, 1045, 1099, 1198, 1258, 1302, 1326, 1327
influenza virus, 1326
infrared lamp, 1037
infrared rays, 965
ingrowing nails, 934
ingrown toenails, 802-3
inguinal canal, 1207, 1304, 1319
inguinal hernia, 752-53
inhalation, 310-11, 337
inhaling dangerous substances, 803-4
inheritance of disease, 804
injection, 804
injection, hormones, 1097
injection, hypodermic, 805
injection technique for insulin, 489
injections, 948
injured, carrying, 546, 547

injuries and accidents, 22-24, 814, 1223
injuries, electrical, 536-37
ink, rotogravure, 977
inner layer, 408
innocent tumor, 1287
innocuous murmur of childhood, 719
innominate bones, 1184, 1185
inoculation, 790, 805
inorganic acids, 26
inorganic salts, 1313
inositol, 1328, 1334
insanity, 805
inscription, 1078
insect bites, 805-6
insect repellents, 805
insecticides, 971, 973, 977, 979
insects, 528, 549
insects, control of, 796
insensible perspiration, 1032
insomnia, 806, 893
instrument makers, diseases of, 901
instrument sterilization, 225
instruments, medical, 883
insulating board bagasse dust, 803
insulin, 487, 765, 774, 804, 806-7, 814, 885, 986, 1005, 1041
insulin injection technique, 489
insulin, NPH, 807
insulin shock, 807, 1178
insulin shock therapy, 807
intellectual grasp, 1085
intelligence, 807-9
intelligence quotient (I.Q.), 809
intercostal nerve, 945
intercourse, sexual, 1177
interest, lack of, 1304
interferon, 1327
intermittent claudication, 809, 852
intermittent hydrathrosis, 818
internal ear, 526
internal organs, nerves for, 943
internal secretion glands, 682-84, 765
internal secretions, 992
internal tympanic cavity, 526
interrupted pregnancy, 20
interstitial cells, 1126, 1251
interstitial keratitis, 447
interstital nephritis, chronic, 409
intertriginous athlete's foot, 149
intertrigo, 251, 809-10

intervertebral disc, 810, 1192, 1322
intervertebral disc syndrome, 810
intestinal bleeding, 1334, 1370
intestinal grippe, 800-1
intestinal tract, 408
intestinal vertigo, 1323
intestinal worms, 951, 1356
intestines, 810-11
intestines, absorption in, 22
intoxication, chronic alcoholic, 811-12
intra-cardiac pressures, 453
intramuscular injection, 805
intraspinal injection, 805
intrauterine devices, 200-1
intravenous injection, 805
intrinsic factor, 84, 86, 1114
introdermic injection, 805
introversion, 1304
intubation tube, 467
intussusception, 19, 811, 812
intussusception, acute, 812
intusussception, chronic, 812
involuntary food restriction, 1302
involuntary muscles, 924, 943
involution, 57
involutional melancholia, 812-13, 896
iodine, 74, 153, 348, 770, 813, 885, 956
iodine, artificially radioactivated, 1106
iodine, radioactive, 153, 689, 770, 1106
iodine, tincture of, 109, 813, 1366
"iodized" salt, 688
iodophthalein, 669
Ipral, 1054
I.Q., 813
iridectomy, 602
iris, 447, 591
iris, prolapse of, 1079
iritis, 602, 813
iron, 348, 813-14, 855, 896, 1107
iron deficiency, 814
iron deposits in lungs, 803
iron, food sources of, 1335
iron, in hemoglobin, 740
iron, replenishment of, 1077
iron supplements, 1219
iron-deficiency anemia, 83, 1111
irradiation, 853
irritability, 1304
irritants, 852
irrumation, 764, 814, 1199

1383

INDEX

Islets of Langerhans, 814-15, 906, 1005
isolated, 1100
isolation, 1193
isolation, complete, 802
isolette, 159-63
isoleucine, 78
isoniazid, 209, 477, 523, 791, 797, 1275, 1284
isonicotinic acid hydrazines, 523
isoproterenol hydrochloride, 718
isosorbide dinitrate, 96
isotope scanning, radioactive, 883
isotopes, radioactive, 152, 305, 1103, 1106
itch, 815
itch mite, 805, 820, 1158
itching, 815, 816
itching skin, 893

J

jail fever, 1290
Japanese river fever, 816, 1165
jaundice, 83, 854, 816-17 1005
jaundice, acute catarrhal, 856
jaundice, acute infectious, 856
jaundice, hemolytic, 83
jaundice, hemorrhagic, 1109
jaundice, obstructive, 1336
jaundiced, 1116
jaw, 817
jaw deformities, 804
jeep disease, 1192
jejunal ulcer, 817
jejunum, 810, 817
Jenner, Edward, 1193
jockey itch, 406, 1151
joint capsule, 818
joint disease, degenerative, 987, 1145
joints, ball-and-socket, 250, 818
joints, disorders, 817-20
joints, inflammation, 819
joints, pain in, 843
joints, tuberculosis of, 1278
Journal of the American Dental Association, 485
jugular veins, 408
Jung, Carl, 1085
jungle rot, 820-21, 871
juvenile myxedema, 931

K

Kahn, Reuben L., 822
Kahn test, 822, 1241, 1342
kala azar, 183, 822, 842
katayama disease, 197, 822

keloides, 822-23
Kenacort, 457
Kendall, E. C. 137
keratin, 933, 1186
keratitis, 823
keratitis, traumatic, 447
keratoconus, 447, 823
kerosene, 971, 973
kerosene poisoning, 1055
ketones, 967
kidney(s), 408, 823-28, 901, 1040, 1313
kidney, artificial, 828-34
kidney, cirrhosis of, 1313
kidney disease, 1114, 1173, 1270
kidney, polycystic, congenital, 232
kidney stone colic, 826
kidney stones, 824-25, 826
kidneys, dialysis of, 828-34
kinesiology, 928
kissing disease, 911, 1351
knee, 818, 834-35
knee jerk, 1117
kneecap, 820, 834
kneecap, broken, 835
knock-knee, 835
Koch, Robert, 169, 403, 1276
Koller, Karl, 89
Koplik's spots, 880
Korsakoff's psychosis, 1240
Korsakoff's syndrome, 1240
Krause's end bulb, 1186
kwashiorkor, 836, 873, 887
Kynex, 1230

L

labia majora, 837, 1130, 1337, 1338
labia minora, 837, 1130, 1337, 1338
labor, 837
laboratory workers, diseases of, 901
laceration, 277, 709, 837, 1365
lacrimal gland, 606
lacteals, 811, 867
lactic acid, 26, 578, 641, 928
lamb, 882
Landsteiner classification, 239
Landsteiner, Karl, 238, 239
large intestine, 252
large intestine, absorption in, 22
laryngeal crisi of locomotor ataxia, 839
laryngeal muscles, paralysis, 838
laryngeal pharynx, 1032
laryngeal tuberculosis, 838, 839
laryngismus stridulus, 466

laryngitis, 837-38, 1206
laryngitis, acute, 837
laryngitis, acute obstructive, 466
larynx, 516, 837, 838-39, 1206, 1258
larynx cancer, 189, 295, 838, 839
laser, 605
L-asparaginase, 308
lasitude, 1360
latah, 80
late adolescence, 897
lateral incisors, 1247
lateral projections, 1322
lateral sclerosis, 839
laughing gas, 89, 975
laughter, 839-40, 1117
laxatives, 323, 840
laxatives, bulk, 884
layette, 351-52
L-DOPA, 1012
lead citrate, soluble, 900
lead line, 900
lead oxide, 973
lead poisoning, 840, 899, 900, 948, 969, 973, 1323
lead poisoning, acute, 840
lead poisoning, chronic, 840
lead salts, 900
lead suphate solution, 840
leafy vegetables, 1334, 1336
learning to walk, child, 356
lechery, 841
lecithin, 197
left auricle, 714
left hypochondrium, 19
left iliac, 19
left lumber, 19
left maxilla, 817
left side, heart, 406
left ventricle, 223, 714
left-handedness, 841
leg, 841, 1184
leg ulcers, 841-42
Leishman, William B., 842
leishmania, 842
leishmania donovani, 822
leishmaniasis, 792, 842
Lempert operation, 992
lens, 842
lenses, contact, 442
leprosy 792, 842
lesbianism, 764, 842
lesions, 1241
lesions, secondary, 1190-91
lettuce, 1335
leucine, 78
leucorrhea, 639, 842-43, 1318
leukemia, 58, 150, 153, 222, 308, 484, 843-46, 1115, 1214, 1215, 1351
leukemia, acute, 843, 1351
leukemia, chronic, 843, 1351

leukocytes, 21, 216, 846
leukocytosis, 846
leukopenia, 846
leukoplakia, 846, 848-49, 1338
leukorrhea, 846
leukotomy, 846, 1088
levodihydroxy-phenylalanine, 1012
Lewisohn, Richard, 238
libido, 846
lice, 789, 805, 846-47, 850-51, 1118
lice, agents for killing, 481
lichens, 1191
ligaments, 250, 847-52, 1218
ligation, 852
light skin, 1038
limbs, artificial, 138
lime, 973
lime liniments, 852
limp, 667
limping, intermittent, 852
linen thread, sterile, 852
liniment, 852-53
liniments, chloroform, 852
liniments, lime, 852
liniments, pain-relieving, 852
linseed oil, 977
lipiodol, 1368
lipoid pneumonia, 427
lipoma, 293, 853, 1286, 1348-49
lip cancer, 853
lips, 853-54
lips, disturbances of, 1332
lips, swelling of, 932
liquids, large quantities of, 802
liquor antisepticus, 484
liquor antisepticus alkalinus, 484
lisping, 1206
Lister, 791
litharge, 973
liver, 337, 408, 487, 682, 817, 854-56, 1004, 1250
liver (as food), 1332, 1333, 1335
liver, abscess, 855
liver, cirrhosis of, 409, 410-11, 954
liver, common diseases, 856-58
liver disease, 85
liver enlargement, 950
liver extracts, 858
liver preparations, 1219
liver spots, 611, 858
lividity, 1302
living matter, characteristic of, 1083
loa loa worm disease, 858
lobar pneumonia, 277, 1049, 1230, 1302
lobes, 256

lobotomy, 858
local infection, 788
lochia, 640
lockjaw, 256-57, 470, 548, 858, 1245-55
lockjaw antitoxin, 548
locomotor ataxia, 148, 572, 667, 858-59, 1243, 1312
locomotor ataxia, laryngeal crisis of, 839
Loeffler's syndrome, 859
Lone Star tick of Texas, 1153
long bones, 247
Long, Crawford W., 89
longevity, 859
lop ears, plastic surgery for, 859-60
lordosis, 860
louse-borne typhus epidemic, 1290
low back pain, 165, 860
low blood pressure, 236-37, 860, 1008
low resistance, 1334
low-carbohydrate diet, 511
lower brain stem, 254
Lower, Richard, 238
low-protein diet, 511
low-salt diet, 235, 507-8, 942
low-salt syndrome, 235
lues, 860
lumbago, 165, 644, 860-61, 1145
lumbar, left and right, 19
lumbar puncture, 329
lumbar vertebrae, 1322
Luminal, 178. 1054
lumpy jaw, 38, 861
lung, abscess, 862-63, 866
lung cancer, 864-65
lung cancer, cigar smoking and, 1197
lung cancer, cigarettes and, 1197
lung fibrosis, 978
lung function test, 453
lung hemorrhage, 546
lung, iron deposits in, 803
lung nodules, 963
lungs, 337, 407, 714, 861-67, 910, 969, 1249
lunula, 867, 963
lupus erythematosus, 423, 511, 573, 867, 868-69
lye, 67, 1055
lymph, 867, 1185
lymph capillaries, 867
lymph glands, tuberculosis of, 1278
lymph nodes, 867, 1352
lymphatic glands, 543, 963
lymphatic system, 867-70

1384

INDEX

lymphatic vessels, 861, 867
lymphocytes, 216, 846, 1350
lymphocytosis, 979
lymphogranuloma venereum, 870
lymphoid tissue, 41
lymphoma, 1115, 1214, 1352
lymphosarcoma, 1352
lysine, 78
Lysol, 870

M

madura foot, 792, 871
maduromycosis, 666
maggots, 952
magnamycin, 101
magnesia products, 1024
magnesium, 840, 956, 1246
magnesium citrate, 871
magnesium silicate, 974, 978
magnesium sulfate, 326
magnesium sulphate heptahydrate, 572
mahuang, 566
maidenhead, 767, 871
malaise, 951, 1099, 1109
malaise, extreme, 799
malaria, 59, 789, 792, 796, 805, 816, 871-72, 910, 915, 948, 1032, 1100, 1108, 1215, 1305
malaria, benign tertian, 109
malaria parasites, 871
male reproductive cells, 1251
male secondary sex characteristics, 1305
malignant, 644
male sex hormone, 1251
male sexual anatomy, 1118
male urethra, 1309
maleness, 1118
malignant, 293
malignant hypertension, 108
malignant melanoma, 602, 887
malignant tumor, 1286, 1287
malnutrition, 872-73, 1020
malocclusion, 986, 1247
Malta fever, 873, 961, 1305
mammary glands, 262, 873, 1187
Mandelamine, 209, 471
mandelic acid, 826
mandible, 817
manganese, 956
manganese poisoning, 973-74
mango fly, 645
mania, 1308

manic-depressive psychosis, 873-74, 896
manustrupration, 874
maple blossom, 704
marasmus, 543, 873, 874
march fracture, 660
Marezine, 108, 349, 889, 916
marihuana, 874-75
marriage, 638, 875
marrow, bone, 248, 1092
Martin, Ancil, 1285
masochism, 875
massage, 138, 875-76 1164
"master" gland, 684
mastitis, 876
mastoid, 526
mastoid antrum, 110, 876-77
mastoidectomy, 400
mastoiditis, 526, 531, 877, 991, 1230
masturbation, 635, 877, 1090, 1338
masturbation, mutual, 764, 1199
mat burn, 1365
maternity corset, 349
matrix, 933
maturation factor, 84
maxilla, 817
maxillary sinus, 110
mean weight, 1345
measles, 277, 474, 505, 530, 704, 792, 837, 877-81, 991 1258, 1318, 1326, 1327
measles, German, 678-79, 680-81, 793, 881, 1326
measles, three-day, 678
meatotomy, 1309
meats, animal 881-83, 1333
meats, edible portions, 882
meatus, 883, 1309
mechanical headache, 706
Meckel's diverticulum, 519
mediastinal emphysema, 562
medical instrumentation, 883
medical terms, key to, xiii-xvi
medicine chest, 883-86
Mediterranean anemia, 886, 1114
Mediterranean fever, 822, 886, 961, 1305
medulla, 52, 1206
medulla, adrenal, 684
medulla, brain, 281
medulla oblongata, 281
meerschaum, 974
megaloblastic anemia, 886, 1111
Meissner's corpuscle, 1186-87
melancholia, 886
melancholia, involutional, 896
melanidrosis, 887

melanin, 61, 886, 1037
melanin pigments, 1185
melanocancers, 887
melanomyces, 887
melanoplakia, 887
melanorrhagia, 887
melanosis, 886-87
melanotonin, 1039
melanuria, 887
membrane, 250, 516
memory, 887-88
Ménière, Prosper, 889
Ménière's disease, 888-89
Ménière's syndrome, 889
meningeal tuberculosis, 1278
meninges, 254, 332, 889, 910
meningioma, 889
meningism, 889
meningitis, 110, 474, 531, 709, 877, 889-92, 921, 1022, 1049, 1191, 1208
meningitis, cerebrospinal, 332
meningococcemia, 890
meningococcus (meningococci), 101, 332, 892, 1230
menopause, 636, 892-93, 993, 1129, 1316
menorrhagia, 893
menstrual cycle, 1223
menstruation, 48, 341, 636, 893-94, 1089, 1092, 1176, 1301, 1313
menstruation, cessation of, 1077
mental abnormalities, 932
mental and emotional health, 896-98
mental attitude, 766
mental defects, 809
mental depression, 894-95
mental diseases and disorders, 623, 898, 1085, 1173
mental disturbances, 1223, 1241
mental retardation, 624, 804, 898
menthol dissolved in alcohol, for itching, 815
mentholated calomine lotion, 805
Mephenesin, 951
mercaptan, 1196
mercaptopurine, 309
Mercurochrome, 109, 885
mercurous chloride, 292
mercury, 505, 853
mercury combinations, 518
mercury fulminate, 972
mercury poisoning, 899, 901, 974, 1056
merthiolate, 1366
merthiolate, tincture of, 109
mesomorphic, 1292

mesothorium, 974
metabolic processes, 1040
metabolism, 898, 1107
metabolism, regulation of, 956
metacarpal bones, 318
metacorten, 41, 761
metal fume fever, 969, 971
metallic poisons, 898-901
metallic taste, 901
Metaphen, 109, 885, 1366
metastases, 294
metastasis, 901-2, 1287
methanol, 974
methanol poisoning, 1356
methemoglobin, 967
methionine, 78
methisozone, 1327
methotrexate, 1085
methyl alcohol, 974
methylene blue, 1055
methyl chloride, 974
methyl violet, 974
metritis, 902
metrorrhagia, 893, 902
metroscope, 902
mica, 975
microfilariae, 645
micro-instrumentation, 1205
microorganisms, 791, 928
microscope, 222
microscope, electron, 1326
micturition, 902, 1312-13
midbrain, 254
middle age change, men, 902-4
middle ear, 526
middle layer, 408
midget, 26
migraine, 549, 707, 904-5, 906-7
migraine, psychological factor in, 905
miliaria, 1078
miliary tuberculosis, 1278, 1285
milibis, 74
milium, 1348-49
milk, 905-9
milk (as antidote), 901
milk (as food), 1190, 1332, 1335, 1336
milk, dried, 908
milk, homogenized, 908
milk of lime, 517
milk of magnesia, 326, 884, 885
milk, pasteurization of, 792
milk secretion, 1041
milk solids, 908
milk sugar, 908
milk teeth, 1247
Miltown, 65
mind, 1162
mineral acids, 26
mineral oil, 192, 323, 884
mineral salt diuretics, 518

minerals, 909, 954, 955-56
miner's nystagmus, 956
minimal, 478
mining, 803
mirbane, oil of, 975
miscarriage, 20, 1335
miscarriage, prevention, 909-10
miscegenation, 910
mite typhus, 1165
mites, 789, 1150, 1165
mitral valve, 714
mixed tumors, 644
moist gangrene, 673
molars, 1247
molds, 663
molestation, simple, 1199
Monday morning fever, 804
mongolism, 520, 910
moniliasis, 666, 910-11
monkshood, 34
monocular, 594
mononucleosis, infectious, 18, 797, 857, 867, 911, 912-13, 1351
monoplegia, 1009
mons pubis, 1337, 1338
mons veneris, 1337
Montgomery's tubercles, 1076
moron(s), 623, 911
morphine, 81, 911-14
morphine and opium poisoning, 914-15
mortality, decline, 915
Morton, William T. G., 89
mosaicism, 521, 915, 1132
mosquito, 54, 482, 871, 872, 915, 1108, 1370, 1371
mother's milk, 905
motion sickness, 318, 916-17, 1199
motor cortex, 256
motor nerve paralysis, 1009
motor nerves, 924
mottling of teeth, 1248
mount of Venus, 1337
mountain sickness, 917
mouth, 917, 1191, 1206, 1227, 1337
mouth cancer, 295
mouth, disturbances of, 1332
mouth dryness, 737
mouth proper, 917
mouth, swollen, 843
mouth-to-mouth breathing, 548
mouth-to-mouth method, 1136
mouth-to-mouth resuscitation, 1136
mucous colitis, 422
mucous material, 799
mucous membranes, 910, 951
mucous membranes, thickening of, 932
mucous patch, 1240
mucilaginous materials, 323

1385

INDEX

mucus, 1198
multiple birth, 205-6
multiple neuritis, 945
multiple paralysis, 968
multiple sclerosis, 148, 917-20, 949
mumps, 530, 789 792, 794, 920-24, 984, 1256, 1326
mumps serum, 984
mumps vaccine, 924
munitions manufacture, 967
murine flea-borne typhus, 1290, 1291
muscarin, 929
muscae volantes, 599
muscle, 924-28, 1218, 1250
muscle cramps, 462-63
muscle cramps, night, 950-51
muscle diseases and disorders, 928-29
muscle fatigue, 928
muscle fibers, 408
muscle tissue, 1344
muscular dystrophy, 925-27, 929, 948
muscle, nonstriated, 924
muscular paralysis, 667
muscular paralysis, pseudohypertrophic, 667, 841
muscular rheumatism, 644, 929
musculature and weight, 1343-44
mushroom poisoning, 929
mushrooms, 663
mussel poisoning, 656
mustard, 852, 929-30
mustard plaster, 930
mutual orgasm, 1177
mutual masturbation, 764, 1199
myasthenia gravis, 930-31
mycins, 797
myelitis, 1208
myocardial infarction, 448-49, 931
myocarditis, 710
myocardium, 318, 450, 710
mycetoma, 871
mycoderma aceti, 641
Mycostatin, 911
myelin sheaths, 949
myoma, 929
myopia, 592, 931
myositis, 928, 1145
myxedema, 85, 464-65, 774, 931-32

N

nail biting, 933
nail, ringworm of, 1352
nail, splinters under, 934
nails, 933-35
naphtha, 968
naphtha jags, 968
naphuride sodium, 543, 645
narcissin, 975

narcissism, 935
narcissus bulbs, 975
narcolepsy, 935
narcosis, 974, 979
narcosynthesis, 773
narcotic addiction, 522, 896, 914-15, 935
narcotic poisoning, 1056
narcotics, 806, 885, 935
nasal cavities, 1191
nasal disorders, 935
nasal duct, 606, 1244
nasal infection, 952
nasal passages, 526
nasal pharynx, 1032
nasal polyp, 1064
nasopharynx, 1199
nates, 935
natural sugar, 908
natural ventilation, 1319-22
nausea, 737, 916, 940, 1024, 1077
nausea and vomiting epidemic, 1326
navel, 1292
navel, diseases, 935-36
nearsightedness, 592, 595, 596, 610, 936
necator americanus, 1360
neck, 1258
neck, broken, 936
neck, tooth, 1246
neck, whiplash injury, 1220-21
necrosis, 937, 976
negative Rh, 1116
negative nitrogen balance, 954
Neisseria gonorrheae, 690
Nembutal, 178
neocortex, 256
Neohetramine, 108, 131, 186
neomycin, 101, 523, 783
neonal, 1054
neostigmine, 931
nephritis, 826, 937-42, 972, 976, 977, 979, 1308, 1312, 1313
nephritis, acute, 938-39, 940
nephritis, chronic interstitial, 409
nephrosis, 941, 942-43
neoprene, 174
nerve(s), 924, 943, 1185, 1191, 1246
nerve block, 80, 1270
nerve cells, 943, 1246
nerve endings, 1185
nerve endings, bare, 1187
nerve endings, specialized, 1186
nerve fibers, bundles of, 943
nerve ganglia, 948
nerve impulses, 943
nerve, inflammation, 945
nerves, injuries and diseases of, 943-45
nerve tissue, 943
nerveless areas, 842
nervous breakdown, 943, 1226

nervous disorders, 815, 943, 1173
nervous prostration, 588
nervous symptoms, 1109
nervous system, 745, 903, 943-45, 1333, 1350
nervous tissue, 1303
nervousness, 1334
neuralgia, 131, 945, 1100
neuralgia, facial, 612, 685
neuralgia, occipital, 960
neuralgia, glossopharyngeal, 685
neuralgia, operation for trigeminal, 1266
neuritis, 131, 945-48, 1009, 1258, 1334
neuritis, cold and, 948
neuritis, multiple, 945
neuritis, optic, 921
neurocirculatory asthenia, 488, 734-35
neurodermatitis, 156
neurological and neuromuscular disorders, 948-49
neurologist, 1212
neuromuscular re-education, 949
neurons, 718, 943
neurosis, 623, 949-50, 1085
neurosis, cardiac, 734-35
neurosyphilis, 1241
neurotic, 1088
neurotropic viruses, 1326
nevus, 202-3
newborn, gonorrheal infection in, 690
newborn, hemolytic disease of, 1116
newborn, jaundice in, 817
Newcastle's disease, 961
niacin, 348, 1190, 1328, 1332
niacin deficiency, 950, 1020
niacin, food sources of, 1332
nickel, 975
nickel carbonyl, 975
nickel rash, 975
nicotinamide, 1020, 1356
nicotine, 153
nicotine poisoning, 962, 979, 1056
nicotinic acid, 1266, 1328, 1332, 1370
nicotinic acid deficiency, 1020
nicotinic acid, food sources of, 1332
Niemann-Pick's disease, 950
night blindness, 477, 1328
night cramps, 950-51
night sweats, 951
night terrors, 951
nine-mile fever, 1099
nipple, 262

nipple, Paget's disease of, 1003
nitric acid, 26, 547, 975
nitrobenzene, 975
nitrocellulose, 975
nitrogen, 954, 1083
nitrogen balance, negative, 954
nitrogen dioxide, 975, 976
nitrogen mustard, 764
nitrogen mustard chemicals, 305
nitrogen oxides, 975-76
nitrogen tetroxide, 975
nitrogenous substances, 1083
nitroglycerin(e), 95, 976
nitrous chloride, 976
nitrous gases, 976
nitrous oxides, 89, 976
nocardiosis 792, 951
nocturnal emission, 951
nodules in lung, 963
noise, 951, 965-66
nonparalytic poliomyelitis, 1057
nonstriated muscle, 924
nontropical sprue, 1218
nor-adrenalin, 226
nor-epinephrine, 226
normal weight, 1292
Norway, 1109
nose, 516, 951-53, 1337
nose, chronic inflammation of, 1238
nose, thickening of skin, 931-32
nosebleed, 545, 571, 917, 921, 953
novocaine, 89, 98, 1270
NPH insulin, 807
nuclear explosions, protection against fallout from, 613-17
nucleus pulposus, 1192, 1193
nuclei, nerve cells, 943
nudism, 589
numbness of hands and feet, 1008
nursing, 953
nursing care, 1099
nursing mothers diet, 369-85
nutrients, chart of key, 955
nutrition, 954-56
nutritional anemias, 83
nutritional deficiencies, 934, 945, 948
nutritional deficiency disorders of small intestine, 1218
nutritional edema, 1300
nuts, 1190
nymphomania, 956, 1157
nystagmus, 889, 956
Nystatin, 106, 911

O

oak blossom, 704
oatmeal extract, 815
obesity, 957-60, 1344
obesity impairment chart, 958
obstructive jaundice, 1336
obstructive laryngitis, acute, 466
occipital bone, 1191
occipital lobes, 256
occipital neuralgia, 960
occlusion, 1223
occupational bifocals, 196
occupational diseases, 100, 436, 787, 899-901
occupational diseases, biological hazards, 960-62
occupational hazards, industry, 962-80
occupational skin diseases, 962
occupational therapy, 980, 1037
ochronosis, 887
oculocardiac reflex, 1117
odors, 980
oil of chenopodium, 1361
oil of mirbane, 975
oiliness of skin, excessive, 1334
ointments, 1164
old age, 980
olfactory bulbs, 984
olfactory nervous system, 980-84
olfactory sense, 980-84, 1196
olfactory tracts, 984
olive or similar oils, 1169
omega-methyl pantothenic acid, 1008
omentum, 984
onanism, 984
onchocercosis, 645
one- and two-year-olds, pictorial guide to needs of, 370-71
onychia, 984
onycholysis, 436-42, 934, 984
onychomycosis, 1152
oophorectomy, 322
Opap, 708
opaque meal of barium, 1368
open fractures, 1191
open heart surgery, 721-29, 1232-36
operation for trigeminal neuralgia, 1266
ophthalmia, 984
ophthalmologist, 1219
ophthalmoscope, 599, 601, 685, 984
opium, 81, 89, 852
opium poisoning, 914-15
optic nerve, 591, 984
optic neuritis, 921
optimal, vitamins, 478
optimum weight averages, 1345-46

1386

INDEX

oral contraceptives (the pill), 200
oral thrush, 910
orbits, of eyes, 1191
orchitis, 984-85, 1256
organ transplants, 985
organic acids, 26
organic phosphates, 977
organisms, invasion by, 791
orgasm, 877, 984, 986, 1022, 1128
orgasm, clitoral, 1338
oriental sore, 842
orinase, 986
orthodontia, 986-87, 1247
orthohydroxydiphenyl, 870
orthopedic surgeons, 251
orthopedists, 1209, 1212
orthoptic training, 598
oscilloscope, cathode-ray, 326-27
osmosis, 310, 1130
ossein, 245
osteitis, 987
osteitis deformans, 987, 1003, 1191
osteitis fibrosa, 1016
osteoarthritis, 136, 250, 617, 817, 987-90
osteoarthritis, chronic, 817
osteoblasts, 245
osteomalacia, 1016, 1335
osteomyelitis, 249, 860, 987, 990
osteopathy, 990-91
osteoporosis, 245, 1016
otitis, 425, 987, 991-92
otitis, acute, 991
otitis, chronic, 991
otitis media, 426, 991
otorhinolaryngologist, 531
otosclerosis, 475, 992
otoscope, 400, 529
Otto, John Conrad, 748
outside coat, 409
ova, 1128
ova, chromosome in, 1131
ovarian infection, 994-95
ovarian ligaments, 993
ovaries, 613, 684, 894, 921, 992-93, 1089, 1128, 1313
overexposure to x-rays or radium radiation, 20
overfeeding, 387
overgrowth of liver, 855
overweight, 235, 766, 1344
overweight, hereditary factors in, 745-48
oviducts, 613, 1128, 1129, 1313

ovulation, 993-96, 1129
ovum, 613, 1128, 1177, 1222
ovum, fertilized, 343, 1372
oxidation, 1262
oxyacetylene gas, 965
Oxycel, 741
oxygen, 212, 268, 996, 1083
oxygen-carrying power of blood, 970
oxygen deficiency, 1116
oxygen, high altitudes, 428
oxygen therapy, high pressure, 996-1002
oxytetracyline, 101
ozena, 1002

P

pacemaker, electronic, 711, 720
pacemakers, implanted, 883
Pacinian corpuscle, 1187
pad, electric, 886
pads, sterile gauze, 885
Paget's disease, 987, 1003
Paget, Sir James, 1003
pain, 470, 1003-4, 1024
pain, abdominal, 17-19
pain, acute, 39
pain in bones and joints, 843
pain relievers, 884-85
pain, sensation of, 943, 1187
painful ankle, 98
painful migratory arthritis, 1138
pain-relieving liniments, 852
painter's colic, 840
palate, 1004, 1199, 1206
palate, cleft, 412, 413, 1206
palate, hard, 917, 1004
palatine arches, 1258
paleocortex, 257
palpitation, heart, 718, 893
palsy, 1004
paludrine, 109
pancreas, 337, 487, 488, 682, 765, 774, 814, 1004-8, 1040, 1041
pancreatitis, acute, 1006-7
pancreas, cancer of, 302-3, 1005
pancreatic cysts, 1005
pancreatic enzymes, 954
pancreatic juice, 1004
pancreatitis, 921
pancreatitis, acute, 1006-7
pancreatitis, chronic, 1005

pancreatitis, advanced hemorrhagic, 1007
pandemia, 1302
pantothenic acid, 956, 1328, 1334, 1370
pantothenic acid deficiency, 1008
Papanicolaou test, 298
papillae, 1267
papilloma, 210
pappataci fever, 1157
papules, 870, 1190
para-amino-benzoic acid, 1008-9, 1328, 1334
para-aminosalicylic acid, 477, 523, 791, 1275, 1284
paradione, 570
paraffin bath, 132
paralysis, 974, 1241
paralysis agitans, 148, 564, 667, 948, 1009-12
paralysis, functions, 257
paralysis, hysterical, 776
paralysis, laryngeal muscles, 838
paralysis, multiple, 968
paralysis, muscular, 667
paralysis, pseudohypertrophic muscular, 667, 841
paralysis, vocal cords, 838
paralytic poliomyelitis, 1057
paranitranilin, 966
paranitraniline red, 977
paranoia, 896, 1012-13
paraphenylendiamine, 962
paraphilia, 1013
paraplegia, 1009, 1013
parasites, 663, 788-89, 815, 857, 866
parasitic infection, 855
parasitic infestations of skin, 850-51
parasympathetic nervous system, 1239
parathion, 977
parathyroid glands, 684, 771, 1013-16, 1036, 1044
parathyroid hormone, 771
paratyphoid fever, 165, 961
parenteral fluids, 1008
paresis, 1016-17
paresis, general, 896, 1241
paretic neurosyphilis, 1016
parietal bones, 1191
parietal lobes, 256
Parkinson's disease, 148, 948, 1012, 1017
Parkinson, James, 1012
paronychia, 934

parotid glands, 648, 917, 921
parotitis, 921, 1017
parrot fever, 1083
parrot infection, 1326
parrot jaw, 817
Parry, Caleb Hillier, 1017
Parry's disease, 1017
partial ague, 59
partial denture, 485
parturition, 1017
passive immunization, 1327
Pasteur, Louis, 169, 761
pasteurella pestis, 1044
pasteurization, 796, 908
patch test, 69, 1017
patella, 820
patellar bursa, 835
pathogens, 169, 788
pathogenic, 169
pathology, 1237
peanuts, 1190, 1333
pederasty, 764, 1017, 1199
pediatrician, 1017
pediatrics, 1017
pediatrist, 1017
pediculoides ventricosus, 972
pediculosis, 25, 847, 1017
pediculus humanus, 243
pellagra, 85, 477, 836, 887, 1017-21, 1190, 1332
pelvimetry, 1021
pelvis, 1021, 1097, 1184, 1207
pemphigus, 1021-22
pemphigus vulgaris, 1021
pendulous breasts, 263-64
penetrating injury, 607
penicillin, 22, 28, 40, 59, 120, 209, 405, 484, 522, 564, 782, 790, 797, 826, 871, 885, 990, 1017, 1022, 1029, 1033, 1052, 1109, 1139, 1159, 1174, 1184, 1225, 1231, 1241, 1259, 1271, 1287
penicillin, crystalline, 1323
penicillium notatum, 1022
penis, 1022-24, 1118, 1126, 1164, 1177, 1309
pentapyrrolidium, 108
pentobarbital, 178, 1054
pentothal sodium, 90, 178
pepsin, 507, 1157
peptic ulcer, 1024-28, 1224
peptic ulcer, bleeding, 814
peptones, 954
perborate of soda, 1323
perforated corneal ulcer, 1079

perforation, acute, 1028
perforation of ulcer, 19
pericarditis, 318, 710, 1028, 1030-31, 1049
pericardium, 318, 710, 910, 1028
perimeter, 602, 685
perineum, 1028-29, 1309, 1338
periodic bloodletting, 1064
periodontal membrane, 1246
periods, 1316
periosteum, 248
periostitis, 976
peripheral arteriosclerosis, 129
peripheral nervous system, 943
peristalsis, 253, 811, 1308
peritoneum, 114, 811, 984, 1029
peritonitis, 22, 114, 118-19, 323, 811, 855, 942, 1029
peritonitis, acute, 812
pernicious anemia, 18, 84, 85-87, 222, 858, 1029, 1114, 1214, 1333
personality, 1304
perspiration, 1029-32, 1187, 1249
perspiration, lack of, 931
pertussis, 795, 1032, 1352-56
pessary(ies), 443, 1079
petit mal, 567
petrolatum, 1352
petroleum jelly, 885
petroleums, 968
pets, allergies to, 71
phagocytes, 217
phagocytosis, 217
phallin, 929
pharmacopsychosis, 40
pharyngeal virus, 112
pharyngitis, 1032, 1199, 1258
pharyngitis, acute, 1032
pharyngitis, atrophic, 1033
pharyngitis, chronic, 1033
pharyngitis, hypertrophic, 1033
pharynx, 516, 1032-33, 1199, 1206, 1224, 1258
phenacitin, 81, 108, 884, 1054
phenindamine tartrate, 108
phenobarbital, 178, 236, 270, 570, 889, 1054, 1353
phenol, 968, 970
phenolated calamine lotion, 805
phenolphthalein, 326, 884, 1033
phenolsulfonephthalein, 209
phenurone, 570
phenylalanine, 78

1387

INDEX

phenyl-thiocarbamide, 745
phenytoin sodium, 570
phlebitis, 1033-36, 1319
phlebotomus fever, 1157
Phlebotomus paptasii, 1157
phobia, 111, 558-59, 622
phobic reaction, 950
phonocardiogram, 719
phonocardiograph, 486
phosgene, 976
phosgene vapors, 977
phosphate, 1036
phosphorus, 348, 956, 976, 1036, 1147, 1245, 1249
phosphorus poisoning, 816
phosphorus, radioactive, 843, 1064, 1115
phosphorus utilization, 1013, 1335
phosphureted hydrogen, 976-77
photophobia, 604
photosynthesis, 311
phototherapy, 739
phrenia, 1162
physical conditioning, 430-31
physiotherapy, 1058-59
phthalates, 1165
phthirius pubis, 462
phthisis, 1036
physical activity, disinclination to, 1301
physical predisposition, 1088
physical therapy, 1036-37
physiological surgery, 1232
physiological weight, 1298
physiology, 1237
physiotherapy, 981-83, 1037, 1119-25
pia mater, 889
pian, 1370
pica, 1037
picrates, 977
picric acid, 977
picric itch, 977
picro toxin, 177
pigment cells, hair, 696
pigmentation, 1037-39, 1185, 1191
pigments, 197, 1313
pigweed, 704
piles, 741-44, 1039
pilonidal cyst, 1039
pimple(s) (acne), 27-33, 529
pinched nail, 934
pine oil, 870
pineal gland, 684, 1039-40
pink disease, 35
pinkeye, 432-33, 600, 1040
pinworm, 788, 1040, 1356-57, 1358-59
pinworm infestation, 1356

pipe smoking and lung cancer, 1197
pitchblende, 1108
pituitary (gland), 20, 34, 53, 137, 174, 247, 255-56, 487, 684, 738, 765, 770, 894, 1040-44
pituitary gland, anterior portion, 1343
pituitary inactivity, 1041
pityriasis rosea, 1042-43, 1044
pivot joints, 250
placenta, 55, 1044, 1130, 1292, 1293
plague, 183, 782, 789, 792, 1044-45, 1100, 1109
planing, 1244
plantar warts, 1045
plasma, 216, 219, 1299
plasma, blood, 219-20
plasma, freezing and packaging, 220, 221
plasminogen, 841
plasmodium, 109
plasmodium vivax, 109
plaster cast, 1180
plastic sponge (contraceptive), 202
plastic teeth, 484
platelets, 216, 1045, 1351
platelets, blood, 217-18, 221, 741, 1092, 1259
platinum, 1108
pleura, 861, 1045
pleurisy, 1045
pleurisy, suppurative, 562
pleurodynia, 486
pneumococcus (pneumococci), 101, 277, 604, 789, 1049
pneumoconiosis, 524
pneumonia, 18, 116, 169, 475, 505, 697, 792, 797, 816, 866, 910, 960, 990, 996, 1022, 1045, 1049-52, 1225, 1286, 1291, 1308
pneumonia, bacterial, 1052
pneumonia, lipoid, 427
pneumonia, lobar, 277, 1049, 1230, 1302
pneumonic influenza, 799
pneumonic plague, 1044, 1052
pneumothorax, artificial, 477, 1285
pneumotropic viruses, 1326
poison ivy, 67, 436, 437-39
poison oak, 436
poison sumac, 436
poisoning, 20, 1052-56
poisons, 866, 1040
poliomyelitis, 781, 782, 789, 792, 794, 841, 924, 945,

1009, 1057-64, 1208, 1326
poliomyelitis, abortive, 1057
poliomyelitis, bulbar, 281
poliomyelitis, paralytic, 1057
poliomyelitis, nonparalytic, 1057
poliomyelitis vaccine, Salk, 1057-64, 1156, 1317
pollen, hay fever-producing plant, 71, 704, 705
polyarteritis nodosa, 422, 423, 1064
polycythemia, 153, 1064, 1115
polycythemia, secondary, 1115, 1169
polycythemia vera, 1115
polymyxin, 106, 783
polyneuritis, 945
polyp, 1064-70
polyp, ear, 1064
polyp, gastric, 1064
polyps, nasal, 952
popliteal vein, 841
pores, 1187
pores, dilated, 1070
pork, and pork products, 882, 1190, 1332
pork tapeworm, 1364
portal circulation, 408
portal vein, 408, 854
positive Rh, 348, 1116
positive skin reaction, 1275
posterior chambers, 591
posterior pituitary, 1040, 1041
postinfection encephalitis, 563
post-natal care of mother. 1070
post-traumatic amnesia, 79
postural hypotension, 236
posture, 1070-75
posture in sleep, 948
potash, 67
potassium, 507, 956
potassium chloride, 931, 935
potassium iodides, 211, 840, 853, 1218
potassium permanganate, 150, 911, 1055
potassium permanganate solution, 1056
potatoes, 1334
Pott's disease, 1278
poultry, 881, 882, 883
predilection to heart damage, 1138
prednisolone, 457
prednisone, 41, 137
prefrontal lobotomy, 1075, 1088
pregnancy, 639-40, 858, 1312

pregnancy and prenatal care, 1075
pregnancy, anemia in, 83
pregnancy, eclampsia in, 532-33
pregnancy, interrupted, 20
pregnancy, signs of, 1075-77
premature babies, 158-64, 1077
premolar, 196
prenatal care, childbirth and, 341-52
prepuce, 409, 1022
presbyopia, 596, 1077-78, 1170
prescription, 1078
pressure, blood, high, 226-36, 605, 755, 1173
pressure, blood, low, 236-37, 860, 1008
pressure, sensation of deep, 1187
pressure stats, 226
pressure-sensitive nerve endings, 226
prevention, eye injuries in industry, 608-9
prickly heat, 1078-79
Priestley, Joseph, 89
primaquine, 109, 872
primary hypotension, 236
primary lesions, 1190-91
primary stage, syphilis, 1240
primary teeth, 1246-47
prime grade meats, 882
primipara, 350
procaine, 89, 1270
proctoscopy, 298
progesterone, 893, 894, 992, 1129
progestin, 910
proglottids, 1361
progressive cancerous growth, 294
projections, on dermis, 1186
projections, on tongue, 1267
prolapse, 1079
prolapse, iris, 1079
prolapse, uterus, 1079
propanolol, 96
propylthiouracil, 770
prostate (gland), 22, 208, 1079-83, 1118, 1126, 1309
prostate cancer, 1080-87
prostate enlargement, 1080-81, 1173
prostatic fluid, 1079
prostatic portion, 1309
prostatitis, 1079
prostatitis, chronic, 1079
prostheses, 138, 1206
prostigmine, 839
protamine-zinc insulin, 807

protective clothing, 100, 312, 394
protective pants, 394
protein(s), 348, 855, 908, 954, 1083, 1298, 1299, 1303
proteins, complete, 1083
protein deficiency, 873, 954
protein, food sources, 1336
protein loss, 1300
protein per pound, meats, 882-83
protective mechanism, pain as, 1003
prothrombin, 218, 219, 221
prothrombin test, 1252-53
prothrombin time, determination of, 218
protoplasm, 1342
protoveratrine, 108
protozoa, 788, 792
pruritis, 815, 1083
pseudoarthrosis, 819
pseudohermaphroditism, 81, 748
pseudohypertrophic muscular paralysis, 667, 841
psittacosis, 792, 1083-84, 1326, 1327
psoriasis, 406, 777, 1084-85, 1086-87
psychasthenia, 588
psychiatry, 1085, 1088
psychoanalysis, 1085-88
psychogenic pain, 1003
psychological factor in migraine, 905
psychology, 1088
psychometric tests of children, 359-62
psychosis, 623, 1088, 1162
psychosis, alcoholic, 896
psychosomatic disorders, 896, 1088
psychosomatic medicine, 558
psychosurgery, 1088
psychotherapy, 783, 956, 1088
psychotic, 950, 1088
psyllium seed, 323
P.T.C., 745
ptomaine poisoning, 1089
puberty, 48, 1089-91
pubis, 636
public health, 1091
puerperal fever, 1225
puerperal mastitis, 876
pulmonary artery, 407, 714, 861
pulmonary circulation 406, 408
pulmonary edema, 975, 976
pulmonary heart disease, 730-31
pulmonary tuberculosis, 1276-77, 1278

1388

INDEX

pulmonary valve, 714
pulmonary veins, 408, 714, 861, 1319
pulmonic stenosis, surgery in, 1091
pulp cavity, 1246
pulse, 586, 1091-92
pump-oxygenator, for heart surgery, 711
puncture wound, 1092
pupil, 591
pupil dilation, 1239
pure food law enforcement, 655, 1093-96
purgative, 323, 1092
purines, 691
purple foxglove, 513
purpura, 953
purpura hemorrhagica, 1092-97, 1214, 1215
purulent, 1097
purulent sinusitis, 425
pus, 799, 1097
pus formation, 991
pustules, 1190
putty, 977
pyelitis, 826, 1097
pyelonephritis, 826, 1097
pyelonephritis, chronic, 232, 937
pyemia, 855, 1097, 1214
pyloric antrum, 110
pyloric canal, 1224
pyloric sphincter, 1224, 1337
pyloric valve, muscle, enlargement, 1224
pylorus, 1097-98, 1337
pyorrhea, 679, 695, 1098, 1248
Pyramidon, 58, 708, 1054
Pyrene, 977
pyrethrotoxic acid, 971
pyrethrum, 663, 971
Pyribenzamine, 108, 131, 186, 239
pyridoxine, 1190, 1328, 1370
pyrogens, 239

Q

Q fever, 792, 796, 1099, 1150
quacks, 337, 441-45, 1099-1100
quadriplegia, 1009
quarantine, 1100, 1193
quartan malaria, 872
quickening, 342, 1076, 1100
quickening of heartbeat, 1239
quinacrine hydrochloride, 148
quinine, 109, 148, 872, 951, 1100-1
quinine compounds, 977
quinine sulphate, 1100

quinidine, 643, 1101
quinsy, 39, 1101
quothane, 157

R

rabbit fever, 1102
rabbit starvation, 124
"rabbit tests," 342
rabies, 97, 519, 549, 782, 792, 1100, 1102-3, 1109, 1326
rabies inoculation, 1103
radial artery, 1091
radiation, 210, 1103-4, 1115, 1270
radiation sickness, 1104-6
radiation therapy, 307-8, 1085
radiation treatment, 910, 948, 952
radical bilateral adrenalectomy, 235
radio iodine, 770
radioactive carbon, 1108
radioactive chromium, 309
radioactive cobalt, 152
radioactive fallout, protection against, 613-17
radioactive gold, 309, 1106
radioactive iodine, 153, 689, 1106
radioactive isotope scanning, 883
radioactive isotopes, 152, 305, 1103, 1106
radioactive phosphorus, 843, 1064, 1115
radioactive selenomethionine, 883
radioactive substances, 964
radioactive thulium, 1106
radioactivity, 1106-8
radiogold, 153
radiographs, 1106
radiography, 1103
radioisotopes, 1106
radiophosphorus, 153
radiosodium, 152
radiostrontium, 155, 1108
radiotherapy, 1104
radiothorium, 974
radium, 210, 964, 1103, 1108-9
radium mesothorium I, 974
radium needles, 210
radium radiation, 20
radium therapy, 823, 887
radium treatment, 304, 846, 1339
radius, 536, 1091
radon, 1108-9
radon seeds, 210
ragweed, 705
râle, 1109
rat, 1291
rat control, 1109-10
rat flea, 1044, 1290
rat poison, 1372

rat tapeworm, 1364
rat-bite fever, 1022, 1109
rats, 797
rattle, 1109
rattlesnake bite, 1197
rauwolfia, 108
rauwolfia serpentina, 236. 1132
ray fungus, 35
Raynaud's disease, 1110, 1112-13
reaction to stimulus, 1117
reading, difficulty in, 917
reading, learning, 48
ready-made sterilized bandages, 885
recipe, 1078
rectal polyp, 1064
rectal syringe, 1242
rectum, 252, 253, 422, 811, 1110
rectum, cancer of, 300-1
red blood cell determination test, 1252-53
red blood cells, 216, 1110, 1351
red blood cells, diseases of, 1110-16
red cells, 216
red-green color blindness, 804
reducing diet, 508-9, 1117
Reed, Walter, 1371
referred pain, 1003
reflex, 1117
reflex actions, 1208
reflexes, hyperactive, 1008
refractive error, measuring, 598
refrigerants, 972, 974, 978
refrigeration workers, 804
regeneration, nerve, 943
regional anesthesia, 87
regional ileitis, 780
regression, 1117
rehabilitation, 1117-18
relapsing fever, 1118
relapsing fever, European, 183
relays of neurons, 943
removal of allergens, 1097
removal of spleen, 1097
removing foreign bodies, eye, 609
renal circulation, 408
renin, 226
rennet, 321
repigmentation, 1337
replenishment of iron, 1097
reproduction system, 1118-32
reproductive cells, 992
reproductive cells, chromosomes in, 1131
reserpine, 1132

reserve power, 903
resin, 978
resistance, low, 1334
respiration, 943
respiration, artificial, 139, 140-41, 1053, 1133
respiratory tract discharges, 799
respiratory diseases, 1132-33
resuscitation, 548, 1133-37
retention cyst, 684
reticulum cell sarcoma, 1352
retina, 147, 591, 1137
retina, detachment, 605, 1137
retina, inflammation, 604-5
retinal camera, 601
retinitis, 967, 1137
retinoblastoma, 602, 1137
retrograde amnesia, 79
retrolental fibroplasia, 1137-38
Rh blood groups, 240
Rh factor, 240, 910, 1145
Rh negative, 240, 348
Rh positive, 348, 1116
Rh system, 1116
rhesus factor, 348
rheumatic diseases, 804
rheumatic fever, 46, 50, 318, 405, 792, 797, 894, 1138-45, 1225, 1270
rheumatic heart disease, 1142-43
rheumatic lesions, 1138
rheumatism, 819, 948, 1145, 1173, 1185
rheumatism, muscular, 644, 929
rheumatoid arthritis, 131, 134-35, 834, 860, 1145
rheumatoid arthritis, chronic, 820
rhinitis, 1145
rhinitis, atrophic, 1002
rhinophyma, 1145
rhinoplasty, 1145
rhubarb, 1145
rhythm method, 202, 443, 1146
riboflavin (vitamin B_2), 348, 882, 908, 1146, 1190, 1328, 1370
riboflavin deficiency, 853, 1332-33
riboflavin, food sources of, 1329
ribs, 337, 1146-47, 1184
rice, 193
rickets, 245, 477, 478, 954, 1032, 1147, 1191, 1247, 1335
rickettsia, 101

Rickettsia acari, 1150
rickettsiae, 789, 792
rickettsial diseases, 1150
rickettsial organism, 1099, 1150
rickettsialpox, 1150
ridges, on dermis, 1186
right auricle, 710
right hypochondrium, 19
right iliac, 19
right lumbar, 19
right lymphatic duct, 867
right maxilla, 817
right side, heart, 406
right ventricle, 714
ringworm, 633, 792, 1109, 1150-53, 1238
ringworm, of beard, 1153
ringworm, body, 1152
ringworm, groin, 1151
ringworm, nail, 1352
ringworm, scalp, 1151
Rio Grande fever, 1153, 1305
RNA, 1328
Rocky Mountain spotted fever, 782, 789, 792, 805, 1150, 1153-55
Rocky Mountain spotted fever group, 1150
rodents, small, 1150
roentgen, 152
roentgen rays, 1103
Roentgen, Wilhelm Konrad, 1368
roentgenography, 1103
roof of skull, 1191
room temperatures, 59-62
root, hair follicle, 1187
roots, tooth, 1246
rotogravure ink, 977
roughage in diet, 509-10
roundworm, 1155, 1357-60
rubber binder, 1353
rubber gloves, wearing of, 1232
rubella, 674, 793, 1155
rubeola, 794, 878-79, 1155
Ruffini's end organs, 1186
rupture, 748-54, 1155
rupture, ear, 528

S

sacral vertebrae, 1156
sacroiliac, 1156
sacroiliac joint, degenerative arthritis of, 860
sacrum, 249, 1156, 1184, 1185, 1239, 1322
sadism, 1156
safety goggles, 603

1389

INDEX

safety rules, eye injuries, 609
St. Anthony's fire, 572, 1222
St. Louis encephalitis, 563
St. Vitus' dance, 148, 405, 696, 1138, 1156, 1205
salicylic acid, 138, 633, 691, 1085, 1118, 1152, 1352
salicylate group, 1144
saline cathartics, 326, 901, 1356
saliva, 1156
saliva, increase in, 901
salivary glands, 682, 917
Salk, Jonas, 1328
Salk poliomyelitis vaccine, 1057-64, 1156, 1317
salmon, 1335
salmonella, 165, 654
salpingitis, 613, 1156
salt, 1156-57
salt-free diet, 511
salts, gold, 137
salt, insufficient, 951
salt loss, 737
salt solution as emetic, 1356
San Joaquin fever, 418, 1157
sandblasting, 803
sandfly fever, 1157
sandstone workers, 803, 977
sanitation, 790, 796
sanitary pads and wicks, 638
sarcoma, 987, 1157, 1286
saprophytes, 663
saturated fats, 620
satyriasis, 1157
saw, 1237
scabies, 850-51, 1157-58
scales (skin lesion), 1191
scalp nerves, 945
scalp, ringworm of, 1151
scalp wound, 546
scalpel, 1237
scanning, 883
scapula, 1185
scarlatina, 795, 1160-61
scarlet fever, 110, 474, 530, 697, 782, 792, 795, 837, 991, 1138, 1158-59, 1160-61, 1225, 1258, 1308, 1318
scars, acne, 29, 32-33
Schaefer technique, 1133
schedule, one-year-old child, 390-91
Schick test, 516, 1252-53
schistosoma, 197, 198
Schistosoma cercariae, 198
Schistosoma haematobium, 197
Schistosoma intercalatum, 198
Schistosoma japonicum, 197

Schistosoma mansoni, 198
schistosomiasis, 198, 1162
schizophrenia, 22, 559, 873, 896, 1162
schizophrenics, mosaicism in, 1132
Schlatter's disease, 818
Schönlein, Johann Lukas, 1152
school-age child, adjustment problems of, 46-48
sciatica, 1145, 1156, 1162
sciatic nerve, 841, 860, 945, 1162, 1163
sciatic neuritis, 1162-64
scissors, 885
sclera, 1301
scleroderma, 423, 1164
sclerosed, 450
sclerosis, 234, 480, 945, 1164, 1191, 1208
sclerosis, lateral, 839
sclerotic coat, 591
scoliosis, 1164, 1208
scorpion bite, 549, 1197
scorpion bite, venomous, 97
scratch test, 69
screw worms, 952
scrotum, 1118, 1126, 1164-65, 1207, 1251, 1304
scrub typhus, 792, 1150, 1165
scurvy, 139, 477, 695, 953, 954, 1165-68, 1190, 1323
scutulum, 1152
sealing wax, 977
seasickness, 1168
seat worm, 1357
sebaceous cyst, 1168, 1350
sebaceous glands, 696, 1168, 1185, 1187
seborrhea, 1168-69
seborrheic dermatitis, 175, 1168, 1169, 1170-71
sebum, 175, 696, 1187, 1350
secobarbital, 178
Seconal, 178, 885, 1054
second childhood, 1117
secondary anemia, 50, 1364
secondary hepatitis, 857
secondary hypotension, 236
secondary jejunal ulcer, 817
secondary infection, 790
secondary lesions, 1190-91
secondary polycythemia, 1115, 1169
secondary sexual characteristics, 1089

secondary shock, 1177
secondary stage, syphilis, 1240-41
security, 897
sedative poisoning, 1053, 1054-55
sedatives, 1085, 1118
sedatives, barbiturate, 948
sedatives, mild, 138
sedimentation test, 1252-53
seeds, 1108
seeing and hearing, child, 356
seeing, difficulty in, 917
segmentation, 811
Seidlitz powder, 884
selenium, 1168
selenium poisoning, 899
selenium sulphide, 175
selenomethionine, radioactive, 1168
self-feeding 391
semen, 1079, 1126, 1169, 1172, 1177, 1309
semen ejaculation, 986
seminal duct, 1126, 1169
seminal vesicle, 1126, 1169, 1172, 1207, 1222, 1251, 1319
semicircular canals, 519
seminiferous tubules, 1126, 1251
Semple vaccine, 1103
senescence, 1172-73
senile cataract, 605
senile psychosis, 896
senile warts, 1342
senility, 559, 1117, 1173-74
sensations, 943, 1103
sensible perspiration, 1032
sensitivity to drugs, 1092
sensitivity to foods and other substances, 815
sensory nerves, 924, 1003
sepsis, 22
septic infection, 817
septic sore throat, 1032, 1174-75, 1225, 1259
septic sore throat epidemic, 1174
septicemia, 790, 1174, 1214
septum, 1198
serious disability, 1109
serous chronic otitis, 991
serum, 418
serum hepatitis, 856
17-B vaccine, 1371
seven-year itch, 1157, 1175
sewer gas, 977
sewer rats, 1109
sex, 1175
sex and weight, 1292
sex behavior, 897
sex chromosomes, 1104, 1130-32

sex education, 1175-77
sex gland, 175, 682, 1040, 1301
sex organs, accessory, 22
sexual characteristics, secondary, 1089
sexual contact, 1240
sexual development, 1040
sexual intercourse, 1177
sexual organs, 765
shaft, hair follicle, 1187
shaking palsy, 148, 948, 1012, 1177
sheath, 443
shellac, 978
shellfish, 1190
Shiga, Kiyoshi, 164
shigella, 164
shingles, 754, 758-59, 792, 1177
ship fever, 1290
shock, 1053, 1177-80
shock, secondary, 1177
shock treatment, 498, 1180
shock treatment, electric, 537
shoes, foot care and, 626-27, 628, 630-31
short and irregular bones, 247
short bones, 247
shortness of breath, 1308
shoulder, 248, 1180-81, 1184
shunting, 238
sick child, 396-97
sick headache, 549, 904
sickle cell anemia, 83, 1114, 1181
sickle cell carriers, 1114
sickle cell hemoglobin, 1114
sickle cell traits, 1114
sideriosis, 803
signa, 1078
signature, 1078
silica, 963
silica, free, 978
silicatosis, 975
silicon dioxide, 803, 968
silicosis, 139, 461, 524, 787, 803, 963, 968, 972, 977, 978
silk thread, sterile, 852
silver nitrate, 124
silver nitrate solution, 690
silver poisoning, 899, 978
silver refining, 901
silver salts, 978
Simmond's disease, 1044, 1181
Simmond's disease and hypogonadism, 1178-79
Simon, Theodore, 199
simple fractures, 1191
simple molestation, 1199

simple goiter, 688, 770-71, 1262
simple tumor, 1287
Simpson, James, 402
sinew, 1251
sino-auricular node, 718
sinus trouble, 991
sinuses, 951, 1064, 1181-84
sinuses, chronic inflammation of, 1238
sinusitis, 426, 799, 1182-83, 1184
sinusitis, purulent, 425
sitz bath, hot, 1082
size and weight, 1292, 1343
skeletal muscle, 924, 1185
skeleton, 245, 246, 1184-85
Skene's glands, 1185, 1337, 1338
skim milk, 1219
skim milk, dried, 908
skin, 1185-91, 1250
skin, allergic diseases of, 440-41
skin, bacterial infections of, 314-15
skin cancer, 1188-89
skin, chemistry of, 336-37
skin, dark, 1038
skin discoloration, 799
skin discoloration, blue, 966-67
skin diseases, occupational, 962
skin disorders, 910
skin, disturbances of, 1332, 1333
skin dryness, sunstroke, 737
skin eruptions, 1334
skin, excessive oiliness of, 1334
skin, fungus infections, 820
skin growths, nonmalignant, 1348-49
skin infections, 1238
skin, light, 1038
skin, parasitic infestations of, 850-51
skualene, 174
skull, 254, 1184, 1191-92
sleep, 1192
sleep, baby, 392-94
sleep, posture in, 948
sleeping bags, baby, 394
sleeping sickness, 563, 789, 1192
sleeplessness, 1192
sleep-producing drugs, 885
sliding joints, 250
slipped disc, 810, 1192-93, 1210-11, 1322
slipped vertebra, 1215
small intestine, 252
small intestine, absorption in, 22
small rodents, 1150
smallpox, 505, 782, 789, 792, 795, 910, 1193-96, 1258, 1326, 1327
smallpox virus, 1326

1390

INDEX

smear test, 1275
smell, 1196
smell, sense of, 804
smoking, 979
smoking and lung cancer, 1196-97
smoking, excessive, 281
snakebite, 97, 110, 549, 1132, 1197
snakebite, venomous, 97
sneezing, 1198
snoring, 1198
snow blindness, 123-24, 706
soap, 852
soap and chapped skin, 336
soap inflammation, 962
social relationships, 897
sodium, 507
sodium bicarbonate (baking soda; bicarbonate of soda), 27, 67, 404, 507, 547, 885, 1198-99
sodium bicarbonate lotion, 815
sodium borate, 251
sodium chloride, 507, 1156
sodium citrate, 238, 900
sodium depletion, 235
sodium fluoride, 485, 652
sodium nitrite injections, 1055
sodium paba, 1164
sodium perborate, 484
sodium phosphate, 884
sodium propionate ointment, 150
sodium, radioactive, 152
sodium sulfate, 326
sodium thiosulphate injections, 1055
sodium urate, 691
sodomy, 1199
soft chancre, 335
soft palate, 1004, 1198, 1258, 1316
soleus, 25
soluble lead citrate, 900
somnambulism, 1199
sore throat, 1032, 1199, 1238
sore throat epidemic, 110
sore throat, septic, 1032, 1174-75, 1225, 1259
sore throat, septic, epidemic, 1174
sore throat, streptococcus, 466
sore tongue, 1334
South African tick-bite fever, 1153
space medicine, 1199-1205
Spanish fly, 309, 1205
spasm, 1205
spasmodic croup, 466
spastic paralysis, 1009

spaying, 322
special tar ointment, 1084
specialized nerve endings, 1186
specks before eyes, 599
speculum, 333
speculum, ear, 529
speech, 1205-6
sperm, 1222, 1251
sperm cells, 1079, 1126
spermatic cords, 1164, 1207, 1319
spermatozoa, 909, 1126, 1169, 1309
spermatozoa, chromosome in, 1131
spermatozoon, 1129, 1131
sphenoid bone, 1191
spherical lens, 842
spherocytosis, hereditary, 748, 1114, 1352
sphincter, 1207, 1312
sphygmomanometer, 224, 719
spider bites, 805, 1207
spider, black widow, 97
spiders, 805
spina bifida, 1207
spinal anesthesia, 87
spinal column, 1192, 1322
spinal cord, 254, 943, 1191, 1207-8, 1239
spinal curvature, 1208-9
spinal fracture, 1209-12
spinal meningitis, 792, 1230
spinal paralysis, infantile, 934
spinal puncture, 329
spinal vertebrae, 337
spine, 1184, 1212-13
spine, curvature of, 1185
spine, tuberculosis of, 1322
spinous process, 1322
spiral bacillus, 1109
spirillum, 789
spirochete, 789, 1118
splanchnic nerves, 1005
spleen, 1213-15, 1260
spleen enlargement, 950, 1214, 1352
spleen, removal of, 1097
spleens, accessory, 1215
splenectomy, 1114, 1115
splenic anemia, 1214
splenic disease, 1215
splint and plaster cast, 1180
split spine, 1207
splinters under nail, 934
splints, 192
splitting, 1162
spondylitis, 1145
spondylolisthesis, 1215, 1322
spontaneous abortion, 20
spontaneous clotting of blood, 1115

sporotrichosis, 666, 792, 961, 1215-18
Sporotrichum schenckii, 1215
spotted fever, 332
sprained ankle, 98
sprains, 818-19, 1178, 1185, 1216-17, 1218
sprue, 18, 85, 1218-19, 1333
sprue, nontropical, 1218
sputum, 589
sputum test, 1275
squint, 1219
stab wound, 1365
stammering, 1206, 1219
standard grade meats, 882
Stanford-Binet test, 1219-22
stapes, 992
staphylococcal diseases, 1022
staphyloccocal infections, 110, 1225
staphylococcal meningitis, 1225
staphylococcus (staphylococci), 176, 654, 789, 876, 987, 1022, 1049, 1230
starches, 348, 1332
startle reflex, 1117
status lymphaticus, 1262
steam inhalation, 1353
sterile, 1305
sterile cotton, 885
sterile gauze bandages, 885
sterile gauze pads, 885
sterility, 797, 1222-23, 1316, 1335
sterility, male, 783
sterilization, 322, 1223-24, 1319
sterilization, instrument, 225
sterilized bandages, ready-made, 885
sternum, 337, 1185
sternutation, 1198
steroid, 443
steroid hormones, 1215
stertor, 1198
stethoscope, 156, 157, 225, 1109, 1237
stimulants, acne and, 28
stimulation, electric, 192
stink damp, 979
stilbine drugs, 211
stimuli, 1103
stomach, 408, 682, 1024, 1097, 1224-25
stomach ache, 1225
stomach cancer, 296-97, 298
stomach cramps, 463
stomach disorder, 505
stomach, distended, 1219
stomach ulcers, 804, 1225
stomach wall, diffuse thickening, 1224

stomatitis, 695, 1225
stones, 209, 1309
stone cutting and polishing, 803
stoppage of flow of gastric juice, 1239
strabismus, 597, 1219
strains, 1216-17
strangulated hernia, 749
stratum corneum, 1186
stratum lucidum, 1186
stratum mucosum, 1185, 1186
strawberry tongue, 1158
streptobacillus of Ducrey, 335
strep throat, 1268-69
streptococcal infections, 797, 993, 1138
streptococci, 39, 101, 277, 876, 940, 1032
streptococcus, 399, 789, 1049, 1159, 1225, 1230, 1259, 1271
streptococcus hemolyticus, 1174
streptococcus infections, 1225
streptococcus sore throat, 466
streptococcus viridans, 564
Streptomyces fradiae, 335
Streptomyces griseus, 1225
Streptomyces halstedii, 101
Streptomyces puniceus, 106
streptomycin, 106, 477, 523, 564, 695, 791, 797, 842, 1022, 1052, 1109, 1225, 1275, 1284, 1286
stress, 1225-26
straited muscle, 924
stricture, 1309
stroke, 112, 1009, 1226-27, 1228-29, 1260
strontium, radioactive, 155, 1108
struck nail, 934
structural disturbances, inheritance of, 804
structure and growth, child, 354-56
structure and mechanism of vision, 590-95
strychnine poisoning, 1056
stuttering, 1206
stuttering and stammering, 1227
sty, 1227
styes, 600-1
styptic, alum as, 73
subacute bacterial endocarditis, 170, 172-73, 564, 1022, 1029
subacute endocarditis, 544
subcutaneous fat, 1344

subcutaneous tissue, 1187-90
subdermis, 1185, 1187
subscription, 1078
sudoriferous glands, 1029
suffocation (asphyxia), 139-41
suffocation, 1227
sugar, acne and, 28
sugars, 348, 854, 908
suicide, 896, 1227-30
sulfa drugs, 319, 405, 782, 797, 853, 870, 892, 990, 993, 1029, 1139, 1159, 1191-92, 1230, 1271
sulfadiazine, 951, 1230
sulfapyridine, 1230
sulfas, 209
sulfhydryls, 174
sulfonamide drugs, 22, 28, 40, 1230-31, 1271
sulfonamides, 211, 426, 543, 790, 826, 871, 876, 1052, 1184, 1230, 1305
sulphone drugs, 842
sulphur, 662, 1083, 1152
sulphur dioxide, 804, 978
sulphur ointment, 1158
sulphur vapor, 517
sulphuric acid, 27, 547
sun, exposure to, 395
sunburn, 1231
sunlight, 1084, 1337
sunshine, 349, 1335
sunstroke, 737, 1231
superfluous hair, 637-38, 699
superior vena cava, 408
superscription, 1078
superstitions about exercise, 587
supplemental air, 269
suppuration, 820, 1003, 1231
suppurative chronic otitis, 991
suppurative pleurisy, 562
suprarenin, 52
surgeon, 1212, 1232
surgery, 192, 304, 307, 770, 928, 985, 1029, 1232-37, 1339
surgery, history of, 1237-38
surgery, older people, 1238
surgical removal, 1082
swallowing reflex, 1117
swayback, 860, 1322
sweat, 1029-32, 1187, 1238
sweat gland deficiency, 804
sweat glands, 682, 1029, 1185, 1187
sweating, 1239
swelling of tissues and face, rapid, 1308

1391

INDEX

swimming, during menstruation, 638
swimming pools, 1238-39
swollen ankle, 98
sycamore, 704
sycosis, 176
sycosis barbae, 176
sycosis vulgaris, 176
sympathectomy, 235, 1239
sympathetic nervous system, 235, 943, 1239-40
sympathetic ophthalmia, 607-8
synapses, 256
syndrome, 1240
synousiology, 1240
synovia, 250, 818
synovial fluid, 818
synovial membrane, 834, 1240
synovitis, 819, 1240
syphilis, 20, 148, 169, 335, 602, 789, 792, 846, 860, 984, 1016, 1022, 1240-42, 1323, 1342, 1370
syphilis, congenital, 447, 1241
syphilis, primary stage, 1240
syringe, 1242
syringe, enema, 886
systemic circulation, 406, 407
systemic poisoning, 968
systolic hypertension, 227
systolic pressure, 223-24

T

T gene, 745
tabes, 1243
tabes dorsalis, 1243
tachycardia, 1092
tachyphage, 1243
tachyphagia, 1243
talc poisoning, 978
Takamine, Jokichi, 52
talipes, 1243
tannic acid, 978, 1056
tantrum, 775
tapeworm, 792, 1109, 1243, 1361-64
tar, 978
tar bath treatments, 1084
tar cancer, 978
tarantula, 97
taste, 804
taste buds, 1267
taste, metallic, 901
tattooing, 1243-44
tear ducts, 606, 1244
tear glands, 1244
teeth, 1206, 1244-49, 1303
teeth, abrasion, 21
teeth, abscess, 1249
teeth, absence of certain, 804
teeth, formation and growth, 1335
teeth, child's, 395-96
teeth, decay of, 483, 931
teeth, discoloration, 1248

teeth, primary, 1246-47
teething, 1246-47
tellurium poisoning, 899
temperature, 1249-51
temperatures, air conditioning and, 59-61
temporal bone, 1191
temporal lobes, 256
temporary teeth, 1247
tendons, 250, 818, 928, 1185, 1218, 1251
tension headache, 905
TEPP, 977
teropterin, 305
terramycin, 28, 40, 59, 74, 75, 101, 120, 564, 695, 870, 885, 1052, 1118, 1286, 1327
tertian malaria, benign, 109
tertiary amyl alcohol, 179
tertiary stage, syphilis, 1241
testes, 684, 921, 1089, 1251-56, 1304
testicles, 309, 984, 1118, 1164, 1169, 1207, 1222, 1251-56, 1304
testicles, undescended, 1306-7
testosterone, 81, 304, 1126, 1251
testosterone propionate, 903
tests, 1256
tests, chart of, 1252-53
tetanus, 110, 169, 782, 792, 817, 964, 1109, 1254-55, 1256-57, 1353
tetanus antitoxin, 470
tetanus bacillus, 1256
tetany, 948, 1013, 1257
tetrachlorethylene, 1361
tetracyline(s), 106, 1017, 1109
tetracyn, 106
tetraethyl lead, 978
tetraethyl-pyrophosphate, 977
tetraiodophthalein, 319
Texas fever, 1257, 1305
textile manufacturing, 977
thalamus, 256
thalassemia, 1114, 1257
thallium, 978
thallium poisoning, 899, 1056
thallium sulfate (sulphate), 1056, 1110
Theiler, Max, 1371
theophylline ethylenediamine, 78
Thephorin, 108
thermometer, 1250, 1257

thiamin(e), 193, 348, 882, 1258, 1328, 1356, 1370
thiamin(e) deficiency, 1257-58, 1329-32
thickening of arteries, 1164
thinking, difficulty in, 917
thiocyanates, 689
thiophos, 977
thiouracil, 689
thonzylamine hydrochloride, 108
thoracic cage, 337
thoracic lymphatic duct, 867
thoracic vertebrae, 1322
thoracoplasty, 1285
thorax, 337
thorium, 974
thorium, radioactive, 974
thorium X, 974
thoron, 974
thought, 888, 943, 1258
threadworm, 1357
three-day fever, 1157, 1258
three-day measles, 678
three-year-olds, pictorial guide to needs of, 372-73
threonine, 78
throat, 1258-59
throat, infection, 1022
throat, sore, 1032, 1199, 1238
throbbing pain, 1003
thrombin, 219, 221, 741
thrombo-angiitis, 280
thrombo-angiitis obliterans, 282-83, 1259
thrombocytes, 216, 900, 1045
thrombocytes, destruction of, 1104
thrombocytocemia, 1214, 1215
thrombocytopenia, 150, 1259-60
thrombocytopenic purpura, 1260
thromboembolism, 1064
thrombophlebitis, 1033, 1260
thromboplastin, 217-18, 221
thrombosis, 1009, 1260-61
thrombus, 1260
thrush, 1261
thrush, oral, 910
thulium, radioactive, 1106
thumb sucking, 358, 363-64, 1261
thymus gland, 684, 1261-62
thyroid cancer, 153
thyroid cartilage, 40
thyroid crises, 589
thyroid gland, 20, 247, 348, 684, 765, 767, 894, 931, 1040, 1041, 1044, 1106, 1262-63, 1301

thyroid gland extract, 932
thyroid heart disease, 1264-65
thyroid hormone, 226
thyrotoxic exopthalmos, 770
thyrotoxicosis, 718
thyroxin, 688, 775, 956, 1262
tibia, 98, 818, 841
tic(s), 46, 696
tic douloureux, 1263-66
tickbite fever, South African, 1153
tickling, 1117
tick(s), 1099, 1118
tick, wood, 1153
tin workers, 979
tincture of benzoin, 886
tincture of green soap, 1151, 1152
tincture of iodine, 109, 813, 1366
tincture of merthiolate, 109
tinea, 1150
tinea barbae, 176
tinea capitis, 1151, 1152
tinea circinata, 1152
tinea cruris, 1151
tinea favosa, 1152
tinea pedis, 149
tinea unguim, 1152
tingling of hands and feet, 1008
tinnitus, 889, 951, 1266
tissue fluid, 408
tobacco, 1266
tobacco workers, 979
toenails, 1266
toes, extra, 804
toes, loss of, 842
toluene, 979
toluol, 979
tomatoes, 1334
tone, muscle, 578
tongue, 917, 1206, 1227, 1266-67
tongue, base of, 1258
tongue, disturbances of, 1332
tongue, projections on, 1267
tongue, sore, 1334
tonic convulsion, 446
tonic spasm, 504, 1205
tonometer, 601, 685
tonsillectomy, 427, 1267, 1270
tonsillitis, 817, 1138, 1199, 1267
tonsillitis, acute, 39-40, 817, 1032, 1268-69, 1308
tonsils, 399-400, 530, 1032, 1199, 1267-70
tooth decay, 483, 931
tooth socket, bleeding, 545
toothpastes, 484
toper's nose, 1145
tophi, 694
topical anesthesia, 87
torch welding, 967
torn ligament, 1178
torticollis, 1270
totaquine, 872

touch, sensation of, 470, 1003, 1187
toumarin, 1110
tourniquet, 545, 1365-66
toxemia, 1270
toxic goiter, 1017
toxic headache, 706-7
toxic hepatitis, 857
toxicity, 1092
toxic substances in industry, 966-80
toxins, 169, 944
trachea, 268, 337, 1270-71
tracheotomy, 467, 1271
trachoma, 603, 792, 1271, 1327
tranquilizing drugs, 944, 1085, 1271
transducers, 883
transfusion, 1114
transfusion, blood, 83, 137, 213-15, 219-20, 238-39, 843, 1219, 1232
transfusion, whole blood, 1097, 1106
translocation, 521
transmissible (transmittable) diseases, 18, 1271
transplantation, corneal, 447, 606-7
transplantation, heart, 985
transplants, organ, 985
transverse colon, 253, 811
transverse processes, 1322
traumatic cataract, 605
traveling, baby, 395
tremors, 901, 948
trench mouth 484, 679, 1022, 1271-74, 1323, 1324-25
Treponema pallidum, 1240, 1370
Treponema pertenue, 1370
trichinae, 1274
Trichinella spiralis, 1274
trichinosis, 789, 792, 928, 961, 1272-73, 1274, 1356
trichlorethylene, 970, 979
trichlorethylene inhalations, 1266
trichloroacetic acid, 25
trichloromethane, 402
trichomonas, 639
Trichophyton schoenleini, 1152
tricuspid valve, 714
tridione, 570
trifocals, 196
trigeminal nerve, 945, 1263
trigeminal neuralgia, 612, 1263-66, 1275
trigeminal neuralgia, operation for, 1266
trinitrophenol, 977
Trional, 885
tripelenamine hydrochloride, 108

1392

INDEX

trismus, 817
trocar, 1237
trombicula irritans, 805
tromexan, 221
tronothane, 157
trophic hormone, 53
tropical sprue, 1218
tropical ulcers, 820
true bacteria 1150
true hypertension, 227
true ribs, 1147
trypanosomiasis, 1275
trypsin, 756
tryptophane, 78
tsutsugamushi, 1165
tsutsugamushi fever, 1275
tt genes, 745
tubal pregnancy, 613
tubercle bacillus, 1275
tubercles, 1275
tubercular infection, 993
tuberculin test, 477, 1252-53, 1275
tuberculosis, 169, 209, 249, 461, 489, 524, 604, 605, 789, 792, 804, 858, 860, 866, 870, 894, 960, 969, 978, 979, 984, 987, 1032, 1045, 1114, 1137, 1244, 1275-85, 1302, 1305
tuberculosis, abdominal region, 1278
tuberculosis, bones, 1278
tuberculosis, joints, 1278
tuberculosis, kidney, 826
tuberculosis, lymph glands, 1278
tuberculosis (tuberculous) meningitis, 797, 890, 1225, 1285
tuberculosis nodules, 842
tuberculosis, pulmonary, 1276-77
tuberculosis, spine, 1322-23
tularemia, 183, 792, 964, 1225, 1285-86
tumescence, 986
tumor(s), 183, 209, 293, 308, 602, 695, 870, 945, 993, 1009, 1016, 1215, 1224, 1244, 1262, 1286
tumor, adenoma, 684
tumors, benign growths or, 293, 1286
tumors, endocrine glands, 232
tumor, fibroid, 1314-15
tumors, internal, 953
tumors, larynx, 839
tumors, mixed, 644
tumor, simple, 1287
tumors, urinary tract, 1310-11
tumorous growth, 1184
tuna fish, 1190, 1335
turgor, 1301
turpentine, 852, 977, 979

turpentine poisoning, 1056
tweezers, 1155
twins, detecting, 486
twins, fraternal, 206
twins identical, 205, 206
type A influenza virus, 799
type AB blood, 240
type B influenza virus, 799
type O blood, 240
type 2 herpes virus, 334
typhoid bacillus, 1287
typhoid carrier, 1287
typhoid fever, 164, 169, 505, 530, 697, 782, 789, 792, 796, 846, 894, 910, 990, 1256, 1287-90, 1305, 1342
typhoid vaccine, 1290
typhus fever, 243, 473, 782, 789, 792, 797, 805, 847, 1109, 1150, 1153, 1290-91, 1303
typhus fever epidemic, 1150
typhus, louse-borne epidemic, 1290

U

ulcer(s), 505, 842, 1292
ulcer, bleeding peptic, 814
ulcer, eye, 604
ulcer, gastric, 674
ulcer, perforated corneal, 1079
ulcer, perforation of, 19
ulcer, secondary jejunal, 817
ulcer stomach, 804, 1225
ulcerating cancer, 1224
ulceration, 841, 1191
ulcerative colitis, 422, 1294-95
ulcerative stomatitis, 1323
ulcers, digestive tract, 1296-97
ulcers, skin, 901
ulcers, stomach, 804
ulna, 536
ultraviolet light, 857
ultraviolet radiation, 1037, 1335
ultraviolet rays, 887, 965, 1084, 1231
ultraviolet rays, artificial, 1337
umbilical cord, 935, 1292, 1293
umbilical region, 19
umbilicus, 935, 1292
underfeeding, 387
undernutrition, harmful, 1304
undernourishment, 894
underweight, 766, 1292-98
underweight, beneficial, 1304
underweight, hazards of, 1292-1304

undescended testes, 1304-5
undescended testicles, 1306-7
undulant fever, 787, 789, 792, 961, 964, 1256, 1305
universal antidote, 1053, 1305
universal donor, 240
universal recipient, 240
unsaturated fats, 620-21
urea, 826, 855, 1313
uremia, 827, 901, 941, 1305-8
uremia, acute, 1308
ureter(s), 208, 1308-9, 1313
urethra, 208, 1022, 1070, 1126, 1169, 1172, 1309-12, 1313
urethral carbuncles, 1312
urethral orifice, 1338
urethral syringe, 1242
urethritis, 1309
uric acid, 26, 691, 826
urinary bladder, 207-8, 1079
urinary infections, 1225
urinary tract infections, 1310-11
urinary tract stones, 824-25
urinary tract tumors and infections, 1310-11
urination, 1312
urine, 208, 1079, 1313
urine test, 1252-53
urologist, 1309
urotropin, 973
urticaria, 760-61, 762-63, 1190, 1316
use of antibiotic drugs, 1106
use of antihistamines, 1097
use of appropriate drugs, 1099
uterine tubes, 1313
uterus, 613, 775, 910, 1128, 1129, 1313-16, 1318
uterus, prolapse of, 1079
uvula, 1032, 1227, 1316

V

vaccination, 790, 1154, 1193, 1317, 1327
vaccine(s), 137, 870, 1184, 1305, 1327
vaccine, anti-cavity, 484
vaccine, concentrated influenza, 802
vagina, 1079, 1126, 1128, 1129, 1177, 1313, 1318, 1338
vaginal bleeding, 21
vaginal douche, 202
vaginal fistula, 648
vaginal foaming tablets, 202

vaginal jellies, creams, and foams, 202
vaginal moniliasis, 910
vaginal orifice, 1337, 1338
vaginal suppositories, 202
vaginismus, 1318
vagus nerve, 718
valetudinarianism, 1318
valine, 78
valley fever, 418, 1318
valvular disease, chronic, 1138
vanadium poisoning, 979
vanadium trioxid, 979
vanilla, 1196
Vapophos, 977
varicella, 337, 793, 1318
varicose veins, 349, 741, 841, 950, 1318, 1320-21
variola, 337, 1193-96, 1319
vas deferens (vasa deferentia), 471, 1126, 1169, 1172, 1207, 1223, 1251, 1319
vasa efferentia, 1319
vasoconstrictors, 427, 1184
vault, 1191
veal, 882
veins, 407, 408, 714, 854, 861, 1319
veins, hepatic, 408
veins, jugular, 408
veins, portal, 408, 854
veins, pulmonary, 408, 714, 861, 1319
veins, varicose, 349, 741, 841, 950, 1318, 1320-21
vena cava, 1319
venae cavae, 714
venereal disease, 1240, 1244, 1319
venereal warts, 1339
venomous scorpion, 97
venomous snake, 97
venous bleeding, 1365
venous blood, 407
venous thrombosis, 1260
ventilation, 1319-22
ventilation, air-conditioning and, 59-61
ventilation, artificial, 1322
ventricle, 406, 710
ventricle, left, 407, 408
ventricle, right, 407
ventricular diastole, 714
ventricular fibrillation, 643
venules, 407
veratrum, 108
veratrum viride, 236
vermiform appendix, 114, 1322
vernal conjunctivitis, 1040

Veronal, 885
vertebra (vertebrae), 249, 818, 1207, 1212, 1322-23
vertebra, slipped, 1215
vertebral column, 1208
vertigo, 1323
vestibule, 917
vesicles, 1190
vibrio, 789
villi, 66, 811
Vincent, Jean H., 1323
Vincent's angina, 484, 1033, 1323-26
Vincent's disease, 679
Vincent's organisms, 821, 1323
vinegar, for insect bites, 805
viomycin, 106, 523
viper bite, 1197
viral hepatitis, 1244
viral hepatitis, acute, 856
virilism, 54
virus(es), 788, 792, 797, 866, 1326-28
virus, adenoidal, 112
viruses, dermatropic, 1326
virus encephalitis, 563
virus pneumonia, 792, 1052, 1099, 1326
viruses, APC, 112
viruses, neurotropic, 1326
viscera, 1326
visceral leishmaniasis, 842
viscerotropic viruses, 1326
vision and retardation, 809
vision, child, 597
vision, disturbance of, 905
vision, double, 520
vision, inherited difficulties, 804
vision, weaknesses and disturbances of, 1332
vital air, 269
vitamin A, 348, 855, 908, 934, 1328-29
vitamin A deficiency, 1190, 1328, 1330-31, 1367
vitamin, antihemorrhagic, 1336
vitamin B, 348, 956
vitamin B complex, 1169, 1328
vitamin B_1, 882, 908, 1328
vitamin B_1 deficiencies, 1329-32
vitamin B_2 (riboflavin), 348, 882, 908, 1146, 1190, 1328, 1370
vitamin B_2 deficiencies, 1190, 1332-33
vitamin B_6, 1328, 1334
vitamin B_6 deficiency, 1190, 1334

1393

INDEX

vitamin B₁₂, 882, 1111, 1169, 1219, 1328, 1333
vitamin C (ascorbic acid), 139, 908, 1328, 1334, 1336
vitamin C deficiency, 1190, 1334
vitamin D (ergosterol), 908, 956, 1147, 1328, 1334-35
vitamin D concentrates, 1335
vitamin D deficiency, 1335, 1343
vitamin deficiency, 20
vitamin disturbances, 954
vitamin E, 1328, 1335-36
vitamin E deficiency, 1335-36
vitamin G, 1328
vitamin K, 1328, 1336, 1356
vitamin K₁, 1097
vitamin P, 1328, 1336
vitamins, 348, 954, 956, 1326-36
vitiligo, 1336-37
vitreous, 604
vitreous body, 591
vocal cords, 1337
vocal cords, paralysis, 838
voice box, 1337
voluntary food restriction, 1302
voluntary muscles, 924, 930, 943
vomiting, 916, 917, 921, 940, 1024, 1077, 1334, 1337
vulva, 1130, 1318, 1337-38
vulva, cancer of, 1338
vulvitis, 1338

W

walk, characteristic, 667
walk, stiff, 932
walking, 350, 632
wandering spleen, 1215
warfarin, 1110
warmth, sensation of, 1186
Warren, John D., 89
warts, 293, 1339-42
warts, senile, 1342
washing soda, 67
Wasserman test, 329, 822, 1241, 1342
waste products, body, 212, 928, 1192
wastes, muscle, 928
water, 197, 518, 1342-43
water, carbonated, 310
water moccasin bite, 1197
water on brain, 766
water on knee, 834, 1240
water requirements, 389
weakened viruses, 1327
weakness, 588, 931, 1099, 1299, 1360
weakness, profound, 799
weight averages, optimum, 1345-46
weight, factors which influence, 1343-45
weight loss, 951, 1334, 1364
weight loss, progressive, 1008
weight-height-age tables, 1345-47

weight, normal for health, 1345-47
weight – regulating machinery of the body, 1347-50
Weil's disease, 816, 1109, 1350
welding occupations, 965
Wells, Horace, 89
wen(s), 1348-49, 1350
"wet" pleurisy, 1045
wetness of working conditions, 963
wheat germ oil, 1335
wheat sensitivity, 327-28, 1350
whiplash injury of neck, 1220-21
whirlpool therapy, 133, 1037
whiskey nose, 1145
white (blood) cell(s), 216, 780, 846, 867, 1350
white (blood) cell determination test, 1252-53
white (blood) cell(s), diseases of, 1350-52
white damp, 979
white matter, 943
whites (leucorrhea), 1318
Whitfield's ointment, 1352
whiting, 977
whole-grain cereals, 1332, 1333, 1335, 1336
whooping cough, 277, 461, 475, 530, 782, 789, 792, 795, 1352-56
Widal test, 1252-53, 1287
will, 888

will, weakness of, 22
Wilm's tumor, 1356
wines, 63
windpipe, 268, 1270-71
wisdom teeth, 1247
witch hazel, 815
womb, 1129, 1313-16, 1356
wood alcohol, 974, 978
wood alcohol poisoning, 1356
wood naphtha, 974
wood spirits, 974
wood tick, 1153
word blindness, 66
working conditions, damp, 963
worms, 19, 792, 951, 952, 1356-64
worms, intestinal, 951
wounds, 547, 1326, 1364-66
wrist, 1091
writing, difficulty in, 917
wry neck, 1270, 1366

XYZ

X chromosomes, 1130-32
xanthoma, 1367
xeroderma, 1367
xerophthalmia, 477, 1328, 1367
xerosis, 1367
xerostoma, 1367-68
x-ray(s), cancer stimulating, 304, 964
x-ray(s), diagnostic use of, 210, 298, 484, 1024, 1237, 1368-70
x-ray(s), overexposure to, 20

x-ray, panoramic, 484
x-ray(s), treatment with, 28, 35, 38, 211, 304, 823, 843, 846, 1339
XX genetic make-up, 1131
XXX genetic make-up, 1132
XY genetic make-up, 1131-32
xylene, 979
xylol, 979
XYY genetic make-up, 1132
Y chromosomes, 1131-32
yaws, 792, 1370
yeast(s), 641, 663, 1332, 1370
yellow fever, 54, 473, 782, 792, 796, 915, 1108, 1326, 1370-72
yellow jaundice, 1372
yellow spots, 1367
Zephiran, 109, 885
zinc, 956, 979, 1372
zinc carbonate, 289, 1372
zinc chills, 967, 979
zinc chloride, 980, 1372
zinc oxide, 979, 1372
zinc oxide ointment, 885
zinc phosphate, 1110
zinc poisoning, 899, 969
zinc silicate, 1372
zinc sulphate, 980
zymogenic cells, 1372
zygoma, 1372
zygomatic arch, 1372
zygote, 1130, 1372
zyme, 1372